Clinical Anesthesia Procedures of the Massachusetts General Hospital

Seventh Edition

Senior Editor
Peter F. Dunn, M.D.

Associate Editors
Theodore A. Alston, M.D., Ph.D.
Keith H. Baker, M.D., Ph.D.
J. Kenneth Davison, M.D.
Jean Kwo, M.D.
Carl E. Rosow, M.D., Ph.D.
Department of Anesthesia and Critical Care
Massachusetts General Hospital
Harvard Medical School
Boston, Massachusetts

Lippincott Williams & Wilkins
a Wolters Kluwer business
Philadelphia · Baltimore · New York · London
Buenos Aires · Hong Kong · Sydney · Tokyo

Acquisitions Editor: Brian Brown
Developmental Editor: Molly Connors, Dovetail Content Solutions
Managing Editor: Nicole T. Dernoski
Marketing Manager: Angela Panetta
Project Manager: Nicole Walz
Senior Manufacturing Manager: Ben Rivera
Design Coordinator: Terry Mallon
Cover Designer: Terry Mallon
Production Services: Techbooks
Printer: R.R. Donnelley–Crawfordsville

Library of Congress Cataloging-in-Publication Data
Clinical anesthesia procedures of the Massachusetts General Hospital /
Department of Anesthesia and Critical Care, Massachusetts General Hospital,
Harvard Medical School.—7th ed. / senior editor, Peter F. Dunn ; associate
editors, Theodore Alston ... [et al.].
     p. ; cm.
    Includes bibliographical references and index.
    ISBN-13: 978-078178-183-1
    ISBN-10: 0-7817-8183-3 (pbk. : alk. paper)
  1. Anesthesiology—Handbooks, manuals, etc.   I. Dunn, Peter F.
II. Alston, Theodore.   III. Massachusetts General Hospital. Dept. of
Anesthesia and Critical Care.
    [DNLM: 1. Anesthesia—methods—Handbooks.   2. Anesthetics—
administration & dosage—Handbooks.   3. Perioperative Care—methods—
Handbooks. WO 39 C639 2006]
   RD82.2.C54 2006
   617.9′6—dc22

                                                                 2006022535

RRC0909

Contents

Preface

The Seventh Edition of *Clinical Anesthesia Procedures of the Massachusetts General Hospital* was written by residents, fellows, and staff of the Department of Anesthesia and Critical Care at the Massachusetts General Hospital. This manual continues to emphasize the clinical fundamentals involved in the safe administration of anesthesia, perioperative care, and pain management. The suggestions reflect current clinical practices at our hospital and represent the foundation of the educational programs in our department's anesthesia residency and critical care, pain, and cardiac anesthesia fellowships.

This handbook complements readings in textbooks and journals and assumes some prior knowledge of anesthesia and critical care. It is designed to be an easily accessible and accurate source of information for practicing anesthesiologists, anesthesia residents, nurse anesthetists, medical students, medical and surgical residents, nurses, respiratory therapists, and other health care professionals involved in perioperative care. The manual is intended to augment experienced clinical teaching and inspire more detailed study. Each chapter contains a suggested reading list for this purpose.

As with previous editions, each chapter has been thoroughly reviewed and updated. Source material from prior editions has been included verbatim where appropriate. The chapters have been highly cross referenced to provide the reader with easy access to related material within the book. With this process, we have been able to eliminate as much redundant information as possible, include new and more detailed discussions of select topics, and still maintain a pocket-sized manual. As our patient population continues to age, the importance of understanding geriatric-specific issues has become even more important and is now a separate chapter. Translated into six languages, *Clinical Anesthesia Procedures of the Massachusetts General Hospital* has been repeatedly edited, revised, and relied upon internationally as a clinical reference for nearly 30 years. More than 200 individuals have contributed to the manual during this time. The authors of this edition are indebted to all of them for their efforts and expertise that contributed to the success of previous editions and established the framework for this edition. The integral contributions of the editors of this handbook are gratefully acknowledged below: Editors of Previous Editions: First Edition (1978): Philip W. Lebowitz, John L. Clark, Daniel F. Dedrick, James R. Zaidan, Robert K. Crone; Second Edition (1982): Philip W. Lebowitz, Leslie A. Newberg, Michael T. Gilette; Third Edition (1988): Leonard L. Firestone, Philip W. Lebowitz, Charles E. Cook; Fourth Edition (1993): J. Kenneth Davison, William F. Eckhardt, III, Deniz A. Perese; Fifth Edition (1997): William E. Hurford, Michael T. Bailin, J. Kenneth Davison, Kenneth L. Haspel, Carl Rosow; Sixth Edition (2002): William E. Hurford, Michael T. Bailin, J. Kenneth Davison, Kenneth L. Haspel, Carl Rosow, Susan A. Vassallo. I thank Ms. Erin K. Murphy for administrative assistance, Ms. Molly Connors of Dovetail Content

Solutions for her editorial assistance, and the staff at Lippincott Williams & Wilkins for their support. Finally, I acknowledge the guidance and support given to early editions by Richard J. Kitz, M.D., and the continuing support of Warren M. Zapol, M.D.

Peter F. Dunn, M.D.

I

Evaluating the Patient Before Anesthesia

1

Evaluating the Patient Before Anesthesia

Mary Kraft and Stephanie L. Roundtree

I. **Overview.** The **preanesthetic evaluation** has specific objectives including establishing a doctor-patient relationship, becoming familiar with the surgical illness and coexisting medical conditions, developing a management strategy for perioperative anesthetic care, and obtaining informed consent for the anesthetic plan. The consultation is detailed in the patient's record and concludes with the anesthetic options and their attendant risks and benefits. The overall goals of the preoperative assessment are to reduce perioperative morbidity and mortality and to allay patient anxiety.

II. **History.** Relevant information is obtained by chart review followed by patient interview. Knowledge of the patient's history when beginning the interview is reassuring to the anxious patient. When the medical record is not available, the history obtained from the patient may be supplemented by direct discussion with the medical and surgical staff. Although patient age and American Society of Anesthesiologists (ASA) Physical Status Classification are more accurate predictors of adverse outcomes, knowledge of patients' activities of daily living, including maximum activity level, may help predict their overall outcome in the perioperative period.

   A. **The anesthetist** should review the symptoms of the present surgical illness, diagnostic studies performed, presumptive diagnosis, initial treatment, and responses. Vital signs should be reviewed and fluid balance estimated.

   B. **Coexisting medical illnesses** may complicate the surgical and anesthetic course. These should be evaluated in a systematic "organ systems" approach with an emphasis on recent changes in symptoms, signs, and treatment (see Chapters 2 through 7). In certain circumstances, preoperative specialty consultation may be advisable. Such consults are most valuable when answering specific questions about the interpretation of unusual laboratory tests, unfamiliar drug therapies, or changes in the patient's baseline status. Consultants should not be asked for a general "clearance" for anesthesia because this is the specific responsibility of the anesthesiologist.

   C. **Medications** used to treat present or coexisting illnesses, their dosages, and schedules must be ascertained. Of special importance are antihypertensive, antianginal, antiarrhythmic, anticoagulant, anticonvulsant, and specific endocrine (e.g., insulin) medications. The decision to continue medications during the preanesthetic period depends on the severity of the underlying illness, the potential consequences of discontinuing treatment, the medication's half-life, and the likelihood of deleterious interactions with proposed anesthetic agents. As a general rule, most medications can be continued up to the time of surgery.

D. Allergies and drug reactions. Unusual, unexpected, or unpleasant reactions to perioperative medications and nonallergic adverse reactions, side effects, and drug interactions are relatively common. True allergic reactions are relatively uncommon. The task of determining the exact nature of specific "reactions" may be difficult. Therefore, it is important to obtain a careful description of the "allergic reaction" experience from the patient.

1. **True allergic reactions.** Any drug reaction that (by direct observation, chart documentation, or description by the patient) produced skin manifestations (pruritus with hives or flushing), facial or oral swelling, shortness of breath, choking, wheezing, or vascular collapse should be considered to be a true allergic reaction.

   a. **Antibiotics,** especially sulfonamides, penicillins, and cephalosporin derivatives are the most common allergens.

   b. **Known allergy to soybean oil and egg yolk components** may preclude the use of some preparations of propofol.

   c. **A history of "allergy" to halothane or succinylcholine** (in the patient or any close relative) warrants special attention because this may represent the occurrence of malignant hyperthermia, halothane hepatitis, or prolonged paralysis caused by an abnormal allele responsible for producing plasma cholinesterase, an enzyme that metabolizes succinylcholine.

   d. **True allergy to the amide-type local anesthetics** (e.g., lidocaine) is exceedingly rare, although a syncopal episode, tachycardia, or palpitations associated with injection of local anesthetic with epinephrine may be falsely labeled as an allergic reaction. Ester-type local anesthetics (e.g., procaine) can produce anaphylaxis (see Chapter 15).

   e. It should be noted that a history to shellfish or seafood has **not** been linked to an allergy to intravenous iodine contrast. However, a history of dermatitis after exposure to topical iodine may preclude the use of intravenous iodine.

2. **Adverse reactions and side effects.** Many perioperative medications can produce memorable and unpleasant side effects (e.g., nausea, vomiting, and pruritus after narcotic administration) in a conscious patient. Droperidol administered alone may result in a "locked in" sensation.

3. **Certain rare but important drug interactions** must be anticipated because of their life-threatening nature. For example, thiopental may precipitate a fatal episode of acute intermittent porphyria, and meperidine may produce a hypertensive crisis when administered to patients treated with monoamine oxidase inhibitors. Newer anticholinesterase treatments for Alzheimer disease (e.g., donepezil, galantamine, and rivastigmine) may prolong the effect of succinylcholine.

B. Anesthetic history

1. **Old anesthesia records** should be reviewed for the following information:

   a. Response to sedative/analgesic premedications and anesthetic agents.
   b. Vascular access and invasive monitoring used, and if any difficulties were encountered.
   c. Ease of mask ventilation, direct laryngoscopy, and size and type of laryngoscope blade and endotracheal tube used.
   d. Perianesthetic complications such as adverse drug reactions, cephalgia, intraoperative awareness, dental injury, protracted postoperative nausea and vomiting, cardiorespiratory instability, postoperative myocardial infarction or congestive heart failure, unexpected admission to an intensive care unit (ICU), and prolonged emergence or reintubation.
   2. Patients should be asked about their experience with prior anesthetics, including common complaints such as postoperative nausea and hoarseness and specific warnings from previous anesthetists describing prior anesthetic problems.
C. Family history. A history of adverse anesthetic outcomes in family members should be evaluated. This history is best obtained with open-ended questions, such as "Has anyone in your family experienced unusual or serious reactions to anesthesia?" Patients should be specifically asked about a family history of malignant hyperthermia.
D. Social history and habits
   1. Smoking. A history of exercise intolerance or the presence of a productive cough or hemoptysis may indicate a need for further pulmonary evaluation or treatment. Eliminating cigarette use for 6–8 weeks before elective surgery may reduce airway hyperreactivity and postoperative pulmonary complications.
   2. Drugs and alcohol. Although self-reporting of drug and alcohol intake typically underestimates use, it is a helpful starting point to define the drugs used, routes of administration, frequency, and timing of most recent use. **Stimulant abuse** may lead to palpitations, angina, weight loss, and lowered thresholds for serious arrhythmias and seizures. **Acute alcohol intoxication** will decrease the anesthetic requirements and predispose to hypothermia and hypoglycemia, whereas withdrawal from ethanol may precipitate severe hypertension, tremors, delirium, and seizures and may markedly increase anesthetic requirements. Routine use of opioids and benzodiazepines may significantly increase the doses needed to induce and maintain anesthesia or to provide adequate postoperative analgesia.
E. Review of systems. Acute or chronic lung disease, ischemic heart disease, hypertension, and gastroesophageal reflux are examples of commonly encountered coexisting conditions that increase the risk of perioperative morbidity and mortality. A minimum review of systems should seek to elicit a history of the following information:
   1. A recent history of an upper respiratory infection, especially in children, which can predispose patients to pulmonary complications including bronchospasm and

laryngospasm during induction of and emergence from general anesthesia.

2. **Asthma,** which may be accompanied by airway mucous plugging and acute bronchospasm after the induction of anesthesia or endotracheal intubation.

3. **Preexisting coronary artery disease (CAD),** which may predispose the patient to myocardial ischemia, ventricular dysfunction, or myocardial infarction with the stress of surgery and anesthesia.

4. **Diabetes,** which may predispose the patient to silent ischemia, especially in those with autonomic nervous system dysfunction. Alterations in autonomic regulation may also lead to gastroparesis and active reflux. In addition, endotracheal intubation may be difficult in some diabetic patients because of arthritis of the temporomandibular joints and cervical spine resulting from glycosylation of synovium.

5. **Untreated hypertension,** which is frequently associated with blood pressure lability during anesthesia. If left ventricular hypertrophy is present, hypertension is associated with a higher incidence of postoperative complications (e.g., stroke, myocardial infarction). Diuretic therapy can produce hypovolemia and electrolyte imbalances, especially in the elderly.

6. **Hiatal hernia with esophageal reflux symptoms,** which increases the risk of pulmonary aspiration and may alter the anesthetic plan (e.g., an awake intubation or a "rapid sequence" induction may be indicated).

7. **Likelihood of pregnancy** and timing of last menses in women of childbearing age because premedications and anesthetic agents may adversely influence uteroplacental blood flow, act as teratogens, or lead to spontaneous abortion.

III. **The physical examination** should be thorough but focused. Special attention is directed toward evaluation of the airway, heart, lungs, and neurologic status. When a regional anesthetic technique is planned, there should be a detailed assessment of the extremities or back.

A. As a minimum, the physical examination should include the following:

1. **Vital signs**
   a. **Height and weight** are useful in estimating drug dosages, and determining volume requirements and the adequacy of perioperative urine output.
   b. **Blood pressure** should be recorded in both arms and any disparity noted (significant differences may imply disease of the thoracic aorta or its major branches). Postural signs should be checked in patients suspected of hypovolemia.
   c. **Resting pulse** should be noted for rhythm, perfusion (fullness), and rate. The pulse may be slow in patients receiving β-adrenergic blockade or rapid and bounding in the patient with fever, aortic regurgitation, or sepsis. Dehydrated patients may have rapid, weak pulses.
   d. **Respirations** should be observed for rate, depth, and pattern while at rest.

2. **Head and neck.** Details of a thorough head and neck examination are outlined in Chapter 13. During the basic preoperative examination, one should:

    a. **Evaluate maximal mouth opening,** the size of the tongue, and the ability to visualize the posterior pharyngeal structures (Mallampati classification).

    b. **Measure thyromental distance.**

    c. **Document loose or chipped teeth,** artificial crowns, dentures, and other dental appliances.

    d. **Note the range of cervical spine motion** in flexion, extension, and rotation.

    e. **Document tracheal deviation,** cervical masses, and jugular venous distention. The presence of carotid bruits is nonspecific but may suggest a need for further workup.

3. **Precordium.** Auscultation of the heart may reveal murmurs, gallop rhythms, or a pericardial rub.

4. **Lungs.** Listen for wheezing, rhonchi, or rales, which should be correlated with observations on the ease of breathing and the use of accessory muscles of respiration.

5. **Abdomen.** Any evidence of distention, masses, or ascites should be noted because these might predispose to regurgitation or compromise ventilation.

6. **Extremities.** Muscle wasting and weakness should be documented as well as general distal perfusion, clubbing, cyanosis, and cutaneous infection (especially over sites of planned vascular cannulation and regional nerve block). Ecchymosis or unexplained injury, especially in children, women, and elderly patients, can be an indication of an abusive relationship.

7. **Back.** Note any deformity, bruising, or infection.

8. **Neurologic examination.** Document mental status, cranial nerve function, cognition, and peripheral sensorimotor function.

IV. **Laboratory studies.** Routine laboratory screening tests are rarely useful. Tests should be selected based on the patient's medical condition and the proposed surgical procedure. A brief review of current guidelines follows:

    A. **Hematological studies** may be indicated if there are concerns about pre- or intraoperative blood loss, anemia, or coagulopathy.

        1. **Recent hematocrit/hemoglobin level.** There is no universally accepted minimum hematocrit before anesthesia. Hematocrits of 25% to 30% are well tolerated by otherwise healthy individuals but could result in ischemia in patients with CAD. Each case must be evaluated individually for the etiology and duration of anemia and the presence of comorbidities. If there is no obvious explanation for anemia, a delay of surgery may be indicated. Healthy patients undergoing minimally invasive procedures do not need a routine hematocrit screen.

        2. **Platelet function** may be assessed by a history of easy bruising, excessive bleeding from gums and minor cuts, and family history. A positive finding in this category warrants additional laboratory evaluation and possibly a consultation with a hematologist.

        3. **Coagulation studies** are ordered only when clinically indicated (e.g., history of a bleeding diathesis, aspirin or anticoagulant use, liver disease, or serious systemic illness) or if postoperative anticoagulation is planned.

B. **Serum chemistry studies** are ordered only when specifically indicated by history and physical examination. For example, measurements of blood urea nitrogen and creatinine are indicated for patients who have chronic renal, cardiovascular, hepatic, or intracranial disease as well as for those with diabetes or morbid obesity. They are also indicated in patients taking diuretics, digoxin, steroids, or aminoglycoside antibiotics.

  1. **Hypokalemia** is common in patients receiving diuretics and is usually readily corrected by preoperative oral potassium supplementation. Mild hypokalemia (2.8 to 3.5 mEq/L) should not preclude elective surgery. Rapid correction with intravenous potassium may lead to dysrhythmias and cardiac arrest. It is reasonable to delay surgery for cautious correction of marked hypokalemia, particularly if the patient is taking digoxin or experiencing dysrhythmias.

  2. **Hyperkalemia** is often seen in patients with end-stage renal disease. In this setting, mild elevations in serum potassium are well tolerated, but it may be prudent to choose replacement fluids that do not contain additional potassium. Large increases in potassium may also predispose to dysrhythmias. Treatment of hyperkalemia is warranted if concentrations exceed 6 mEq/L or if electrocardiogram (ECG) changes are seen.

C. **An ECG** is advised for any patient with risk factors for CAD. It may also be useful for detecting new dysrhythmias and evaluating the stability of known abnormal rhythms. It is suggested that men >45 years and women >55 years obtain an ECG before surgery. Although the resting ECG is not a sensitive test for occult myocardial ischemia, an abnormal ECG mandates correlation with history, physical examination, and prior ECGs. It may require further workup and consultation with a cardiologist before surgery.

D. **Chest radiography** should be performed only when clinically indicated (e.g., heavy smokers, the elderly, and patients with pulmonary symptoms or major organ system disease including malignancy and symptomatic heart disease).

E. **Pulmonary function tests** may be useful to evaluate the severity of lung disease and the response to bronchodilators. These tests are often used in patients who will be undergoing thoracic surgery, especially in cases that will involve the resection of lung parenchyma (see Chapters 3 and 21).

V. **Anesthesiologist–patient relationship**

A. **The perioperative period is emotionally stressful** for many patients who may have fears about surgery (e.g., cancer, physical disfigurement, postoperative pain, and even death) and anesthesia (e.g., loss of control, fear of not waking up, waking up during surgery, postoperative nausea, confusion, pain, paralysis, and headache). The anesthesiologist can alleviate many of these fears and foster trust by doing the following:

  1. **Conducting an unhurried organized interview** in which you convey to the patient that you are interested and understand his or her fears and concerns.

  2. **Reassuring patients** that you will see them in the operating room. If the physician performing the assessment is not the anesthetizing physician, patients should be advised and reassured that their concerns and needs will be competently relayed and addressed.

3. **Informing the patient** of the events of the perioperative period including the following:

a. The time after which the patient must have nothing to eat or drink (nulla per os [NPO]).

b. The estimated time of surgery.

c. Medications to be continued on the day of surgery. In general, antihypertensives (beta-blockers, calcium channel blockers, clonidine), anticonvulsants, antiarrhythmic agents, inhaled bronchodilators, antireflux medications, and steroids and hormonal supplements should be continued. Angiotensin converting enzyme inhibitors and angiotensin receptor blocking agents are sometimes discontinued, because they can cause refractory hypotension intraoperatively. See Chapter 6 for management of insulin regimens and hormonal supplements.

d. The need for premedications (see section VIII.B).

e. The need for autologous blood donation. This usually is indicated for only a limited number of surgical procedures such as total joint arthroplasty, radical prostatectomy, extensive spine surgery, and certain tumor resections.

f. Management of aspirin and nonsteroidal anti-inflammatory drug (NSAID) therapy. Modest inhibition of platelet function is not a problem in many surgeries, and NSAIDs do not significantly increase the risk for bleeding from spinal or epidural anesthesia. Complete reversal of aspirin effects requires 1 to 2 weeks for new platelet synthesis, while the effect of NSAIDS like ibuprofen disappears in 3 or 4 half-lives. Celecoxib does not need to be discontinued before surgery.

g. Procedures that will occur on the day of surgery before the start of surgery (e.g., placement of IV or arterial catheters, placement of routine monitors, epidural catheters) with reassurance that supplemental IV sedation and analgesia will be provided as necessary during this period.

h. Plans for postoperative recovery in the postanesthesia care unit or ICU for closer observation.

i. Plans for postoperative pain control.

j. **Note:** The above discussion should be restricted to those endeavors specific to anesthesia; opinions about the surgical diagnosis, prognosis, and issues of surgical technique should be conveyed by the surgeon.

B. **Informed consent** involves discussing the anesthetic plan, alternatives, and potential complications in terms understandable to the layperson. It is preferable that this discussion be conducted in the patient's native language. Furthermore, written forms should also be available in the patient's native language. There may not be an on-site interpreter for some rare languages. In this setting, it may be necessary to conduct the interview with the assistance of an interpreter via the telephone.

1. **Certain aspects of anesthetic management are outside the realm of common experience** and must be explicitly defined and discussed beforehand. Examples include endotracheal intubation, mechanical ventilation, invasive hemodynamic monitoring, regional anesthesia techniques, blood product transfusion, and postoperative ICU care.
2. **Alternatives** to the suggested management plan should be presented because they may become necessary if the planned procedure fails or if there is a change in clinical circumstances.
3. **Risks associated with anesthesia-related procedures** should be disclosed in a way that a reasonable person would find helpful in making a decision. In general, disclosure applies to complications that occur with a relatively high frequency, not to all remotely possible risks. The anesthetist should familiarize the patient with the most frequent and severe complications of common procedures including the following:
   a. **Regional anesthesia:** headache, infection, local bleeding, nerve injury, drug reactions, and possible failure of regional anesthesia to provide adequate anesthesia. General anesthesia and its attendant risks should also be discussed, because general anesthesia, as an alternative plan, may be necessary.
   b. **General anesthesia:** sore throat, hoarseness, nausea and vomiting, dental injury, allergic reactions to drugs administered. The possibility of intraoperative awareness, pulmonary or cardiac injury, stroke or death, postoperative intubation, or ICU admission should be discussed when appropriate.
   c. **Blood transfusion:** fever, infectious hepatitis, HIV infection, and hemolytic reactions.
   d. **Vascular cannulation:** peripheral nerve, tendon, or blood vessel injury; hemothorax; pneumothorax; and infection.
   e. **Note:** In cases in which the risk has not been objectively defined, the patient should be so informed.
4. **Extenuating circumstances.** Anesthesia procedures may proceed without informed consent in emergency situations.
5. **Consents should never be obtained with the use of young children as interpreters. If family members serve as interpreters the patient should sign a waiver of disclosure.**

VI. **Anesthesia consultant's note.** The preoperative anesthesia note is a medicolegal document in the permanent hospital record. As such, it should contain the following:
   A. **A concise legible statement** of the date and time of the interview, the planned procedure, and a description of any extraordinary circumstances about the anesthesia (e.g., location outside the operating room).
   B. **Relevant positive and negative findings** from the history, physical examination, and laboratory studies including a list of allergies and relevant medications.
   C. **A problem list** that delineates all disease processes, their treatments, and current functional limitations.

D. **An overall impression** of the complexity of the patient's medical condition with assignment to one of the **ASA Physical Status classes:**
   1. Class 1. A healthy patient (no physiologic, physical, or psychologic abnormalities).
   2. Class 2. A patient with mild systemic disease without limitation of daily activities.
   3. Class 3. A patient with severe systemic disease that limits activity but is not incapacitating.
   4. Class 4. A patient with incapacitating systemic disease that is a constant threat to life.
   5. Class 5. A moribund patient not expected to survive 24 hours with or without the operation.
   6. Class 6. A brain-dead patient whose organs are being removed for donor purposes.
   7. **Note:** If the procedure is performed as an emergency, an E is added to the previously defined ASA Physical Status.

E. **The anesthesia plan** in the hospital record is used to convey a general management strategy. At a minimum, the plan should include the following:
   1. **An assessment of the need for premedication.** Many patients scheduled for surgery have a significant level of apprehension and anxiety. The depth and breadth of anxiety are exceptionally variable among patients. Thus, the dose and type of anxiolytics should be tailored to each patient.
   2. **An evaluation of the need for invasive monitoring.** ASA I patients undergoing minimally invasive surgery need only standard ASA monitors. However, if the patient may experience large hemodynamic fluctuations, invasive monitoring should be considered (e.g., central venous pressure for volume monitoring, arterial line for potential hemodynamic instability).
   3. **A review of anesthetic options.** Numerous methods are available for providing anesthesia, analgesia, and hemodynamic stability for any given type of surgery. General anesthesia, regional anesthesia, and combinations thereof should be reviewed and options appropriate for the patient listed in the final assessment.
   4. **Plan for postoperative pain control.** Some patients may have disease states (e.g., cancer, osteoarthritis, Crohn disease, disc herniations) that require chronic pain therapy. A review of patients' current pain regimen with their input about the efficacy of prior pain regimens may be useful in choosing appropriate analgesics and assessing the need for adjunctive therapies (e.g., epidurals and regional blocks).
   5. **Note:** If the interviewer will not be caring for the patient on the day of surgery, the patient should understand that final details of the anesthetic plan will be determined by the anesthesia team providing care. The anesthesia consultant's note should detail the discussion that occurred with the patient including anesthetic options, particular risks, monitoring needs, and postoperative plans. Direct communication between the interviewer and the anesthesia team should occur if important comorbid problems are present.

Table 1.1. ASA guidelines for NPO status preoperatively

Age	Clear Liquids	Breast Milk	Nonhuman Milk/ Light Snack	Fried Fatty Foods/Meat
Infant	2 hours	4 hours	6 hours	8 hours
Child	2 hours	4 hours	6 hours	8 hours
Adult	2 hours	N/A	6 hours	8 hours

VII. Guidelines for NPO status. The current ASA guidelines for NPO status before the start of surgery are as shown in Table 1.1.

VIII. Premedication

    A. Preexisting medical conditions should be controlled or stabilized before surgery. Many of the complications associated with these conditions may be prevented by thoughtful administration of standard medications.

        1. Untreated **hypertension** (HTN) can cause end-organ damage in the perioperative period. Acute treatment of chronic HTN may be indicated in patients with systolic blood pressures (SBP) greater than 20% of their baseline. If HTN persists despite treatment or if the diastolic blood pressure (DBP) is greater than 115 mm Hg, elective surgery should be postponed until the patient's blood pressure can be controlled.

        2. Patients with known **coronary artery disease** (CAD) (history of previous coronary artery bypass grafting/PTCA, previous myocardial infarction, or angina and ischemia on stress-testing) or at risk for CAD (age $\geq$65 years, HTN, diabetes mellitus, hypercholesterolemia, family history of CAD, current smokers) may benefit from premedication with **beta-blockers.** Treatment with beta-blocker therapy before and after surgery has been shown to decrease the risk of perioperative myocardial ischemia. Patients on chronic beta-blocker therapy should continue their medication until the day of surgery. If a patient has a heart rate greater than 60 beats/min and a SBP greater than 110 mm Hg, metoprolol 5 mg intravenously may be administered before the induction of anesthesia.

        3. Asthma. Patients with moderate to severe asthma or patients with symptoms despite optimal medical management may require treatment with albuterol or ipratropium (two puffs via metered dose inhaler in the induction area). Pretreatment with albuterol may reduce the incidence of wheezing and bronchospasm intraoperatively.

        4. Diabetes mellitus. Patients may be hyperglycemic or hypoglycemic preoperatively and intraoperatively. Hyperglycemia can predispose the patient to a hyperosmolar state that can result in impaired enzyme function (e.g., nitric oxide synthase, leukocyte elastase, and amylase and lipase), diabetic ketoacidosis, or hyperosmolar hyperglycemic nonketotic state. The signs and symptoms of hypoglycemia in patients who have taken insulin or hypoglycemic agents can be masked by general anesthesia. A fingerstick blood test for glucose level should be obtained preoperatively and treatment with either a glucose infusion or insulin should be started if needed (see Chapter 6).

5. **Guidelines for prophylaxis for pulmonary aspiration** have been recommended by the ASA and should be considered for patients at high risk for aspiration pneumonitis, including parturients, patients with hiatal hernia and reflux symptoms, with difficult airways, with ileus, with obesity, or with central nervous system depression. Routine use of aspiration prophylaxis in patients without risk factors is not recommended. The following medications are effective in reducing the amount of gastric acid, but there is little conclusive evidence that they decrease the frequency of pulmonary aspiration or reduce morbidity and mortality in patients who aspirate gastric contents:

a. **Histamine (H2) antagonists** produce a dose-related decrease in gastric acid production. **Cimetidine** (Tagamet), 200 to 400 mg orally, intramuscularly or intravenously, and **ranitidine** (Zantac), 150 to 300 mg orally or 50 to 100 mg intravenously or intramuscularly, significantly reduce the volume and the acidity of gastric secretions. Multidose regimens (i.e., the night before and the morning of surgery) are the most effective, although parenteral administration may be used to achieve a rapid (<1 hour) onset. Cimetidine prolongs the elimination of many drugs, including theophylline, diazepam, propranolol, and lidocaine, potentially increasing the toxicity of these agents. Ranitidine has not been associated with such side effects.

b. **Proton pump inhibitors** like omeprazole are highly effective in reducing acid production but do not work quickly enough to be used in the immediate preoperative period. Patients taking these medications chronically should receive a dose the night before surgery.

c. **Nonparticulate antacids.** Colloidal antacid suspensions effectively neutralize stomach acid but can produce a serious pneumonitis if aspirated. A nonparticulate antacid, such as Bicitra (30 to 60 mL, 30 min before induction), is less effective in raising gastric pH but is less harmful if aspirated.

d. **Metoclopramide** (Reglan) enhances gastric emptying by increasing lower esophageal sphincter tone and simultaneously relaxing the pylorus. An oral dose of 10 mg is given 1 to 2 hours before anesthesia. The intravenous dose should be given in the induction area. When administered intravenously, it should be given slowly to avoid abdominal cramping. Like all dopamine antagonists, the drug can produce dystonia and other extrapyramidal effects.

B. The goals for administering **sedatives and analgesics** before surgery are to allay the patient's anxiety; prevent pain during vascular cannulation, regional anesthesia procedures, and positioning; and facilitate smooth induction of anesthesia. It has been shown that the requirement for these drugs can be reduced by a thorough preoperative visit by an anesthesiologist.

1. Doses of sedatives and analgesics should be reduced or withheld in patients who are elderly, debilitated, or acutely intoxicated and in patients with upper airway obstruction or trauma, central apnea, neurologic deterioration, or severe pulmonary or valvular heart disease.

2. Patients addicted to opioids and barbiturates and patients on chronic pain therapy should receive sufficient premedication to overcome tolerance and to prevent withdrawal during or shortly after surgery.

3. **Benzodiazepines** facilitate γ-aminobutyric acid (see Chapter 11) and are highly effective for the treatment of anxiety.

   a. **Midazolam** (Versed), 1 to 3 mg intravenously or intramuscularly, is a short-acting benzodiazepine that provides excellent amnesia and sedation.

   b. **Lorazepam** (Ativan) may also be used (1 to 2 mg orally or intravenously) but can cause more prolonged amnesia and postoperative sedation. It should not be given intramuscularly.

4. **Barbiturates** such as pentobarbital (Nembutal) are rarely used for preoperative sedation. However, they are occasionally used by nonanesthetists for sedation during diagnostic procedures (e.g., endoscopy, magnetic resonance imaging, and computed tomography).

5. **Opioids** are not usually given as premedication unless the patient has significant pain. A hospital in-patient may have the normal dose of morphine, hydromorphone, or meperidine. The outpatient taking oral opioids like oxycodone may take a dose that will provide comfort until the time of surgery. Intravenous fentanyl is appropriate for use immediately before induction because its effects are rapid and intense but short-lived.

C. **Anticholinergics** are not frequently used as premedicants. **Glycopyrrolate** (0.2–0.4 mg intravenously for adults and 10 to 20 μg/kg for pediatric patients) or **atropine** (0.4 to 0.6 mg for adults and 0.02 mg/kg for pediatric patients) is given during ketamine induction as an antisialogogue. Occasionally, this drying effect is desirable during oral surgery or during bronchoscopy.

D. **Antiemetic agents** can be given before induction or intraoperatively to prevent postoperative nausea and vomiting (PONV; see Chapter 35). Risk factors for PONV include female gender, a history of motion sickness or PONV, nonsmoking, and the use of postoperative opioids. Prophylactic antiemetic agents should be considered for patients with at least two risk factors. Patients at high risk for PONV should receive two agents with different mechanisms of action (Table 1.2). The efficacy of all antiemetic agents is similar. Therefore, the first-line agent should be the safest and least expensive drug.

IX. **Delaying surgical procedures.** Occasionally, it is in the best interest of the patient to delay elective surgical procedures for further medical evaluation and optimization of the patient. Some conditions can significantly increase morbidity and mortality if not appropriately evaluated and treated:

A. **Myocardial infarction** within 6 months requires an evaluation of the patient's current potential for ischemia and may require

Table 1.2.   Antiemetic agents

Antiemetic Agent	Mechanism of Action	Side Effects	Dose
Ondansetron	5-HT3 receptor antagonist	Dizziness, headache, QTc prolongation	4 mg intravenously
Droperidol[a]	Dopamine (D2) receptor antagonist	Dystonia, prolong QTc, decrease seizure threshold	0.5–1.25 mg intravenously
Haloperidol	D2 receptor antagonist	Dystonia, prolong QTc, decrease seizure threshold	1 mg i.v.
Dexamethasone	Unknown	Anal/vulvar pruritus, hyperglycemia	4 mg intravenously
Metoclopramide	Dopamine receptor antagonist	GI upset with abdominal cramping, dystonia	10 mg intravenously
Promethazine	Antihistamine	Sedation, decrease seizure threshold	6.25 mg intravenously
Scopolamine	Anticholinergic	Dry mouth, blurred vision, confusion, urinary retention	1.5 mg Transderm

[a] Food and Drug Administration restrictions now emphasize risk of QTc prolongation and Torsades and require 2 to 3 hours of ECG monitoring after dose.

cardiac consultation to determine whether further interventions are needed before proceeding with surgery.

B. New unstable cardiac rhythm. New-onset atrial fibrillation, atrial flutter, supraventricular tachycardia, sustained ventricular tachycardia (10 beats or more), and second or third degree heart block should be evaluated with an ECG, rhythm strip, electrolyte replenishment, and a cardiology consultation.

C. Coagulopathy can predispose the patient to potentially enormous blood loss and can be due to multiple causes including liver dysfunction, medications, and sepsis. Possible causes should be thoroughly investigated and treated before surgery.

D. Hypoxia of unclear etiology should be investigated before surgery. There are many causes of hypoxia that can range from decreased fraction of inspired oxygen to a large ventricular septal defect. The work-up should begin with an arterial blood gas and a chest xray (CXR) and can lead to a vast array of other diagnostic studies depending on the possible etiology of the hypoxia.

E. Administrative uncertainties may warrant postponing surgery. The Jehovah's Witness patient undergoing elective surgery should have a clear plan that is understood and agreed to by the patient and the entire surgical team. The same considerations apply to the patient with "do not resuscitate" orders.

SUGGESTED READING

American Society of Anesthesiologists. Practice guidelines for preoperative fasting and the use of pharmacologic agents to reduce the risk of pulmonary aspiration: application to healthy patients undergoing elective procedures. A report by the Task Force on Preoperative Fasting and the Use of Pharmacologic Agents to Reduce the Risk of Pulmonary Aspiration. http://www.asahq.org/practice/npo/npoguide.html.

American Society of Anesthesiologists. Basic standards for preanesthetic care. http://www.asahq.org/publicationsAndServices.

American Society of Anesthesiologists. Statement of routine preoperative laboratory and diagnostic screening. http://www.asahq.org/publications and Services.

Apfel CC, Korttila K, Abdalla M, et al. A factorial trial of six interventions for the prevention of postoperative nausea and vomiting. *N Engl J Med* 2004;350: 2441–2451.

Eagle KA, Berger PB, Calkins H, et al. ACC/AHA guideline update for perioperative cardiovascular evaluation for noncardiac surgery update: a report of the American College of Cardiology/American Heart Association Task Force on Practice Guidelines (Committee to Update the 1996 Guidelines on Perioperative Cardiovascular Evaluation for Noncardiac Surgery). 2002. American College of Cardiology Web site. Available at http://www.acc.org/clinical/guidelines/perio/update/periupdate_index.htm. Accessed Feb. 23, 2006.

Egan TD, Wong KC. Perioperative smoking cessation and anesthesia: a review. *J Clin Anesth* 1992;4:63–72.

Egbert LD, Batttit GE, Turndorf H, et al. The value of the preoperative visit by an anesthetist. A study of doctor-patient rapport. *JAMA* 1963;185: 553–555.

Fleischer LA, Barash PG. Preoperative cardiac evaluation for noncardiac surgery: a functional approach. *Anesth Analg* 1992;74:586–598.

Klafta JM, Roizen MF. Current understanding of patients' attitudes toward and preparation for anesthesia: a review. *Anesth Analg* 1996;83:1314–1321.

Mangano DT, Layug EL, Wallace A, et al. Effect of atenolol on mortality and cardiovascular morbidity after noncardiac surgery. *N Engl J Med* 1996;335:1713.

Raith K, Hochhaus G. Drugs used in the treatment of opioid tolerance and physical dependence: a review. *Int J Clin Pharmacol Ther* 2004;42:191–203.

Smetana GW. Preoperative pulmonary evaluation. *N Engl J Med* 1999;340:937.

Vealnovich V. The value of routine preoperative laboratory testing in predicting postoperative complications: a multivariate analysis. *Surgery* 1991;109:236–243.

White PF. Pharmacologic and clinical aspects of preoperative medication. *Anesth Anal* 1986;65:963–974.

2

Specific Considerations with Cardiac Disease

Johnica A. Eyvazzadeh and Hovig V. Chitilian

I. **Ischemic heart disease.** Coronary artery disease (CAD) afflicts approximately 10 million Americans. CAD increases in prevalence with age: 4 in 1,000 for ages 15 to 44, 48 in 1,000 for ages 45 to 65, and 80 in 1,000 for those over age 65. Nearly 10 million noncardiac surgical patients are at risk annually for perioperative morbidity and mortality from ischemic cardiac events. These include 1 million with diagnosed CAD (angina or Q waves on electrocardiogram [ECG]), 2 to 3 million with two or more coronary risk factors, and 4 million older than age 65. Perioperative cardiac events, including myocardial infarction (MI), unstable angina, congestive heart failure (CHF), and serious dysrhythmias, are the leading cause of perioperative deaths.

A. **Physiology**

1. **Oxygen supply–demand balance.** Myocardial ischemia occurs when oxygen demand exceeds delivery.

a. **Supply.** The myocardium is perfused via coronary arteries. The **left coronary artery** branches into the **left anterior descending** and the **circumflex** to supply most of the left ventricle (LV), interventricular septum (including atrioventricular [A-V] bundles), and left atrium. The **right coronary artery** supplies the interventricular septum, including the sinoatrial and A-V nodes. Coronary arteries are end arteries with minimal collateralization. **Myocardial oxygen supply** depends on coronary artery diameter, LV diastolic pressure, aortic diastolic pressure, and arterial oxygen content.

(1) **Coronary blood flow** is dependent on the aortic root to downstream coronary pressure gradient. Most coronary blood flow occurs during diastole. Coronary artery blood flow in normal individuals is controlled primarily through local mediators. Patients with significant coronary diseases may be maximally dilated at rest.

(2) **Heart rate** is inversely proportional to the length of diastole. Faster heart rates decrease the duration of maximal coronary perfusion.

(3) **Blood oxygen content** is determined by hemoglobin concentration, oxygen saturation, and dissolved oxygen. Increasing inspired oxygen fraction and/or hemoglobin concentration increases blood oxygen content.

b. **Demand.** Myocardial oxygen consumption ($M\dot{V}O_2$) is increased by increases in ventricular wall tension and heart rate (velocity of shortening) and, to a lesser degree, contractility.

(1) **Ventricular wall tension** is modeled by Laplace's law: wall tension equals transmural ventricular pressure multiplied by the cardiac radius divided by twice wall thickness. Changes in these parameters affect oxygen demand.

(2) **Heart rate.** Tachycardia is well tolerated in normal hearts. Atherosclerotic coronary arteries may not adequately dilate to meet increased demands of faster heart rates.

(3) **Contractility** increases with the increased chronotropy, myocardial stretch, calcium, and catecholamines. Increasing contractility increases oxygen consumption.

c. **Supply and demand balance.** Atherosclerosis is the most common etiology for supply–demand imbalances. Conditions such as aortic stenosis, systemic hypertension, and hypertrophic cardiomyopathy, which are characterized by marked ventricular hypertrophy and high intraventricular pressures, may also increase $M\dot{V}O_2$ and create imbalances, even in the setting of normal coronary arteries. The goal of treatment is to improve the supply–demand balance.

(1) **Increase supply**

(a) **Increase coronary perfusion pressure** with administration of volume or α-adrenergic agonists to increase aortic diastolic pressure.

(b) **Increase coronary blood flow** with nitrates and calcium channel antagonists to dilate coronary arteries.

(c) **Increase oxygen content** by raising hemoglobin concentration or oxygen partial pressure.

(2) **Decrease demand**

(a) **Decrease heart rate** either directly with β-adrenergic antagonists or indirectly by decreasing sympathetic tone with opioids and anxiolytics.

(b) **Decrease ventricular size** (decrease wall tension) by decreasing preload with nitrates, calcium channel antagonists, or diuretics. Occasionally, increasing inotropy may decrease demand by decreasing ventricular size and wall tension.

(c) **Decreasing contractility** may decrease $M\dot{V}O_2$ if ventricular size and wall tension do not increase excessively. Calcium channel blockers and volatile anesthetics may decrease contractility.

(d) **Intra-aortic balloon counter pulsation** increases coronary perfusion pressure by augmenting diastolic pressure. It also reduces resistance to LV ejection, thereby reducing LV size and wall tension.

B. **Preoperative cardiovascular evaluation for noncardiac surgery.** The American College of Cardiology and American Heart

Association (ACC/AHA) have developed joint guidelines for preoperative cardiovascular evaluation of patients undergoing noncardiac surgery. The initial evaluation consists of obtaining a patient's history with specific emphasis on cardiac status and conducting a focused physical examination. It is suggested that patients with known cardiovascular disease obtain blood urea nitrogen and creatinine levels, chest radiograph, and ECG. Preoperative ECGs should be obtained for men over 40 and women over 50 years of age. Hemoglobin levels should be obtained for males over 65 and females of any age, or if significant blood loss is expected. Based on a patient's clinical history, functional status, and the nature of the surgical procedure, the ACC/AHA guidelines provide a stepwise approach for identifying patients that may benefit from further cardiovascular testing.

1. **Initial screening**
   a. The need for **emergency surgery** preempts further cardiac workup.
   b. In the absence of any change in symptoms, further cardiac testing is usually unnecessary if a patient has undergone **coronary revascularization within the past 5 years** or has had a favorable **coronary evaluation within the past 2 years.**
   c. In all other circumstances, further cardiac evaluation is guided by the patient's **clinical predictors, functional status,** and the **risk of surgery.**
2. **Clinical predictors**
   a. **Major clinical predictors** are an acute (<7 days) MI, recent (<1 month before surgery) MI, unstable angina, decompensated heart failure, severe valvular disease, and significant dysrhythmias (high-grade A-V block, symptomatic dysrhythmias in the presence of underlying heart disease, or supraventricular dysrhythmias with uncontrolled ventricular rate).
   b. **Intermediate clinical predictors** are mild angina pectoris, a remote MI (>1 month before surgery), compensated heart failure, preoperative creatinine ≥2.0 mg/dL, and diabetes mellitus.
   c. **Minor clinical predictors** are advanced age (>65 years), abnormal ECG, rhythm other than sinus, low functional capacity, history of stroke, and uncontrolled systemic hypertension.
3. **Functional capacity** can be expressed in metabolic equivalent (MET) values. A single MET represents oxygen consumption at rest.
   a. **Poor functional capacity** is defined as an exercise capacity of less than 4 METs. Activities requiring fewer than 4 METs include cooking, slow-dancing, golfing with a cart, and walking 1 to 2 blocks on level ground at 2 to 3 miles per hour.
   b. **Moderate or excellent functional capacity** is defined as an exercise capacity greater than 4 METs. Activities that correspond to moderate functional capacity include climbing a flight of stairs, walking on level ground at 6.4 km/hour, running a short distance, scrubbing floors, or playing a game of golf without a cart. The ability to

participate in strenuous sports such as swimming, singles tennis, or football corresponds to excellent functional capacity.

4. **Surgery-specific risk** is categorized as high, intermediate, or low.

   a. **High-risk** procedures have a reported risk of perioperative cardiac morbidity of greater than 5%. These procedures include major emergency surgery, aortic and major vascular surgery, peripheral vascular surgery, and procedures that are associated with large fluid shifts and/or blood loss.

   b. **Intermediate-risk** surgery includes procedures with a reported cardiac risk of less than 5%, such as otherwise uncomplicated intraperitoneal and intrathoracic surgery, carotid endarterectomy, head and neck surgery, orthopedic surgery, and prostate surgery.

   c. **Low-risk** surgery has a reported cardiac risk of less than 1%. These procedures include endoscopic surgery, superficial procedures, breast surgery, and cataract surgery.

5. **ACC/AHA guidelines for preoperative cardiovascular evaluation**

   a. Patients with **major clinical predictors** should have elective surgery delayed pending further evaluation and optimization of their cardiac condition. Further cardiovascular evaluation, including invasive and noninvasive tests (see section I.C.), should be tailored to the patient's specific condition.

   b. Patients with **intermediate clinical predictors** should have additional evaluation before **high-risk surgical** procedures. Those with **poor functional capacity** also need evaluation before **intermediate-risk surgical procedures.**

   c. Patients with **minor clinical predictors** do not require further evaluation unless they have **poor functional capacity** and are undergoing a **high-risk surgical** procedure.

C. **Specific cardiovascular tests**

1. **Noninvasive studies.** Specific situations may warrant one or more of the following:

   a. **Exercise stress testing** gives an estimate of functional capacity along with the ability to detect ECG changes and hemodynamic response. Exercise stress tests are highly predictive when ST segment changes are characteristic of ischemia (>2 mm, immediate, sustained into recovery, and/or associated with hypotension).

   b. **Radionuclide imaging** is a safe and effective method to assess myocardial perfusion, infarction, and function.

      (1) **Thallium 201** is a radioactive tracer that is injected intravenously and avidly extracted as a potassium analogue by cardiac muscle. Myocardial distribution of thallium is closely related to regional myocardial blood flow. Areas of thallium redistribution upon delayed imaging are considered to represent myocardium at risk. A fixed defect (unchanged distribution with time) is believed to represent scar tissue (an old MI). Coronary stenoses of >90% likely produce perfusion abnormalities at rest, whereas stenoses of

50% or greater may be detected only with increased stress or exercise.

(2) **Technetium-99^m sestamibi** is injected intravenously and accumulated in myocardium in proportion to blood flow. Using a first-pass technique, multiple ventricular images synchronized to the cardiac cycle are acquired at rest and during exercise. The occurrence of regional wall motion abnormalities and the inability to increase LV ejection fraction during exercise suggest myocardial ischemia.

(3) **Pharmacologic stress test with radionuclide imaging** may be useful in patients who are unable to complete an exercise-based test. Dipyridamole or adenosine is used for coronary dilation. The presence of areas of redistribution correlates well with increased perioperative cardiac risk. Specificity is reduced when the test is used as a general screening examination.

c. **Echocardiography** is used to evaluate global and regional ventricular function, pericardial effusions, and congenital abnormalities. Transthoracic and/or transesophageal views may be obtained. Transesophageal echocardiography may provide a better view of valvular function, mural or atrial thrombi, and aortic aneurysms and is often used intraoperatively to evaluate valve function (e.g., during mitral valve reconstruction) and wall motion. Stress echocardiography may be useful if a prior stress ECG is nondiagnostic, if there is an abnormal baseline ECG, or if atypical symptoms are present. Dobutamine can be used in patients who are unable to exercise. Contrast echocardiography may be useful in quantifying regional myocardial perfusion patterns.

d. **Continuous ECG monitoring** may be useful for detecting arrhythmias or periods of ischemia and correlating the findings with symptoms.

2. **Cardiac catheterization** is considered the "gold standard" for evaluating cardiac disease. Information obtained includes anatomy with visualization of direction and distribution of flow, hemodynamics, and overall function of the heart (see Chapter 23).

3. **Cardiac consultation** may be helpful in determining which tests will be useful and can expedite the process and interpret the results. The consultant can help optimize the patient's preoperative medical therapy and provide follow-up in the postoperative period. Such follow-up is crucial with the initiation of new drug therapies.

D. **Preanesthetic considerations**

1. Patients are likely to be anxious. Reassurance during the preoperative visit has been shown to be useful in decreasing anxiety. **Anxiolytics** may blunt rises in sympathetic tone and may be invaluable.

2. **Cardiac medications** are usually continued preoperatively. Possible exceptions include angiotensin-converting enzyme inhibitors (due to prolonged vasodilation), slow-release or long-acting medications, and diuretics.

a. **Beta blockers** have been shown to decrease the risk of perioperative ischemia and infarction. Patients receiving β-adrenergic blockers should continue to receive them. In the absence of any contraindications (i.e., previous adverse reaction, symptoms of CHF, or bronchospasm), consider initiating perioperative beta blockers for patients with increased risk of cardiac events undergoing a high-risk surgical procedure. The benefit of perioperative beta blockade for high-risk patients undergoing low- and intermediate-risk surgical procedures is unknown.

b. **Clonidine.** Small preoperative doses of clonidine may confer cardioprotective effects.

c. **Statins.** Based on observational studies, the perioperative use of statins may be associated with reduced mortality in patients undergoing vascular surgery.

3. **Supplemental oxygen** should be provided to all patients with significant risk of ischemia, especially when sedation is being ordered preoperatively.

4. **Monitoring** is discussed in Chapter 10.

5. **Perioperative issues**

a. **General versus regional anesthesia.** No convincing outcome data support the superiority of either general or regional anesthesia with regard to cardiac outcome. Reasons other than the cardiac issues should guide the choice of anesthetic technique.

b. **Site of surgery** may predict perioperative cardiac morbidity. Patients undergoing thoracic, upper abdominal, and major vascular surgery have a severalfold increased risk of cardiac and other perioperative complications.

II. **Noncoronary cardiac disease**

A. **Bacterial endocarditis prophylaxis.** Transient bacteremia after surgical and dental procedures may cause endocarditis. Blood-borne bacteria can lodge on damaged or abnormal valves or tissues. Antibiotic prophylaxis is recommended for patients with prosthetic cardiac valves, previous history of endocarditis, most congenital malformations, rheumatic valvular disease, hypertrophic cardiomyopathy, and mitral valve regurgitation. See Chapter 7 (section V.B.) for discussion of appropriate prophylactic antibiotic choices. Prophylaxis is not recommended for patients with permanent pacemakers, implantable defibrillators, and mitral valve prolapse without regurgitation. Patients with subacute bacterial endocarditis may experience dysrhythmias secondary to nodal abscesses and inflammation; pacing capabilities should be considered preoperatively.

B. **Aortic stenosis**

1. **The etiology** is usually progressive calcification and narrowing of a normal or bicuspid valve. A valve area <1.0 cm^2 defines severe stenosis and results in a marked increase in obstruction to LV ejection, leading to an increased wall tension. Critical aortic stenosis is defined as a valve area ≤ 0.75 cm^2.

2. **Symptoms** appear late in the disease process. In the absence of surgical intervention, life expectancy is 5 years after the onset of angina and 2 years after the development of CHF.

3. The **ventricle** becomes **hypertrophied** and stiff in response to the increased pressure load. Coordinated atrial contraction becomes critical to maintaining adequate ventricular filling and

stroke volume. The ventricle is susceptible to ischemia due to increased muscle mass and decreased coronary perfusion in the setting of increased intraventricular pressure.

4. **Anesthetic considerations.** Aortic stenosis is the only valvular lesion directly associated with an increased risk of perioperative ischemia, MI, and death.

    a. **Normal sinus rhythm** and adequate **volume status** should be maintained. Hypotension, tachycardia (decreasing filling and increasing oxygen demands), and severe bradycardia (decreasing cardiac output) are poorly tolerated and should be aggressively treated to maintain coronary perfusion pressure.

    b. **Cardiac pacing** capabilities should be considered to treat bradycardia. Supraventricular tachydysrhythmias should be treated aggressively with direct current cardioversion.

    c. **Pulmonary artery catheters** may be useful to assess baseline filling pressures, ventricular function, and response to pharmacologic interventions, fluid therapy, and changes of heart rate and rhythm.

    d. **Nitrates** and **peripheral vasodilators** should be administered with extreme caution because small reductions of ventricular volume can markedly reduce cardiac output.

    e. The **treatment of ischemia** in these patients is directed at increasing oxygen delivery by raising coronary perfusion pressure and decreasing oxygen consumption (usually by lowering heart rate).

C. **Hypertrophic cardiomyopathy** is a genetic cardiac disorder characterized by **asymmetric LV hypertrophy.** Although most patients with hypertrophic cardiomyopathy do not have an increased LV outflow tract gradient at rest, many of them develop **dynamic outflow tract obstruction** with increased cardiac output. The mechanism of subaortic LV outflow tract obstruction is systolic anterior motion of the mitral valve leaflets leading to ventricular septal contact.

1. Factors that **worsen the outflow obstruction** include decreased arterial pressure, decreased intraventricular volume, increased contractility, and increased heart rate.

2. **Clinical implications** and treatment are similar to those for aortic stenosis.

3. **Anesthetic considerations** include the following:

    a. Maintain normal sinus rhythm.

    b. Consider cardioversion for supraventricular tachycardia.

    c. Continue β-adrenergic and calcium channel blocker therapy.

    d. Maintain normal volume status.

    e. Correct vasodilation with α-adrenergic agonists to avoid tachycardia and marked changes in contractility.

    f. Use inotropes with caution because they may exacerbate the outflow obstruction.

    g. Use nitrates and peripheral dilators only with extreme caution.

D. **Aortic regurgitation**

1. **Etiologies** include rheumatic heart disease, endocarditis, trauma, collagen vascular diseases, and processes that dilate the aortic root (e.g., aneurysm, Marfan disease, and syphilis).

2. **Pathophysiology**
   a. Acute aortic regurgitation may cause sudden LV volume overload with increased LV end-diastolic pressure and pulmonary capillary occlusion pressure. Manifestations include decreased cardiac output, CHF, tachycardia, and vasoconstriction.
   b. Chronic aortic regurgitation leads to LV dilation and eccentric hypertrophy. Symptoms may be minimal until late in the disease process when left heart failure occurs.
3. **Anesthetic considerations**
   a. Maintain a normal to slightly increased heart rate to minimize regurgitation and maintain aortic diastolic and coronary artery perfusion pressure.
   b. Maintain adequate volume status.
   c. Improve forward flow, decrease LV end-diastolic pressure and myocardial wall tension with vasodilators.
   d. Avoid peripheral arterial constrictors. They may worsen regurgitation.
   e. Consider pacing. These patients have an increased frequency of conduction abnormalities.

E. **Mitral stenosis**
   1. **The etiology** is almost always rheumatic.
   2. **Pathophysiology**
      a. Increased left atrial pressure and volume overload increases left atrial size and may produce **atrial fibrillation.**
      b. **Elevated left atrial pressure** increases pulmonary venous pressure and pulmonary vascular resistance. In turn, right ventricular (RV) pressure is increased for a given cardiac output. Chronic pulmonary hypertension produces pulmonary vascular remodeling.
      c. **Pulmonary hypertension** may lead to tricuspid regurgitation, RV failure, and decreased cardiac output.
      d. **Tachycardia** is poorly tolerated because it decreases diastolic filling time, decreases cardiac output, and increases left atrial pressure.
   3. **Anesthetic considerations**
      a. **Avoid tachycardia.** Control ventricular response pharmacologically or consider cardioversion for patients with atrial fibrillation. Continue digoxin, calcium channel blockers, and β-adrenergic blockers perioperatively.
      b. **Avoid pulmonary hypertension.** Hypoxia, hypercarbia, acidosis, atelectasis, and sympathomimetics increase pulmonary vascular resistance. Oxygen, hypocarbia, alkalosis, nitrates, prostaglandin E_1, and inhaled nitric oxide decrease pulmonary vascular resistance.
      c. **Hypotension** may be caused by hypovolemia; however, one must have a high suspicion for RV failure. Inotropes and agents that decrease pulmonary hypertension may be useful (e.g., dopamine, dobutamine, milrinone, amrinone, nitrates, prostaglandin E_1, and inhaled nitric oxide).
      d. A **pulmonary artery catheter** may assist in perioperative evaluation of volume status, intracardiac pressures, and cardiac output.

e. **Premedication** should be adequate to prevent anxiety and tachycardia. Exercise caution in patients with hypotension, pulmonary hypertension, or low cardiac output.

F. **Mitral regurgitation**
  1. **Etiologies** include mitral valve prolapse, ischemic heart disease, endocarditis, and post-MI papillary muscle rupture. Mitral regurgitation allows blood to be ejected into the left atrium during systole. The amount of regurgitant flow depends on the ventricular–atrial pressure gradient, size of the mitral orifice, and duration of systole.
  2. **Pathophysiology**
    a. **Acute mitral regurgitation** usually occurs in the setting of MI. Acute volume overload of the left heart leads to LV dysfunction with increased wall tension.
    b. **Chronic mitral regurgitation** causes gradual left atrial and LV overload and dilation with compensatory hypertrophy.
    c. **Measurement of ejection fraction** does not quantify forward versus backward flow, because the incompetent valve permits immediate bidirectional ejection with systole.
  3. **Anesthetic considerations**
    a. **Relative tachycardia** is desirable to decrease ventricular filling time and ventricular volume. Bradycardia is associated with increased LV volume and regurgitation.
    b. **Afterload reduction** is beneficial. Intra-aortic balloon counterpulsation may be life-saving. Increased systemic vascular resistance will increase regurgitation.
    c. **Maintain preload.**
    d. **Careful titration** of myocardial depressants is indicated.

G. **Mitral valve prolapse** has a prevalence of 5% to 10%.
  1. **Clinical features** include atypical chest pain, a midsystolic click, palpitations, anxiety, dyspnea, and nonspecific ECG changes. Associated pathologic conditions include conduction abnormalities, supraventricular dysrhythmias, mitral regurgitation, and endocarditis.
  2. **Diagnosis** is confirmed by echocardiography.
  3. **Subacute bacterial endocarditis** prophylaxis is recommended if mitral regurgitation is present (see section II.A. and Chapter 7, section VI.B.).
  4. **Anesthetic considerations** are those appropriate for the patient's coexisting diseases.

III. **Congenital heart disease (CHD).** With improved survival of CHD patients, anesthesiologists are encountering them with greater frequency as adults in noncardiac surgical settings. Depending on the underlying lesion, an adult with a history of CHD may have an **uncorrected** lesion or may have undergone a **reparative** or **palliative** procedure in the past. Furthermore, as the medical and surgical management of these conditions continues to evolve, different patients with the same original congenital defect may have undergone significantly different procedures and as a result may differ in their anatomy and physiology. Transferring patient care to institutions with extensive experience in managing these disorders should be considered.

A. **General considerations**
  1. A thorough understanding of the patient's **cardiac anatomy and physiology** (i.e., presence, type, and degree of shunts), as

well as **functional status,** and the **physiologic stresses** associated with the surgical procedure is essential.

2. **Myocardial dysfunction** may be present as a long-term consequence of the physiology of the original lesion or the subsequent reparative or palliative procedure. It may also be a consequence of chronic hypoxemia.

3. **Dysrhythmias** are common in this patient population and may be due to the pathophysiology of the cardiovascular defect or the scarring from surgery. Intra-atrial reentrant tachycardia and ventricular tachycardia are commonly encountered in this patient population.

4. **Cyanotic patients** are often polycythemic and at risk for stroke and thrombosis. Intravenous hydration is important. Hemodilution may be considered in the instance of a preoperative hematocrit greater than 60%.

5. **Abnormal hemostasis,** usually mild in severity, has been noted in patients with cyanotic CHD. Abnormalities of the extrinsic and intrinsic coagulation pathways as well as platelet function are possible.

6. **Systemic air emboli** are a constant danger in the presence of bidirectional or right-to-left shunts. Intravenous lines must be purged of air bubbles, and the use of air filters should be considered.

7. **Bacterial endocarditis prophylaxis.** Patients with prosthetic heart valves, complex CHD, surgically constructed conduits, and mitral valve prolapse with mitral regurgitation are at moderate to high risk for developing infective endocarditis (see section II.A. and Chapter 7, section VI.B.).

8. Specific considerations with selected lesions are presented below. For a more thorough treatment of the subject, the reader is referred to the Suggested Readings.

B. **Atrial septal defect**
   1. **Physiologic consequences** depend on the **size** of the defect and the **degree of shunting.**
   2. **Left-to-right shunts** produce RV overload, increased pulmonary blood flow, and pulmonary hypertension.
   3. Patients may present with a flow murmur, dysrhythmias, atrial fibrillation, CHF, or a stroke.
   4. Most atrial septal defects in adults can be closed by percutaneous catheter-based techniques.

C. **Ventricular septal defect (VSD)**
   1. Most undergo spontaneous closure.
   2. Physiologic consequences depend on the size of the defect and the balance between the pulmonary and systemic vascular resistances.
   3. Chronic left-to-right shunting across moderate-sized defects leads to RV overload, increased pulmonary vascular resistance, and, ultimately, reversal of shunt flow (Eisenmenger syndrome). RV failure carries a poor prognosis.
   4. Surgical repair of VSDs is associated with injuries to the bundle of His and heart block. Percutaneous catheter-based closure may be an option.

D. **Tetralogy of Fallot**
   1. Consists of a large **VSD, RV outflow tract obstruction** (usually infundibular), **RV hypertrophy,** and an **overriding aorta.**

   2. After surgical correction, most patients have **residual RV dysfunction** and **right bundle branch block.** Patients may also have reduced exercise tolerance. Some show **residual RV outflow obstruction** or **pulmonic stenosis,** which may lead to RV failure and ventricular arrhythmias.
   3. **Pulmonary regurgitation** is common and may require pulmonic valve replacement later in life.
   4. A few patients have residual VSDs or LV dysfunction.
   5. There is an increased incidence of ventricular tachydysrhythmias and sudden death.

E. **Fontan physiology**
   1. Certain defects such as **tricuspid atresia** and **hypoplastic left heart syndrome** are treated with a multistaged surgical approach with the goal of establishing a single-ventricle circulation.
   2. The **Fontan procedure** is the final procedure in the pathway. It is performed in patients who have already undergone a bidirectional Glenn (superior vena cava to main pulmonary artery) shunt. The procedure connects the inferior vena cava to the main pulmonary artery via an atrial (intra- or extra-atrial) conduit. Thus, total venous return passively flows directly to the pulmonary arteries, travels through the pulmonary circulation and into the single ventricle, and is ejected into the systemic circulation. The conduit is often fenestrated. The fenestration allows blood to bypass the pulmonary circulation and be shunted to the systemic ventricle in the event of a rise in the pulmonary vascular resistance, preserving cardiac output and systemic perfusion at the expense of oxygenation.
   3. **Hypovolemia** and **increases in pulmonary vascular resistance** are poorly tolerated by patients who have had a Fontan procedure.
   4. **Long-term complications** include progressive **hepatic dysfunction** with the development of a **coagulopathy** and an increased risk for **thromboembolism, protein-losing enteropathy,** and **arrhythmias.**

IV. **Cardiac transplant patient**
A. More than 2,000 cardiac transplants, including 225 pediatric transplants, are performed each year with a 90% 1-year survival rate and a 70% 5-year survival. Increasingly, these patients present for noncardiac surgery.
B. Postcardiac transplant patients typically require surgery related to underlying vascular disease or complications of chronic steroid or immunosuppressive therapy.
C. **Physiology of the transplanted heart**
   1. Sympathetic reinnervation may occur over time. Parasympathetic reinnervation does not occur.
   2. Transplanted hearts exhibit accelerated graft atherosclerosis and are at increased risk for myocardial ischemia.
   3. **Hemodynamics of the transplanted heart**
      a. Cardiac impulse formation and conduction are normal, although the resting heart rate is increased.
      b. The Frank-Starling mechanism remains intact. Transplanted hearts respond normally to circulating catecholamines.
      c. Autoregulation of coronary blood flow is intact.

    d. Due to autonomic denervation, the transplanted heart meets the demand for increased cardiac output initially by increasing stroke volume and subsequently by increasing heart rate in response to circulating catecholamines.

  4. Drug effects

    a. Drugs that act via the autonomic system (e.g., atropine and digoxin) are ineffective.

    b. Direct-acting agents are effective. Isoproterenol may be used to increase heart rate. Norepinephrine or phenylephrine may be used to increase blood pressure.

    c. β-Adrenergic receptors are intact and may be present in increased density.

D. Anesthetic considerations

  1. The patient's activity level and exercise capacity should be determined. A cardiology consultant may provide data concerning cardiac function and anatomy as measured by echocardiography and catheterization.

  2. Underlying CAD may be asymptomatic. Evidence of ischemia may include a history of dyspnea, signs of reduced cardiac function, and dysrhythmias.

  3. A baseline 12-lead ECG should be obtained and may demonstrate multiple P waves and right bundle branch block.

  4. A chest radiograph may be useful.

  5. To assess the effect of immunosuppression and concomitant drug therapy, baseline laboratory studies should include complete blood count, electrolytes, blood urea nitrogen, creatinine, glucose, and liver function tests.

  6. Strict aseptic technique is required for all interventions (e.g., intravenous access, intubation), because the patient may be receiving long-term immunosuppression.

  7. Monitoring. Invasive monitoring is used when indicated by the patient's cardiopulmonary status and the proposed surgical procedure. The right internal jugular vein is often the access site for repetitive endocardial biopsies and may need to be reserved for this purpose.

  8. Anesthesia

    a. General, regional, and spinal anesthesia have been administered to cardiac transplant patients. Selection of anesthesia may be guided by issues other than the history of cardiac transplant.

    b. Hemodynamic goals

      (1) Maintain preload.

      (2) Avoid sudden vasodilation. Initial compensatory changes in cardiac output depend on the Frank-Starling mechanism because of the delayed heart rate response.

      (3) If sudden hypotension occurs, administer volume and direct-acting vasopressors such as phenylephrine and norepinephrine.

V. Pacemakers

  A. A standardized five-letter code is used to describe the function of each pacemaker.

    1. The first letter designates the **chamber paced** (O, none; A, atrium; V, ventricle; D, dual [both atrium and ventricle]).

2. The second letter describes the **chamber sensed** (O, none; A, atrium; V, ventricle; D, dual).

3. The third letter describes the **pacemaker's response** to sensed events (O, none; I, inhibition of pacemaker output; T, triggering of pacemaker output; D, dual response: spontaneous atrial and ventricular activity inhibit atrial and ventricular pacing and atrial activity triggers a ventricular response).

4. The fourth letter indicates the presence or absence of **rate modulation** (O, no rate modulation; R, rate modulation present).

5. The fifth letter specifies the presence and type of multisite **pacing** (O, none; A, more than one stimulation site in either atrium, stimulation sites in each atrium, or a combination of the two; V, more than one stimulation site in either ventricle, stimulation sites in each ventricle, or a combination of the two; D, any combination of A and V).

6. For example, a **VVI** pacemaker will sense and pace the ventricle yet will be inhibited and not fire if an R wave is detected. A **DDD** pacemaker is known as a universal, with the ability to sense and pace both atrium and ventricle. A VVIRV pacemaker has ventricular inhibitory pacing with rate modulation and multisite ventricular pacing. This mode is often used in patients with heart failure, chronic atrial fibrillation, or intraventricular conduction delay. A **DDDRD** pacemaker has dual-chamber pacing with rate modulation and multisite pacing in both the atrium (or atria) and ventricle(s).

B. **Indications.** See ACC/AHA/North American Society of Pacing and Electrophysiology (NASPE) practice guidelines (see Suggested Readings) for additional information.

1. Third degree (complete) A-V block

2. Type II, second degree A-V block

3. Symptomatic bradycardia

4. Cardiac resynchronization therapy. A relatively new indication in which the weight of the evidence is in favor of usefulness. It consists of biventricular pacing to improve the timing of RV and LV depolarization in patients with symptomatic heart failure who also have an intraventricular conduction abnormality. Such therapy has been shown to reduce hospitalization and mortality in patients who are otherwise optimally medically managed.

C. **Preoperative evaluation of patients with permanent pacemakers**

1. Determine the **indication** for the pacemaker and **device dependency.**

2. Determine the **location** of the pulse generator. Most are currently placed in the upper chest. Older models may be located in the abdomen.

3. Determine the **model** and programmed **mode** of the pacemaker. If the information is not readily available, the manufacturer and model number may be obtained from a radiograph of the generator. The manufacturer of the device must be known to be able to program the pacemaker, as each manufacturer has a unique programming device. Determine whether rate modulation is active. Also, determine the magnet response of the device.

4. Determine proper functioning of the device by patient history, electrophysiology clinic follow-up records, and ECG. Formal interrogation of the pacemaker is not routinely required before surgical procedures if the patient has received regular follow-up for the device, has experienced no problems with the device in the interim, and if the presence of pacing impulses, along with their ability to create a paced beat, can be confirmed.

5. If central access is required, consider placement under fluoroscopic guidance to avoid dislodging a lead if the pacemaker has been placed within 6 weeks.

D. **Intraoperative management**

1. **Modern pacemakers** are extremely resistant to electromagnetic interference (**EMI**) associated with the use of electrocautery. If interference does occur, the pacemaker output may be inhibited or the pacemaker may be reset to a committed pacing mode (i.e., DOO or VOO).

2. Applying a common donut **magnet** to any pacemaker will cause it to function temporarily in the magnet mode, which is an asynchronous mode. This will prevent pacemaker output inhibition by EMI associated with electrocautery use. Normal pacemaker function is restored upon removal of the magnet. Use of a magnet during surgical procedures is necessary only if inhibition of pacemaker output is noted coincident with EMI. If used, the magnet should be placed directly over the pacemaker. It is best to tape the magnet in place to avoid inadvertent dislodgment.

3. **Resetting of pacemakers** by EMI will produce asynchronous (i.e., "competitive") pacing that can be noted on the ECG.

4. Intraoperative exposure of the device to EMI can be reduced by placing the current return pad ("**grounding pad**") so that the **current from the electrocautery does not pass near the pulse generator.** Other measures include the use of **short, intermittent bursts** at the lowest possible energy level and the use of a **bipolar electrocautery** system or an **ultrasonic (harmonic) scalpel.** Consider inactivating rate-responsive features during the procedure.

5. **Monitor heart rate** during electrocautery with a precordial or esophageal stethoscope, pulse oximeter, arterial line, or a finger on the pulse.

6. **Postoperative evaluation of pacemaker function** is recommended when there is evidence that the pacemaker has been reset (i.e., asynchronous pacing is present) on the postoperative ECG. Routine postoperative interrogation of the pacemaker is not necessary.

E. **Perioperative pacing options**

1. **Transcutaneous.** External pacing can be performed via large pads placed on the anterior and posterior thorax. This is an easy and inexpensive method of ventricular pacing.

2. **Transvenous**
   a. A temporary pacing electrode can be inserted via a central vein into the heart.
   b. Various pulmonary artery catheters exist that have pacing options (see Chapter 10).

3. **Transesophageal.** The left atrium can be paced with a pacing probe placed in the esophagus.

VI. The implantable cardioverter defibrillator (ICD) has dramatically changed the treatment of patients at high risk for sudden cardiac death.

    A. Electrical countershock is the only reliable treatment for ventricular fibrillation.

    B. The ICD is implanted in the abdominal or chest wall and connected to two defibrillating electrodes (patches) or transvenous leads. A separate electrode is used for pacing and sensing. This electrode can sense ventricular tachycardia or fibrillation and deliver a counter shock of 20 to 30 joules for up to four consecutive attempts.

    C. All ICDs are exquisitely sensitive to EMI associated with electrocautery. EMI is detected by the ICD as ventricular fibrillation and may result in spurious shocks.

    D. All ICDs are specifically designed to suspend detection in response to a magnet application. Magnet application therefore will prevent misinterpretation of EMI as ventricular fibrillation. Magnet application does not affect the pacing functions of the ICD. Most ICDs are designed to resume functioning upon removal of the magnet. Some ICDs may be programmed to turn off permanently after magnet application. These ICDs are reactivated by removing and reapplying the magnet. Consult with the patient's cardiologist or the manufacturer of the ICD to determine the magnet response of the device.

    E. Intraoperative magnet application, rather than deactivation of the ICD, is preferred: If ventricular tachycardia or ventricular fibrillation occurs intraoperatively, simply removing the magnet will cause the ICD to resume detection and deliver therapy, typically in less than 10 seconds. This is more certain and faster than any possible human response (such as external defibrillation).

    F. ICD failure during anesthesia may occur as a result of changes in defibrillation thresholds. An external defibrillator should be available, and some advocate placing external defibrillator pads preoperatively.

    G. Patients with an ICD should not enter a room with a magnetic resonance imaging machine because of the potential for ICD dysfunction.

SUGGESTED READING

Appleton CP, Hatle LK. The natural history of left ventricular filling abnormalities: assessment of two-dimensional and Doppler echocardiography. *Echocardiography* 1992;9:437–456.

ASA Task Force on Perioperative Management of Patients with Cardiac Rhythm Management Devices. Practice advisory for the perioperative management of patients with cardiac rhythm management devices: pacemakers and implantable cardioverter-defibrillators. *Anesthesiology* 2005;103:186–198.

Ballal RS, Kapadia S, Secknus MA, et al. Prognosis of patients with vascular disease after clinical evaluation and dobutamine stress echocardiography. *Am Heart J* 1999;137:469–475.

Bernstein AD, Daubert J-C, Fletcher RD, et al. The revised NASPE/BPEG generic code for antibradycardia, adaptive-rate, and multisite pacing. *Pacing Clin Electrophysiol* 2002;25:260–264.

Bode RH, Lewis KP, Zarich SW, et al. Cardiac outcome after peripheral surgery: comparison of general and regional anesthesia. *Anesthesiology* 1996;84:3–13.

Child JS. Stress echocardiographic techniques. *Echocardiography* 1992;9:77–84.

Coley CM, Field TS, Abraham SA, et al. Usefulness of dipyrimidole-thallium scanning for preoperative evaluation of cardiac risk for nonvascular surgery. *Am J Cardiol* 1992;69:1280–1285.

Danjani AS, Bisno AL, Chung KJ, et al. Prevention of bacterial endocarditis. Recommendations of the American Heart Association. *JAMA* 1990;264:2919–2922.

Deutch N, Hantler CB, Morady F, Kirsch M. Perioperative management of the patient undergoing automatic internal cardioverter defibrillator implantation. *J Cardiothorac Anesth* 1990;4:236–244.

Eagle KA, Berger PB, Calkins H, et al. ACC/AHA guideline update for perioperative cardiovascular evaluation for noncardiac surgery—executive summary. A report of the American College of Cardiology/American Heart Association Task Force on Practice Guidelines (Committee to update the 1996 Guidelines on Perioperative Cardiovascular Evaluation for Noncardiac Surgery). *Circulation* 2002;105:1257–1267.

Gregoratos G, Abrams J, Epstein AE, et al. ACC/AHA/NASPE 2002 guideline update for implantation of cardiac pacemakers and antiarrhythmia devices—summary article. *J Am Coll Cardiol* 2002;40:1703–1719.

Lovell A. Anaesthetic implications of grown-up congenital heart disease. *Br J Anaesth* 2004;93:129–139.

Mangano DT. Perioperative cardiac morbidity. *Anesthesiology* 1990;72:153–184.

Mangano D, Goldman L. Preoperative assessment of patients with known or suspected coronary disease. *N Engl J Med* 1995;333:1750–1756.

Palda VA, Detsky AS. Perioperative assessment and management of risk from coronary artery disease. *Ann Intern Med* 1997;127:313–328.

Poldermans D, Boersma E, Bax JJ, et al. The effect of bisoprolol on perioperative mortality and myocardial infarction in high risk patients undergoing vascular surgery. Dutch Echocardiographic Cardiac Risk Evaluation Applying Stress Echocardiography Study Group. *N Engl J Med* 1999;341:1789–1794.

Roizen MF. Cost effective preoperative laboratory testing. *JAMA* 1994;271:319–320.

Wallace A, Layug B, Tateo I, et al., for the McSPI Research Group. Prophylactic atenolol reduces postoperative myocardial ischemia. *Anesthesiology* 1998;88:7–17.

Zelzman CH, Miller SA, Zimmerman MA, et al. The case for beta-adrenergic blockade as prophylaxis against perioperative cardiovascular morbidity and mortality. *Arch Surg* 2001;136:286–290.

Specific Considerations with Pulmonary Disease

Ricardo R. Rivera and Kenneth E. Shepherd

I. **General considerations.** The incidence of postoperative pulmonary complications is second only to cardiovascular complications as a cause of perioperative mortality. These complications are related to the type and severity of respiratory disease; the site, duration, urgency, and magnitude of the surgical procedure; coexisting extrapulmonary diseases; and postoperative events.

A. Patients with significant chronic pulmonary disease are at greater risk for postoperative respiratory failure than the general population because anesthesia and surgery more easily produce hypoventilation, hypoxemia, retention of secretions, and pneumonia in such patients.

B. Patients with moderate to severe chronic lung disease and those having thoracic and upper abdominal operations have an increased morbidity and mortality rate.

C. Postoperative morbidity and mortality can be reduced by identifying patients at risk for perioperative respiratory complications, optimizing their medical therapy, and instituting a program of chest physiotherapy before and after surgery.

II. **Classification of pulmonary disease**

A. **Obstructive airway diseases** are characterized by abnormal expiratory gas flow rates. The **airflow limitation** can be structural or functional.

1. **Chronic obstructive pulmonary disease** (COPD) is airflow obstruction attributable to emphysema ("pink puffer") or chronic bronchitis ("blue bloater").

a. **Emphysema** is due to abnormal permanent enlargement of the airspaces distal to the terminal bronchioles accompanied by destructive changes of the alveolar wall. This leads to loss of the normal elastic recoil of the lung with subsequent premature airway closure at higher than normal lung volumes during exhalation.

b. **Chronic bronchitis** is defined as the presence of productive cough for at least 3 months in each of 2 successive years in a person in whom the excessive secretions are not due to other diseases. The most common precipitant is cigarette smoking.

2. **Asthma** is defined as episodic variable airflow obstruction. Asthma is an inflammatory disease in which a complex cascade of cellular and chemical mediators leads to increased airway tone, edema, mucus secretions, and increased airway responsiveness to a variety of stimuli that include exercise, cooling, drying and/or instrumentation of the airways, infection, medications, and occupational exposure.

3. **Cystic fibrosis** involves the secretion of highly viscous mucus. This results in airway obstruction, fibrosis, chronic pulmonary infection, and cachexia. Late changes include pneumothorax and bronchiectasis with hemoptysis, hypoxemia, carbon dioxide retention, and respiratory failure.

4. **The mechanism of hypoxemia** in obstructive disease is primarily through regional mismatching of ventilation and perfusion (**$\dot{V}/\dot{Q}$ mismatch**). **Dyspnea,** a major symptom, is multifactorial in origin but is in large part related to loading of the respiratory muscles.

B. **Restrictive pulmonary disease** is characterized by a decrease in lung compliance and may be intrinsic or extrinsic. Airway resistance is usually normal, whereas lung volumes and diffusing capacity are reduced.

1. **Intrinsic**
   a. **Pulmonary edema** occurs when fluid accumulates in the interstitium and alveoli by hydrostatic, cardiogenic (e.g., congestive heart failure [CHF]), or "noncardiogenic" (e.g., acute respiratory distress syndrome [ARDS]) mechanisms.
   b. **Pulmonary interstitial disease** causes inflammation/fibrosis of interstitium, alveoli, or vascular beds. The latter may lead to pulmonary hypertension and cor pulmonale. Examples include sarcoidosis, chronic hypersensitivity pneumonitis, and radiation fibrosis.

2. **Extrinsic**
   a. **Pleural disease,** either fibrosis or effusion.
   b. **Chest wall deformity,** such as kyphoscoliosis, ankylosing spondylitis, pectus excavatum, trauma, or burns.
   c. **Diaphragmatic compression** by obesity, ascites, pregnancy, or from retraction during abdominal surgery.

3. As in obstructive disease, the primary cause of hypoxemia in restrictive states is $\dot{V}/\dot{Q}$ mismatch. Often patients have multiple reasons for pulmonary dysfunction as well as mixed obstructive and restrictive defects. Proper diagnosis requires a careful history and physical examination. Pulmonary function testing may be required to differentiate obstructive from restrictive defects and can be used to assess a patient's response to therapy.

C. **Pulmonary hypertension** is characterized by a mean pulmonary artery pressure of more than 25 mm Hg at rest (or >30 mm Hg with exercise) with a normal pulmonary capillary wedge pressure. It can result in right atrial and right ventricular dilatation, hypertrophy, and failure.

1. **Primary pulmonary hypertension** occurs due to idiopathic fibrin deposition in the pulmonary capillaries and arterioles accompanied by increased thrombogenesis. The total cross-sectional area of the pulmonary vasculature may be markedly decreased.

2. **Secondary pulmonary hypertension** occurs due to any disease process that
   a. **Increases capillary or pulmonary venous pressures** (e.g., mitral regurgitation);
   b. **Increases pulmonary artery blood flow** (e.g., patent ductus arteriosus); or

      c. **Decreases the cross-sectional area of the pulmonary vasculature** (e.g., acute causes such as pulmonary embolus or chronic causes such as pulmonary fibrosis).

   3. **Cor pulmonale** is right ventricular failure secondary to conditions that reduce the cross-sectional area of the pulmonary vasculature. Polycythemia, $\dot{V}/\dot{Q}$ mismatch, and right ventricular failure with displacement of the interventricular septum to the left occur with advanced disease.

III. **Identification of the patient at risk**

  A. **History**

    1. Symptoms of respiratory disease such as cough, expectoration, hemoptysis, wheezing, dyspnea, and chest pain should be elicited. Preexisting lung and systemic diseases, occupational exposures, symptoms of disordered breathing during sleep, medications, and recent changes in clinical status should be defined.

    2. **Chronic cough** may suggest bronchitis or asthma. If cough is productive, sputum should be examined for evidence of infection and, if appropriate, sent for Gram stain, culture, or cytology.

    3. **Smoking history** should be quantified in pack-years (number of packs smoked per day multiplied by the number of years smoked). The risks of malignancy, COPD, and postoperative pulmonary complications are directly proportional to the smoking history.

    4. **Dyspnea** is an uncomfortable sensation of breathing. The activity level should be defined; severe dyspnea (occurring at minimal activity or at rest) may be a predictor of both poor ventilatory reserve and the need for postoperative ventilatory support.

  B. **Physical findings**

    1. **Body habitus** and general appearance.

      a. **Obesity, pregnancy, and kyphoscoliosis** reduce lung volumes (functional residual capacity [FRC], total lung capacity) and pulmonary compliance and predispose to atelectasis and hypoxemia.

      b. **Cachectic malnourished patients** have blunted respiratory drive and decreased muscle strength and are predisposed to pneumonia.

      c. **Cyanosis** requires a minimum reduced hemoglobin concentration of 5 g/dL. The appearance of cyanosis depends on many factors, including cardiac output, oxygen uptake by the tissue, and hemoglobin concentration. Cyanosis suggests hypoxemia but can be unreliable.

    2. **Respiratory signs.** Respiratory rate and pattern, diaphragmatic coordination, and the use of accessory muscles should be assessed.

      a. **Tachypnea,** a respiratory rate greater than 25 breaths/min, is usually the earliest sign of respiratory distress.

      b. **Respiratory pattern**

        (1) **Pursed-lip breathing, tripoding,** and visible expiratory effort may indicate airway obstruction.

        (2) **Accessory muscle use** increases with load and dysfunction of the diaphragm and intercostal muscles.

        (3) **Asymmetry of chest wall expansion** may result from unilateral bronchial obstruction, pneumothorax, pleural effusion, lung consolidation, or unilateral phrenic nerve injury (causing an elevated hemidiaphragm).

        (4) **Tracheal deviation** may suggest pneumothorax or mediastinal disease with tracheal compression. Severe cases may cause difficulty during intubation or airway obstruction during induction of general anesthesia.

        (5) **Inspiratory paradox.** Normally the abdominal wall should move outward with the chest wall during inspiration. Inspiratory paradox occurs when the abdomen collapses as the chest wall expands during inspiration and suggests paralysis or severe dysfunction of the diaphragm.

    c. Auscultation

        (1) **Diminished breath sounds** may indicate local consolidation, pneumothorax, or pleural effusion.

        (2) **Rales,** usually in dependent portions, may indicate atelectasis or CHF.

        (3) **Wheezing** may indicate obstructive airway disease.

        (4) **Stridor** may indicate upper airway narrowing.

3. Cardiovascular signs

    a. Pulsus paradoxus is defined as a fall in systolic blood pressure of greater than 10 mm Hg during inspiration. It is probably due to selective impairment of left ventricular filling and ejection secondary to the negative pleural pressure generated during spontaneous ventilation. Pulsus paradoxus can also been seen with pericardial tamponade and superior vena cava obstruction, but the physiological mechanism is different than it is with asthma.

    b. Pulmonary hypertension occurs as a result of elevated pulmonary vascular resistance.

        (1) **Physical signs** may include splitting of the second heart sound with an accentuated pulmonic component, jugular venous distention, hepatomegaly, hepatojugular reflux, and peripheral edema.

        (2) **Factors that may acutely increase pulmonary vascular resistance** include hypoxia, hypercarbia, acidosis, pulmonary embolism, ARDS, and the application of high levels of positive end-expiratory pressure (PEEP).

C. Laboratory studies

  1. Chest radiograph

    a. Hyperinflation and decreased vascular markings are characteristic of COPD.

    b. Pleural effusion, pulmonary fibrosis, and skeletal abnormalities (kyphoscoliosis, rib fractures) may predict restrictive disease states.

    c. Air space disease, including CHF, consolidation, atelectasis, lobar collapse (bronchial obstruction), and pneumothorax, is an important predictor of V/Q mismatch and hypoxemia.

      d. **Specific lesions,** including pneumothorax, emphysematous blebs, and cysts, may preclude the use of nitrous oxide.

      e. **Tracheal narrowing or deviation** may occur as a result of mediastinal compression or masses. Further workup with computed tomography or magnetic resonance imaging may be of value in detailing the precise location and degree of obstruction of tracheal and bronchial lesions.

2. **Electrocardiogram.** Electrocardiographic signs of significant pulmonary dysfunction include the following:

      a. **Low voltage and poor R-wave progression** attributable to hyperinflation.

      b. **Signs of pulmonary hypertension and cor pulmonale,** such as

          (1) Right-axis deviation.

          (2) P pulmonale (P waves greater than 2.5 mm in height in lead II).

          (3) Right ventricular hypertrophy (R/S ratio >1 in lead V_1).

          (4) Right bundle branch block.

3. **Arterial blood gas tensions**

      a. **Partial pressure of oxygen (PaO_2).** Hypoxemia is considered severe when PaO_2 is less than 55 mm Hg. Patients with severe hypoxemia at rest have significant pulmonary dysfunction and are at increased risk for postoperative pulmonary complications.

      b. **Partial pressure of carbon dioxide ($PaCO_2$).** Hypercarbia occurs when $PaCO_2$ is greater than 45 mm Hg. Patients who chronically retain carbon dioxide often have end-stage lung disease with little or no reserve and are at increased risk for postoperative pulmonary complications.

      c. **Measurement of pH** in conjunction with $PaCO_2$ allows determination of acid-base disturbances.

4. **Pulmonary function tests** (PFTs) measure pulmonary mechanics and functional reserve and provide an objective assessment of lung function. PFTs help make decisions on management of lung resection candidates. In this context, they are used to estimate residual lung function after pulmonary resection, as measured by split-function studies (which quantify dysfunction in each lung). The impact of preoperative PFTs in predicting the risk of clinically important postoperative pulmonary complications in other surgical procedures is not as clear. The use of preoperative PFTs in evaluating these patients must be individualized. Normal values for a 70-kg adult male include total lung capacity (TLC), 5.5 L; vital capacity (VC), 4 L; FRC, 2.5 L; residual volume (RV), 1.5 L; and forced expiratory volume in the first second (FEV_1), 3.2 L, which is 80% of VC. **Obstructive defects** are characterized by elevated TLC, FRC, and RV with reduced FEV_1 ($<80\%$). **Restrictive defects** are characterized by proportional decreases in all lung volumes with a normal or increased FEV_1/FVC ratio.

IV. Effects of anesthesia and surgery on pulmonary functio[...] eral anesthesia decreases lung volumes and promotes $\dot{V}/\dot{Q}$ mis[...] and atelectasis formation. Many anesthetic drugs blunt the ven[...] tory response to hypercarbia and hypoxia. Postoperatively, atelec[...] sis and hypoxemia are common findings, especially in patients with preexisting pulmonary disease. Pulmonary function is further compromised by postoperative pain, which can limit coughing and lung expansion.

A. Respiratory mechanics and gas exchange

1. **General anesthesia and the supine position decrease FRC.** Atelectasis occurs when lung volumes during tidal breathing fall below the volume at which airway closure occurs (closing capacity). PEEP can minimize this effect. The supine position causes a cephalad movement of the diaphragm and a reduction in FRC.

2. **Positive-pressure ventilation compared with spontaneous breathing leads to $\dot{V}/\dot{Q}$ mismatching.** During positive-pressure ventilation, nondependent portions of the lung receive a greater proportion of ventilation than do dependent portions. In contrast, pulmonary blood flow tends to be increased in dependent portions of the lung; its distribution is affected by gravity and the anatomical distribution of pulmonary vessels. The result is a variable increase in both $\dot{V}/\dot{Q}$ mismatch and physiologic dead space.

B. Regulation of breathing

1. **The ventilatory response to hypercarbia is reduced by inhalation anesthetics, propofol, barbiturates, and opioids.** $Paco_2$ is elevated with spontaneous ventilation during general anesthesia, as is the **apneic threshold** (the $Paco_2$ at which patients who have had hyperventilation to apnea again resume spontaneous ventilation).

2. **The ventilatory response to hypoxia may also be blunted by inhalation anesthetics, propofol, barbiturates, and opioids.** This effect may be particularly important in patients with severe chronic lung disease who normally retain carbon dioxide and depend more on hypoxic drive to increase ventilation.

3. The respiratory depressant effects of anesthetic and analgesic drugs may be more pronounced in patients with obstructive sleep apnea.

C. Effect of surgery. Postoperative pulmonary function is affected by the site of surgery. The ability to cough and breathe deeply is reduced after abdominal operations compared with peripheral procedures and appears to be related to diaphragm dysfunction and to the pain produced by coughing and deep breathing. Vital capacity can be reduced by up to 75% after upper abdominal procedures and by approximately 50% after lower abdominal or thoracic operations. Recovery of normal pulmonary function may take several weeks. Peripheral procedures have little impact on vital capacity or the ability to clear secretions.

D. Effect on ciliary function. The upper respiratory tract normally warms and humidifies inspired air, providing an ideal environment for normal function of respiratory tract cilia and mucus. General anesthesia, often conducted with unhumidified gases at

ites, dries secretions and can easily damage respiratory
Endotracheal intubation exacerbates this problem
the nasopharynx. Secretions become thickened, cil-
is reduced, and the patient's resistance to pulmonary
decreased.

...ment in pulmonary disease. The goals of preop-
... treatment are to improve aspects of disease that may be reversible.

A. **Cessation of smoking** for 12 hours before surgery may reduce
nicotine and carboxyhemoglobin levels, promoting better tissue
oxygen transport. Cessation of smoking for longer periods (at
least several weeks) does reduce the risk of wound infection and
may reduce the risk of postoperative pulmonary complications
by improving ciliary function and reducing airway secretions and
irritability.

B. **Acute bacterial infection** should be treated before elective
surgery. Therapy is guided by sputum Gram stain and culture.
Recent viral respiratory infections, especially in children, may
predispose the patient to bronchospasm or laryngospasm.

C. **Hydration and humidification of inspired gases aid clearance
of bronchial secretions.**

D. **Chest physiotherapy** (voluntary deep breathing, coughing, incentive spirometry, and chest percussion and vibration combined
with postural drainage) improves mobilization of secretions and
increases lung volumes, reducing the incidence of postoperative
pulmonary complications.

E. **Medical treatment**
   1. **Sympathomimetics,** or β_2-adrenergic agonist drugs, cause
   bronchodilation via cyclic AMP-mediated relaxation of
   bronchial smooth muscle. See Table 3.1 for some commonly
   used agents.
      a. **Drugs with β_2-adrenergic selectivity** are generally se-
      lected. These are classified as those that are short acting
      and those with prolonged action.
         (1) **Short-acting β_2-agonists** by inhalation are used
         for prophylaxis before instrumentation of the air-
         ways and for episodes of acute bronchospasm.
         (2) **Long-acting β_2-agonists** are used in combination
         with an inhaled cortisteroid for maintenance ther-
         apy. They are not indicated for treating acute ex-
         acerbations of bronchoconstriction.
      b. **Drugs with mixed β_1- and β_2-adrenergic effects**
      include **epinephrine** (Adrenalin) and **isoproterenol**
      (Isuprel). The chronotropic and arrhythmogenic poten-
      tial of these drugs is a concern in patients with car-
      diac disease. The intravenous (IV) use of low doses of
      epinephrine (<1 μg/min) may be considered for severe
      medically refractory bronchospasm. At low doses (0.25
      to 1.0 μg/min), β_2-adrenergic agonist effects predom-
      inate, with an increase in heart rate attributable to β_1-
      adrenergic stimulation. At higher doses of epinephrine,
      α-adrenergic effects become predominant, with increases
      in systolic blood pressure.
   2. **Parasympatholytics.** Anticholinergics have a direct bron-
   chodilating effect by blocking the action of acetylcholine

Table 3.1. Some commonly inhaled β_2-adrenergic drugs

Drug	Trade Name	Administration	Initial Adult Dose	Interval (h)
Albuterol	Proventil	MDI (90 μg)	2 puffs	4–6
	Ventolin	Nebulizer (5 mg/mL)	0.5 mL	
Levalbuterol	Xopenex	Nebulizer (0.21 mg/mL)	3–6 mL	6–8
Terbutaline	Brethaire	MDI (200 μg)	2–3 puffs	4–6
Metaproterenol	Alupent	MDI (650 μg)	2–3 puffs	3–4
	Metaprel	Nebulizer (50 mg/mL)	0.2–0.3 mL	
Isoetharine mesylate	Bronkosol	MDI (340 μg)	1–2 puffs	4–6
		Nebulizer (10 mg/mL)	0.25–0.5 mL	
Pirbuterol	Maxair	MDI (200 μg)	2 puffs	4–6
Salmeterol	Serevent	DPI (50 μg)	1 inhalation	12
Formoterol	Foradil	DPI (12 μg)	1 inhalation	12
Bitoterol	Tornolate	MDI (270 μg)	2 puffs	6–8
		Nebulizer	1–2 mg	

Initial adult doses are for spontaneously breathing adults. Increased doses are required for patients who are tracheally intubated. MDI, metered-dose inhaler; DPI, dry-powder inhaler.

ond messengers, such as cyclic guanine monophos-
They may improve the FEV_1 in patients with
when administered by inhalation. Specific agents

   tropium bromide (Atrovent) is a short acting drug
   by metered-dose inhaler (MDI) or by nebulizer.

- **v.** **Tiotropium (Spiriva)** is a long-acting drug administered by dry powder inhaler for maintenance therapy.
- **c.** **Glycopyrrolate** (Robinul), 0.2 to 0.8 mg by nebulizer.
- **d.** **Atropine sulfate,** which has considerable systemic absorption, may cause tachycardia and thus has limited usefulness.

3. **Methylxanthines** (e.g., aminophylline and theophylline).

- **a.** Methylxanthines cause bronchodilation by multiple mechanisms, including activating histone deacetylases, blocking adenosine receptors, releasing endogenous catecholamines, and increasing the intracellular concentration of cyclic AMP through nonspecific inhibition of phosphodiesterase enzymes. They are also thought to affect direct stimulation of the diaphragm.

- **b.** Some patients with bronchial asthma or COPD receive chronic therapy with oral **theophylline.** Serum theophylline levels should be checked and the dosage adjusted to keep levels at 10 to 20 μg/mL. These medications should be continued until the morning of surgery. The use of methylxanthines in patients who have an acute exacerbation should be individualized. For patients not currently taking theophylline, a loading dose of 5 to 6 mg per kg of body weight IV (aminophylline) may be given over 20 min followed by infusion rates of 0.5 to 0.9 mg/kg per hour. Smokers and adolescents may require higher doses, reflecting rapid metabolism. Patients who are elderly, who have CHF or liver disease, or who are taking cimetidine, propranolol, or erythromycin should receive reduced doses, reflecting slower drug metabolism. Serum drug levels should be checked.

- **c.** **Continuation of methylxanthines during general anesthesia** is rarely indicated. Bronchodilation can be achieved more safely and predictably with volatile anesthetics or β_2-adrenergic agonists. Oral theophylline preparations can be restarted once enteral intake of medications is tolerated.

- **d.** **Patients who will remain on "nothing by mouth" status for an extended period** may receive IV theophylline or aminophylline (a soluble ethylenediamine salt containing 85% theophylline by weight). For such patients who are already taking theophylline, an infusion rate may be estimated based on the patient's total daily requirement, divided by 24 (divided again by 0.85 if aminophylline is used, because theophylline dose = 0.85 × aminophylline dose).

- **e.** **Toxicity** occurs frequently when drug levels exceed 20 μg/mL; symptoms and signs include nausea, vomiting, headache, anxiety, tachycardia, arrhythmias, and seizures.

4. **Corticosteroids** are often used in patients not responding to bronchodilators. Their mechanisms of action are complex and not completely understood; however, they appear to reduce airway inflammation and responsiveness, edema, mucus secretion, and smooth muscle constriction. Although they are useful for acute severe exacerbations, their clinical effect may take several hours.

    a. **Steroids** are preferably administered by inhalation (e.g., Flunisolide [Aerobid] by MDI, two puffs every 6 hours) because of decreased systemic side effects.

    b. Commonly used IV steroids include **hydrocortisone** (Solu-Cortef), 100 mg IV every 8 hours, and **methylprednisolone** (Solu-Medrol), up to 0.5 mg/kg IV every 6 hours in asthmatic bronchitis and often higher doses in an exacerbation of severe asthma. Perioperative regimens are usually tapered in dose, frequency, and route of administration as dictated by clinical response.

    c. **"Stress dose"** replacement may be needed in patients currently or recently taking corticosteroids (see Chapter 6).

5. **Cromolyn** is an inhaled medication used as prophylactic therapy for asthma. Its precise mechanisms of action remain unknown, but it appears to act by stabilizing mast cell membranes and blunting the acute release of preformed bronchoactive mediators. It is of no utility in the acute treatment of bronchospasm.

6. **Mucolytics**

    a. **Acetylcysteine** (Mucomyst), administered by nebulizer, can decrease the viscosity of mucus by breaking the disulfide bonds in mucoproteins.

    b. **Hypertonic saline** is sometimes used to decrease mucus viscosity. When it is given by nebulizer, an osmotic shift of water to mucus enhances mucus volume and promotes clearance. Inhalation of hypertonic saline, like acetylcysteine-and even occasionally β-adrenergic agonists, anticholinergics, and steroid preparations—may increase airway resistance.

    c. **Recombinant deoxyribonuclease** (DNase or Pulmozyme), 10 to 40 mg inhaled daily, is used in some patients with cystic fibrosis to decrease the viscosity of bronchial secretions by cleaving DNA strands in sputum. This improves airway clearance and pulmonary function by 5% to 20% in many patients with cystic fibrosis.

7. **Leukotriene (LT) modifying drugs** have anti-inflammatory effects that act by blocking LT receptors (Zafirlukast and Montelukast). These are approved currently for prophylaxis and maintenance therapy of chronic asthma. A specific benefit in the perioperative period has not yet been determined. Potential adverse reactions include liver function abnormalities and eosinophilic vasculitis (Churg-Strauss syndrome).

8. **Anti-IgE antibody (Omalizabab),** by injections, is used as a maintenance therapy for asthmatic patients with a strong allergic component and poorly controlled symptoms despite otherwise maximal therapy.

9. **Ketamine** is a bronchial smooth muscle relaxant. The mechanism is thought to be sympathomimetic and/or antagonism of spasmogenic carbachol and histamine. Ketamine has been used for medically unresponsive bronchospasm, or status asthmaticus.

VI. **Premedication.** The goals of premedication are to allay anxiety, minimize reflex bronchoconstriction to airway irritants (dry gases and instrumentation), and facilitate the smooth induction of anesthesia.

A. **Oxygen therapy,** if required preoperatively, should be continued while the patient is being transported to the operating room and clearly written as a preoperative "order."

B. **If the patient is taking inhaled β-adrenergic agonists or anticholinergics,** these should accompany the patient to the operating room; their preoperative use may decrease airway responsiveness.

C. **Anticholinergics** are often indicated by inhalation to prevent bronchospasm secondary to vagal stimulation caused by airway manipulations such as laryngoscopy and endotracheal intubation. Some of these agents can be given parenterally. Parenteral administration, however, may cause drying of secretions, increasing the viscosity of mucus.

D. **Histamine (H_2) antagonists** (cimetidine, ranitidine) may exacerbate bronchospasm in patients with asthma, because blockage of H_2 receptors may result in unopposed H_1-mediated bronchoconstriction. Coadministration of an H_1 blocking agent (diphenhydramine, 25 mg IV) should be considered.

E. **Benzodiazepines** are effective anxiolytics but may cause excessive sedation and respiratory depression in compromised patients, especially when used with opioids.

F. **Opioids** provide analgesia and sedation but must be carefully titrated to avoid respiratory depression, especially in patients with severe pulmonary dysfunction and/or obstructive sleep apnea.

VII. **Anesthetic technique**

A. **Peripheral nerve blockade or local anesthesia** may be the best choice of anesthetic for patients with pulmonary disease when the site of operation is peripheral, such as eye or extremity procedures.

B. **Spinal or epidural anesthesia** is a reasonable choice for lower extremity surgery. Patients with severe COPD depend on accessory muscle use, including intercostals for inspiration and abdominal muscles for forced exhalation. Spinal anesthesia may be deleterious if motor blockade decreases FRC, reduces a patient's ability to cough and clear secretions, or precipitates respiratory insufficiency or failure. **Combined epidural and general anesthetic techniques** ensure airway control, provide adequate ventilation, and prevent hypoxemia and atelectasis. Prolonged peripheral procedures are probably best performed with a general anesthetic or a combined technique.

C. **General anesthesia,** often in combination with epidural anesthesia, is indicated for upper abdominal and thoracic procedures.

1. Most volatile agents provide bronchodilation and an adequate depth of anesthesia to decrease the hyperreactivity of sensitive airways. However, Desflurane can cause airway irritation and coughing with inhalation and is not an optimal choice in patients with reactive airways.

2. Dynamic lung hyperinflation (**auto-PEEP**) is also important to avoid during general endotracheal anesthesia in patients with reactive airways or elevated lung compliance (severe COPD). **Auto-PEEP,** which can result in hypotension and decreased cardiac output, often occurs when not enough expiratory time is given to completely empty the lungs.

3. The use of a laryngeal mask airway (LMA) reduces but does not eliminate the risk of bronchospasm, as laryngoscopy or instrumentation of the larynx alone can elicit a laryngo-bronchospastic response in these patients. An additional risk of using the LMA is the inability to ventilate during bronchospasm as inspiratory pressure may exceed the sealing force of the LMA in the larynx. The ProSeal LMA was recently developed to overcome this limitation and can be considered.

VIII. Postoperative care. Chest physiotherapy and suctioning should be immediately available to all patients who are identified as high risk. The possibility of ventilatory support should be anticipated and discussed with the patient. Postoperative pain management is critical to decreasing respiratory complications.

SUGGESTED READING

Arozullah AM, Daley J, Henderson WG, Khuri SF. Multifactorial risk index for predicting postoperative respiratory failure in men after major noncardiac surgery. *Ann Surg* 2000;232:242–253.

Arozullah AM, Shukri SF, Henderson WG, et al. Development and validation of a multifactorial risk index for predicting postoperative pneumonia after major noncardiac surgery. *Ann Intern Med* 2001;135(10):847–857.

Blaise G, Langleben D, Hubert B. Pulmonary arterial hypertension. *Anesthesiology* 2003;99:1415–1432.

Duggan M, Kavanagh BP. Pulmonary atelectasis: a pathogenic perioperative entity. *Anesthesiology* 2005;102(4):838–854.

Fisher DW, Majumdar SR, McAlister FA. Predicting pulmonary complications after non-thoracic surgery: a systematic review. *Am J Med* 2002;112:219–225.

Loadsman JA, Hillman DR. Anaesthesia and sleep apnoea. *Br J Anaesth* 2001;86:254–266.

McAlister FA, Bertsch K, Man J, et al. Incidence of and risk factors for pulmonary complications after nonthoracic surgery. *Am J Respir Crit Care Med* 2005;171(5):514–517.

Shepherd KE, Hurford WE. Preoperative evaluation of the patient with pulmonary disease. In: Sweitzer BJ, ed. *Handbook of preoperative assessment and management.* Philadelphia: Lippincott, Williams & Wilkins, 2000:97–125.

Thompson JS, Baxter T, Allison JG, et al. Temporal patterns of postoperative complications. *Arch Surg* 2003;138:596–603.

Warner DO. Perioperative abstinence from cigarettes. Physiologic and clinical consequences. *Anesthesiology* 2006;104:356–367.

Warner DO. Preventing postoperative pulmonary complications. *Anesthesiology* 2000;92:1467–1472.

4

Specific Consideration with Renal Disease

Jason M. Isa and Ward Reynolds Maier

I. **General considerations.** Approximately 5% of the population has renal disease, with a trend toward increasing prevalence with age. Perioperative renal dysfunction complicates patient management and results in increased morbidity and mortality. Aside from optimizing intravascular volume status, there is no definite consensus on prophylaxis for the development of acute renal failure (ARF). However, morbidity and mortality may be decreased by a thorough understanding of considerations related to renal disease.

II. **Physiology.** Blood flow to the kidneys is regulated by intrinsic autoregulatory mechanisms, which help maintain volume and composition of body fluids and aid in excretion of metabolites and toxins and retention of nutrients. The kidneys maintain a stable internal balance despite large fluctuations in fluid and solute intake. They regulate intravascular volume, osmolality, and acid-base and electrolyte balance, and they excrete hormones as well as the end products of metabolism and drugs.

A. **Regulation of blood flow**

1. The kidneys receive 20% of total cardiac output, with the renal cortex receiving 94% of total blood flow. The renal medulla receives only 6% of total renal blood flow but extracts approximately 80% of the oxygen that it receives, making it very susceptible to ischemia, particularly the medullary thick ascending loop of Henle.

2. **Renal blood flow** is autoregulated between mean arterial pressures of 60 to 150 mm Hg by intrinsic mechanisms balancing afferent and efferent arteriolar tone. Extrinsic factors such as sympathetic vasoconstrictor innervation, dopaminergic receptors, and the renin-angiotensin system can also alter renal blood flow. Autoregulation can be impaired in states of severe sepsis, ARF, and possibly cardiopulmonary bypass. The kidney is largely devoid of β-2 receptors.

B. **Fluid regulation**

1. **Total body water** (TBW) is approximately 60% of body weight. In obese patients, it may be more precise and practical to calculate TBW based on ideal body weight.

   a. Two-thirds of TBW is **intracellular.**

   b. One-third of TBW is **extracellular.**

   (1) Two-thirds of extracellular fluid is **interstitial** and one-third is **intravascular.**

   (2) **Estimated blood volume** is 70 mL/kg with an estimated plasma volume of 50 mL/kg.

2. The cells of the **macula densa** of the thick ascending limb are chemoreceptors that sense the tubular concentration of sodium and can help to regulate volume status.

3. **Hypovolemia** is managed by the activation of vasoconstrictor and salt-retaining neurohormonal systems including the following:

   a. **Renin-angiotensin-aldosterone system**

      (1) The **juxtaglomerular apparatus** of the kidney secretes renin in response to renal hypoperfusion, decreased sodium chloride delivery to the distal nephron, and increased sympathetic activity. Renin cleaves angiotensinogen to form angiotensin I, which is then converted to angiotensin II by angiotensin-converting enzyme (ACE) in the lung and other tissues.

      (2) **Angiotensin II** produces arteriolar vasoconstriction and stimulates aldosterone release.

      (3) **Aldosterone** is a mineralocorticoid released by the adrenal cortex in response to angiotensin II, increased potassium levels, decreased sodium content, and adrenocorticotropic hormone. Aldosterone acts on the distal tubules to increase resorption of sodium in exchange for potassium and protons.

      (4) **Diuretics** abolish the kidneys' ability to concentrate urine by washing out the renal medullary concentration gradient. Acute tubular necrosis (ATN) presents early as an inability to concentrate urine caused by the breakdown of the Na^+/K^+-ATPase pump in the medullary thick ascending loop of Henle because of a loss of cell polarity.

   b. **Arginine vasopressin** (AVP) (also called antidiuretic hormone [ADH]) is released by the posterior pituitary gland in response to increased osmolality, decreased extracellular volume, positive pressure ventilation, and surgical stimuli, including pain. AVP increases the permeability of the collecting duct to water through insertion of water channel "aquaporins." Thus, ADH conserves water and concentrates urine.

4. **Hypervolemia**

   a. **Atrial natriuretic peptide,** a neuropeptide, is the predominant salt-excreting stimulus along with decreases in angiotensin II and sympathetic activity resulting in decreased sodium resorption producing a dilute urine (300 mOsm/kg) and abundant urine sodium (80 mEq/L). Loop diuretics may produce a similar picture even in the face of hypovolemia.

   b. **Kinins** are converted from kininogens by kallikreins and are regulated by salt intake, renin release, and hormone levels. They cause renal vasodilatation and natriuresis.

5. **Osmotic equilibrium**

   a. The **medullary interstitium** is kept hypertonic by the countercurrent multiplier effect of the loop of Henle.

   b. **Calculated osmolality** (mOsm/kg) = $2[Na^+]$ + ([blood urea nitrogen](mg/dL)/2.8) + ([glucose](mg/dL)/18). Normal osmolality = 290 mOsm/kg.

   c. **Osmolal gap** = Osm (measured) − Osm (calculated) is normally <10. An increased osmolal gap occurs when osmotically active but unmeasured substances (e.g., ethanol, mannitol, methanol, sorbitol) are present in the blood.

6. **Daily adult water intake** is approximately 2,600 mL:1,400 mL in liquids, 800 mL in solid food, and 400 mL from metabolism. The minimum water intake to excrete solute load is about 600 mL/day.

C. **Electrolyte balance**

1. **Disorders of sodium homeostasis**

a. **Hyponatremia:** plasma sodium concentration less than 134 mEq/L.

(1) **Total body water** may be high, low, or normal (usually a sign of free water excess).

(2) **Hyponatremia** often results in reduced plasma osmolality.

(3) **Pseudohyponatremia** from hyperglycemia (uncontrolled diabetes mellitus), hyperlipidemia, or hyperproteinemia (multiple myeloma) should be ruled out to avoid mistreatment.

(4) **Clinical features** vary with the degree of hyponatremia and the rapidity of onset. Symptoms generally do not appear until the sodium concentration falls below 125 mEq/L.

(a) **Moderate hyponatremia or gradual onset:** confusion, muscle cramps, lethargy, anorexia, and nausea.

(b) **Severe hyponatremia or rapid onset:** seizures, coma.

(5) Generally, acute normalization of the serum $[Na^+]$ is not necessary. It should be **corrected at a rate of 0.5 mEq/L per hour** until 120 mEq/L is reached to prevent complications from rapid correction (e.g., cerebral edema, central pontine myelinolysis, seizures). At this point, the patient should be out of danger, and the $[Na^+]$ should be normalized slowly over a period of days. Treatment depends on the volume status of the patient.

(a) **Hypervolemic hyponatremia** due to renal failure, congestive heart failure, cirrhosis, or nephrotic syndrome is treated by sodium and water restriction and possibly with diuresis.

(b) **Hypovolemic hyponatremia** from diuretics, vomiting, or bowel preparations is treated with normal saline. For severe hypovolemic hyponatremia, the $[Na^+]$ may be partially corrected to 125 mEq/L or a serum osmolality of 250 mmol/L over 6 to 8 hours with 3.5% hypertonic saline. Hypertonic saline is dangerous in volume-expanded salt-retaining states such as congestive heart failure.

(c) **Normovolemic hyponatremia** from the syndrome of inappropriate ADH secretion, hypothyroidism, drugs that impair renal water excretion, or water intoxication is treated by fluid restriction.

b. Hypernatremia: plasma sodium concentration >144 mEq/L. Usually caused by impairment of thirst or the ability to obtain water.

(1) **Total body water** may be high, low, or normal (usually a sign of free water deficit).

(2) **Clinical features** vary with degree of hypernatremia and rapidity of onset, ranging from tremulousness, weakness, irritability, and mental confusion to seizures and coma.

(3) **Treatment** depends on determining the volume status of the patient. Rapid correction can induce cerebral edema, seizures, permanent neurologic damage, and death. Plasma [Na^+] should be corrected at a maximum rate of 0.5 mEq/L per hour. The water deficit, if present, can be calculated as follows:

Volume to be replaced (L) =
$$[(0.6 \times \text{body weight [kg]}) \times ([Na^+] - 140)/140]$$

(a) **Hypervolemic hypernatremia** occurs secondary to Na^+ overload from mineralocorticoid excess, dialysis with hypertonic solutions, or treatment with hypertonic saline or sodium bicarbonate ($NaHCO_3$). The excess total body Na^+ (i.e., volume) may be removed by dialysis or with diuretic therapy and the water loss replaced with 5% dextrose in water (D5W).

(b) **Hypovolemic hypernatremia** occurs secondary to water loss exceeding Na^+ loss (e.g., diarrhea, vomiting, osmotic diuresis) or inadequate water intake (e.g., impaired thirst mechanism, altered mental status). If **hemodynamic instability or evidence of hypoperfusion** is present, initial volume therapy should consist of 0.45% or even 0.9% NaCl. **After volume replenishment,** the remaining free water deficit should be replaced with D5W until the Na^+ concentration decreases. Then, 0.45% saline may be substituted.

(c) **Normovolemic hypernatremia** is typically the result of diabetes insipidus in patients with a normal thirst response. Therapy consists of treating the underlying etiology, correcting the free water deficit with D5W, and using exogenous vasopressin in neurogenic diabetes insipidus.

2. Disorders of potassium homeostasis

a. Hypokalemia: plasma [K^+] <3.3 mEq/L.

(1) Serum [K^+] is a poor index of **total body potassium** stores, because 98% of body potassium is located intracellularly. Thus, large [K^+] deficits must be present before seeing a decrease in serum [K^+]. In a 70-kg man with normal pH, a fall in serum [K^+] from 4 to 3 mEq/L reflects a deficit of 100 to

200 mEq. Below 3 mEq/L, each decrease of 1 mEq/L reflects an additional deficit of 200 to 400 mEq.

(2) **Etiologies**

(a) **Total body K$^+$ deficit.**

(b) **Shifts in distribution** of K$^+$ (extracellular to intracellular.)

(3) **[K$^+$] loss** may be from the following:

(a) **Gastrointestinal tract** (e.g., vomiting, diarrhea, nasogastric suctioning, chronic malnutrition, or obstructed ileal loops).

(b) **Kidney** (e.g., diuretics, mineralocorticoid and glucocorticoid excess, some types of renal tubular acidosis).

(4) Changes in **K$^+$ distribution** occur with alkalosis (H$^+$ shifts to the extracellular fluid and K$^+$ moves intracellularly). Thus, rapid correction of acidosis, by hyperventilation or NaHCO$_3$ administration, may produce undesirable hypokalemia.

(5) **Clinical features** rarely appear unless [K$^+$] is less than 3 mEq/L or the rate of fall is rapid.

(a) **Signs** include weakness, augmentation of neuromuscular block, ileus, and disturbances of cardiac contractility.

(b) Hypokalemia increases excitability and predisposes the patient to **arrhythmias** that may be refractory to treatment unless the hypokalemia is resolved. Electrocardiographic (ECG) changes include flattened T waves, U waves, increased PR and QT intervals, ST segment depression, and atrial and ventricular dysrhythmias. Ventricular ectopy is more likely with concomitant digitalis therapy.

(c) Serum [K$^+$] <2.0 mEq/L is associated with vasoconstriction and rhabdomyolysis.

(6) **Treatment.** Rapid replacement of K$^+$ may cause more problems than hypokalemia. There is no need to correct chronic hypokalemia ([K$^+$] $\geq$2.5 mEq/L) before induction of anesthesia. Hypokalemia-induced conduction disturbances or diminished contractility can be treated with K$^+$ (0.5 to 1.0 mEq intravenously [IV] every 3 to 5 min) until resolution. Serum [K$^+$] must be closely followed during correction.

b. **Hyperkalemia:** plasma [K$^+$] >4.9 mEq/L.

(1) Certain conditions and drugs can worsen hyperkalemia such as catabolic stress, acidosis, nonsteroidal anti-inflammatory drugs (NSAIDs), ACE-I, potassium-sparing diuretics, and beta-blockers.

(2) **Etiologies**

(a) **Decreased excretion** (e.g., renal failure, hypoaldosteronism).

(b) **Extracellular shift** (e.g., acidosis, ischemia, rhabdomyolysis, tumor lysis syndrome, and drugs such as succinylcholine). Acidosis increases the serum $[K^+]$ by 0.5 mEq for every 0.1 unit decrease in the pH.

    (c) Administration of blood, potassium penicillins, and salt substitutes to renal failure patients.

    (d) **Pseudohyperkalemia** from a hemolyzed specimen.

  (3) **Clinical features** are more likely with acute changes than with chronic elevation.

    (a) **Signs and symptoms** include muscle weakness, paresthesias, and cardiac conduction abnormalities, which become dangerous as K^+ levels approach 7 mEq/L. Bradycardia, ventricular fibrillation, and cardiac arrest may result.

    (b) Hyperkalemia suppresses electrical conduction. **ECG findings** include high peaked T waves, ST segment depression, prolonged PR interval, loss of the P wave, diminished R-wave amplitude, QRS widening, and prolongation of the QT interval.

  (4) **Treatment** depends on the nature of ECG changes and serum levels.

    (a) **ECG changes** are treated with slow IV administration of 0.5 to 1.0 g of calcium chloride ($CaCl_2$). The dose may be repeated in 5 min if changes persist.

    (b) **Hyperventilation and NaHCO$_3$** administration shifts K^+ intracellularly. Between 50 and 100 mEq of $NaHCO_3$ may be given IV over 5 min, with a repeated dose in 10 to 15 min.

    (c) **Insulin** also shifts K^+ intracellularly. Regular insulin (10 units) is given IV simultaneously with 25 g of glucose (one ampule of a 50% solution) over 5 min. Check glucose 30 min later to avoid hypoglycemia.

    (d) The above therapies are short-term measures to decrease $[K^+]$ via cellular shifts. Cation exchange resins (sodium polystyrene sulfonate [Kayexalate], 20 to 50 g with sorbitol) given orally or rectally will slowly remove K^+ from the body and should be used as soon as possible. Serum $[K^+]$ can also be lowered by dialysis.

D. Extrarenal regulatory and metabolic functions

  1. **Erythropoietin** is produced to stimulate red blood cell production. Treatment of patients with exogenous recombinant erythropoietin can prevent the anemia of chronic renal failure (CRF) and its sequelae.

  2. **Vitamin D** is converted to its most active form, 1,25-dihydroxy-vitamin D by the kidney.

  3. **Parathyroid hormone** acts on the kidney to conserve calcium, to inhibit phosphate resorption, and to increase conversion of vitamin D by the kidney.

  4. Peptides and protein hormones such as insulin are metabolized, accounting for the generally decreased insulin requirements as renal failure progresses.

III. **Renal failure.** Definition varies but has been reported as an increase in serum creatinine by 0.5 mg/dL, increase in serum creatinine by 50%, or serum creatinine >2 mg/dL.

A. **Acute renal failure.** Incidence varies according to etiology, definition, and type of surgery but is 4% to 24% with mortality rates as high as 60% to 90%. Postoperative renal dysfunction is associated with higher incidence of gastrointestinal bleeding, respiratory infection, sepsis, longer ICU and hospital length of stay.

1. **Epidemiology.** From 2% to 5% of hospitalized patients; increases with age.

2. **Etiology**
   a. **Prerenal.** Due to decreased circulating volume (hypovolemia) or a perceived decrease in circulating volume (decreased cardiac output or hypotension). Early correction of the underlying cause usually results in rapid reversal of renal dysfunction, but continued renal hypoperfusion may result in intrinsic renal damage.
   b. **Intrarenal.** The most common cause is ATN due to ischemia (see section III.C). Other intrarenal causes include toxins, acute glomerulonephritis, and interstitial nephritis.
   c. **Postrenal.** Obstructive lesions result in disrupted emptying and can be caused by renal calculi, neurogenic bladder, prostatic disease, or an encroaching tumor. Unilateral obstruction rarely causes ARF.

3. **Diagnosis.** Clinical features occurring late in the course of the disease include hypervolemia due to an impaired ability to excrete water and sodium with resultant hypertension and peripheral edema, potential hypovolemia due to lack of urine concentrating ability, potassium retention, impaired excretion of drugs and toxins, and potential progression to CRF. Results of urine and serum indices can help to distinguish pre-/intra-/postrenal etiologies (Table 4.1).

4. **Prevention.** Mainly based on tradition, anecdotes, or extrapolation from animal models. A modest goal is to keep urine output >0.5 mL/kg/hour and avoid hypovolemia, hypoxia or decreased O_2 delivery, renovascular constriction, increased renal O_2 demand, and maintenance of renal vasodilation and renal tubular blood flow along with attenuation of renal ischemic reperfusion injury.

Table 4.1.   Urine and serum diagnostic indexes

	Prerenal	Renal	Postrenal
Urine (Na)	<10 mEq/L	>20 mEq/L	>20 mEq/L
Urine (Cl)	<10 mEq/L	>20 mEq/L	
FE_{Na}	<1%	>2%	>2%
Urine osmolarity	>500	<350	<350
Urine/serum (creatinine)	>40	<20	<20
Renal failure index	<1%	>2%	>2%
Urine/serum (urea)	>8	<3	<3
Serum (BUN)/creatinine	>20	=10	=10

BUN, Blood urea nitrogen; FE_{Na}, fractional excretion of sodium.

5. **Treatment**
   a. **Medications** such as diuretics and dopamine and fenoldopam can be used to increase urine output, treat hypertension, and manage electrolyte, fluid, and acid-base disturbances but have not been proven to prevent or treat ARF (see sections IV.A. and IV.B).
   b. **Hemodialysis.** Incidence of ARF patients requiring dialysis varies depending on the underlying surgical operation (e.g., coronary artery bypass grafting 1.1% versus general surgery 0.6%).
      (1) **Hemodialysis** uses an artificial semipermeable membrane that separates the patient's blood from dialysate and allows the exchange of solutes by diffusion. Vascular access (via central venous catheters or a surgically created arteriovenous fistula) and systemic or regional anticoagulation are often required. Hemodialysis typically is performed three times a week, and serum electrolyte and volume abnormalities are corrected by adjusting the dialysis bath fluid. Blood samples taken immediately after dialysis will be inaccurate, because redistribution of fluid and electrolytes takes about 6 hours. Continuous arteriovenous or venovenous hemodialysis may also be performed. Complications include arteriovenous fistula infection or thrombosis, dialysis disequilibrium or dementia, hypotension, pericarditis, and hypoxemia.
      (2) **Hypotension** can occur during hemodialysis with changes in preload, electrolyte changes, acid-base abnormalities, hemodynamic effects of buffering drugs, and impaired sympathetic response.
      (3) **Indications** for dialysis in ARF and CRF include hyperkalemia, acidosis, volume overload, uremic complications (pericarditis, tamponade, encephalopathy), and severe azotemia.
      (4) **Ultrafiltration** and **hemofiltration** allow for the removal of volume with minimal removal of waste products. These techniques are useful in volume-overloaded patients. As with standard hemodialysis, anticoagulation may be required.
         (a) **Ultrafiltration** uses hemodialysis equipment to create a hydrostatic driving force across the membrane without a dialysate on the opposing side. Thus, an ultrafiltrate of serum is removed and this volume is not replaced. If large volumes of fluid are removed rapidly, hypotension may ensue.
         (b) **Hemofiltration** uses the same principle as ultrafiltration; however, replacement fluid is given to the patient either before or after the membrane filter and solutes/electrolytes are removed by convection. Volume shifts are minimized so that patients can tolerate longer periods of continuous filtration.

Table 4.2. **National Kidney Foundation classification of CKD**

Stage	Description	GFR	U.S. prevalence (%)
Stage I	Normal	≥ 90	3.3
Stage II	Mild	60–89	3.0
Stage III	Moderate	30–59	4.3
Stage IV	Severe	15–29	0.2
Stage V	Failure	<15	0.1

  c. **Continuous renal replacement therapy (CRRT)** refers to any continuous mode of extracorporeal solute or fluid removal. Indications in addition to ARF include fluid clearance, electrolyte imbalances, and managing metabolic acidosis. Slower blood flow rates with CRRT improve hemodynamic stability compared with regular hemodialysis.

B. **Chronic kidney disease (CKD)** is defined by kidney damage (structural or functional abnormalities of the kidney) for ≥ 3 months as manifested by abnormalities in the composition of blood or urine, abnormalities in imaging tests, or a glomerular filtration rate (GFR) <60 mL/min/1.73m^2 for ≥ 3 months.

 1. **Epidemiology.** CKD affects more than 20 million adults in the United States (Table 4.2).

 2. **Etiology.** Common causes include hypertension, diabetes mellitus, chronic glomerulonephritis, tubulointerstitial disease, renovascular disease, and polycystic kidney disease.

 3. **Clinical features**

  a. **Hypervolemia and hypertension,** sometimes resulting in congestive heart failure and edema.

  b. **Accelerated atherosclerosis,** which may increase the risk of coronary artery disease.

  c. **Uremic pericarditis and pericardial effusions,** which may cause cardiac tamponade.

  d. **Hyperkalemia, hypermagnesemia, and hyponatremia** may occur.

  e. **Hypocalcemia and hyperphosphatemia** due to elevated parathyroid hormone, resulting in renal osteodystrophy.

  f. **Metabolic acidosis** due to retained sulfates and phosphates and an inability to excrete products of metabolism.

  g. **Chronic anemia** secondary to decreased erythropoietin production and decreased red blood cell survival.

  h. **Platelet dysfunction,** which can be temporarily treated with desmopressin acetate.

  i. **Increased gastric volume, acid production, and delayed gastric emptying** resulting in increased incidence of nausea, vomiting, and peptic ulceration.

  j. **Increased susceptibility to infection.**

  k. **Central nervous system changes** range from mild changes in mentation to severe encephalopathy and coma. Peripheral and autonomic neuropathies are common.

  l. **Glucose intolerance, hypertriglyceridemia.**

4. **Treatment.** When needed, 85% receive hemodialysis and 15% receive peritoneal dialysis. Transplantation is the preferred method of treatment for most CRF patients.

    a. **Hemodialysis (see section IV.A.5.d.)**

    b. **Peritoneal dialysis** uses the capillaries of the peritoneum as a semipermeable exchange membrane with the dialysate infused into the peritoneal cavity via an indwelling peritoneal catheter. Advantages over hemodialysis include less hypotension or disequilibrium and no need for heparin treatment. However, peritoneal dialysis is less efficient and limited in catabolic states compared with hemodialysis. Complications include infection, hyperglycemia from the dextran in the dialysate, and increased protein loss into the dialysate.

C. **Specific causes of renal failure**

1. **ATN** may be produced by ischemic or toxin injuries and is the major intrinsic form of ARF. ATN is the most common cause of perioperative renal failure, and its development is associated with high mortality. The major risk factors for ATN are a history of preexisting renal insufficiency, administration of radiocontrast agents or aminoglycoside antibiotics, and advanced age. Anesthetic management of patients who are at risk for developing ATN includes meticulous management of fluids and hemodynamics with the goal of maintaining euvolemia, normal renal perfusion, and urinary output. No specific therapies have proved consistently beneficial in preventing or treating perioperative ATN.

2. **Glomerulonephropathies** are a diverse family of diseases that may present insidiously or more acutely with fulminant renal failure. Nephrotic syndrome may be the initial presentation with severe proteinuria (>3.5 g/day), hypoalbuminemia, hyperlipidemia, and edema. Anesthetic concerns include depleted intravascular volume and protein, accelerated atherosclerotic disease, and increased risk of infection. Glomerulonephropathy may be secondary to autoimmune diseases such as systemic lupus erythematosus or vasculitides such as Wegener granulomatosis. Therapy may include glucocorticoids and cytotoxic agents.

3. **Hypertensive nephrosclerosis** is a major etiology in the development of end-stage renal disease (ESRD) and may account for up to 30% of patients beginning dialysis. Treatment of diastolic hypertension reduces disease progression and the associated morbidity and mortality.

4. **Diabetic nephropathy** is the single largest cause of ESRD in the United States, affecting one-half of all adult patients with insulin-dependent diabetes mellitus. The nephropathy presents with proteinuria and there is a progressive decline in renal function over 10 to 30 years after the initial diagnosis. Diabetic nephropathy often manifests itself as a type IV renal tubular acidosis (hyporeninemic hypoaldosteronism) or as papillary necrosis. There is a high correlation between renal dysfunction and diabetic retinopathy. Aggressive control of blood glucose and blood pressure may forestall the development and prevent progression of nephropathy.

5. **Tubulointerstitial diseases** primarily affect the renal tubules and interstitium and include acute and chronic forms of interstitial nephritis.

    a. **Acute interstitial nephritis** is most commonly caused by drugs (e.g., penicillins, cephalosporins, sulfonamides, rifampin, and NSAIDs) in adults. Systemic infections are the most common etiologies in children. Acute interstitial nephritis usually presents as oliguric renal failure with a variable degree of proteinuria. Symptoms of an inflammatory response, such as fever, rash, eosinophilia, and eosinophiluria, are suggestive of the diagnosis of acute interstitial nephritis. Treatment is supportive and includes discontinuation of suspect drugs.

    b. **Chronic interstitial nephritis** is most commonly due to obstruction of urine flow or reflux, analgesic abuse, or heavy metal intoxications. Early in the disease, patients lose the ability to concentrate urine and have polyuria and nocturia. Later manifestations depend on the specific anatomic lesions. Involvement of the proximal convoluted tubule results in a Fanconi-like syndrome (HCO_3^- wasting and renal tubular acidosis with glucose, phosphate, and amino acid wasting). Involvement of the distal convoluted tubule and collecting ducts will cause loss of acid secretion, acidemia, and salt wasting with resultant hyperkalemia. The only specific therapy for chronic interstitial nephritis is treatment of the underlying cause.

6. **Polycystic kidney diseases** are autosomal dominant diseases responsible for 5% to 8% of adult ESRD. Approximately 25% of patients at 50 years of age and 50% of patients at 75 years of age will manifest ESRD. Cystic disease may also affect the liver. Also, there is an association with intracranial and aortic aneurysms. Tuberous sclerosis and von Hippel-Lindau disease may also present as cystic renal disease.

IV. **Pharmacology and the kidney**

A. **Diuretics** are used to increase urine output (Table 4.3), treat hypertension, and manage electrolyte, fluid, and acid-base disturbances. The use of diuretics (e.g., furosemide) has been shown to decrease the duration of oliguria and the need for hemodialysis but has no effect on mortality or recovery from ARF.

B. **Dopamine and fenoldopam** dilate renal arterioles, increase renal blood flow, and augment natriuresis and the GFR. Low-dose dopamine (0.5 to 3 μg/kg/min) has been proposed to prevent and treat ARF, but efficacy has never been demonstrated. Low-dose fenoldopam, a specific dopamine-1 receptor agonist, may preserve renal function without the toxicity of dopamine.

C. **Anesthetic effects on the kidney.** Patients with normal kidney function experience transient postanesthetic alterations in renal function. These alterations may occur despite insignificant changes in blood pressure and cardiac output, suggesting that changes in intrarenal distribution of blood flow are responsible. With brief exposures to anesthesia, the observed changes in renal function are reversible (renal blood flow and GFR return to baseline within a few hours). With extensive surgery and prolonged anesthesia, impaired ability to excrete a water load or concentrate urine may last for several days.

Table 4.3. Diuretics

	Primary Site of Action	Primary Effect	Side Effects	Comments
Nonosmotic				
Loop (furosemide, edercrin, bumetanide)	Thick ascending loop of Henle, active Na^+Cl pump	Moderate to severe natriuresis, chloruresis	Hypokalemia, alkalosis, volume contraction	Interferes with both urinary concentration and dilution
Thiazides (chlorothiazide, dyazide, metolazone)	Distal tubules (Na^+-H^+, Na^+-K^+ exchange)	Mild to moderate natriuresis	Hyponatremia, hypokalemia, alkalosis, volume contraction	Interferes with urinary dilution, tends to be ineffective in renal failure and CHF
Carbonic anhydrase inhibitors (acetazolamide)	Proximal tubule Na^+-H^+ exchange)	Mild natriuresis	Hyperchloremia, hypokalemia	Used primarily for ophthalmology; self-limiting renal effect
Potassium sparing (aldactone, triamterene, amiloride)	Collecting duct, Na^+-K^+, Na^+-H^+ exchange	Mild to moderate natriuresis	Hyperkalemia	Used in conjunction with K^+ losing diuretics or in hyperaldosterone states
Osmotic				
Mannitol	Intratubular osmotic load	Moderate to severe diuresis	Early: vasodilation, volume expansion Late: hyperosmolality, volume contraction	Draws intracellular fluid into intravascular space

CHF, congestive heart failure.

1. **Indirect effects.** All inhalational agents and many induction agents cause myocardial depression, hypotension, and a mild-to-moderate increase in renal vascular resistance, leading the decreased renal blood flow and GFR. Compensatory catecholamine secretion causes redistribution of renal cortical blood flow. AVP levels do not change during halothane or morphine anesthesia but increase with the onset of surgical stimulation. Hydration before the induction of anesthesia attenuates the rise in AVP produced by painful stimuli. Spinal and epidural anesthesia produce decreases in renal blood flow, GFR, and urine output.

2. **Direct effects.** The direct toxicity of fluorinated agents is of concern, because fluoride (F^-) inhibits metabolic processes, affects urine-concentrating ability, and can cause proximal tubular swelling and necrosis. The magnitude of F^- elevation depends on the concentration and duration of the anesthetic.

   a. **Isoflurane** and **desflurane** are not associated with significant release of F^-.

   b. Only 2% of absorbed **enflurane** is metabolized to F^-, thus producing low levels of F^- (typically <15 μmol/L). There is a theoretical concern that use of enflurane in patients with renal dysfunction may lead to F^- accumulation and additional nephrotoxicity.

   c. **Sevoflurane** is also metabolized to F^-. Strong bases that accumulate in the CO_2 absorbent at low gas flows can degrade sevoflurane to a nephrotoxic by-product. Nephrotoxicity has been observed in rats. The Food and Drug Administration warns against using low inspired gas flows with sevoflurane. Some have warned against use in patients with preexisting renal disease.

   d. **Halothane** metabolism results in very low F^- levels.

V. **Pharmacology and renal failure.** Many common anesthetic drugs may be affected by renal dysfunction due to changes in compartment volumes, electrolytes, pH (acidemia resulting in a higher percentage of nonionized drug), decreased serum protein concentration resulting in increased bioavailability of protein-bound drugs, and impaired biotransformation and rates of excretion.

   A. **Lipid-soluble drugs** generally are poorly ionized and must undergo metabolism by the liver to water-soluble forms before elimination by the kidney. With few exceptions, the metabolites have little biologic activity.

   1. **Benzodiazepines and butyrophenones** are metabolized in the liver to both active and inactive compounds, which are then eliminated by the kidney. Benzodiazepines are 90% to 95% protein bound. Great care must be used with diazepam because of its long half-life and its active metabolites. Accumulation of benzodiazepines and their metabolites may occur in severe renal failure. Benzodiazepines are not appreciably removed by dialysis.

   2. **Barbiturates, etomidate, and propofol** are highly protein bound, and in hypoalbuminemic patients a much greater proportion will be available to reach receptor sites. Acidosis and changes in the blood-brain barrier will further reduce

induction requirements. Lower initial doses are recommended in renal failure.

3. **Opioids** are metabolized in the liver but may have a more intense and prolonged effect in patients with renal failure, particularly in hypoalbuminemic patients, in whom protein binding will be reduced. Active metabolites of morphine and meperidine may prolong their actions and accumulation of normeperidine may cause seizures. The pharmacokinetics of fentanyl, sufentanil, alfentanil, and remifentanil are unchanged in renal failure.

B. **Ionized drugs.** Drugs that are highly ionized at physiologic pH tend to be eliminated unchanged by the kidney, and their duration of action may be prolonged by renal dysfunction.

1. **Muscle relaxants.** Neuromuscular blocking drugs that have a more predictable duration and may be preferable for patients with renal dysfunction include mivacurium, cisatracurium, and rocuronium.

2. **Cholinesterase inhibitors.** With impaired renal function, elimination of the reversal drugs is decreased and their half-lives are prolonged. Prolongation is similar or greater than the duration of blockade from pancuronium or *d*-tubocurarine, so the return of muscle relaxation after adequate reversal (recurarization) is rarely seen.

3. **Digoxin** is excreted in the urine and patients with renal failure are at increased risk of digitalis toxicity.

C. **Vasoactive agents** have certain properties that merit concern in the patient with renal disease.

1. **Catecholamines** with α-adrenergic effects (norepinephrine, epinephrine, phenylephrine, ephedrine) constrict the renal vasculature and may reduce renal blood flow.

2. **Isoproterenol** also reduces renal blood flow but to a lesser extent.

3. **Sodium nitroprusside** contains cyanide and is metabolized by the kidney and excreted as thiocyanate. Toxicity, primarily neurologic, from excessive accumulation of thiocyanate is more likely in renal failure patients.

VI. **Anesthetic management**

A. **Preoperative assessment.** The etiology of renal disease should be elucidated (e.g., diabetes mellitus, glomerulonephritis, polycystic kidney disease). Elective surgery should be postponed pending resolution of acute disease processes. The degree of residual renal function is best estimated by creatinine clearance (see section VI.A.3.e) and is the most important consideration for anesthetic management. A thorough, systems-based history and physical should be performed (see Chapter 1).

1. **History**

a. **Signs and symptoms** of polyuria, polydipsia, dysuria, edema, and dyspnea should be sought.

b. **Relevant medications** should be detailed: diuretics, antihypertensives, potassium supplements, digitalis, and nephrotoxic agents (NSAIDs, aminoglycosides, exposure to heavy metals, and recent radiographic dye).

c. **Schedule of hemodialysis** should be noted and coordinated with elective procedures.

2. **Physical examination**
   a. Patients should be thoroughly examined for the stigmata of renal failure as described in section III.B.3.
   b. **Arteriovenous fistula** should be evaluated for patency (by the presence of a thrill or bruit). IV access and blood pressure determinations should be performed on the opposite limb.
3. **Laboratory studies**
   a. **Urinalysis** provides a qualitative assessment of general renal function.
      (1) Findings suggestive of renal disease include abnormal pH, proteinuria, pyuria, hematuria, and casts.
      (2) The kidney's ability to concentrate urine is often lost before other changes become apparent. A specific gravity of 1.018 or greater after an overnight fast suggests that concentrating ability is intact. However, radiographic dye and osmotic agents will elevate specific gravity and invalidate this test.
   b. **Urine electrolytes,** osmolality, and urine creatinine can help determine volume status and concentrating ability and are used to help differentiate between prerenal and intrarenal disease (see Table 4.1).
   c. **Blood urea nitrogen** is an insensitive measure of GFR, because it is influenced by volume status, cardiac output, diet, and body habitus. The ratio of blood urea nitrogen to creatinine is normally 10 to 20 to 1; disproportionate elevation of the blood urea nitrogen may reflect hypovolemia, low cardiac output, gastrointestinal bleeding, or steroid use.
   d. **Serum creatinine** normally is 0.6 to 1.2 mg/dL but is affected by the patient's skeletal muscle mass and activity level. Creatinine concentration is inversely proportional to GFR so that a doubling of the creatinine generally corresponds to a 50% reduction in GFR.
   e. **Creatinine clearance** is used to estimate GFR and provides the best estimate of renal reserve. It is normally 80 to 120 mL/min. A gross estimate of creatinine clearance can be calculated with the following equation:

   $$\{[140 - \text{age (years)}] \times \text{weight (kg)}\}/[72 \times \text{serum creatinine (mg/dL)}]$$

   Multiply by 0.85 for women. In obese individuals, ideal body weight should be used to estimate creatinine clearance. This formula is invalid in the presence of gross renal insufficiency or changing renal function. Medications such as trimethoprim, H2-receptor antagonists, and salicylates block secretion of creatinine and may elevate serum creatinine and decrease creatinine clearance.
   f. Serum Na^+, K^+, Cl^-, and HCO_3^- concentrations usually will be normal until renal failure is advanced. Careful consideration of the risk and benefit of proceeding with elective surgery should be made if $[Na^+]$ is <131 or >150 mEq/L or $[K^+]$ is <2.5 or >5.9 mEq/L, because these

abnormalities may exacerbate arrhythmias and compromise cardiac function.

g. Serum Ca^{2+}, PO_4^-, and Mg^{2+} concentrations are altered.

h. **Hematologic studies** should assess anemia and coagulation abnormalities (see section II.D.1.).

i. **ECG** may reveal myocardial ischemia or infarction, pericarditis, and the effects of electrolyte abnormalities (see section II.C)

j. **Chest radiographs** may reveal evidence of fluid overload, pericardial effusion, infection, uremic pneumonitis, or cardiomegaly.

4. **Risk assessment.** Risk factors for postoperative renal dysfunction are as follows:

   a. **Preexisting renal insufficiency**

   b. **Diabetes mellitus,** types 1 and 2 (see section III.C.4)

   c. **Age >65 years** due to an age-related decline in renal reserve and GFR.

   d. **Congestive heart failure**

   e. **High-risk surgery** such as renal artery surgery, thoracic and abdominal aortic surgery, and prolonged (>3 hours) cardiopulmonary bypass.

   f. Recent exposure to **toxins**

      (1) **Contrast media** cause a decrease in O_2 supply, by causing intrarenal vasoconstriction and a decreased medullary blood supply, and an increase in O_2 demand. The osmotic load increases work to the medullary nephrons.

      (2) Bile pigments

      (3) Endotoxemia

      (4) Aminoglycoside antibiotics

      (5) NSAID

   g. **Prolonged renal hypoperfusion** resulting from shock, sepsis, nephritic syndrome, and cirrhosis

5. **Optimization**

   a. Patients on hemodialysis should be dialyzed before surgery, allowing time between dialysis and surgery to permit equilibration of fluids and electrolytes (see section IV.A.5.d.1).

   b. If the patient is on CRRT, the decision to continue intraoperatively must be based on the underlying reason for the CRRT, the duration of the procedure, and the type of procedure. Most patients will be able to tolerate discontinuation of CRRT before surgery and reinstitution afterward. However, certain patients may not be able to tolerate even a short period off CRRT, usually because of increased K^+ or acidosis, and one may need to decide whether the surgery can be postponed or to arrange for CRRT in the operating room or even during transport to the operating room. Major surgical procedures or prolonged surgical procedures may also dictate the need for intraoperative CRRT.

   c. It may be prudent to postpone major elective vascular surgery for a few days after contrast media exposure. In addition, pretreatment with **N-acetylcysteine** (NAC) and **sodium bicarbonate infusion** (SBI) before radiographic contrast administration may prevent contrast-induced nephropathy.

(1) **NAC** 20% (200 mg/mL) 600 mg orally is given every 12 hours, on the day before and on the day of contrast administration, for a total of 2 days.

(2) **SBI** of 150 mEq/L of sodium bicarbonate (three ampules of 50 mEq sodium bicarbonate in 1 L of D5W or freewater [FW]) is administered at 3 mL/kg/hour for 1 hour before contrast administration and followed by an infusion of 1 mL/kg/hour for 6 hours after the procedure.

B. **Intraoperative management.** Either general or regional anesthesia with standard monitoring is acceptable. When regional anesthesia is considered, coexisting neuropathies should be determined (and documented) and the coagulation profile checked for coagulopathies.

1. **Premedication** should be administered carefully because renal failure patients may have increased sensitivity to central nervous system depressants especially if significant uremia is present (see section III.A.1).

2. The dose of **induction agents** may need to be reduced and their rate of administration slowed to avoid hypotension. Serum potassium should be checked before administration of succinylcholine (see section III.A.2).

3. Most anesthetics cause peripheral vasodilation and myocardial depression with the need for vasoconstrictors or fluid replacement to compensate. Angiotensin II increases efferent arteriolar vasoconstriction to maintain glomerular filtration pressure. However, in patients taking ACE-I or angiotensin receptor blocker (ARBs), this compensatory mechanism may be decreased, which could cause a decrease in renal perfusion pressure and urine production.

   a. **Narcotics** increase ADH release, which may further reduce urine output (UOP) (see section III.A.3).

   b. Halogenated **volatile anesthetics** may have direct renal toxicity (see section IV.C.2).

4. Surgical stimulation results in an increase in circulating catecholamine, catabolic hormones, and cytokines that increase ADH. Stimulation increases aldosterone as well as glucocorticoids, which result in sodium/water retention and potassium loss.

5. **Positioning** should be done carefully because these patients are prone to fractures secondary to renal osteodystrophy (see section II.D.3.).

6. **Fluid replacement** should take into account maintenance fluid requirements, evaporative/insensible losses (e.g., open abdominal procedures with losses up to 10 mL/kg/hour), extravasation/third-space losses of fluids, and intravascular/blood loss.

   a. Fluid replacement should proceed cautiously with isotonic crystalloids. Potassium-containing fluids should be avoided in anuric patients.

   b. Large volumes of 0.9% sodium chloride administration may result in a hyperchloremic metabolic acidosis.

        c. For more extensive procedures, a central venous pressure or pulmonary artery catheter may help guide fluid management (see Chapter 10).

C. Postoperative management

    1. Postoperative fluid replacement should take into account effusions and drainage tube losses and mobilization of third-space fluid back into the vascular compartment.

        a. Replacement fluid should consist of isotonic fluid and dextrose until the patient is able to take adequate fluid orally.

    2. Hypertension is a common postoperative problem and is aggravated by fluid overload. For those not on dialysis, diuretics and short-acting antihypertensives are effective. For those on dialysis, postoperative dialysis may be required.

SUGGESTED READING

Colson P, Ryckwaert F, Coriat P. Renin angiotensin system antagonists and anesthesia. *Anesth Analg* 1999;89:1143–1155.

Merten GJ, et al. Prevention of contrast induced nephropathy with sodium bicarbonate. *JAMA* 2004;291:2328–2334.

Petroni KC. Continuous renal replacement therapy: anesthetic implications. *Anesth Analg* 2002;94:1288–1297.

Petroni KC, Cohen NH. Continuous renal replacement therapy: anesthetic implications. *Anesth Analg* 2002;94:1288–1297.

Sadovnikoff N. Perioperative acute renal failure. *Int Anesthesiol Clin* 2001;39(1): 95–109.

Sear JW. Kidney dysfunction in the postoperative period. *Br J Anaesth* 2005;95: 20–32.

Sladen RN. Renal physiology. In: Miller R, ed. *Anesthesiology*, 6th ed. New York: Churchill Livingstone, 2005:777–811.

Sladen RS. Anesthetic considerations for the patient with renal failure. *Anesthesiol Clin North Am* 2000;18(4):863–881.

Tepel M. Prevention of radiographic contrast agent induced reductions in renal function by acetylcysteine. *N Engl J Med* 2000;343:180–184.

Weldon BC, Monk TG. The patient at risk for acute renal failure. *Anesthesiol Clin North Am* 2000;18(4):705–737.

5

Specific Considerations with Liver Disease

Stacey Lynn Remchuk and Wilton C. Levine

I. **Hepatic anatomy**
   A. **Hepatic blood supply.** The liver composes only 2% of the total body mass but it receives 20% to 25% of the cardiac output.
   1. The **hepatic artery** supplies 20% to 25% of the total liver blood flow and 45% to 50% of the liver's oxygen requirement.
   2. The **portal vein** drains the stomach, spleen, pancreas, and intestine. It supplies 75% of the hepatic blood flow and 50% to 55% of hepatic oxygen supply. Portal venous blood has a low oxygen content but contains a rich supply of nutrients (carbohydrates, lipids, amino acids) and hormones (insulin, glucagon, gastrin, vasoactive intestinal peptide). It also contains drugs and toxins absorbed from the intestine.
   3. **Total hepatic blood flow** depends greatly on venous return from the preportal organs. Flow in the hepatic artery is regulated by sympathetic tone and local adenosine concentration and is inversely related to portal vein flow (PVF). For example, a reduction in PVF leads to increased adenosine concentrations in the liver. This causes local arteriole dilation and an increase in hepatic artery flow. Total hepatic blood flow may be reduced in diseases causing increased hepatic vascular resistance (e.g., cirrhosis, infiltrative disease, Budd-Chiari syndrome).
   B. **Liver structure**
   1. The anatomic unit of the liver is the **lobule.** The lobule is composed of hexagonal plates of hepatocytes and portal triads (terminal portal vein, hepatic artery, bile duct branch) surrounding a central hepatic vein.
   2. The functional microvascular unit of the liver is the **acinus.** Here the portal triad is central and surrounded by hepatocytes with centrilobar veins at the periphery. These hepatocytes are classified by their position in relation to the triad. Those closest to the triad are labeled **Zone 1 cells.** These cells receive the most oxygen and nutrients and are responsible for most nitrogen metabolism, oxidation, and glycogen synthesis. **Zone 2** is a transitional area. **Zone 3 hepatocytes** are the farthest from the triad and are at the greatest risk for ischemic injury.

II. **Hepatic function**
   A. **Synthesis and storage**
   1. **Proteins.** Nearly all plasma proteins are synthesized by hepatocytes with the exception of gamma globulins and hemoglobin. The normal adult liver produces 2 to 15 g of protein per day including the following:
      a. **Albumin** is manufactured exclusively in the liver and has a half-life of approximately 20 days. It comprises 50% of

all circulating plasma proteins and is the most important drug-binding protein (especially for organic acids such as penicillins and barbiturates). Albumin contributes to oncotic pressure and also serves as a carrier protein for bilirubin and hormones.

b. α_1-**Acid glycoprotein** is an "acute phase reactant" and is responsible for binding basic drugs such as amide local anesthetics, propranolol, and opioids.

c. **Pseudocholinesterase,** also known as butyrylcholinesterase or nonspecific cholinesterases, is responsible for the degradation of succinylcholine, mivacurium, and ester-type local anesthetics. In the presence of severely depressed hepatocellular function or a genetically mediated enzyme deficiency, a low plasma level of this enzyme may become clinically relevant. During pregnancy, serum pseudocholinesterase levels are decreased by 20% but clinical relevance is variable.

d. All proteinaceous **clotting factors** are produced in the liver with the exception of factor VIII, which is produced in the vascular endothelium. Synthesis of factors II, VII, IX, and X; protein C; and protein S is vitamin K dependent.

2. **Carbohydrates.** Homeostatic regulation of plasma glucose levels depends on normal hepatic function. The liver is responsible for **glycogen synthesis** and **gluconeogenesis.** The normal liver can store enough glycogen to provide glucose during a fast of 12 to 24 hours. After that time, glucose is derived by gluconeogenesis from amino acids, glycerol, and lactate. Release of stress hormones (e.g., epinephrine, norepinephrine, cortisol, and glucagon), as is common during the perioperative period, promotes gluconeogenesis and hyperglycemia.

3. **Lipids.** Most of the body's lipoproteins, as well as cholesterol and phospholipids, are formed in the liver.

4. **Heme/bile**

a. The liver is the primary erythropoietic organ of the fetus and continues to be a major site of hematopoiesis until approximately 2 months of age. In healthy adults, the liver is responsible for 20% of heme production.

b. The liver forms approximately 800 mL of bile per day. **Bile** contains mostly electrolytes and bile salts (from cholesterol and hemoglobin breakdown). Bile salts are detergents that aid in absorbing, transporting, and excreting lipids. Bile also carries metabolic waste products and drug metabolites to the intestine from the liver. As an emulsifier, bile facilitates fat absorption by the small intestine. Failure to manufacture or release bile causes jaundice and an inability to absorb fat and fat-soluble vitamins (A, D, E, and K) and can result in steatorrhea, vitamin deficiencies, and possibly coagulopathy.

c. Abnormalities in **heme synthesis** can result in porphyria (see Chapter 6).

B. **Degradation**

1. **Proteins.** The liver is the major site of protein degradation. Acinar Zone 1 cells are responsible for most of the deamination of amino acids generating urea for the elimination of ammonia. Patients with liver disease may lack the ability to form urea, resulting in rapidly rising plasma ammonia levels and hepatic encephalopathy.

2. **Steroid hormones.** Cholesterol is degraded principally by the liver, and its by-products serve as a substrate for the production of bile salts, steroid hormones, and cell membranes. Because the liver is also the major site of steroid hormone degradation, **hepatic failure results in steroid excess.** Elevations of serum aldosterone and cortisol result in increased resorption of sodium and water and loss of potassium in the urine, contributing to the edema, ascites, and electrolyte abnormalities frequently seen with liver disease. Decreased metabolism of estrogens and impaired conversion to androgens causes other clinical stigmata of liver disease, including spider angiomata, gynecomastia, palmar erythema, and testicular atrophy.

3. **Heme/bile.** Albumin binds and delivers bilirubin to the hepatocytes where it then undergoes conjugation with glucuronic acid to its water-soluble form. These products are excreted within bile and eliminated via the feces or urine.

C. **Drug metabolism**

1. **Hepatic extraction ratio** (HER) is defined as the fraction of the drug concentration flowing into the liver that is removed through hepatic elimination or metabolism.

2. **Hepatic clearance** is the product of the hepatic blood flow rate and HER. Some drugs are extensively metabolized by the liver and have an HER close to 1.0 (propofol). Because the metabolic capacity of the liver is so extensive in this case, hepatic metabolism depends predominantly on blood flow and moderate changes in hepatic function have little effect on clearance. Other drugs have an HER much <1.0 and clearance depends heavily on hepatic metabolic capacity and is minimally affected by changes in blood flow.

3. **Protein binding.** Only free, unbound drug is pharmacologically active and available to the hepatocytes for conversion to a less active form. The degree of protein binding depends on the specific drug's protein binding affinity and the protein concentration. Decreased concentrations of plasma proteins, as often seen in liver disease, will result in a greater proportion of unbound drug. This may result in a higher apparent potency of that drug. The larger the unbound fraction of a drug, the more rapid its hepatic elimination.

4. **Volume of distribution** is often increased in patients with liver disease and **portal-systemic shunting** permits orally administered drugs to bypass the liver, reducing the first-pass effect. Both of these phenomena can alter drug effects and metabolism.

5. **Enzyme induction/cytochrome P450** enzymes are produced in the liver and are responsible for much drug metabolism. Certain drugs such as barbiturates, ethanol, and phenytoin induce cytochrome P450 enzymes. Induction of cytochrome P450 increases tolerance to a drug's effect and tolerance to other drugs that are also metabolized by the cytochrome P450 system.

6. Two steps are involved in **hepatic drug elimination.**
    a. **Phase I** reactions change a compound's structure via oxidation, reduction, or hydrolysis mostly by a family of enzymes called the cytochrome P450 enzymes. The products of this phase may be metabolically active. Drugs that have a high affinity for the P450 complex (e.g., cimetidine) may decrease the metabolism of concurrently administered drugs.
    b. **Phase II** reactions may or may not follow Phase I reactions and are enzymatically enhanced conjugations with glucuronide, sulfate, taurine, or glycine. These conjugations increase the water solubility of the metabolite for excretion via the urine.

III. **Metabolism of anesthetics**
   A. **Volatile anesthetics** are metabolized minimally (<5%) by the cytochrome P450 system (Table 5.1). By-products of halothane metabolism may lead to the formation of neoantigens, resulting in the development of immune hepatitis known as "halothane hepatitis." Hepatitis related to isoflurane, sevoflurane, and desflurane has not been reported in the literature.
   B. **Intravenous anesthetics**
      1. **Induction agents**
         a. **Propofol** is metabolized by the liver (HER = 1) to water-soluble compounds that are excreted by the kidneys. Extrahepatic metabolism of propofol also contributes to total propofol clearance.
         b. **Barbiturates.** Long- and intermediate-acting barbiturates have a duration of action that is determined by hepatic metabolism and therefore may have prolonged effects in patients with liver failure. Short-acting barbiturates have a duration of action that is determined by redistribution. Hypoalbuminemia seen in liver failure reduces protein binding and increases the free, active fraction of these drugs. Therefore, all barbiturates must be titrated carefully in liver disease.
         c. **Ketamine** is metabolized by the hepatic microsomal enzyme system to norketamine, which has approximately 30% of the activity of the parent drug. Ketamine has an HER near 1, so clearance approximates hepatic blood flow.
         d. **Etomidate** is metabolized by the liver through ester hydrolysis to inactive metabolites. Etomidate has a high HER, so clearance is affected by conditions that reduce

Table 5.1. Minimum alveolar concentration (MAC) values and the extent of metabolism for various volatile anesthetics

	MAC with Oxygen	% Metabolized
Halothane	0.74	20
Enflurane	1.68	2
Isoflurane	1.15	0.2
Desflurane	6.0	0.02–0.2
Sevoflurane	2.05	2–5

blood flow. Recovery from an initial induction dose is primarily due to rapid redistribution.

2. **Benzodiazepines and opioids** are metabolized primarily by the liver and have significantly increased half-lives in patients with liver disease. Additionally, they have increased potency due to hypoalbuminemia. Both may confound the clinical picture of hepatic encephalopathy and should be used cautiously.

3. **Neuromuscular blocking agents.** Patients with liver disease often demonstrate resistance to nondepolarizing neuromuscular blockers, probably because of increased volume of distribution or increased neuromuscular receptors. However, a slower elimination time may decrease the requirement for maintenance dosing.

   a. **Long-acting neuromuscular blockers** (e.g., doxacurium, pancuronium) are excreted primarily in the urine. Approximately 30% of pancuronium is eliminated through hepatobiliary mechanisms, and its effect may be prolonged in patients with biliary obstruction or cirrhosis.

   b. **Intermediate-acting neuromuscular blocking drugs, vecuronium** and **rocuronium,** are highly dependent on hepatobiliary excretion and metabolism (both are excreted >50% unchanged in the bile). This translates to a decreased clearance and a prolonged effect in patients with liver disease. **Cisatracurium** is degraded via Hofmann elimination and is unaffected by liver disease.

   c. **The short-acting neuromuscular blocking drugs. Mivacurium,** like succinylcholine, is completely metabolized in the plasma by pseudocholinesterase. Cholinesterase production may be depressed in severe liver disease, and the duration of action of mivacurium and succinylcholine may be prolonged in patients with hepatic dysfunction.

IV. **Liver disease**
   A. **Liver disease** is classified by time course and severity.
      1. **Parenchymal**
         a. **Acute hepatocellular injury** has many etiologies, including viral infection (hepatitis A, B, C, D, and E; Epstein-Barr virus; cytomegalovirus; herpes simplex virus; Echo virus; and Coxsackie virus), drugs, chemicals and poisons (including alcohol, halothane, phenytoin, propylthiouracil, isoniazid, tetracycline, and acetaminophen), and inborn errors of metabolism (e.g., Wilson disease and α_1-antitrypsin deficiency).

         b. **Chronic parenchymal disease** may be associated with varying degrees of functional impairment. **Cirrhosis** may result from many insults, including chronic active hepatitis, alcoholism, hemochromatosis, primary biliary cirrhosis, and congenital disorders. End-stage hepatic fibrosis causes significant resistance to portal blood flow, leading to portal hypertension and esophageal varices. Further complications from the combination of portal hypertension and decreased hepatic synthetic and metabolic function include ascites, coagulopathy, gastrointestinal bleeding, and encephalopathy. Many patients present for procedures aimed at reducing these manifestations of portal hypertension (splenorenal shunt, transjugular intrahepatic portocaval shunt, LeVeen shunt, and orthotopic liver transplantation).

2. **Cholestasis** occurs most frequently in cholelithiasis and acute or chronic cholecystitis. Primary biliary cirrhosis and primary sclerosing cholangitis also begin as cholestatic diseases, ultimately leading to parenchymal damage and liver failure. **Hyperbilirubinemia** is an important marker for hepatobiliary disease. **Unconjugated hyperbilirubinemia** is due to excess bilirubin production (e.g., massive transfusion, absorption of large hematomas, or hemolysis) or impaired uptake of unconjugated bilirubin by the hepatocyte (e.g., Gilbert syndrome). **Conjugated hyperbilirubinemia** generally occurs with hepatocellular disease (e.g., alcoholic or viral hepatitis, cirrhosis), disease of the small bile ducts (e.g., primary biliary cirrhosis, Dubin-Johnson syndrome), or obstruction of the extrahepatic bile ducts (e.g., pancreatic carcinoma, cholangiocarcinoma, gallstones).

B. **Manifestations of liver disease**
   1. **Central nervous system.** Hepatic dysfunction can lead to **encephalopathy.** Although the exact pathogenesis is unclear, impaired neurotransmission, presence of intrinsic γ-aminobutyric acid-ergic substances, and altered cerebral metabolism may be involved in its pathogenesis. **Ammonia levels** are often elevated in encephalopathic patients but do not correlate with the severity or outcome of encephalopathy. Signs may vary from sleep disturbances and the presence of asterixis to coma. Patients with severe acute liver failure often present with a rapidly progressive encephalopathy complicated by **cerebral edema.** Elevated intracranial pressure must be aggressively managed to prevent cerebral ischemia. Extreme hyponatremia or its overly aggressive treatment may lead to fatal **central pontine myelinolysis.** Changes in mental status and increased sensitivity to sedatives mandates caution in dosing premedications.
   2. **Cardiovascular system**
      a. Patients with advanced liver disease exhibit a **hyperdynamic circulatory state** with an elevated **cardiac output,** resting tachycardia, and **decreased systemic vascular resistance.** Elevated levels of nitric oxide, glucagon, and prostaglandins are thought to be responsible for arteriolar vasodilation. Multiple **arteriovenous shunts,** such as spider angiomata in the skin, can be present in almost all vascular beds.
      b. Patients with advanced liver failure also have a reduced effective intravascular volume due to vasodilation and portosystemic shunting. In addition, hypoalbuminemia, increased levels of aldosterone, and inappropriate secretion of antidiuretic hormone all lead to increased **total body fluid volume** and worsen ascites and edema/anasarca.
      c. **Alcoholic cardiomyopathy** should always be considered in patients with a history of alcohol abuse.

3. **Respiratory system**
   a. **Airway protection** is a major concern in patients with altered mental status. Patients with the stigmata of advanced liver disease such as ascites (increased abdominal pressure) should be considered at increased risk for aspiration. Definitive airway protection with rapid sequence induction and intubation is frequently advisable when general anesthesia is required.
   b. **Chronic hypoxemia** results from many causes. Massive ascites and pleural effusions lead to atelectasis and restrictive lung physiology. Diminished hypoxic pulmonary vasoconstriction results in ventilation perfusion mismatch and intrapulmonary shunting can be significant (10% to 40%). Pulmonary hypertension can coexist with portal hypertension and can produce right heart failure. Platypnea-orthodeopia, characterized by dyspnea and deoxygenation after a change to sitting or standing from the recumbent position, may be seen.
4. **Gastrointestinal system**
   a. The increased resistance to portal blood flow results in **portal hypertension,** splenomegaly, and splanchnic venous congestion. This increases collateral circulation, which is manifested as hemorrhoids, esophageal varices, and dilated abdominal wall veins (caput medusae). **Ascites** is due to splanchnic venous congestions coupled with hypoalbuminemia and decreased oncotic pressure.
   b. **Variceal bleeding** can progress rapidly to hemorrhagic shock. After volume resuscitation, treatment consists of vasopressin, somatostatin, β-adrenergic blockade, sclerotherapy, or endoscopic ligation.
5. **Renal system**
   a. Intravascular volume depletion may produce **prerenal azotemia.** The blood urea nitrogen level may be deceptively low because of the liver's inability to synthesize urea from ammonia.
   b. **Water and electrolyte balance** is complicated by frequent use of diuretics. Metabolic alkalosis, hypokalemia, and hyponatremia (despite total body sodium overload) are common in patients with hepatic disease.
   c. **Hepatorenal syndrome** is characterized by increased renal vascular resistance, oliguria, and renal failure in the presence of hepatic failure. Its exact etiology is unknown but may include abnormal prostaglandin metabolism. The sequelae include decreased renal blood flow, sodium retention, and increased sensitivity to nonsteroidal antiinflammatory medications. Normal renal function returns after liver transplantation or if liver failure resolves.
6. **Coagulopathy** is caused by several factors.
   a. **Synthesis of clotting factors** (II,VII, IX, X) as well as that of endogenous anticoagulants (proteins C and S) is impaired in liver failure.
   b. **Cholestasis** causes impaired absorption of fat and fat-soluble vitamins (A, D, E, and K). **Vitamin K,** produced in the intestinal mucosa, is an important cofactor in the synthesis of clotting factors II, VII, IX, and X.

      c. **Thrombocytopenia** secondary to hypersplenism, alcohol-induced bone marrow failure, and consumption is frequently seen and impairs clot formation.

      d. **Preoperative correction of clotting abnormalities** with fresh frozen plasma or vitamin K should be performed as necessary. Regional anesthesia may not be appropriate in the setting of liver failure or anticipated liver failure. The potential for postoperative coagulopathy should be taken into account before placing an epidural. Invasive monitoring can help evaluate and guide volume status, and blood bank support is necessary. The importance of adequate venous access for intraoperative infusion of crystalloid, colloid, blood products, and vasoactive drugs should not be underestimated.

  7. **Nutritional deficiency** as manifested by marasmus and kwashiorkor can be part of liver disease, especially in alcoholics. Nutritional deficiency is a risk factor for increased morbidity and mortality postoperatively. If surgery is not urgent, nutritional status should be optimized preoperatively.

  8. **Glycemic control** depends heavily on the liver. **Hypoglycemia** may occur in end-stage hepatic insufficiency, during the anhepatic phase of liver transplantation, or in liver failure that may accompany an episode of severe circulatory shock. Close monitoring of blood glucose levels should be performed frequently and glucose-containing solutions should be administered as necessary. Severe hepatic insufficiency leads to diminished **glycogen** stores, requiring gluconeogenesis to maintain normoglycemia. **Gluconeogenesis** is also impaired in severe liver disease and alcoholism.

V. Surgical risk in patients with liver disease

  A. Risk assessment

    1. Historical perspective: In the 1960s, **Child and Turcotte** noted five consistent clinical variables common to patients with liver disease who did poorly during surgery for portal decompression to treat bleeding esophageal varices. They developed a risk stratification system for perioperative morbidity and mortality **ascites, bilirubin level, albumin level, nutritional status, and encephalopathy.** Approximately 10 years later, Pugh added the **prothrombin time** as an additional element and assigned numeric values so that a total score could be classified (Table 5.2). The Child-Pugh system is one of the best current predictors of surgical morbidity and mortality. Grade A Child-Pugh classification system correlates with a 100% and 85% 1- and 2-year survival, respectively; Grade B correlates with an 80% and 60% 1- and 2-year survival; Grade C correlates with a 45% and 35% 1- and 2-year survival, respectively.

    2. Other predictors of perioperative risk include **type of surgery,** presence of **sepsis, reoperation,** and elective versus **emergent** surgery.

    3. The **MELD score** is a statistical model predicting overall survival in patients with cirrhosis. Its primary use is to prioritize selection of patients for liver transplantation. It has not been validated to assess risk outside of transplantation.

Table 5.2.   Modified Child-Pugh Score

| | Points | | |
Parameter	1	2	3
Albumin (g/dL)	>3.5	2.8–3.5	<2.8
Bilirubin (mg/dL)[a]	<2.0	2.0–3.0	>3.0
Ascites	Absent	Slight	Moderate
Encephalopathy	Absent	Grades I and II	Grades III and IV
PT prolongation (s)	<4.0	4.0–6.0	>6.0

Class A, 5 to 6 points; class B, 7 to 9 points; class C; 10 to 15 points; PT, prothrombin time.
[a]For primary biliary cirrhosis: one point for bilirubin <4.0 mg/dL, two points for bilirubin 4–10 mg/dL, and three points for bilirubin >10 mg/dL.

    B.   Preoperative assessment
        1.   Screening liver function with lab tests has not proven to be useful when applied to a general surgical population.
        2.   A careful **history** and **physical exam** are the best screening tools in the preoperative period. Symptoms of concern include a history of jaundice, pruritis, malaise, and anorexia. Exposure to drugs, alcohol, and other toxins should be considered. Physical examination may reveal stigmata of liver disease such as hepatosplenomegaly, ascites, peripheral edema, spider angiomata, testicular atrophy, caput medusae, hemorrhoids, asterixis, gynecomastia, and temporal wasting.
        3.   **Laboratory tests** should be considered for the patient in whom liver disease is suspected (bilirubin, transaminases, alkaline phosphatase, albumin, total protein, prothrombin time, and hepatitis serologies).
        4.   EKG, chest radiograph, and evaluation of myocardial function should be considered when indicated based on age, disease severity, and duration. In patients with end-stage liver disease, a dobutamine stress echocardiogram is the test of choice as it appears to be more sensitive (but less specific) for coronary artery disease than dipyridamole or adenosine nuclear imaging in this population.
        5.   **Duration** and severity of liver disease have general prognostic implications and **percutaneous liver biopsy** may be indicated to establish a diagnosis before elective surgery.
    C.   Every effort should be made to **correct abnormalities before surgery,** including coagulopathy, poorly controlled ascites, volume and electrolyte imbalances, renal function, encephalopathy, thrombocytopenia, and nutritional status.
VI.   Anesthesia in patients with liver disease
    A.   Planning the anesthetic must take into account the surgical procedure, type and severity of liver disease, and alterations to hepatic blood flow due to anesthetics. Meticulous attention must be paid to **maintain adequate hepatic perfusion** and oxygen delivery. Both **general and regional anesthesia** techniques can decrease total hepatic blood flow. **Isoflurane** and **sevoflurane** in concentrations up to 2 times MAC have minimal effects on hepatic blood

flow in experimental animals. Episodes of perioperative hepatic ischemia (due to surgical manipulation or anesthetics) can exacerbate preexisting liver disease. Hypotension, hemorrhage, and vasopressors can compromise hepatic oxygenation delivery, resulting in increased postoperative hepatic dysfunction. Positive pressure ventilation and positive end-expiratory pressure may cause deleterious effects in hepatic venous pressure, resulting in decreased cardiac output and total hepatic blood flow. **Hyperventilation** should be avoided because hypocarbia can independently reduce hepatic blood flow.

B. Caution must be exercised when **regional anesthesia** is considered in a patient with liver disease. Coagulopathy and thrombocytopenia put these patients at a higher risk for epidural bleeding and hematoma formation. In a patient with well-compensated liver disease and a reasonably normal coagulation profile and platelet count, regional anesthesia may be appropriate but this must be considered on a case-by-case basis. Surgical traction and patient positioning can lend to compromise of hepatic blood flow.

C. Sufficient **venous access** is of paramount importance, especially in surgery involving the liver parenchyma. **Large-bore peripheral intravenous cannulas** are inserted before or after induction of anesthesia for major surgery (often 12-gauge or larger). In patients with insufficient peripheral access, **large-bore central venous catheters** (8.5 to 9.5 French single-lumen or 12 French double-lumen catheters) may be inserted. Universal precautions are mandatory given the high incidence of viral disease in this patient population.

D. Invasive monitoring is also an important component of anesthetic planning. An **arterial catheter** facilitates blood sampling for monitoring serial blood gases, glucose, and electrolytes and for measuring arterial blood pressure. It is considered routine in major surgery for patients with end-stage liver disease. **Central venous catheterization** is indicated for pressure monitoring and rapid drug administration into the central circulation. **Pulmonary artery catheters** may help guide fluid and vasopressor therapy in some patients. Skillful line placement is important in coagulopathic patients. Ultrasonographic visualization of the vein before or during cannulation will reduce the incidence of carotid arterial puncture and the number of needle passes needed to cannulate the jugular vein.

E. A low threshold for performing a **rapid sequence induction** should exist for these patients given their elevated intra-abdominal pressure and increased risk of aspiration.

F. Other physiologic variables that should be taken into consideration include urine output, body temperature, blood sugar levels, electrolyte disturbances, and coagulation status.

G. Proper **postoperative care** and timing of **extubation** for patients presenting with severe comorbidities should also be considered.

H. **Surgical considerations for the anesthesiologist during procedures on the liver.** Excessive bleeding and transfusion requirements have been correlated with increased postoperative morbidity. Newer surgical techniques for hepatic resection and other procedures on the liver have been developed to decrease blood loss. **Total hepatic vascular exclusion** (TVE), the **Pringle maneuver** (PM), and **low central venous pressure anesthesia** are three such techniques.

1. TVE consists of clamping the hepatic inflow vessels (portal vein and hepatic artery) to the liver as well as the outflow vessels (inferior vena cava and suprahepatic inferior vena cava). This can have profound deleterious effects on venous return and the hemodynamics of the patient. This also results in a significant amount of warm ischemic time to the liver and may increase postoperative hepatic dysfunction.

2. The PM consists of intermittent clamping of the hepatic inflow vessels (portal vein and hepatic artery). There can be significant back bleeding through the hepatic veins and vena cava.

3. **Low central venous pressure (CVP) anesthesia.** A low CVP facilitates control of bleeding from hepatic veins and the inferior vena cava during parenchymal dissection. This anesthetic technique has been correlated with decreased blood loss and transfusion requirements in small studies. To date, no randomized controlled trials have been published on this technique. Likewise, the possibility of complications related to maintaining a low CVP is real but they occur infrequently.

VII. **Postoperative liver dysfunction** after surgery and anesthesia is common and can range from mild enzyme elevations to fulminant hepatic failure. There are many etiologies for postoperative hepatic dysfunction.

A. **Surgical causes** include maneuvers that impair hepatic blood flow or obstruct the biliary system (clamped vessels, retraction, or direct injury). Postoperative elevations of hepatocellular enzymes or bilirubin also can be caused by increased bilirubin loads after massive transfusion, resorption of hematoma, or hemolysis. Overt hepatic failure can occur during or after shock of any etiology.

B. **Nonsurgical** causes of hepatic dysfunction include undiagnosed cases of preoperative viral hepatitis, alcoholism, and cholelithiasis. Drug therapy in the perioperative period must also be evaluated as a cause of jaundice.

C. **Halothane hepatitis** is clinically indistinguishable from viral hepatitis. The diagnosis is one of exclusion. The availability of isoflurane, desflurane, and sevoflurane generally eliminates the need for halothane administration. Halothane hepatitis is now recognized as two distinct types of halothane-induced hepatic dysfunction.

1. One is caused by **hepatotoxic lipoperoxidases** generated during reductive metabolism of halothane in a hypoxic environment. This can occur with a single exposure to halothane.

2. The more fulminant form is due to an **immunologic phenomenon** when an oxidative metabolite of halothane, **trifluoroacetyl chloride,** binds to hepatocytes, creating a neoantigenic structure to which antibodies may be generated. Hepatocellular damage then occurs on subsequent exposure to halothane.

3. The Massachusetts General Hospital has established restrictive guidelines for the use of halothane in adults. There are no restrictions on the use of halothane in pediatric patients; however, it has not been used in many years. Halothane use in adults may be considered in patients with severe airway compromise or bronchospasm, but sevoflurane appears to be a preferable alternative. If halothane use is anticipated,

informed consent should specifically include the indications for its use and the possible risks.

SUGGESTED READING

Badalamenti S, Graziani G, Salerno F, et al. Hepatorenal syndrome. New perspectives in pathogenesis and treatment. *Arch Intern Med* 1993;153:1957–1967.

Carton EG, Plevak DJ, Kranner PW, et al. Perioperative care of the liver transplant patient. Part 2. *Anesth Analg* 1994;78:382–399.

Carton EG, Rettke SR, Plevak DJ, et al. Perioperative care of the liver transplant patient. Part 1. *Anesth Analg* 1994;78:120–133.

Chen H, Merchant NB, Didolkar MS. Hepatic resection using intermittent vascular inflow occlusion and low central venous pressure anesthesia improves morbidity and mortality. *J Gastrointest Surg* 2000;4:162–167.

Child CG, Turcotte JG. Surgery and portal hypertension. *Major Probl Clin Surg* 1964;1:1–85.

Cook RC. Pharmacokinetics and pharmacodynamics of nondepolarizing muscle relaxants. In: Park GR, Kang Y, eds. *Anesthesia and intensive care for patients with liver disease.* New York: Butterworth-Heinemann, 1995:79–88.

Dershwitz M, Hoke JF, Rosow CE, et al. Pharmacokinetics and pharmacodynamics of remifentanil in volunteer subjects with severe liver disease. *Anesthesiology* 1996;84:812–820.

Jones RM, Moulton CE, Hardy, KJ. Central venous pressure and its effect on blood loss during liver resection. *Br J Surg* 1995;85:1058–1060.

Kamath PS. Clinical approach to the patient with abnormal liver test results. *Mayo Clin Proc* 1996;71:1089–1095.

Melendez JA, Arslan V, Fisher ME, et al. Perioperative outcomes of major hepatic resections under low central venous pressure anesthesia: blood loss, blood transfusion, and the risk of postoperative renal dysfunction. *J. Am Coll Surg* 1998;187:620–625.

Parks DA, et al. Hepatic physiology. In: Miller RD, ed. *Anesthesia*, 5th ed. New York: Churchill Livingstone, 2000:647–662.

Patel T. Surgery in the patient with liver disease. *Mayo Clin Proc* 1999;74:593–599.

Scott VL, Dodson SF, Kang Y. The hepatopulmonary syndrome. *Surg Clin North Am* 1999;79:23–41.

Wiklund RA. Preoperative preparation of patients with advanced liver disease. *Crit Care Med* 2004;32:S106–S115.

6

Specific Considerations with Endocrine Disease

Robin Kelly Guillory, Robert A. Peterfreund, and Stephanie L. Lee

I. Diabetes mellitus

A. **Diabetes mellitus** (DM) is a chronic systemic disease characterized by an absolute or relative lack of insulin. DM is the most common endocrinopathy encountered in the perioperative period.

B. **Physiology of DM.** Insulin is synthesized in pancreatic beta cells. Glucose, β-adrenergic agonists, arginine, and acetylcholine stimulate insulin secretion; α-adrenergic agonists and somatostatin inhibit insulin secretion. Insulin facilitates glucose and potassium transport across cell membranes, increases glycogen synthesis, and inhibits lipolysis. Peripheral tissues resist the effects of insulin during times of stress (e.g., surgery, infection, and cardiopulmonary bypass). Low-level insulin production continues during fasting periods, preventing catabolism and ketoacidosis. The liver and kidney metabolize insulin. As a result, renal insufficiency may produce clinically significant prolongation of insulin action.

C. **Types of DM**

1. **DM type 1** (formerly known as juvenile-onset or insulin-dependent diabetes). Patients have autoimmune destruction of beta cells and an absolute insulin deficiency. They are generally thin, diagnosed at a younger age, sensitive to small amounts of insulin, and prone to ketosis. Management is with insulin.

2. **DM type 2** (formerly known as adult-onset or non–insulin-dependent diabetes) represents 90% of all diabetics. Patients have peripheral resistance to insulin and require high insulin levels to maintain euglycemia. They are generally older, obese, ketosis resistant, and prone to hyperosmolar complications. Patients are initially managed with diet and exercise alone. Oral hypoglycemic agents, insulin sensitizers, and/or insulin are added as needed. Type 2 diabetics frequently have metabolic syndrome, a combination of obesity, hyperlipidemia, hypertension (HTN), and insulin resistance.

3. **Gestational DM.** Between 2% and 5% of pregnancies are complicated by gestational DM. More than 50% of parturients with gestational DM will develop DM type 2 later in life.

4. **Secondary DM** is due to other causes of absolute or relative insulin insufficiency. Pancreatic insulin hyposecretion is seen with pancreatic destruction due to cystic fibrosis, pancreatitis, hemochromatosis, cancer, and after pancreatic surgery. Glucose intolerance may result from glucagonoma,

pheochromocytoma, thyrotoxicosis, acromegaly, or glucocorticoid excess.
  D. **Outpatient therapy for DM**
    1. **Oral hypoglycemic agents (Table 6.1)**
       a. **Sulfonylureas** increase pancreatic insulin release. **Glyburide,** the longest acting of the currently used sulfonylurea agents, can induce hypoglycemia up to 50 hours after administration. Chlorpropamide can cause hyponatremia and a disulfiram-like effect. Sulfonylureas increase the effectiveness of thiazide diuretics, barbiturates,

Table 6.1.   Non-insulin agents used to treat DM

Agent		Onset (hours)	Duration (hours)
Sulfonylurea	Tolbutamide (Orinase, Oramide)	1	6–12
	Glipizide (Glucotrol)	1	6–12
	Glipizide XL	1–4	10–24
	Acetoheximide (Dymelor)	1	8–12
	Tolazamide (Tolinase)	4–6	10–15
	Glyburide (Micronase, DiaBeta)	1–4	10–24
	Glimepiride (Amaryl)	1	18–24
	Chlorpropramide (Diabinase)	1	24–72
Alpha glucosidase inhibitor[a]	Acarbose (Precose)	Immediate	<0.3
	Miglitol (Glyset)	Immediate	<0.3
Biguanide[a]	Metformin (Glucophage, Glumetza, Riomet, Fortamet)	1	8–12
Thiazolidinedione[a]	Pioglitazone (Actos)	1	24
	Rosiglitazone (Avandia)	1	24
Meglitinide	Repaglinide (Prandin)	≤0.25	6–7
D-Phenylalanine derivative	Netaglinide (Starlix)	<0.25	3–4
Exenatide[a,b]	Byetta	<0.25	6–12
Amylin analogs[a]	Pramlintide (Symlin)	<0.25	2–4

[a] When used as the sole agent for treatment, hypoglycemia while NPO is unlikely.
[b] GLP-1 analog.

and anticoagulants by displacing these drugs from albumin. Because of their ability to produce hypoglycemia, sulfonylureas should be held while the patient is fasting (NPO).

b. **Meglitinides and D-phenylalanine derivatives** act via a nonsulfonylurea receptor pathway to rapidly increase insulin release from the pancreas. They are given before meals and should be held while the patient is NPO.

c. **Biguanides** increase sensitivity to insulin. Although biguanides will not produce hypoglycemia when used as single agent therapy for diabetes, they should be held the day of surgery because of their association with lactic acidosis, especially in patients with congestive heart failure, shock, or renal or hepatic dysfunction. Diarrhea is a common side effect.

d. **Thiazolidinediones** increase sensitivity to insulin. They do not cause hypoglycemia and may be given the morning of surgery. Side effects include edema, abdominal obesity, anemia and hepatotoxicity.

e. **α-Glucosidase inhibitors** delay carbohydrate digestion and reduce postprandial hyperglycemia. Although these medications will not induce hypoglycemia, they are ineffective when patients are NPO. Side effects include malabsorption, flatulence, and diarrhea.

f. **Amylin** is a peptide made in pancreatic beta cells. Amylin analogs suppress postprandial glucose release from the liver and reduce appetite by delaying gastric emptying. Amylin analogs do not cause hypoglycemia, but they may increase gastric fluid volumes, especially when used with other medications that slow gastrointestinal transit.

g. **GLP-1,** a member of the incretin family of peptides, stimulates insulin secretion only if there is hyperglycemia. There is no risk for hypoglycemia during fasting with GLP-1 analogs. GLP-1 analogs slow gastric emptying and may increase gastric fluid volumes, especially when used with other medications that slow gastrointestinal transit.

2. **Insulin (Table 6.2).** Short-acting insulins are given just before meals to prevent postprandial hyperglycemia. Intermediate acting insulins are often given several times a day to provide basal and peaking levels. Long-acting insulins are given once daily to mimic basal insulin secretion.

E. **Acute complications of diabetes.** Diabetic ketoacidosis (DKA) and hyperglycemic, hyperosmolar, nonketotic state (HONK) are the result of insulin deficiency, resistance to insulin during stress (e.g., infection, surgery, myocardial infarction [MI], dehydration, trauma), or medications.

1. **DKA** occurs almost exclusively in DM type 1. It may be the initial presentation of DM type 1.

a. **DKA** is associated with depressed myocardial contractility, decreased vascular tone, anion gap acidosis due to ketones, electrolyte abnormalities, hyperglycemia, and hyperosmolarity. Patients are often profoundly hypovolemic because of the forced diuresis of hyperglycemia, emesis, and reduced oral intake with illness. Total body

Table 6.2. SC insulin preparations used to treat DM

Class	Agent	Onset (hours)	Peak Effect (hours)	Duration (hours)
Short acting				
	Lispro (Humalog)	≤0.25	1–2	4–6
	Aspart (NovoLog)	≤0.25	1–2	4–6
	Regular	0.25	2–4	6–10
	Glulisine (Apidra)	≤0.25	1–2	4–6
Intermediate acting				
	NPH	0.5–3	6–12	12–18
	Lente	2–4	6–15	22–28
Long acting				
	Ultralente	1–6	10–30	≥36
	Glargine (Lantus)	2–8	No peak	20–24
	Detemir (Levemir)	2–4	No peak	20–24

Note: When regular insulin is administered IV, the onset of action is immediate. The duration of action is ~1 hour. The preparations semilente insulin and protamine zinc insulin are no longer available.

K^+ is depressed (3 to 10 mEq per kg of body weight), but serum levels are falsely normal or elevated because acidosis shifts K^+ out of cells. Measured Na^+ concentrations are artifactually lowered 1.6 mEq/L for every 100 mg/dL that the glucose is elevated. Hypophosphatemia and hypomagnesemia from osmotic diuresis are common. Patients may present with nausea, vomiting, abdominal pain, polyuria, polydipsia, weakness, renal failure, shock, deep rhythmic (Kussmaul) breathing, a fruity odor, or mental status changes.

  b. **Treatment of DKA** is with volume replacement, insulin, correction of electrolyte abnormalities, identification and treatment of underlying stressors or precipitants (MI, infection, etc.), and supportive care.

  (1) Begin treatment with saline at 5 to 10 mL/kg/hour. Monitor hemodynamics and urine output. Consider invasive monitoring.

  (2) Treat hyperglycemia and insulin deficiency with regular intravenous (IV) insulin. First bolus 0.1 unit (U)/kg IV or 10 U, and then start an infusion at ~0.1 U/kg/hour. Monitoring should include hourly glucose and electrolyte determinations and frequent measures of pH, osmolarity, and ketones to guide adjustment of insulin dose and electrolyte replacement. If serum glucose falls <10% after 1 hour or the anion gap and pH are unchanged, double the insulin infusion rate. Once glucose is <250 mg/dL, reduce the insulin infusion rate to 2 to 3 U/hour and add 5% dextrose to the IV fluids. Continue the insulin infusion until the anion gap and serum bicarbonate are normal. Premature cessation of the insulin infusion may result in recrudescence of DKA.

        (3) Replace potassium, magnesium, and phosphate as needed once normal renal function and urine output have been verified. Consider bicarbonate therapy only for severe acidosis (pH <7), hemodynamic instability, or rhythm disturbances.

        (4) Patients with altered mental status may require intubation for airway protection.

2. HONK may be the initial presentation of DM type 2.

  a. HONK is often associated with glucose levels exceeding 500 mg/dL, electrolyte abnormalities, central nervous system (CNS) dysfunction (depressed sensorium, seizure, coma), and severe hyperosmolarity, hypovolemia, and hemoconcentration from osmotic diuresis. Typical water deficit may be 8 to 10 L. Patients may present with blurred vision, neurologic deficits, weight loss, leg cramps, polydipsia, or polyuria. Although insulin levels are inadequate to prevent hyperglycemia, they are sufficient to block lipolysis, ketogenesis, and ketoacidosis.

  b. Treatment of HONK

        (1) Vigorous volume replacement with normal saline can reduce plasma glucose load up to 50% over several hours. Urinary fluid losses in HONK are similar in composition to $\frac{1}{2}$ normal saline (NS) + KCl at 40 mEq/L. Initial fluid administration is with NS to support the circulation. Once the circulation has been restored, administer $\frac{1}{2}$ NS. NS (1 to 2L) is an appropriate fluid bolus in a patient with adequate cardiac and renal function and a serum osmolarity <320 milliosmoles (mOsm)/L. Larger fluid boluses may be required if the serum osmolarity exceeds 320 mOsm/L. Hypotensive patients not responding to aggressive crystalloid administration should be treated with colloids or vasopressors. Typical adult replacement is with NS: first hour, 2 to 3 L; second and third hours, 1 L/ hour; after 3 hours, 0.5 to 1 L/hour. Adjusting infusion rates and switching to $\frac{1}{2}$ NS should be guided by careful monitoring of volume status and electrolytes, especially in elderly patients with cardiovascular or renal disease. Consider invasive monitoring. Approximately 50% of the fluid deficit should be given over the first 12 hours, with the remainder administered more slowly over the following 24 to 36 hours. After the initial resuscitation, correct severe hyperglycemia and hyperosmolarity gradually over 24 hours to reduce the risk of cerebral edema.

        (2) Administer regular insulin (10 U IV bolus followed by a continuous insulin infusion starting at ~0.1 U/kg/hour IV). Double the insulin infusion rate if the glucose concentration is unchanged after 1 to 4 hours. Titrate insulin infusion rates to maintain glucose levels at <250 mg/dL until cardiovascular, electrolyte, and metabolic parameters are normal.

(3) Measure glucose and electrolyte levels hourly. Electrolyte replacement may be necessary, but the absence of acidosis decreases the likelihood of severe potassium depletion.

(4) It is important to search for and treat precipitants. Patients with altered mental status may require intubation for airway protection. Consider venous thrombosis prophylaxis, as these patients are at high risk for thrombotic events.

F. **Anesthetic considerations in the patient with DM** focus on risk reduction, maintenance of euglycemia, avoidance or treatment of acute complications of DM, and prevention of perioperative complications related to chronic complications of DM.

1. **DKA, HONK and metabolic abnormalities** should be treated before elective surgery and actively managed in the operating room if surgery is urgent.

2. **Glycemic management** is simplified when patients are scheduled for surgery in the morning. Glucose and insulin management should maintain serum glucose levels between 120 and 180 mg/dL and prevent DKA, HONK, and hypoglycemia. Perioperative hyperglycemia is undesirable. It decreases white blood cell chemotaxis and function, increases infection rates, impairs wound healing, leads to dehydration from osmotic diuresis, and promotes a hyperviscous and possibly thrombogenic state. Hyperglycemia is also associated with increased rates of renal allograft rejection and worse outcomes after MI, stroke, burn, traumatic brain injury, and spinal cord injury.

a. **Oral hypoglycemic agents** and insulin sensitizers that can cause hypoglycemia should be held the day of surgery. (See section I.D.1). Metformin should be held from the day of surgery until normal postoperative renal function has been confirmed. Patients with well-controlled DM type 2, who are having a minor surgery and have held their oral hypoglycemics, can often be managed without insulin. However, glucose levels should be monitored in all patients to prevent undiagnosed hypo- or hyperglycemia. Patients who have taken their oral hypoglycemics may require a glucose infusion, and poorly controlled patients or patients having major surgery may require insulin treatment.

b. **Insulin-treated type 2 diabetics.** Insulin should be continued through the night before surgery. For patients having minor procedures of short duration in the morning (e.g., in the ambulatory care setting), give half of the long or intermediate acting, but none of the short-acting morning insulin until the patient is alert postoperatively and able to eat. Check the glucose level by finger stick immediately before and after the procedure to assess a need for therapy. For more substantial procedures, patients should receive $\sim^{1}\!/_{2}$ of their total normal morning dose of intermediate- or long-acting insulin in a subcutaneous dose. Substituting the dose with glargine, a peakless insulin, will minimize the risk of hypoglycemia. Short-acting insulins should be held. Start a glucose-containing infusion (5% dextrose, 1.5 mL/kg/hour) as soon as possible (with the morning insulin dose for hospitalized patients and on arrival to the hospital for same-day admit patients). Patients scheduled for surgery later in the day should arrive early to facilitate glucose and insulin management while they are NPO. The blood glucose should be checked frequently (every 2 to 4 hours). If glucose drops below 120 mg/dL, the glucose infusion rate should be increased. If glucose rises above 180 mg/dL, an infusion of regular insulin should be started and continued throughout the perioperative period. Because of unreliable subcutaneous absorption, IV insulin dosing is preferable during surgery, especially in the presence of hypothermia, hemodynamic instability, or a requirement for vasopressors. A guideline for managing intraoperative infusions of regular insulin is presented in Table 6.3. During therapy with IV insulin, glucose should be checked at least every hour until stable and every 2 hours thereafter. Monitor potassium levels during insulin infusion. Decrease the insulin infusion rate and avoid potassium administration if renal insufficiency develops.

c. **Type 1 DM. These patients must always receive some insulin to prevent ketoacidosis.** Simultaneous infusion of a glucose-containing solution may be necessary to

Table 6.3. Guidelines for routine regular IV insulin infusions

Begin regular insulin infusion at 0.5 to 1 unit/hour (25 units/ 25 mL of saline). Check glucose at least hourly until stable and adjust infusion as appropriate. Then check glucose at least every 2 hours.

Adjustment of Regular Insulin Infusion Rate, units/hour

Blood glucose (mg/dL)	Infusion Change	Other Treatment
<70	Hold 30 min	Administer 15–20 mL D50. Recheck glucose after 30 min. Repeat D50 administration until glucose >70 mg/dL.
70–120	−0.3 U/hour	
121–180	No change	
181–240	+0.3 U/hour	
241–300	+0.6 U/hour	
>300	+1.0 U/hour	

Note: Guidelines assume the patient is fasting and not in DKA or HONK. Dosing must be individually titrated based on frequent blood glucose monitoring.
D50 is a solution of 50% dextrose in water.

prevent hypoglycemia. Perioperative insulin management for the type 1 diabetic on an insulin pump or patients receiving the newer intensive regimens of three or more daily insulin injections should be discussed in advance with the physician responsible for managing the patient's diabetes. See section I.F.2.b above and Table 6.3 for guidelines on insulin management.

d. **Fixed ratio insulin combinations** (e.g., 70/30 NPH/regular or 75/25 NPH/Lispro) are prescribed for the outpatient management of some diabetics. In consultation with the physician managing the diabetes, these patients should be switched to preparations of individual insulins in the immediate preoperative period. An appropriately reduced dose (~50%) of only the long-acting insulin can then be taken on the morning of surgery as described above.

3. **Vascular Disease.** Diabetic patients have a strong predisposition to all types of vascular disease. Macrovascular disease (coronary artery, cerebrovascular, and peripheral vascular) and microvascular disease (retinopathy and nephropathy) occur more frequently, more extensively, and at an earlier age than in the general population. Ischemic heart disease is the most common cause of perioperative morbidity in diabetic patients. Cardiac ischemia may be silent because of autonomic neuropathy. Risk reduction with perioperative β-blockade and a high index of suspicion are mainstays of treatment. DM and HTN are often comorbid diseases. Patients may be hypovolemic due to chronic anti-HTN treatment, resulting in significant hypotension postinduction. This may be exacerbated in patients with autonomic neuropathy due to an inability to compensate for vasodilation. DM is the most common cause of chronic renal insufficiency requiring hemodialysis. Avoid nephrotoxins and consider renal protective treatments in patients exposed to IV contrast loads.

4. **Neuropathy.** Autonomic neuropathy is present in 20% to 40% of patients with longstanding DM. It may result in symptomatically silent cardiac ischemia, decreased lower esophageal sphincter tone, gastroparesis, bladder atony, and labile blood pressure. There is an increased risk of sudden cardiac death because of autonomic cardiac dysfunction and a diminished central ventilatory response to hypoxia. Patients with autonomic neuropathy may have more intraoperative hypothermia, be at higher risk of aspiration due to increased gastric volumes, and be less able to compensate for the sympathectomy of regional anesthesia. Signs of cardiac autonomic neuropathy include resting tachycardia, orthostatic hypotension, and decreased beat-to-beat variability with deep breathing. Metoclopramide, 10 mg IV preoperatively, may increase gastric emptying in patients with gastroparesis. If the gastroparesis is severe, consider placing the patient on a clear liquid diet 1 to 2 days preoperatively. Peripheral neuropathies may cause pain and/or numbness. Patients with peripheral neuropathy are more vulnerable to positioning injuries and should be padded carefully. Document neuropathies before initiating regional anesthesia.

5. **Airway management**
   a. **Stiff joint disease** may complicate airway management. Approximately 30% of type 1 diabetics are considered "difficult intubations" because of decreased temporomandibular joint and cervical spine mobility.
   b. **Obesity,** sleep apnea, and redundant pharyngeal tissue are common in patients with metabolic syndrome.
6. **Protamine.** Diabetic patients receiving NPH insulin are at increased risk for protamine reactions.

II. **Hypoglycemia**
   A. **Etiologies.** Although extremely rare, when present hypoglycemia may be due to pancreatic adenoma (insulinoma) or carcinoma, cirrhosis, hypopituitarism, adrenal insufficiency, hepatoma, sarcoma, ethanol ingestion, renal failure, or therapy with insulin or oral hypoglycemic agents.
   B. **Signs and symptoms.** Adrenergic excess produces tachycardia, diaphoresis, palpitations, HTN, and tremulousness. Neuroglycopenia is accompanied by symptoms of excess adrenergic tone and also produces irritability, headache, confusion, stupor, seizure, and coma. These are masked by general anesthesia. **Hypoglycemic unawareness** occurs when patients with long-standing DM and previous episodes of hypoglycemia lose the sympathetic response to hypoglycemia. Hypoglycemic unawareness is more common in patients with excellent glucose control.
   C. **Anesthetic considerations** include providing a continuous glucose infusion and periodically checking the serum glucose. Glucose levels may fluctuate with surgical stress and with insulinoma manipulation.

III. **Thyroid disease** is the second most common endocrine disease encountered perioperatively, occurring in ~1% of the adult population. The female to male ratio is 5 to 10:1.
   A. **Physiology.** Thyroid hormones are major regulators of metabolic activity. They alter the speed of biochemical reactions, total body oxygen consumption, and heat production. Thyroid-stimulating hormone (TSH) from the anterior pituitary stimulates the thyroid gland to take up iodine and produce the hormones triiodothyronine (T_3) and L-thyroxine (T_4); 80% of T_3 is produced by conversion from T_4 by peripheral tissues. T_3 is 20-50 times more potent than T_4 but has a shorter half-life. T_3 and T_4 are extensively (>99%) bound to plasma proteins, but only the free (unbound) thyroid hormone is biologically active.
   B. **Evaluation and laboratory studies.** In ambulatory patients, serum TSH is currently the best initial screen for determination of thyroid function. TSH levels rise in hypothyroidism and fall in thyrotoxicosis. Evaluation of thyroid function is complex in sick patients. The TSH level may be lowered by starvation, glucocorticoids, stress, dopamine, and fever. As a result, total T_4, free thyroxine index, and total T_3 may aid diagnosis in sick patients.
   C. **Thyrotoxicosis**
      1. **Etiologies of thyrotoxicosis,** in order of decreasing frequency, include Graves disease, toxic multinodular goiter, subacute thyroiditis (acute phase), toxic adenoma, TSH receptor stimulation from β-human chorionic gonadotropin overproduction due to pituitary or placental tumors, and ovarian tumors secreting thyroid hormone (struma ovarii).

Ingestion of excess thyroid hormone, excess iodine, or amiodarone can also lead to thyrotoxicosis.

2. **Thyrotoxicosis is a hypermetabolic state.** Patients present with nervousness, heat intolerance, fatigue, diarrhea, insomnia, increased perspiration, muscle weakness, tremors, irregular menses, and weight loss. Cardiovascular signs include arrhythmias (sinus tachycardia, atrial fibrillation), palpitations, HTN, and high output or ischemic congestive heart failure. Patients may have leukopenia, anemia, or thrombocytopenia. Low clotting factor concentrations from increased metabolism result in increased sensitivity to anticoagulation therapy. Ophthalmic disease occurs only with Graves' hyperthyroidism. **Thyroid storm** is a state of physiologic decompensation due to severe thyrotoxicosis. Surgery and other stressors, excess iodine, or IV contrast may precipitate this condition, But thyroid storm may occur 6 to 18 hours postoperatively. Manifestations include diarrhea, vomiting, and hyperpyrexia (38 to 41°C) leading to hypovolemia, tachycardia, congestive heart failure, shock, weakness, irritability, delirium, and coma. Thyroid storm may mimic malignant hyperthermia, neuroleptic malignant syndrome, sepsis, hemorrhage, pheochromocytoma crisis, or transfusion/drug reaction.

3. **Treatment of thyrotoxicosis.** Chronic thyroid hormone excess is treated by gland ablation with surgery or radioactive iodine or by inhibition of hormone production with specific antithyroid drugs (e.g., propylthiouracil [PTU] and methimazole). Two to 6 weeks of drug therapy may be required to normalize hormone levels. The most serious side effects of antithyroid agents are hepatitis and agranulocytosis. Urticaria is a more frequent side effect of antithyroid therapy. **Mandatory therapy for thyroid storm,** an endocrine emergency (Table 6.4), includes active cooling, meperidine to attenuate heat-producing shivering, vigorous hydration, β-adrenergic blockade, steroids if there is any indication of adrenal insufficiency (including cardiovascular collapse), and drugs (PTU and iodine) to block thyroid hormone synthesis and release. PTU must be given **at least 1 hour before** treatment with iodine to avoid worsening thyrotoxicosis.

4. **Anesthetic considerations.** Only emergency surgery should be performed in thyrotoxic patients. Antithyroid drugs, pharmacologic iodine doses, and β-antagonist medications should continue through surgery.

   a. In an emergent situation, thyrotoxic patients can be prepped for surgery in <1 hour with high-dose propranolol or esmolol (100 to 300 μg/kg/min IV until heart rate is <100 beats/min).

   b. Generous sedative premedication should be considered, unless there is concern for airway compromise. Avoid sympathetic stimulation (pain, ketamine, pancuronium, local anesthetics with epinephrine).

   c. Regional anesthesia may be beneficial in thyrotoxic patients, because it blocks sympathetic responses, but the addition of epinephrine to the local anesthetic should be avoided because of the risk of worsening tachycardia

Table 6.4.   Treatment of thyroid storm

Block Sympathetic Response

Propranolol	1–2 mg IV (repeat as needed) or 40–80 mg orally every 6 hours
Verapamil	5–10 mg IV (repeat as needed)
Esmolol	50–100 μg/kg/min IV

Block Thyroid Hormone Synthesis (Thionamides)

PTU	200 mg orally every 4–6 hours
Methimazole	20 mg orally or per rectum every 4 hours

Block Thyroid Hormone Release

Iopanoic acid[a]	500 mg orally twice a day
Dexamethasone	2 mg orally every 6 hours

Block T_4 to T_3 Conversion

Propranolol, PTU, Iopanoic acid,
Steroids (Hydrocortisone 100 mg orally/IV every 8 hours or dexamethasone 2 mg orally/IV every 6 hours)

Supportive Therapy

Fluids, cooling (with meperidine to block shivering), electrolyte replacement, antipyretics (no aspirin), treatment of precipitating illness and congestive heart failure, oxygen, nutrition, consider plasmapheresis and airway support

---

[a] Give iopanoic acid >1 hour after PTU or methimazole to avoid a hormone surge.

and HTN. Thrombocytopenia sometimes occurs in thyrotoxicosis. Consider checking the platelet count before initiating regional anesthesia.

d. Patients may be hypovolemic due to HTN, diarrhea, and perspiration. Hypotension should be treated with direct-acting agents and fluids. The tachycardic response to anticholinergics may be brisk.

e. The proptotic eyes of patients with Graves disease should be well protected from exposure.

f. Drug metabolism and anesthetic requirements appear to be increased because of rapid metabolism. However, myasthenia gravis may be seen in some patients with Graves disease (30-fold increased incidence), so relaxants should be titrated carefully.

g. Large goiters may displace and compress the trachea, compromising the airway. In addition, emergent tracheostomy may be difficult in patients with goiter.

h. Some surgeons perform recurrent laryngeal nerve testing and request that intraoperative neuromuscular blockade be avoided.

i. Postoperative complications of thyroid surgery include recurrent laryngeal nerve palsy, hypothyroidism, hypoparathyroidism, phrenic nerve injury, pneumothorax, thyroid storm, and tracheal compression from bleeding, edema, or preexisting tracheomalacia.

D. **Hypothyroidism**
   1. **Etiologies of hypothyroidism.** Hypothyroidism may be congenital, result from thyroid gland damage (surgery, radioiodine, radiation), or be secondary to pituitary disease. Other causes include Hashimoto thyroiditis, iodine deficiency, drug therapy (lithium, amiodarone, or phenylbutazone), and late-phase subacute thyroiditis. Hashimoto thyroiditis is the most common cause of hypothyroidism in adults and can be associated with other autoimmune processes (systemic lupus, rheumatoid arthritis, primary adrenal insufficiency, pernicious anemia, DM type I, or Sjögren syndrome).
   2. **Clinical features of hypothyroidism** include lethargy, cold intolerance, facial edema with an enlarged tongue, weight gain, hoarseness, paresthesias, irregular menses, depression, diastolic hypertension, impaired mentation, pericardial effusion, ascites, anemia, coagulation abnormalities, constipation, and an adynamic ileus with delayed gastric emptying. There may be autoimmune adrenal destruction with decreased cortisol and aldosterone production and hyponatremia with decreased water excretion, congestive heart failure from reduced GFR, and the syndrome of inappropriate antidiuretic hormone secretion (SIADH). There may also be bradycardia, hypovolemia, a reversible cardiomyopathy, EKG changes with conduction abnormalities, and diminished baroreceptor reflexes. **Myxedema coma** (profound hypothyroidism) is a clinical diagnosis. Surgery, drugs, trauma, and infection initiate this decompensated state in a severely hypothyroid patient. It is defined by decreased mental status associated with hyporesponsiveness to CO_2, congestive heart failure, hypothermia, and exaggerated symptoms of hypothyroidism.
   3. **Treatment of hypothyroidism.** Chronic treatment involves oral supplementation with thyroid hormone. T_4 is administered once daily and requires 7 to 10 days to have initial effects; 3 to 4 weeks of therapy are needed to achieve a stable state. T_4 dosing is usually adjusted every 4 to 6 weeks based on serum TSH levels. Oral T_3 begins to have an effect in 6 hours but must be dosed two or three times daily. T_3 is not used as routine therapy for hypothyroidism. Cautious IV or oral thyroid hormone loading will hasten recovery. IV thyroid hormone should be given with caution in patients with coronary artery disease because the increased metabolic state and oxygen consumption may induce cardiac ischemia. Myxedema coma is treated with T_3, 25 μg IV every 12 hours, passive rewarming, supportive care (which may include intubation/ventilation), correction of electrolyte abnormalities, hydrocortisone (50 mg IV every 8 hours or by continuous infusion), and management of hypotension, congestive heart failure, effusions, and the precipitating cause (such as MI, CVA, or infection).
   4. **Anesthetic considerations.** Only severe hypothyroidism requires postponing elective surgery.

      a. Securing the airway may be difficult because of an enlarged tongue, relaxed oropharyngeal tissues, goiter, and poor gastric emptying.

      b. Patients may be prone to hypotension due to hypovolemia and blunted baroreceptor reflexes (especially with cardiac depressants and vasodilators).

      c. These patients also manifest CO_2 insensitivity and increased sensitivity to CNS-depressant and paralytic medications.

      d. Corticosteroid supplementation may be necessary.

      e. There is an increased susceptibility to congestive heart failure, hypothermia, hypoglycemia, hyponatremia, and delayed emergence.

IV. Calcium metabolism and parathyroid disease

  A. Physiology. Parathyroid hormone (PTH) and vitamin D maintain the extracellular calcium concentration within a narrow range. PTH increases intestinal calcium absorption, increases osteoclastic release of calcium and phosphorus from bone, decreases renal clearance of calcium, and enhances formation of 1,25-dihydroxyvitamin D by the kidney. Levels of ionized calcium and magnesium determine secretion of PTH. Vitamin D augments the effects of PTH and is necessary for calcium absorption from the gastrointestinal tract. Calcitonin from thyroid "C" cells lowers calcium and phosphorous concentrations by inhibiting renal calcium reabsorption and osteoclast activity but has a limited physiologic role in humans.

  B. Calcium is essential for neuromuscular excitability, cardiac automaticity, mitotic division, coagulation, muscle contraction, neurotransmitter and hormone secretion and action, and the activity of many enzymes. At normal pH, phosphate, citrate, and other anions complex about 6% of total calcium. The remainder is equally divided between protein bound (primarily to albumin) and unbound (free, ionized). Hypoalbuminemia produces a decrease in total calcium of approximately 0.8 mg/dL for each g/dL of albumin below normal (4.0 g/dL). Ionized calcium, the physiologically important form, can be measured easily in whole blood, but improper sample handling can lead to nonreproducible measurements. Acidosis increases, and alkalosis decreases, ionized calcium due to alterations in albumin binding. Thus, signs and symptoms of hypocalcemia may be precipitated by hyperventilation and respiratory alkalosis.

  C. Hypercalcemia

    1. Etiologies of hypercalcemia include hyperparathyroidism (>50% of cases), malignancy, immobilization, granulomatous diseases, vitamin D intoxication, familial hypocalciuric hypercalcemia, thyrotoxicosis, drugs (lithium, thiazides, calcium, vitamin A, theophylline), Paget disease, renal disease, AIDS, and adrenal insufficiency. **Hyperparathyroidism** is characterized by hypercalcemia and hypophosphatemia with an elevated intact PTH level, usually caused by a parathyroid adenoma. Four-gland parathyroid hyperplasia causes only 10% of cases of hyperparathyroidism. Parathyroid hyperplasia can be associated with pituitary adenoma and pancreatic tumors in multiple endocrine neoplasia (MEN) type I or medullary thyroid carcinoma and pheochromocytoma

Table 6.5. Hypercalcemia: signs and symptoms

Gastrointestinal	Osteopenia/osteoporosis
• Nausea/vomiting	
• Anorexia	**Weakness/atrophy/fatiguability**
• Constipation	
• Pancreatitis	**Central nervous system**
• Peptic ulcers	• Seizures
• Abdominal pain	• Disorientation/psychosis
	• Mermory loss
Hemodynamic	• Sedation/lethargy/coma
• Dehydration	• Anxiety/depression
• Hypertension	
• EKG/conduction changes	**Renal**
• Digitalis sensitivity	• Polyuria
• Dysrhythmias	• Nephrolithiasis
• Catecholamine resistance	• Decreased renal blood flow
	• Oliguric failure (late)
Hematologic	
• Anemia	
• Thrombosis	

in MEN type IIa. Parathyroid carcinoma is a rare cause of hyperparathyroidism and hypercalcemia. **Hypercalcemia of malignancy** is due to release of a PTH-like molecule (PTH-related protein) from tumors and cytokine-mediated or direct bony destruction resulting in resorption of calcium from the skeleton.

2. **Clinical features of hypercalcemia** are summarized in Table 6.5. Mild hypercalcemia is usually asymptomatic. When total serum calcium (corrected for albumin level) is >13mg/dL, there is increased risk of end-organ calcification, renal calculi, and nephrocalcinosis. A calcium level >14 to 15 mg/dL is considered an endocrine emergency as patients may have uremia, coma, cardiac arrest, or death.

3. **Treatment of hypercalcemia**
   a. Treatment includes limiting oral intake of calcium, hydration with normal saline IV (6 to 10 L/day), and diuresis with furosemide (for a urine output goal of 3 to 5 L/day). The patient must be monitored for fluid overload, hypokalemia, and hypomagnesemia. In patients with hypercalcemia and renal or cardiac failure, dialysis should be considered. Goals should also include treatment of the underlying cause of hypercalcemia. ICU care may be necessary.
   b. Bisphosphonates (Pamidronate 60 to 90 mg IV over 4 hours or Zoledronate 4 mg IV over 15 min every 2 to 3 weeks) decrease bone resorption and are the treatment of choice in severe (>13.5 mg/dL) or life-threatening (>15 mg/dL) hypercalcemia and in humoral hypercalcemia of malignancy. Side effects include renal insufficiency, fever, and myalgias. Lower bisphosphonate doses are used in patients with renal insufficiency.

    c. Administration of oral phosphate (1 to 2 g/day) limits intestinal absorption and increases skeletal reuptake of calcium. Although effective, oral phosphate is reserved for life-threatening hypercalcemia, because it causes diarrhea; elevations in serum phosphorus (>5 mg/dL) may result in soft tissue calcification and should be avoided.

    d. Mithramycin (5 to 25 μg/kg IV over 4 to 6 hours) will correct hypercalcemia in 48 hours, but risks of thrombocytopenia, hepatotoxicity, and nephrotoxicity limit its use to emergencies.

    e. Hypercalcemia may temporarily respond to salmon calcitonin (4 to 8 international units [IU]/kg subcutaneously [SC] every 12 hours).

    f. Glucocorticoid therapy (Prednisone 40 to 100 mg/day for 3 to 5 days) is effective in some cases of multiple myeloma, vitamin D toxicity, and granulomatous diseases, although not in other causes of hypercalcemia.

  4. **Anesthetic considerations.** Hypercalcemia warrants correction. Intravascular volume and other electrolyte abnormalities should be normalized and monitored. Hypercalcemia has an unpredictable effect on neuromuscular blockade, so relaxants should be carefully titrated. Careful positioning is required because patients can be osteoporotic. Patients with hypercalcemia are predisposed to digitalis toxicity and may have conduction abnormalities. Avoid hypoventilation because acidosis increases free calcium levels. Thyroid and parathyroid surgery can be done under local or regional anesthesia. Complications after parathyroid surgery are similar to complications after thyroid surgery.

D. **Hypocalcemia** is serum calcium <8.5 mg/dL in the absence of hypoalbuminemia or abnormalities in pH.

  1. **Etiologies of hypocalcemia.** Hypoparathyroidism is due to underproduction of PTH or, rarely, resistance to its effects by end-organ tissues. PTH underproduction may occur after gland damage during neck surgery. Symptoms may be seen in the immediate postoperative period or days to weeks later. Other causes include radiation, hemosiderosis, infiltrative processes (malignancy, amyloidosis), severe hypomagnesemia (<1 mg/dL), and severe vitamin D deficiency. Extensive burns, fat emboli, and pancreatitis cause sequestration of calcium. **Massive transfusion** (>30 mL/kg/hour), especially in patients with liver failure, results in hypocalcemia when citrate binds to calcium. Furosemide, hyperphosphatemia, and antiepileptic drugs can cause hypocalcemia.

  2. **Clinical features of hypocalcemia.** Patients are usually asymptomatic until calcium <7.5 mg/dL, especially if onset is insidious. Bedside demonstration of facial nerve irritability to percussion (Chvostek sign) or carpal spasm with tourniquet ischemia for 3 min (Trousseau sign) indicates a need for supplementation. However, 10% to 15% of normocalcemic patients will have a positive Chvostek sign.

    a. Chronic hypocalcemia causes lethargy, muscle cramps, a prolonged QT interval, renal failure, cataracts, and personality changes.

   b. Acute hypocalcemia produces neuromuscular irritability with muscle cramps and hand, foot, and circumoral paresthesias.

   c. Severe hypocalcemia results in stridor, laryngospasm, tetany, apnea, coagulopathy, hypotension with catecholamine resistance, psychosis/confusion, and seizures unresponsive to conventional therapy.

3. **Treatment of hypocalcemia**

   a. Severe or symptomatic hypocalcemia should be treated with IV calcium. Calcium IV irritates veins; administer calcium centrally whenever possible. A 10-mL ampule of calcium gluconate contains 93 mg of elemental calcium, and a 10-mL ampule of calcium chloride contains 273 mg of calcium. For urgent therapy, two ampules of calcium gluconate or one ampule of calcium chloride may be given IV over 10 to 20 min. Less urgent situations are treated with a 15-mg/kg infusion of elemental calcium IV over 8 to 12 hours. During parenteral therapy, calcium levels, creatinine, EKG, and hemodynamic status must be monitored. Therapeutic goals are serum calcium near 8 mg/dL and a low urinary calcium level. Evaluate phosphorus, potassium, and magnesium levels and correct abnormalities. Treat elevated phosphorus levels with oral phosphate binders; treat low magnesium levels (<1 mg/dL) with parenteral magnesium sulfate.

   b. Mild to moderate hypocalcemia may be treated with oral calcium and vitamin D. Patients require elemental calcium at 1.5 to 3 g/day (3,750 to 7,500 mg of calcium carbonate) and 1,25-dihydroxyvitamin D (calcitriol 0.25 to 3.0 μg/day) in divided doses.

   c. For chronic replacement, patients either take calcitriol or the parent hormone vitamin D (ergocalciferol 50,000 IU, 1 to 3 times/week), with calcium.

4. **Anesthetic considerations.** Correct calcium and other electrolyte abnormalities. Respiratory or metabolic alkalosis, hypothermia, rapid infusions of blood products (especially with hepatic insufficiency), and renal dysfunction can worsen hypocalcemia. Follow coagulation status. Patients may have hypotension with insensitivity to β-adrenergic agonists, a prolonged QT interval, advanced atrial-ventricular block, and digitalis insensitivity. Response to neuromuscular blocking drugs is unpredictable. Careful positioning is required, as patients may be osteoporotic.

V. **Adrenal cortical disease**

   A. **Physiology.** The adrenal gland consists of a cortex that secretes glucocorticoids, mineralocorticoids, and androgens and a medulla that secretes catecholamines. These hormones act to maintain homeostasis in states of stress.

   1. **Glucocorticoids.** Cortisol is the principal hormone of this class. About 10 to 20 mg of cortisol is produced daily in a diurnal manner in response to adrenocorticotropic hormone (ACTH) from the anterior pituitary. Stress stimulates increased cortisol release. Cortisol is required for converting norepinephrine to epinephrine in the adrenal medulla and for producing angiotensin II. It acts as an anti-inflammatory

agent and has multiple effects on carbohydrate, protein, and fatty acid metabolism. Cortisol is metabolized by the liver and is filtered and excreted unchanged by the kidney.

2. **Mineralocorticoids.** Aldosterone is the principle hormone of this class and the major regulator of extracellular fluid volume and potassium homeostasis. Its production is regulated by the renin-angiotensin system and blood potassium concentration (see Chapter 4). Aldosterone causes reabsorption of Na^+ and excretion of K^+ and H^+ in the distal tubule.

   a. Aldosteronoma causes HTN and electrolyte abnormalities. This condition is treated with adrenalectomy.

   b. Aldosterone excess from bilateral adrenal hyperplasia is treated medically. The standard treatment has been with spironolactone, an aldosterone receptor inhibitor. There is less clinical experience with Eplerenone, a new agent approved by the Food and Drug Administration, but limited studies suggest it has fewer antiandrogenic side effects than spironolactone. In patients who are intolerant to aldosterone receptor antagonists, amiloride may be used for its potassium-sparing properties along with other antihypertensive medications.

   c. Conn syndrome (hypoaldosteronism) causes hypotension and electrolyte abnormalities. Management is with fludrocortisone supplementation.

3. **Androgens.** Abnormalities in androgen secretion are rarely pertinent to anesthetic management.

B. **Pharmacology.** Synthetic steroids are available with different potencies and ratios of glucocorticoid to mineralocorticoid effect (Table 6.6).

C. **Adrenal cortical hyperfunction (Cushing syndrome)**

1. **Etiologies.** Eighty percent of cases are secondary to adrenal hyperplasia from excess ACTH secretion from pituitary (Cushing disease), carcinoid, pancreatic, or lung tumors. Other causes include adrenal adenoma, bilateral adrenal

Table 6.6.   Glucocorticoid and mineralocorticoid hormones

Steroid	Relative Potency		Equivalent Dose (mg)	Duration (hours)
	Gluco-corticoid	Mineralo-corticoid		
Short-acting				8–12
Cortisol	1.0	1.0	20	
Cortisone	0.8	0.8	25	
Aldosterone	0.3	3,000	—	
Intermediate-acting				12–36
Prednisone	4.0	0.8	5	
Prednisolone	4.0	0.8	5	
Methylprednisolone	5.0	0.5	4	
Fludrocortisone	10.0	125	—	
Long-acting				>24
Dexamethasone	25–40	0	0.75	

micronodular hyperplasia (BAMH), or exogenous steroid administration.

2. **Clinical features.** Patients present with truncal obesity, moon face, gastroesophageal reflux disease, HTN, hypernatremia, excess intravascular volume, hyperglycemia, hypokalemia, red or purple cutaneous striae, poor wound healing, muscle wasting and weakness, osteopenia/osteoporosis, hypercoagulability with thromboembolism, mental status changes and emotional lability, aseptic osteonecrosis, pancreatitis, benign intracranial hypertension, peptic ulceration, glaucoma, or infection.

3. **Anesthetic considerations.** Patients often exhibit hypertension refractory to treatment. Excess intravascular volume can be reduced with diuretics, but potassium must be replaced. Monitor serum glucose levels and treat as needed. Osteoporosis makes careful positioning necessary. Patients may have unrecognized coronary artery disease. Consider venous thrombosis prophylaxis. Adrenalectomy is performed for adrenal adenoma or BAMH and may be open or laparoscopic. Glucocorticoid replacement should begin postoperatively for both unilateral and bilateral adrenalectomy. Mineralocorticoid replacement is necessary only after bilateral adrenalectomy. Excess ACTH secretion is treated by excision of the secreting tumor. Anesthesia for trans-sphenoidal pituitary surgery is discussed in Chapter 24.

D. **Adrenal cortical hypofunction**

1. **Etiologies.** Idiopathic hypofunction, autoimmune destruction, surgical removal, radiation, metastatic destruction, infection (e.g., fungus, tuberculosis, human immunodeficiency virus, cytomegalovirus), hemorrhage (septicemia, Waterhouse-Friderichsen syndrome, anticoagulant therapy), drugs (ketoconazole, rifampin, metyrapone), granulomatous infiltration, vasculitis, adrenal vein thrombosis, or loss of ACTH stimulation can produce adrenal cortical hypofunction. Exogenous steroid administration may suppress the hypothalamic-pituitary-adrenal axis for up to 12 months after treatment has stopped.

2. **Clinical features.** Lack of glucocorticoids may produce episodic fever, abdominal pain, and hypotension that are difficult to distinguish from an acute surgical abdomen. Mineralocorticoid deficiency will lead to decreased urinary sodium conservation, decreased response to circulating catecholamines, and hyperkalemia.

   a. **Primary adrenal insufficiency (Addison disease)** is associated with both low cortisol and low aldosterone levels, resulting in weight loss, headache, weakness, fatigue, anorexia, nausea/vomiting, abdominal pain, postural hypotension, diarrhea or constipation, and hyperpigmentation.

   b. **Secondary adrenal insufficiency,** precipitated by abnormalities in ACTH secretion, results in low cortisol levels but normal aldosterone function. Patients with secondary adrenal insufficiency may have panhypopituitarism with symptoms of TSH, growth hormone (GH), or gonadotropin deficiency.

3. **Treatment.** Under basal conditions, the hydrocortisone replacement is 10 to 20 mg daily (10 to 15 mg upon awakening and 5 to 10 mg at 4 PM) or prednisone at 4 to 7.5 mg once daily. During times of stress, the glucocorticoid dose must be increased. Acute adrenal insufficiency (Addisonian crisis) is a medical emergency. Patients present with hypotension unresponsive to fluid and tachycardia. Fever, abdominal pain, and intractable nausea/vomiting may occur. Treatment includes fluids (5% dextrose in normal saline), steroid replacement (hydrocortisone 100 to 150 mg IV or dexamethasone 6 mg IV, and then hydrocortisone 30 to 50 mg IV every 8 hours or as a continuous infusion), inotropes as necessary, and electrolyte correction. Patients may be hypoglycemic and have changes in mental status. Precipitating causes must be sought and treated. Hydrocortisone dosage may be decreased by 50% every 1 to 2 days, depending on the clinical status. In primary adrenal insufficiency, daily fludrocortisone (Florinef), 0.05 to 0.1 mg orally, is required once the hydrocortisone dose is below 50 to 75 mg daily.

4. **Anesthetic considerations.** Evaluate and treat volume, hemodynamic, glucose, and electrolyte status as necessary. Avoid etomidate in the hypoadrenal patient because of the potential for further adrenal suppression. Patients with adrenal hypofunction may exhibit marked sensitivity to sedative, anesthetic, or vasoactive drugs. Titrate drug doses carefully to avoid cardiovascular depression. Other endocrinopathies may be present and affect anesthetic management. Perioperative steroid replacement is controversial and should be individualized. Any patient who has received more than a 14-day course of supraphysiologic steroid dosing in the past year may need glucocorticoid supplementation perioperatively. Following is one recommendation for perioperative IV hydrocortisone dosing:

   a. **Minor surgery** (inguinal herniorrhaphy, minor urologic or gynecologic procedures, oral or minor plastic surgery), 25 mg or usual daily steroid dose (whichever is higher) preoperatively. Resume usual regimen on postoperative day 1.

   b. **Moderate surgery** (open cholecystectomy, joint replacement, extremity revascularization), 50 to 75 mg or usual daily steroid dose (whichever is higher) preoperatively, 50 mg every 8 hours intraoperatively, 20 mg every 8 hours on postoperative day 1. Resume usual regimen on postoperative day 2.

   c. **Major surgery** (thoracotomy, cardiac or major abdominal surgery), 100 to 150 mg or usual daily dose (whichever is higher) within 2 hours preoperatively, 50 mg every 8 hours until postoperative day 2 or 3, and then reduce by 50% daily until preoperative regimen is reached.

VI. **Adrenal medullary disease**

A. **Physiology.** Preganglionic fibers of the sympathetic nervous system stimulate release of catecholamines from the adrenal medulla. Peripheral effects of catecholamines include chronotropic and inotropic stimulation of the heart, vasomotor changes, enhanced hepatic glycogenolysis, and inhibition of insulin release. Catecholamines are biotransformed in the kidney and liver to metanephrine, normetanephrine, and vanillylmandelic acid.

B. Pheochromocytoma

1. **Epidemiology.** Pheochromocytomas are functionally active catecholamine-secreting tumors of the adrenal medulla; 10% occur extra-adrenally, 10% are bilateral, 10% are metastatic, and 10% to 25% are familial (occur as part of MEN IIa and MEN IIb with medullary thyroid cancer, hyperparathyroidism, and marfanoid habitus or are associated with neurofibromatosis, tuberous sclerosis, von Hippel-Landau or Sturge-Weber syndrome). Pheochromocytoma is a rare cause of hypertension (0.1%). Most tumors secrete epinephrine, norepinephrine, and dopamine. Secretion is independent of neurogenic control.

2. **Clinical features.** Signs and symptoms are due to excess catecholamine release. The classic presentation includes palpitations, headache, and diaphoresis in an episodically HTN patient, but 10% do not have HTN. Other symptoms include anxiety, tremor, hyperglycemia, orthostatic hypotension, and weight loss. Patients with pheochromocytoma are usually dehydrated and hemoconcentrated. A 24-hour urine collection for catecholamines and their metabolites is the routine screening test. Preoperative diagnosis is important, as intraoperative diagnosis is associated with a mortality approaching 50%. Treatment is with excision.

3. **Preoperative evaluation and preparation.** Preoperative recognition of end-organ damage is important for optimization. Catecholamine-induced dilated or hypertrophic cardiomyopathy occurs in 20% to 30% of patients. Congestive heart failure, hypovolemia, intracranial hemorrhage, hyperglycemia, and renal failure are other potential concerns. Comorbid endocrinopathies should be sought and treated. Goals of preoperative treatment are to restore intravascular volume and reduce the end-organ effects of catecholamines.

   a. α-Receptor blockade is often started with oral phenoxybenzamine, a long-acting irreversible α_1- and α_2-adrenergic blocker (starting with 20 to 30 mg/day and increasing to 60 to 250 mg/day until blood pressure is controlled), or prazosin (1 to 6 mg orally four times a day) or doxazosin (4 to 12 mg orally per day), shorter-acting competitive α_1 blockers. Achieving adequate α-receptor blockade may require 14 days. Clinical endpoints that suggest a patient is ready for surgery include blood pressure <165/95, postural hypotension (but blood pressure >80/45), a maximum of one PVC every 5 min, no changes on ECG for 1 to 2 weeks, and nasal stuffiness. Prazosin/doxazosin and phenoxybenzamine should be stopped approximately 12 and 48 hours preoperatively, respectively.

   b. Adequate volume repletion is reflected by weight gain and decreasing hematocrit.

   c. Beta blockade is instituted with caution (due to potential cardiomyopathy) and *only* after the onset of adequate alpha blockade (to prevent unopposed vascular alpha stimulation and worsening HTN).

d. A less common preoperative management is to deplete the adrenal medulla of stored catecholamine with metyrosine, a catecholamine synthesis inhibitor (1 to 4 g/day). Clinical endpoints are the same as with prazosin, doxazosin, and phenoxybenzamine.

4. Anesthetic considerations. The goal is to avoid hypotension or sympathetic outflow, as either scenario can produce adrenergic crisis. Preoperative sedation may be helpful. Avoid sympathomimetic, vagolytic, or histamine-releasing drugs as well as sympathetic responses to induction, intubation, pneumoperitoneum, and surgical stimulation. A combined technique using an epidural is effective in ablating sympathetic responses (but not catecholamine surges), but hypotension should be actively avoided.

a. Blood pressure should be measured directly. The need for other invasive monitoring depends on the patient's medical status.

b. Magnesium blocks catecholamine receptors and catecholamine release from the adrenal medulla and peripheral adrenergic nerve terminals. It can be a useful adjunct (40 to 60 mg/kg IV loading dose, infusion 2 g/hour, 20-mg/kg boluses prn), but it may delay awakening and cause muscle weakness.

c. Dysrhythmias and severe hypertension (hypertensive crisis) may occur intraoperatively. Treatment options include IV boluses of NTP, 50 to 100 μg; nicardipine, 1 to 2 mg; magnesium, 20 mg/kg; or phentolamine, 1 to 5 mg. Beta blockade with labetalol or esmolol may be required after HTN has been treated.

d. Once the tumor's venous supply is ligated, a sudden decrease in blood pressure may occur due to the decrease in circulating catecholamine levels and residual alpha and beta blockade. Vigorous volume support and treatment with a direct-acting vasopressor such as phenylephrine is customary. Vasopressin may be helpful.

e. Glucose should be monitored perioperatively, as patients may have hyperglycemia preoperatively and hypoglycemia postoperatively.

f. Endogenous catecholamine levels should return to normal within a few days after tumor removal. ICU care may be required in the postoperative period. Patients undergoing bilateral adrenalectomy will require glucocorticoid and mineralocorticoid replacement therapy.

VII. Pituitary disease

A. Anterior pituitary gland

1. Physiology. By producing TSH, ACTH, follicle-stimulating hormone, luteinizing hormone, GH and prolactin, the anterior pituitary regulates the thyroid and adrenal glands, the ovaries and testes, growth, and lactation through a negative feedback system. Pituitary tumors are usually benign adenomas, but they may secrete hormones or produce visual disturbances, epilepsy, or increased ICP through mass effect. Secreting adenomas may lead to hormone excess but rarely cause pituitary insufficiency. Large, usually non-secreting, adenomas may cause anterior pituitary destruction and hypopituitarism. Rarely, a large tumor erodes through the sphenoid sinus into the posterior pharynx and impedes intubation.

2. **Anterior pituitary hyperfunction.** Most hyperfunctioning adenomas do not affect anesthetic management. The hyperthyroidism of a TSH-secreting adenoma and the hyperadrenalism of an ACTH-secreting adenoma are treated as described above (see sections III and V). The anatomic and physiologic changes seen with GH-secreting tumors warrant careful consideration.

   a. **Acromegaly (excess GH)**

      (1) **Clinical features.** GH stimulates bone, cartilage, and soft tissue growth, leading to prognathism, soft tissue overgrowth of the lips, tongue, epiglottis, and vocal cords, and subglottic narrowing of the trachea. Connective tissue overgrowth can cause recurrent laryngeal nerve paralysis, carpal tunnel syndrome, and other peripheral neuropathies. These patients often develop glucose intolerance, muscle weakness, arthritis, osteoporosis, HTN, obstructive sleep apnea (OSA), congestive heart failure, and arrhythmias, and they have an increased incidence of coronary artery disease and colon carcinoma. The primary treatment is surgical removal of the tumor. Surgery is often unsuccessful because of the large size of the tumor at time of diagnosis. Medical management for persistent disease after surgery includes dopamine agonists (bromocriptine, cabergoline), somatostatin analogs (octreotide), and GH receptor antagonists (pegvisomant). Excision of GH-secreting pituitary adenomas is often performed trans-sphenoidally (see Chapter 24).

      (2) **Anesthetic considerations.** Patients should be evaluated for other endocrinopathies preoperatively. Conventional mask airways are often difficult to achieve, and endotracheal intubation can be challenging. Small-diameter endotracheal tubes and awake intubation is often chosen. Advanced airway and tracheostomy equipment should be available. Serum glucose levels should be carefully maintained and muscle relaxants titrated using a peripheral nerve stimulator. Patients may be osteoporotic and have increased susceptibility to peripheral neuropathies. Careful positioning is necessary. Patients with OSA are at high risk for postoperative obstruction. Cardiac status may affect management and should be evaluated before surgery.

3. **Anterior pituitary hypofunction** (panhypopituitarism)

   a. **Etiologies.** Sheehan syndrome is a condition of pituitary failure in which hemorrhagic shock causes vasospasm and subsequent pituitary necrosis in postpartum patients. Other causes of pituitary failure include trauma, radiation, pituitary apoplexy, tumors, infiltrative disease, and surgical hypophysectomy.

   b. Anesthetic considerations. Adrenal insufficiency develops over 4 to 14 days after destruction of the pituitary. Perioperative glucocorticoid supplementation may be necessary. Because the half-life of thyroid hormone is 7 to 10 days, symptomatic hypothyroidism does not occur until 3 to 4 weeks after pituitary surgery or apoplexy. Management of hypothyroid patients is discussed in section III.D.

B. Posterior pituitary gland

1. **Physiology.** The posterior pituitary is composed of the nerve terminals of neurons originating in the hypothalamus. Antidiuretic hormone (ADH; vasopressin) and oxytocin are stored in the posterior pituitary. ADH regulates plasma osmolarity and extracellular fluid volume and facilitates renal tubular resorption of water. Intravascular hypovolemia, pain from trauma or surgery, nausea, and positive airway pressure stimulate ADH secretion. Oxytocin stimulates uterine contraction in labor and milk ejection in lactation.

2. **Diabetes insipidus (DI)**

   a. Etiologies. DI results from insufficient ADH secretion by the posterior pituitary (central DI) or failure of the renal tubules to respond to ADH (nephrogenic DI). Causes of central DI include intracranial trauma, hypophysectomy, hypophysitis, metastatic disease to the pituitary or hypothalamus, and infiltrative diseases. Causes of nephrogenic DI include hypokalemia, hypercalcemia, sickle cell anemia, chronic myeloma, obstructive uropathy, chronic renal insufficiency, and lithium therapy. It may be seen in the third trimester of pregnancy. Nephrogenic DI may also be congenital.

   b. Clinical features include polydipsia and polyuria. The urine is inappropriately dilute, and serum osmolarity is high. Urine output is >2 L/day.

   c. Anesthetic considerations. Mild DI (daily urinary volumes of 2 to 6 L in patients with an adequate thirst mechanism) does not require treatment. In patients who cannot drink, initial therapy should be with isotonic fluids (normal saline) to reverse shock. Once osmolality <290 mOsm/kg, hypotonic fluids (half normal saline) are necessary. Total body water deficit can be estimated as follows:

$$\text{Water deficit (L)} = [0.6 \times \text{body weight (kg)}]$$
$$\times [([\text{Na}^+] - 140)/140]$$

Body weight is the initial weight before dehydration. Careful monitoring and titration of urine output and plasma volume, sodium, and osmolarity are necessary.

   (1) Central DI may be treated with the synthetic vasopressin analog desmopressin, DDAVP, at 1 to 2 μg (0.25 to 0.5 mL) SC or IV every 6 to 24 hours as needed (or with an infusion intraoperatively). Side effects of DDAVP include hyponatremia, hypertension, and coronary artery vasospasm.

    (2)   **Nephrogenic DI** is associated with failure of vasopressin to reduce urinary volume. Adequate oral or parenteral hydration must be assured. Chlorpropamide (an oral hypoglycemic) potentiates the effects of ADH on renal tubules and may be helpful. Inhibition of prostaglandin synthesis (by ibuprofen, indomethacin, or aspirin) or mild salt depletion with a thiazide diuretic may reduce urine volume.

  3. **SIADH** is persistent secretion of ADH in the absence of an osmotic stimulus.

    a.   SIADH can be caused by malignancy, CNS disorders (trauma, infection, tumor), pulmonary disorders (tuberculosis, pneumonia, positive pressure ventilation, chronic obstructive pulmonary disease), and drugs (nicotine, narcotics, chlorpropamide, clofibrate, vincristine, vinblastine, cyclophosphamide, serotonin reuptake inhibitors). Other etiologies include lupus, human immunodeficiency virus, Guillain-Barre, hypothyroidism, Addison disease, congestive heart failure, cirrhosis, or porphyria. SIADH is associated with urine osmolality > serum osmolality (with a low serum osmolality), urine sodium >20 mEq/L, and serum sodium <130 mEq/L. If serum sodium falls below 110 mEq/L, cerebral edema and seizures may result.

    b.   Fluid restriction (800 to 1,000 mL daily) is the primary treatment for the mild hyponatremia of SIADH. Chronic hyponatremia without symptoms has virtually no mortality. Thus, resuscitation with sodium-containing solutions is reserved for symptomatic, severe hyponatremia (serum Na^+ <120 mEq/L). Hyponatremia should be corrected no faster than 0.5 mEq/L/hour, because overly aggressive correction may produce central pontine myelinolysis, an irreversible neurologic disorder (see Chapter 4). Demeclocycline antagonizes the effects of ADH on renal tubules and may be helpful.

VIII. **Carcinoid**

  A. **Carcinoid tumors.** Most carcinoid tumors arise in the gastrointestinal tract (appendix, ileum, rectum), but they can also be seen in the lungs and elsewhere. Carcinoid tumors are capable of secreting substances that affect vascular, bronchial, and gastrointestinal smooth muscle tone. Serotonin and histamine are the most commonly secreted hormones, but carcinoid tumors are capable of secreting >35 peptides and hormones, including bradykinin, prostaglandins, kallikrein, and others. Stimuli for the release of mediators include catecholamines, histamine, hypotension, and tumor manipulation. Patients develop carcinoid syndrome when substances produced by the tumor reach the systemic circulation. Substances secreted from gastrointestinal tumors are metabolized in the liver (preventing carcinoid syndrome) until secretion overwhelms the liver's neutralizing ability, either because of the quantity produced or because of decreased liver activity from metastases. Tumors located outside the gastrointestinal tract may produce the syndrome by direct release of mediators into the systemic circulation; 40% to 50% of small bowel and proximal colon carcinoids produce carcinoid syndrome. Symptoms are less frequent with carcinoids of the bronchus, rarely seen with appendiceal carcinoids, and never seen with rectal carcinoid tumors. Carcinoid tumors can also produce symptoms from local effects (hemoptysis, bowel obstruction, or ischemia).

B. **Carcinoid syndrome** is seen in 2% to 5% of patients with carcinoid tumors. Clinical features of carcinoid syndrome depend on which mediators a tumor releases. Common symptoms include flushing, bronchoconstriction, gastrointestinal hypermotility, and hypo- or hyperglycemia. Peripheral vasodilation and vasoconstriction can produce profound hypotension and HTN. Right-sided valvular lesions resulting in tricuspid regurgitation and pulmonic stenosis are seen in 20% to 40% of patients with carcinoid syndrome. Left-sided valvular disease is unusual.

C. **Treatment** is by surgical removal of the tumor. Liver metastases may be surgically resected or embolized. Medical treatment is used in preparation for surgery or embolization, in patients with unresectable disease, and in patients who are not surgical candidates. In the past, medical treatment used a host of mediator blockers (aprotinin to block bradykinin/kallikrein, diphenhydramine, ketanserin, and cyproheptadine for histamine and serotonin blockade, ranitidine to block gastrin, etc.). Now octreotide, a long-acting somatostatin analog, is the mainstay of treatment. Somatostatin is naturally produced by cells of the gastric antrum and pancreas and inhibits release and peripheral actions of *many* hormones.

D. **Anesthetic considerations**
   1. Hypovolemia and glucose and electrolyte abnormalities should be treated preoperatively. Patients should be evaluated for valvular heart disease and may require endocarditis prophylaxis. Octreotide at 50 to 100 μg SC is usually given preoperatively. Peak levels are achieved in 30 min. Preoperative sedation may be helpful to minimize mediator release due to anxiety.
   2. Large blood loss should be expected as tumors are vascular, and there may be liver dysfunction or metastases. Invasive blood pressure monitoring should be used, as large blood pressure swings are anticipated. Central venous pressure monitoring may help differentiate the cause of hypotension (hypovolemia versus carcinoid crisis).
   3. Triggers of mediator release should be avoided (hypotension, anxiety, pain, hypoxia, hypercarbia, tumor compression, drugs that cause histamine or catecholamine release, or sympathetic stimulation). Intraoperative mediator release should be anticipated and treated with octreotide boluses (25 to 50 μg IV, diluted to 10 μg/mL) or infusion (50 to 100 μg/hour IV). If a carcinoid crisis occurs with bronchoconstriction, hypotension, or HTN, the patient should be treated with octreotide, fluids, and direct-acting vasoconstrictors as needed (phenylephrine). Conventional therapies for these conditions (ß agonists, epinephrine, nitroprusside) can stimulate mediator release and exacerbate symptoms.

4. Patients with carcinoid syndrome may have delayed awakening due to excess serotonin. Postoperative ICU care may be appropriate, especially if an octreotide taper is required.

IX. Porphyrias

A. **Etiology.** Heme, a molecule in hemoglobin, myoglobin, and cytochromes, is made from iron and porphyrins. The porphyrias result from defects in the heme biosynthetic pathway, resulting in accumulation of porphyrin precursors proximal to the abnormality in the biosynthetic chain. There are a variety of forms, depending on where the biochemical aberration occurs in the pathway. When an environmental or physiologic trigger stimulates heme production, porphyrins accumulate and cause symptoms via an unknown mechanism. Known porphyric triggers include fasting, dehydration, infection, stress, alcohol intake, hormonal variation, and many drugs. Porphyria is an autosomal dominant disease with incomplete penetrance. It is essential to identify patients at risk preoperatively (via family history, ancestry, or symptomatology) to prevent causing a life-threatening porphyric crisis by giving a patient with porphyria a triggering agent.

B. **Classification of the porphyrias.** Porphyrias are classified as hepatic or erythropoietic, depending on where the enzymatic defect occurs. Porphyrias are also classified as acute or nonacute, depending on their ability to produce an acute porphyric crisis in response to an environmental or physiologic trigger. This classification is more relevant to anesthesiologists, as only acute porphyrias are of significant perioperative concern.

1. **The acute porphyrias** include acute intermittent porphyria, variegate porphyria, hereditary coproporphyria, and the rare plumboporphyria. These are also classified as hepatic porphyrias. Hallmarks of an acute attack are abdominal pain, nausea/vomiting, autonomic disturbances with sweating, tachycardia, and sustained hypertension, and neurologic manifestations including seizures and neuromuscular weakness. Attacks can be life-threatening and neurologic manifestations may be permanent.

2. **The nonacute porphyrias** include porphyria cutanea tarda (a hepatic porphyria), congenital erythropoietic porphyria, and erythropoietic protoporphyria. Although patients may have liver disease, splenomegaly, anemia, increased infection risk, photosensitivity, and cutaneous manifestations, attacks with neurovisceral manifestations precipitated by drugs or physiologic stresses are unlikely in the nonacute porphyrias.

C. **Photosensitivity** is a feature of erythropoietic protoporphyria, congenital erythropoietic porphyria, porphyria cutanea tarda, variegate porphyria, and hereditary coproporphyria. Light at the visible wavelengths, 400 to 410 nm and 580 to 650 nm, interacts with the heme compounds accumulated in the skin to precipitate cutaneous changes, including blistering and a burning sensation. Clinical equipment, including operating room lights, may generate light at these wavelengths. Care should be taken to avoid burns in photosensitive patients.

D. **Anesthetic implications.** Initiation or exacerbation of a porphyric crisis should be actively avoided. Hypovolemia and electrolyte abnormalities should be treated. Avoid fasting. Aim to provide 2,000 calories/day enterally or via 10% dextrose IV. Respiratory muscle weakness or mental status changes may necessitate preoperative intubation and ventilation or prevent postoperative extubation. Although regional anesthesia may be used, patients are prone to neuropathies and significant autonomic instability.

1. **Commonly used local anesthetics,** with the possible exception of cocaine, mepivacaine, and ropivacaine, are likely to be safe.

2. **Propofol,** ketamine, muscle relaxants, opioids, and nitrous oxide are thought to be safe. Neuromuscular blockade reversal agents, droperidol, the phenothiazines, and most vasoactive agents (with the possible exception of hydralazine, nifedipine, and phenoxybenzamine) are likely to be safe.

3. **Firm data** about the safety of volatile anesthetics does not exist.

4. **Ondansetron,** ranitidine, and metoclopramide should be used cautiously.

5. **Lists of contraindicated drugs** (including etomidate, barbiturates, antiepileptic drugs, and many benzodiazepines) are available and should be consulted. Minimizing the number of drugs and using shorter-acting drugs reduces the risk. Administer all drugs with caution and with attention to the possible acute presentation of signs and symptoms consistent with an attack of porphyria.

E. **Acute attacks** should be managed with supportive care, treatment or withdrawal of any precipitants, carbohydrate loading, and treatment of hypovolemia, pain, and cardiovascular and electrolyte abnormalities. Consider infusing Hematin, 3 to 4 mg/kg IV, over 20 min. Risks of hematin therapy include renal failure, coagulopathy, and thrombophlebitis.

SUGGESTED READING

General

Breivik H. Perianaesthetic management of patients with endocrine disease. *Acta Anaesthesiol Scand* 1996;40:1004–1015.

Graham GW, Unger BP, Coursin DB. Perioperative management of selected endocrine disorders. *Int Anesthesiol Clin* 2000;38:31–67.

Schiff RL, Welsh GA. Perioperative evaluation and management of the patient with endocrine dysfunction. *Med Clin North Am* 2003;87:175–192.

Diabetes

Coursin DB, Connery LE, Ketzler JT. Perioperative diabetic and hyperglycemic management issues. *Crit Care Med* 2004;32:S116–S125.

Glister BC, Vigersky RA. Perioperative management of type 1 diabetes mellitus. *Endocrinol Metab Clin North Am* 2003;32:411–436.

Inzucchi SE. Glycemic management of diabetes in the perioperative setting. *Int Anesthesiol Clin* 2002;40:77–93.

Magee MF, Bhatt BA. Management of decompensated diabetes—diabetic ketoacidosis and hyperglycemic hyperosmolar syndrome. *Crit Care Clin* 2001;17: 75–106.

McAnulty GR, Robertshaw HJ, Hall GM. Anaesthetic management of patients with diabetes mellitus. *Br J Anaesth* 2000;85:80–90.

Thyroid

Edwards R. Thyroid and parathyroid disease. *Int Anesthesiol Clin* 1997;35:63–83.

Farling PA. Thyroid disease. *Br J Anaesth* 2000;85:15–28.

Langley RW, Burch HB. Perioperative management of the thyrotoxic patient. *Endocrinol Metab Clin North Am* 2003;32:519–534.

Stathatos N, Wartofsky L. Perioperative management of patients with hypothyroidism. *Endocrinol Metab Clin North Am* 2003;32:503–518.

Calcium

Aguilera IM, Vaughan RS. Calcium and the anaesthetist. *Anaesthesia* 2000;55: 779–790.

Ariyan CE, Sosa JA. Assessment and management of patients with abnormal calcium. *Crit Care Med* 2004;32:S146–S154.

Mihai R, Farndon JR. Parathyroid disease and calcium metabolism. *Br J Anaesth* 2000;85:29–43.

Adrenals

Axelrod L. Perioperative management of patients treated with glucocorticoids. *Endocrinol Metab Clin North Am* 2003;32:367–383.

Connery LE, Coursin DB. Assessment and therapy of selected endocrine disorders. *Anesthesiol Clin North Am* 2004;22(1):93–123.

Ganguly A. Primary aldosteronism. *N Engl J Med* 1998;339:1828–1834.

Nicholson G, Burrin JM, Hall GM. Peri-operative steroid supplementation. *Anaesthesia* 1998;53:1091–1104.

Oelkers W. Adrenal insufficiency. *N Engl J Med* 1996;335:1206–1212.

Orth DN. Cushing's syndrome. *N Engl J Med* 1995;332:791–803.

Sheeran P, O'Leary E. Adrenocortical disorders. *Int Anesthesiol Clin* 1997;35: 85–98.

Pheochromocytoma

Kinney MAO, Bradly JN, Warner MA. Perioperative management of pheochromocytoma. *J Cardiovasc Anesth* 2002;16:359–369.

O'Riordan JA. Pheochromocytomas and anesthesia. *Int Anesthesiol Clin* 1997;35: 99–127.

Prys-Roberts C. Phaeochromocytoma-recent progress in its management. *Br J Anaesth* 2000;85:44–57.

Pituitary

Ben-Shlomo A, Melmed S. Acromegaly. *Endocrinol Metab Clin North Am* 2001;30: 565–583.

Nemergut EC, Dumont AS, Barry UT, Laws ER. Perioperative management of patients undergoing transsphenoidal pituitary surgery. *Anesth Analg* 2005;101: 1170–1181.

Nemergut EC, Zuo Z. Airway management in patients with pituitary disease: a review of 746 patients. *J Neurosurg Anesthesiol* 2006;18:73–77.

Singer I, Oster JR, Fishman LM. The management of diabetes insipidus in adults. *Arch Intern Med* 1997;157:1293–1301.

Smith M, Hirsch NP. Pituitary disease and anaesthesia. *Br J Anaesth* 2000;85:3–14.

Vance ML. Hypopituitarism. *N Engl J Med* 1994;330:1651–1662.

Carcinoid

Kulke MH, Mayer RJ. Carcinoid tumors. *N Engl J Med* 1999;340:858–868.

Vaughan DJA, Brunner MD. Anesthesia for patients with carcinoid syndrome. *Int Anesthesiol Clin* 1997;35:129–142.

Porphyria

James MFM, Hift RJ. Porphyrias. *Br J Anaesth* 2000;85:143–153.

Jensen NF, Fiddler DS, Striepe V. Anesthetic considerations in porphyrias. *Anesth Analg* 1995;80:591–599.

7

Infectious Diseases and Infection Control in Anesthesia

Rebecca Aslakson and Judith Hellman

I. **General.** Anesthetists play an important role in many aspects of infection control in the operating room (OR).
   A. **Infection control-related responsibilities of anesthetist**
      1. **Prevention of transmission** of infectious agents between patients, between patients and operating personnel, and between OR personnel and patients.
      2. **Prevention of infectious complications** resulting from invasive procedures such as placement of intravenous, intra-arterial, and regional anesthetic catheters; nerve blocks; and spinal anesthetics.
      3. **Avoidance of anesthesia-related complications** that can predispose to infection, such as aspiration during induction and intubation.
      4. **Participation in preventing surgical wound infections**
         a. Timely and proper administration of perioperative antibiotics.
         b. A recent study reported a lower incidence of surgical site infections in colorectal surgery patients treated intraoperatively with a higher inspired fraction of oxygen (FIO_2 0.8 versus 0.3). However, another study reported an increased incidence of wound infections in general surgery patients treated with higher FIO_2. Thus, additional studies are required to determine whether manipulating the FIO_2 will benefit patients undergoing different surgical procedures.
   B. **Routes of infection transmission in the OR**
      1. **Physical contact** between the host and a contaminated object or a colonized or infected person is the most common mechanism of infection transmission.
      2. **Droplet transmission** results from deposition of large microorganism-containing droplets that are produced by an infected individual by coughing, sneezing, and talking. The droplets travel short distances and are deposited on the mucous membranes of the new host or on surfaces and then are transmitted by direct contact.
      3. **Airborne transmission** results from inhalation of small particles that contain microorganisms and are suspended in the air by coughing, sneezing, and talking. Unlike larger droplets, these particles may remain suspended in the air and can be spread by air currents.
      4. **Blood and body fluids** can be a source of infected material, which can be transmitted through breaks in the host's skin or mucosa when there is contact between the infected body fluid and the host. Routine testing of blood products for some common blood-borne pathogens (human immunodeficiency

virus [HIV], hepatitis B virus [HBV], hepatitis C virus [HCV]) has dramatically reduced the incidence of transfusion-related infections.

II. **Infection control in the OR**

A. **Infection control measures** must be undertaken to prevent transmission of pathogens from patients to OR staff and vice versa, to prevent surgical wound infections, and to prevent introduction of microorganisms during invasive procedures such as placement of central venous, pulmonary artery, and epidural catheters. Adherence to **isolation precaution** guidelines reduces the occupational risk of contracting infectious diseases and decreases transmission of infections in the hospital.

B. **Standard precautions** are intended to limit transmission of microorganisms by decreasing microbial colonization of surfaces, equipment, clothing, and hands and by preventing occupational exposure to blood and other potentially infected body fluids. Routine **handwashing** is essential to control the spread of infection.

1. **Minimize colonization of OR surfaces and OR equipment**

   a. **Clean the OR,** including the anesthesia machine and anesthesia monitoring devices, with a bactericidal agent between cases.

   b. **Limit flow of traffic** through the OR.

   c. **Sterilize reusable equipment** (e.g., laryngoscopes, bronchoscopes, surgical instruments).

   d. **Air exchanges** in the OR should be a minimum of 15 total exchanges per hour. In addition, the OR should be maintained at positive pressure relative to adjacent areas.

   e. **Other** (not always used): laminar flow ventilation, ultraviolet radiation, high-efficiency particulate air filtration.

2. **Minimize transmission through contact with patients**

   a. **Wash hands** with antiseptic-containing solutions before and after contact with each patient or after contact with contaminated materials.

   b. **Wear gloves** when hands are likely to come in contact with blood or other body fluids. Gloves must be changed (and hands washed) before and after contact with each patient.

   c. **Wear lint-free OR attire,** including cap, mask, suit, and shoe covers or properly and regularly cleansed dedicated OR shoes.

3. **Minimize the likelihood of infections related to anesthesia and anesthetic procedures**

   a. **Use sterile technique** for placement of catheters, nerve blocks, and spinal anesthesia. Sterile gloves and drapes should be used, and the insertion site should be carefully inspected and cleaned with antiseptic solution. Indwelling catheters should not be placed through areas that appear infected or inflamed. A sterile gown should be worn for placing central venous and pulmonary artery catheters. Peripheral intravenous catheters may be placed after cleaning the insertion site with 70% isopropyl alcohol or povidone iodine.

   b. **Cover catheter sites with sterile transparent dressings.** Catheter sites should be regularly inspected postoperatively for signs of infection.

   c. **Administer drugs using a sterile technique.**

4. **Universal precautions** apply to all patients, regardless of underlying diseases. Barrier precautions are required when there is potential for contact with blood and other bodily secretions and fluids, because they may harbor infectious agents. Barriers include gloves, protective eyewear or face shields, and gowns.

C. **Transmission-based precautions.** Specialized precautions, including **contact, airborne,** and **droplet precautions,** apply to patients who are suspected or are known to be infected or colonized with particular microorganisms. Different precautions apply to different microorganisms. When special precautions are in effect, **signs** are placed at the entrance to the patient's room indicating the type of precaution and required procedures to enter and exit the room. These guidelines should be followed in the OR and postanesthesia care unit (PACU), and signs should be placed on the door(s) to the OR and near the patient in the PACU.

1. **Contact precautions** apply in many situations, including (but not limited to) colonization or infection with various antibiotic-resistant bacteria, such as methicillin-resistant *Staphylococcus aureus* (MRSA) and vancomycin-resistant enterococcus (VRE), some viral infections, and *Clostridium difficile.*
   a. **Wear gloves and a gown** when entering the room.
   b. **Remove gowns and gloves** and wash hands upon exiting the room.
   c. **Medical record.** Leave charts and flow sheets outside the room and do not allow them to be in contact with the patient or contaminated bedding. Place records in a plastic bag during transport.
   d. **Placement after PACU.** A private room is preferred. A semiprivate room shared with a patient who is colonized or infected with the same microorganisms is acceptable.
   e. **Cessation of contact precautions.** Guidelines for when contact precautions may be stopped vary among infectious organisms and among hospitals. For example, contact precaution cessation protocols for MRSA may be different than those for VRE. Moreover, some hospitals may require two negative cultures from the previously infected site, whereas others require a series of negative nasal cultures. The Massachusetts General Hospital policy requires the following:
      (1) That the patient is off all antibiotics for at least 48 hours.
      (2) That there are negative cultures of the infected site if possible, and three negative cultures from different days of swabs of the most common sites of colonization for the organism (e.g., the rectal swabs for VRE and nasal swabs for MRSA).
      (3) If criteria (1) and (2) are not met, the patient should continue to be on contact precautions. For example, ambulatory surgery patients with a previously documented MRSA infection and without documented subsequent negative cultures should be placed on contact precautions.

2. **Droplet precautions** are used to limit the spread of infectious agents that are present in larger droplets produced by

coughing, sneezing, and talking. *Neisseria meningitidis, Haemophilus influenzae, Mycoplasma pneumoniae,* adenovirus, and rubella virus are examples of infectious agents that are transmitted through droplets.

   a. **Wear a surgical mask** when within 3 feet of an infected individual. Discard the mask upon exiting the room and wash hands after discarding the mask.

   b. **Transport.** The infected patient should wear a surgical mask during transportation.

   c. **Placement after PACU.** A private room is preferred. A semiprivate room shared with a patient who is colonized or infected with the same microorganisms is acceptable.

3. **Airborne precautions** are used to limit the spread of infectious agents in particles that remain suspended in the air. *Mycobacterium tuberculosis* (MTB), varicella zoster virus (VZV), Ebola virus, severe acute respiratory syndrome (SARS)-associated coronavirus, and rubeola (measles) are examples of microorganisms that are transmitted through airborne particles.

   a. **Specialized masks (N95 respirators)** are designed to filter out very small particles.

      (1) **Respirators,** and not standard surgical masks, should be worn by all persons entering rooms of patients who require airborne precautions for tuberculosis and by persons who must enter the room who are not immune to VZV or rubeola.

      (2) Personnel using respirators must be **fit-tested** before use to ensure an adequate seal.

   b. **A private room with negative-pressure isolation is required for all patients on airborne precautions.**

   c. **Transport.** The patient should wear a surgical mask for transport. Intubated patients should be transported with a bacterial filter in place on the endotracheal tube.

4. The **PACU (or intensive care unit)** and the floor where the patient will be going should be informed of any special isolation precautions in advance.

D. **Preventing exposure to infected blood and body fluids**

1. **Occupational exposure** to blood-borne pathogens such as HIV, HBV, and HCV are of particular concern to anesthetists who routinely perform procedures that involve needles and blood. Exposure can occur through needlesticks but may also occur as a result of exposure through open cuts, splashes into eyes and other exposed areas, and contact with sharp contaminated objects other than needles (e.g., scalpels, cracked ampules).

2. **Preventive measures**

   a. **Hand washing, gloves, protective eyewear** as above.

   b. **Do not recap used needles or remove used needles from syringes.** Needlestick injuries most often occur during recapping of used needles. Used needles should be discarded without recapping. A number of devices have been developed that protect the used needle tip without requiring recapping.

   c. **Dispose of used needles immediately.** All needles should be discarded in special puncture-proof receptacles.

   d. **Administer parenteral drugs using needleless systems.**

e. **Do not place syringes with attached needles in pockets.**

E. **Management of exposure to infected blood and bloody fluids**
1. **Wash areas of contact.** Use soap and water or sterile saline for skin; flush mucous membranes with water or sterile saline. Washing with caustic agents such as bleach is not recommended.
2. **Immediately report exposure** to hospital occupational/employee health or an equivalent service. The Occupational Safety and Health Administration requires that all health care institutions have protocols for assessing and managing occupational exposures that include the following:
   a. **Serologic testing** (HIV, HBV, and HCV) of the source (if known) and the health care worker.
   b. Consideration of **postexposure prophylaxis (PEP)** for HIV and HBV exposures.
   c. **Counseling.**

III. **Microorganisms of concern to anesthetists.** The Centers for Disease Control and Prevention (CDC) Web site (www.cdc.gov) has current reviews of potential pathogens, including all the microorganisms reviewed here, and their treatment.
A. **Viruses**
1. **HIV**
   a. **Transmission.** HIV is transmitted through percutaneous or mucosal exposure to infected blood or body fluids through needlestick and other sharp injury, blood transfusion, and sexual contact. Perinatal transmission of HIV from an infected mother to the neonate also occurs.
   b. **Occupational risk of HIV.** The risk of occupationally acquired HIV in health care workers is low. Most documented cases of seroconversion have occurred after percutaneous exposure; mucosal exposure is believed to be low risk.
      (1) **The risk of seroconversion is 0.3%** after percutaneous exposure to blood from an HIV-infected person.
      (2) **The risk of HIV transmission** is increased with deep injury, visible patient blood on the device causing injury, needle placed in a vein or artery of the source patient, the patient in the terminal stages of HIV infection, and possibly larger-bore hollow needles.
   c. **PEP.** The CDC has published guidelines for management of HIV-exposed health care workers. These guidelines are frequently updated as additional studies become available; the reader is directed to the CDC Web site (www.cdc.gov/) and to the National Clinicians' Post-Exposure Prophylaxis Hotline (888-448-4911) for up-to-date information on PEP. Multiple factors are considered in deciding whether to initiate PEP and in choosing the PEP regimen. Basic and extended regimens may be considered based on the type of exposure, the volume of the exposure source blood or body fluid, the HIV status of the exposure source, and, if known, the sensitivity of the virus to antiretroviral drugs. Persons taking PEP should be monitored for side effects and drug toxicity. The CDC guidelines stress the

importance of institutional protocols for early reporting of exposure to HIV and timely administration of PEP and recommend that practitioners with expertise in antiretroviral therapy be involved in PEP management.

2. **HBV.** Acute HBV hepatitis usually resolves without sequelae. Ten percent of infected individuals become chronic HBV carriers and are at risk of developing chronic active hepatitis, cirrhosis, and hepatocellular carcinoma. The severity and chronicity of infection varies among people; those infected with HBV can remain infectious throughout their lifetime. Approximately 250 health care workers die each year from sequelae of occupationally transmitted HBV infection. Vaccination against HBV is an effective and safe means for preventing hepatitis B infection.

   a. **Transmission of HBV** is through percutaneous or mucosal exposure to infected blood or body fluids caused by needlestick and other sharp injury, blood transfusion, sexual contact, or during the perinatal period. Some health care workers who develop HBV infection have no recollection of exposure to blood or body fluids of infected patients.

   b. **The occupational risk of contracting HBV** depends on the amount of inoculate as well as the hepatitis B e antigen (HBeAg) status of the source patient. Hollow, large-bore needle inoculation carries a higher risk than exposure of a mucous membrane to potentially infectious saliva. If a source patient is both hepatitis B surface antigen (HBsAg) and HBeAg positive, the risk of clinical hepatitis via needle inoculation is 22% to 31%. However, if a source patient is HBsAg positive but HBeAg negative, the risk of clinical hepatitis is merely 1% to 6%.

   c. **Vaccination against HBV.** A recombinant HBV vaccine is recommended for all health care workers having contact with blood or bloody body fluids. The vaccine series consists of three vaccinations over 6 months that should be completed before potential contact with contaminated blood or body fluids. Standard vaccination is effective at least 90% of the time. Antibody levels should be checked after completion of the vaccination series. Twenty-five percent of initial nonresponders will respond to repeating the vaccination series.

   d. **PEP** may be indicated after exposure to blood or body fluids if the source is known to be HBsAg positive or if the HBsAg state of the source is unknown. The decision depends on the immune statues of the exposed individual. PEP usually involves a combination of passive immunization with hepatitis B immunoglobulin (HBIg) and active immunization against HBsAg (antibody to HBsAg [anti-HBs]). PEP should be administered as early as possible after exposure. According to the CDC guidelines,

      (1) **Previously unvaccinated individuals** should begin the vaccine series in any instance of exposure, regardless of the HBsAg state of the source. If the source is known to be HBsAg positive, HBIg is also recommended in a single dose.

    (2) **Vaccinated individuals** should be evaluated for adequacy of anti-HBs response. **Nonresponders** (anti-HBs <10 mIU/mL) are treated with HBIg and, in some cases, revaccinated if the source is known to be HBsAg positive or if the HBsAg status is of the source is unknown and they are believed to be high risk. **Responders** (anti-HBs ≥10 mIU/mL) require no additional treatment.

3. **HCV.** Health care workers with occupational exposure to blood are at risk of contracting HCV. Chronic HCV infection and chronic hepatitis occur in 85% and 75%, respectively, of those infected with HCV.

  a. **Transmission in the hospital setting** generally occurs through large volume or repeated percutaneous exposure to blood, although transmission has been reported through blood splashing into the conjunctivae.

  b. **Risk of HCV transmission.** The rate of HCV seroconversion after a needlestick or other sharp injury involving infected blood has been reported to average 1.8%.

  c. **PEP.** There are no guidelines for PEP in HCV. Although interferon is approved for treating chronic hepatitis C, it has not been extensively studied as a prophylactic agent and is not currently recommended for PEP.

4. **Herpes simplex viruses (HSV) I and II**

  a. **Transmission of HSV** is via direct contact between an infected individual or infected secretions and mucosa or damaged skin. HSV can be shed by asymptomatic individuals. HSV can be transmitted by health care workers.

  b. **Herpetic whitlow** is HSV infection of the finger and can be caused by occupational exposure to HSV I or HSV II. Lesions are painful and inflamed and may be accompanied by fever and localized lymphadenopathy. Anesthetists may acquire herpetic whitlow (primarily HSV I) through contact with oral secretions of an infected source. Persons with active herpetic whitlow can transmit HSV and should avoid contact with patients during the period of transmissibility.

5. **Cytomegalovirus (CMV)** is a herpesvirus. Although usually asymptomatic, certain situations predispose to life-threatening CMV infection, including infections that occur in utero and in hosts who are severely ill or are immunocompromised. Infection can result from reactivation of latent infection lying dormant in the host and from exposure to an external source such as a blood transfusion or organ transplantation.

  a. **Transmission** occurs via direct contact between the susceptible host and the infected source and through blood transfusion or transplantation of infected organs.

  b. **Blood products commonly contain CMV.** To reduce the chance of CMV transmission, CMV-negative immunosuppressed patients and CMV-negative parturients should receive blood from CMV-seronegative donors if transfusion is necessary.

6. **VZV** causes chickenpox and herpes zoster (shingles).

  a. **Transmission.** VZV is highly contagious and is spread through direct contact or through airborne routes via respiratory secretions. Anesthetists may be exposed to VZV when caring for patients with a primary infection or who have shingles. Infected health care workers can transmit VZV to other health care workers and to patients.

b. **Infection** is extremely common in children who generally have an uncomplicated course. Severe infection can occur in adults and in immunocompromised persons. Infection during pregnancy can have disastrous effects on the fetus.

c. **Nonimmune health care workers** who are likely to be in contact with high-risk patients should receive VZV vaccination. They should not have patient contact during the contagious stage of active infection and should not have direct patient contact between 10 and 21 days after significant exposure to active VZV.

7. **Influenza virus** outbreaks occur annually. Influenza virus causes more severe manifestations than most other viral respiratory infections. Generally, infection is not life threatening, but roughly 20,000 deaths are attributable to influenza virus per year. Severe infections usually occur in elderly, debilitated, and chronically ill persons.

a. **Transmission.** Influenza virus spreads through virus-containing droplets that are produced by coughing or sneezing. Anesthetists may acquire and then spread influenza virus because of their close involvement with respiratory secretions.

b. **Annual vaccination** is recommended for health care workers caring for patients who are at risk of severe influenza-related complications.

8. **Prion diseases,** such as **Creutzfeldt-Jakob disease** and **kuru,** are caused by an unusual group of protein-containing infectious particles (prions). Prions can cause slowly progressive fatal neurodegenerative disorders. **Transmission** appears to result from direct inoculation of infected material into a host. There are numerous reports of transmission through transplantation of dura. The long incubation time has made epidemiologic evaluation of the occupational risk of prion diseases difficult. Nevertheless, the risk of transmission to health care workers is believed to be low, and transmission via transfused blood has not been reported. In addition to the universal precautions that apply to all patients, reusable equipment (such as laryngoscopes) should be completely sterilized before reuse.

9. **SARS.** SARS is caused by a novel coronavirus, SARS-associated coronavirus (SARS-CoV), and leads to a febrile severe lower respiratory illness. From the winter of 2002 through the spring of 2003, the World Health Organization received >8,000 reports of SARS cases, primarily in China, Taiwan, and Canada. Many cases involved health care workers who had cared for patients with SARS. At the time of this publication, the SARS virus has not been detected, and it is uncertain whether there will be future SARS epidemics. Mortality from SARS is high, reported between 6% and 55%, depending on the country, with a general rate of 6% to 20%. No clinical or laboratory test is specific for SARS.

a. **SARS is transmitted** via droplets or airborne particles.

   b. Precautions. According to current CDC guidelines, in the absence of person-to-person transmission of SARS-CoV in the world, patients with severe pneumonia and one SARS risk factor should be placed on droplet precautions. SARS risk factors include recent travel to a previously SARS-affected area or close contact with such a traveler, close contact with pneumonia patients, and employment in an occupation at risk for SARS-CoV exposure including health care workers with patient contact and/or workers in laboratories containing live SARS-CoV. When there is person-to-person transmission of SARS-CoV in the world or when the clinician has a strong suspicion for SARS, the patient should be placed on contact precautions and airborne infection isolation. The Massachusetts General Hospital's policy also includes use of a powered air purifying respirator, instead of a standard N95 respirator, for high-risk procedures such as bronchoscopy, airway intubation, and other procedures that are likely to generate uncontained aerosols of respiratory secretions.

   c. Treatment is supportive. The role of medications such as steroids or ribovarin is uncertain.

B. Bacteria

1. MTB causes tuberculosis (TB). MTB infection usually is localized to the lungs, but it can also cause extrapulmonary disease. TB infection frequently is asymptomatic and the bacteria become inactive. Nevertheless, the bacteria remain alive and eventually can become active and cause disease. Active disease usually occurs in patients who are chronically ill, debilitated, or immunocompromised. Antibiotic-resistant strains of TB are problematic.

   a. Transmission is through inhalation of aerosolized MTB-containing droplets that are suspended in the air after an infected host coughs, sneezes, or talks. Health care workers who routinely deal with respiratory secretions are at significant risk for contracting MTB.

   b. Preventing transmission

   (1) Respiratory precautions should be used in all cases of known or suspected TB until it is confirmed that the sputum does not contain acid-fast bacilli.

   (2) Health care workers should be routinely screened for TB by skin testing. Recent conversion can be treated with isoniazid.

   (3) Specialized face masks (N95 respirators) should be worn. These are designed to filter out very small particles (see section II.C.3.a).

2. Antibiotic-resistant bacteria have become a major problem in hospitalized patients and can severely limit the treatment options for serious infections. Frequent and prolonged use of antibiotics contributes significantly to the emergence of antibiotic-resistant bacteria.

   a. Transmission can occur through physical contact with contaminated health care workers or equipment.

   b. Contact precautions are required for patients who are colonized or infected with **MRSA** or **VRE** and sometimes with highly resistant Gram-negative bacteria.

Contact precautions should be maintained through the OR and PACU.

IV. Antibiotics in the OR

Tables 7.1 and 7.2 include guidelines for perioperative antibiotic prophylaxis and endocarditis.

A. Indications for antibiotics in the OR

1. **Prophylaxis** against surgical wound infections and endocarditis.
2. **Continuation of treatment** for active infection.

B. Basic principles of antibiotic prophylaxis

1. **The Partners Healthcare Guidelines** for routine perioperative antibiotic prophylaxis are summarized in Table 7.1.
2. **Indications** for antibiotic prophylaxis include surgical procedures with a high risk of postoperative infection, procedures involving implantation of foreign materials, and if the consequences of postoperative infection would be disastrous. Prophylactic antibiotics are not necessary for all surgical procedures in all patients.
3. **The timing and duration of perioperative antibiotics are extremely important.**
   a. **Preoperative intravenous antibiotics** should be given within 30 to 60 min of incision to ensure adequate antibiotic levels at the time of incision.
   b. **Repeated intraoperative dosing** should be considered for longer surgeries. For example, cefazolin is often administered every 4 to 8 hours in the OR. The more frequent dosing (every 4 hours) is done when surgery is accompanied by large blood losses and/or volume requirements.
   c. **Postoperatively,** antibiotics usually are continued for 24 to 48 hours. Prolonged administration is not recommended because of lack of benefit and the risk of colonization and subsequent infection with antibiotic-resistant bacteria.
4. **Adverse effects of antibiotics**
   a. **Hypersensitivity reactions** can occur with virtually any class of antibiotic and can vary in severity from rash to anaphylaxis.
   b. **Hypotension** may result from histamine release (e.g., vancomycin) or anaphylaxis.
   c. **Neuromuscular blockade and potentiation of neuromuscular blocking drugs** can occur with aminoglycosides, clindamycin, polymyxins, and tetracyclines. Rarely, profound and prolonged weakness of the respiratory muscles occurs.
   d. **Hypernatremia** can be result from the large sodium load associated with administration of penicillin derivatives such as ticarcillin and piperacillin.
   e. **Nephrotoxicity** (e.g., aminoglycosides) and **ototoxicity** (e.g., aminoglycosides and vancomycin).
   f. **Bleeding** can result from platelet dysfunction (e.g., ticarcillin, piperacillin) or impaired production of vitamin K-dependent clotting factors (e.g., cefotetan).
5. **Rate of infusion.** Some antibiotics can be rapidly administered without difficulty. Others, such as vancomycin,

Table 7.1. Partners Health Care Guidelines for routine perioperative antibiotic prophylaxis for procedures involving incision of skin or mucosa

Procedure or Site	Preoperative Antibiotic	For Allergy	Postoperative Antibiotic
Appendix or esophagus	Cefazolin 1 g and metronidazole 500 mg	#1	Same q8h × 2
Colon or rectum	2 days and 1 day before surgery: oral neomycin 500 mg and erythromycin base 250 mg at 7 AM, 12 n, 6 PM, & bedtime. Preop: cefazolin 1 g and metronidazole 500 mg	#1	Cefazolin 1 g and metronidazole 500 mg q8h × 2
Biliary tract or other gastrointestinal	Cefazolin 1 g	#1	Cefazolin q8h × 2
Open gynecologic	Cefazolin 1 g	#1	Cefazolin q8h × 2
Thoracic or head and neck	Cefazolin 1 g when procedure involves the oropharynx or esophagus add metronidazole 500 mg	#3	None
Cardiac	Cefazolin 1 g[a]	#3	Cefazolin q8h × 3–5
Vascular	Cefazolin 1 g	#3	Cefazolin q8h × 3–5
Neurosurgery	Cefazolin 1 g	#2	Cefazolin q8h × 2
Orthopedic Includes joint replacement and other procedures	Cefazolin 1 g	#3	Cefazolin q8h × 2
Plastic	Cefazolin 1 g	#3	None
Breast	Cefazolin 1 g	#3	None

Pacemaker/automatic internal cardiac defibrillator insertion	Cefazolin 1 g	#3	None
Other clean surgery	Cefazolin 1 g at surgeon's discretion	#3	None
Genitourinary			
Transurethral prostatectomy, sterile urine	None		
Open surgery, sterile urine	Cefazolin 1 g	#2	Cefazolin q8h × 2

Prophylaxis should be given shortly before the start of surgery. The drug should be redosed if the elapsed time from the start of administration until incision is more than 90 min for cefazolin or 150 min for vancomycin.

Intraoperative redosing: cefazolin should be redosed every 4 hours intraoperatively.

Vancomycin should be redosed after 8 hours intraoperatively.

Patients with open wounds and those at risk for endocarditis may require additional antibiotic therapy. Patients undergoing genitourinary surgery who have nonsterile urine require additional therapy.

Patients at extremes of weight and age and those with abnormal renal or hepatic function may require alterations of dose or frequency.

[a] For prosthetic valve surgery, vancomycin may be substituted for cefazolin. Use 1 g, repeat every 12 hours for 3–5 doses.

For allergy to cephalosporins or history of immediate-type hypersensitivity, exfoliation, or other life-threatening reaction to penicillin:

1. Clindamycin 600 mg every 8 hours and gentamicin 5 mg/kg × 1.
2. Vancomycin 1,000 mg every 12 hours and gentamicin 5 mg/kg × 1.
3. Vancomycin 1,000 mg preoperative dose; if postoperative dosing is indicated, then repeat every 12 hours for 3–5 doses.

Table 7.2. Endocarditis prophylaxis regimens recommended by the American Heart Association for dental and surgical procedures

Surgical Site	Endocarditis Risk	Standard Regimen		Alternative for Penicillin Allergy[b]	
		Antibiotic (Route)	Dose[a] and Timing Relative to Surgery	Antibiotic (Route)	Dose* and Timing Relative to Surgery
Mouth Pharynx Respiratory tract Esophagus	High and Moderate	Amoxicillin (oral)	Adults: 2 g Children: 50 mg/kg 1 hour before	Clindamycin (oral)	Adults: 600 mg Children: 20 mg/kg 1 hour before
				Cephalexin or Cefadroxil (oral)	Adults: 2 g Children: 50 mg/kg 1 hour before
				Azithromycin or clarithromycin (oral)	Adults: 500 mg Children: 15 mg/kg 1 hour before
		Ampicillin[c] (intravenous or intramuscular)	Adults: 2 g Children: 50 mg/kg Within 30 min before	Clindamycin (intravenous)	Adults: 600 mg Children: 20 mg/kg Within 30 min before
				Cefazolin (intravenous)	Adults: 1 g Children: 25 mg/kg Within 30 min before

Situation	Risk	Agent[b]	Regimen[a]	Penicillin-allergic agent	Regimen[a]
Genitourinary tract GI tract (other than esophagus)	High	Ampicillin (intravenous) and Gentamicin (intravenous)	Adults: ampicillin 2 g, gentamicin 1.5 mg/kg (up to 120 mg) Children: ampicillin 50 mg/kg, gentamicin 1.5 mg/kg (up to 120 mg) Within 30 min before. Second dose of ampicillin recommended 6 hours after initial dose[d]	Vancomycin (intravenous) and Gentamicin (intravenous or intramuscular)	Adults: vancomycin 1 g, gentamicin 1.5 mg/kg (up to 120 mg) Children: vancomycin 20 mg/kg, gentamicin 1.5 mg/kg (up to 120 mg) Complete within 30 min before; administer vancomycin over 1–2 hours
Genitourinary tract GI tract (other than esophagus)	Moderate	Amoxicillin (oral)	Adults: 2 g Children: 50 mg/kg 1 hour before	Ampicillin (intravenous) Adults: 2 g Children: 50 mg/kg Within 30 min before	Vancomycin (intravenous) Adults: 1 g Children: 20 mg/kg Complete within 30 minutes before; administer vancomycin over 1–2 hours

[a] Maximum dose for children = adult dose.

[b] Cephalosporins should not be used if there is a history of anaphylaxis, urticaria, or angioedema with penicillins.

[c] For patients unable to take oral prophylaxis.

[d] Second dose of amoxicillin (adults, 1 g; children, 25 mg/kg) or ampicillin (adults, 1 g; children, 25 mg/kg) recommended 6 hours after the initial dose.

aminoglycosides, and clindamycin, should be given more slowly to prevent adverse effects.

C. **Postoperative surgical infections.** Many factors influence the development and severity of postoperative infections. Prophylactic measures are effective in preventing wound infections. Bacteria that cause wound infections reflect the site of origin of the infection and are altered by recent treatment with antibiotics, prolonged preoperative hospitalization, and coexisting diseases. Severe wound infections that occur in the first 48 hours after surgery can be caused by *Clostridium* or group A streptococcus (*Streptococcus pyogenes*), which can require emergent surgical debridement in addition to intensive antibiotic therapy.

1. **Surgical wound classifications** may be helpful in guiding antibiotic therapy.

   a. **Clean.** No entry into internal organs that harbor bacteria. Clean surgical wound infections are most often caused by aerobic Gram-positive bacteria that colonize the skin, such as *S. aureus,* coagulase-negative *Staphylococcus,* and *Streptococcus* spp.

   b. **Contaminated.** Bacteria causing contaminated wound infections reflect the origin of contamination (respiratory, gastrointestinal [GI], or genitourinary tract) and often include enteric Gram-negative bacteria and anaerobic bacteria such as *Bacteroides.*

      (1) **Clean-contaminated.** Organs are entered without spillage of contents.

      (2) **Contaminated.** Spillage of organ contents without formation of pus.

      (3) **Dirty.** Spillage of organ contents with pus formation.

2. **Pathogens.** Infections after "clean" surgeries tend to be caused by Gram-positive bacteria, such as *S. aureus* and streptococci. Infections after "contaminated surgeries" may be polymicrobial, involving aerobic and anaerobic Gram-positive and Gram-negative bacteria. Many factors influence the colonizing flora, including length of hospitalization, use of antacids and histamine-2 blockers, recent use of antibiotics, GI dysmotility or obstruction, and the immune status of the host.

D. **Commonly used antibiotics**

1. **β-Lactams** include penicillins, cephalosporins, carbapenems (such as meropenem), and monobactams (such as aztreonam).

   a. **Cefazolin,** a first-generation cephalosporin, is widely used for prophylaxis because it is active against most Gram-positive and many Gram-negative bacteria that are likely to cause infections of clean wounds in the early postoperative period. Second-generation cephalosporins, such as **cefoxitin** and **cefotetan,** provide additional Gram-negative and anaerobic coverage and may be used for "contaminated" surgeries, particularly those involving the GI tract. Third- and fourth-generation cephalosporins, such as **ceftriaxone, ceftazidime,** and **cefepime,** are usually administered as continuation of preoperative treatment for a known or suspected Gram-negative bacterial infection. **Penicillin** is often used as prophylaxis for dental surgery.

  b. **Adverse reactions**
    (1) **Hypersensitivity reactions** ranging from rash to anaphylaxis. Between 5% and 10% of penicillin-allergic patients are allergic to cephalosporins.
    (2) **Bleeding** (see section IV.B.4.f).
    (3) **Volume overload or hypernatremia** (see section IV.B.4.d).
    (4) **Interstitial nephritis** (especially nafcillin).
    (5) **Central nervous system toxicity.**
  2. **Vancomycin** is used as an alternative to β-lactams in allergic patients or in patients who are colonized with antibiotic-resistant Gram-positive bacteria such as MRSA. Additional antibiotics are required if coverage of Gram-negative organisms is needed.
  a. **Adverse reactions**
    (1) **Red man syndrome** is characterized by flushing of the face, neck, and trunk and variable degrees of hypotension. It results from histamine release and is not allergic in nature. Red man syndrome can be minimized by delivering the drug in a large volume and slowing the rate of infusion.
    (2) **Hypersensitivity reactions** ranging from rash to anaphylaxis.
    (3) **Ototoxicity** can be permanent and occurs more frequently in patients receiving vancomycin and an aminoglycoside.
    (4) **Nephrotoxicity** used to be a major concern with vancomycin but does not appear to be significant with current preparations.
  3. **Aminoglycosides** include gentamicin, amikacin, and tobramycin. In the OR, aminoglycosides may be used in combination with other agents, such as a β-lactam and an antianaerobic agent, particularly when there has been spillage of bowel contents.
  a. **Adverse reactions**
    (1) **Nephrotoxicity** is the most common adverse effect and is usually mild, nonoliguric, and reversible. Risk factors include advanced age, debilitation, baseline renal insufficiency, hypotension, hypovolemia, and concomitant administration of other nephrotoxins such as intravenous contrast agents.
    (2) **Ototoxicity** can produce vertigo and deafness. Slow rates of administration have been suggested to potentially decrease the risk of ototoxicity.
    (3) **Weakness and potentiation of neuromuscular blockade** (see section IV.B.4.c).
  4. **Clindamycin** may be used for prophylaxis in head and neck surgery or as an alternative to β-lactams in patients who are allergic. Clindamycin is active against most anaerobes and Gram-positive aerobes. **Adverse reactions** include GI upset, rash, and elevated liver enzymes. Clindamycin is notorious as a cause of *C. difficile* colitis. Rapid administration of clindamycin may have adverse side effects, such as an unpleasant metallic taste and perineal pain; there have been reports of rapid infusion causing profound hypotension and even cardiac arrest. Thus,

clindamycin should be infused slowly, at a rate not to exceed 30 mg/min (~20 min/600-mg dose).

5. **Metronidazole** may be used in combination with other agents, such as a β-lactam and an aminoglycoside, particularly when there has been spillage of bowel contents. Metronidazole is active only against anaerobic bacteria. **Adverse reactions** are uncommon and include GI symptoms (metallic taste, anorexia, nausea) and neurologic dysfunction (peripheral neuropathy, seizures, ataxia, vertigo).

V. **Miscellaneous considerations**

A. **Aspiration pneumonia**

1. Infectious and noninfectious complications can result from **aspiration of gastric contents** during induction and intubation or at other times in the perioperative period.

a. **Aspiration pneumonitis** (Mendelson syndrome) is a **noninfectious** chemical pneumonitis caused by aspiration of sterile gastric contents.

b. **Aspiration pneumonia** is an infectious process resulting from aspiration of oropharyngeal or nonsterile gastric secretions that contain pathogenic bacteria. The chest radiograph often shows an infiltrate in dependent portions of the lung (often the right lower lobe).

2. **Microbiology.** Aspiration pneumonia is caused by Gram-positive bacteria such as *S. aureus,* Gram-negative bacteria such as *Pseudomonas aeruginosa, Escherichia coli, Klebsiella pneumoniae,* and sometimes anaerobes.

3. **Risk factors for development of aspiration pneumonia** include large-volume aspiration, impaired immunity, colonization of oropharyngeal secretions with pathogenic bacteria, and poor dentition (lower likelihood in edentulous individuals).

4. **Antibiotics and aspiration.** Unnecessary use of antibiotics should be avoided to decrease the chance of colonization with antibiotic-resistant bacteria.

a. Antibiotics should not be used routinely in the initial management of **witnessed aspiration of gastric contents.** Exceptions are situations that predispose to colonization of the usually sterile stomach, such as bowel obstruction and antacid or histamine 2 receptor blocker use. Antibiotics should be considered if pneumonitis fails to improve after 48 hours.

b. **Antibiotics are indicated for aspiration pneumonia.** The choice of antibiotics depends on multiple factors, including the presence of periodontal disease, allergies, and recent antibiotic therapy. Initial therapy targets Gram-negative and Gram-positive bacteria and possibly anaerobic bacteria. Subsequent antibiotic choices should be guided by Gram stain and culture of lower respiratory tract secretions.

B. **Endocarditis.** Patients with congenital and acquired cardiac abnormalities are at risk of developing infective endocarditis after certain surgical and dental procedures and may require perioperative antibiotic endocarditis prophylaxis.

1. **Risk of postoperative endocarditis.** Endocarditis is an uncommon disease and very few cases of bacterial endocarditis are caused by surgery.

2. **Endocarditis prophylaxis.** The American Heart Association has published guidelines for endocarditis prophylaxis that include risk stratification based on the underlying cardiac abnormality and the surgical or dental procedure being performed (Table 7.2).

3. **The risk of endocarditis** depends on the cardiac abnormality.

    a. **Prophylaxis is recommended for high-risk** conditions, including prosthetic valve, complex congenital heart disease, surgically placed systemic pulmonary shunts and conduits, and prior endocarditis.

    b. **Prophylaxis is also recommended for moderate risk** conditions including less complex congenital heart disease (e.g., coarctation of the aorta), bicuspid aortic valve, acquired valvular disease, hypertrophic cardiomyopathy, and mitral valve prolapse with regurgitation.

    c. **Routine prophylaxis is not recommended for negligible risk** conditions including less complex congenital heart disease such as isolated secundum atrial septal defect, mitral valve prolapse without regurgitation, cardiac pacemakers and defibrillators, and innocent heart murmurs.

4. **Bacterial pathogens in postoperative endocarditis** include *Streptococcus, Staphylococcus,* and *Enterococcus.*

5. **Endocarditis prophylaxis is recommended** for procedures that cause bacteremia. Provided that the skin has been appropriately cleaned before incision, surgeries that do not invade viscera or cross mucosal barriers do not produce significant bacteremia. Bacteremia may occur with procedures that cross mucosal barriers or enter an internal viscus such as the GI tract. Antibiotic prophylaxis is recommended for dental and intraoral procedures that may result in significant bleeding such as dental extractions, periodontal surgery, root canal work, and placement of dental implants.

C. **Immunocompromised patients** are at increased risk of community-acquired, nosocomial, and opportunistic infections. **Causes of immunocompromise** include immunosuppressive therapy such as for solid organ and bone marrow transplants, burns, malignancy, HIV infection, chemotherapy, corticosteroids, and severe malnutrition.

1. **Elective surgery** should be delayed, if possible, in patients who are severely immunocompromised (such as total neutrophil count <500 cells/mm^3).

2. **Personnel with respiratory infections** should not be involved in the care of severely immunocompromised patients. If this is not possible, then the provider should wear a surgical mask during contact with the patient.

3. Strict adherence to **sterile technique** is essential in preventing infectious complications.

4. **Antibiotic prophylaxis** is used in organ transplant recipients for short-term prophylaxis against postoperative wound infection and for long-term prevention of opportunistic infections. Some antibiotics have significant interactions with immunosuppressive agents. Cyclosporine metabolism may be altered (with fluoroquinolones, erythromycin, fluconazole, rifampin, isoniazid) and toxicity increased (with aminoglycosides,

amphotericin B, vancomycin, pentamidine, trimethoprim/ sulfamethoxazole) by concomitant administration of various antibiotics. Cyclosporine levels should be monitored in patients receiving these agents.

5. It may be appropriate for immunocompromised patients to wear masks during transport.

D. **Intravascular catheter-related infections** may involve any type of intravenous access but are particularly related to central venous and pulmonary artery catheters. Infection may be localized to the catheter site (site infections) or disseminated (catheter-related bloodstream infections).

1. **Bacterial pathogens** typically include coagulase-negative *Staphylococcus* and *Streptococcus* but may also include a variety of Gram-negative and other Gram-positive bacteria. *Candida* spp. account for about 10% of catheter-related infections.

2. **Risk factors** include total parenteral nutrition and prolonged catheterization.

3. **Clinical manifestations** can include fever and leukocytosis. Although there may be erythema at the catheter insertion site, localized signs of infection are often absent. Patients may develop septic physiology.

4. **Diagnosis.** Cultures of the blood, sputum, and urine should be obtained before initiating antibiotics but should not delay antibiotic administration. Blood cultures should be obtained from two different sites. Often central venous catheters are removed when catheter-related bloodstream infection (CRBSI) is suspected. However, if CRBSI is suspected in a patient with limited vascular access potential, or in whom for other reasons it may be particularly undesirable to remove the catheter, diagnosis may be assisted by obtaining simultaneous quantitative blood cultures from a peripheral vein and the hub of the central venous catheter. A 5- to 10-fold higher colony count in the central line culture versus the peripheral vein culture supports the diagnosis of CRBSI.

5. **Treatment** includes removal of the line and antibiotic administration. Initial empiric coverage should target potential pathogen(s) and should then be tailored to cover the organism(s) cultured from the blood.

   a. **Line removal** protocols vary among institutions and ICUs. At the Massachusetts General Hospital, potentially infected lines are usually replaced at a fresh site unless there are specific mitigating circumstances, such as thrombosis of other central vessels. However, at other institutions, suspected line infections are managed by changing the catheter over a guidewire, analyzing blood cultures and quantitative cultures on the catheter tip, and replacing the line at a fresh site only if the quantitative tip cultures or blood cultures are positive.

   b. **Antibiotic choice** should be guided by the clinical situation and available culture data. Empiric therapy may be necessary if the patient shows symptoms of line infection before defining the causative organism. Antibiotics should be modified to cover appropriate pathogens based on the results of the culture. For uncomplicated catheter-related bacterial infections, antibiotics are continued for

7 to 14 days. However, immunocompromised hosts, particularly those with fungal infections, may require longer courses of treatment.

6. **Prevention** of line infections involves using strict sterile technique during line insertion, including sterile drapes, sterile gloves, sterile gown, cap, and mask. Appropriate skin antisepsis before line placement is also crucial. Studies have shown 2% chlorhexidine to be superior to 10% povidine-iodine and 70% ethanol in preventing catheter-related infections. Finally, a sterile, occlusive dressing should be present on the line insertion site at all times and should be replaced regularly.

7. **Replacement** protocols may vary among institutions and even among different ICUs at the same institution. There has been no demonstrable benefit from routine replacements of catheters, yet many practitioners change central lines after approximately 1 week.

SUGGESTED READING

Belda FJ, Aguilera, de la Garcia A, et al. Supplemental perioperative oxygen and the risk of surgical wound infection: a randomized controlled trial. *JAMA* 2005;294:2035–2042.

Bratzel DW, Houck PM. Antimicrobial prophylaxis for surgery: an advisory statement from the national surgical infection prevention project. *Clin Inf Dis* 2004;38:1706–1715.

Cardo DM, Culver DH, Ciesielski CA, et al. A case-control study of HIV seroconversion in health care workers after percutaneous exposure. *N Engl J Med* 1997;337:1485–1490.

Centers for Disease Control and Prevention. Guidelines for preventing the transmission of Mycobacterium tuberculosis in health care facilities, 1994. *MMWR Morb Mortal Wkly Rep* 1994;43:1–132.

Centers for Disease Control and Prevention. Immunization of health care workers. *MMWR Morb Mortal Wkly Rep* 1997;46:1–42.

Centers for Disease Control and Prevention. Recommendations for prevention and control of hepatitis C virus (HCV) infection and HCV-related chronic disease. *MMWR Morb Mortal Wkly Rep* 1998;47:1–15.

Centers for Disease Control and Prevention. Updated US Public Health Service guidelines for the management of occupational exposures to HBV, HCV, and HIV and recommendations for postexposure prophylaxis. *MMWR Morb Mortal Wkly Rep* 2001;50(RR11):1–42.

Cheng EY, Numphius N, Hennen CR. Antibiotic therapy and the anesthesiologist. *J Clin Anesth* 1995;7:425–439.

Dajani AS, Taubert KA, Wilson W, et al. Prevention of bacterial endocarditis: recommendations by the American Heart Association. *JAMA* 1997;277:1794–1801.

Ludwig KA, Carlson MA, Condon RE. Prophylactic antibiotics in surgery. *Annu Rev Med* 1993;44:385–393.

Marik PE. Aspiration pneumonitis and aspiration pneumonia. *N Engl J Med* 2001;344:665–671.

Moran GJ. Emergency department management of blood and body fluid exposures. *Ann Emerg Med* 2000;35:47–62.

Osmon DR. Antimicrobial prophylaxis in adults. *Mayo Clin Proc* 2000;75:98–109.

Pryor KO, Fahey TJ, Lien CA, and Goldstein PA. 2004. Surgical site infection and the routine use of perioperative hyperoxia in a general surgical population: a randomized controlled trial. *JAMA* 2004;291:79–87.

II

Administration of Anesthesia

8

Safety in Anesthesia

Sara N. Goldhaber-Fiebert and Jeffrey B. Cooper

I. **The risk of anesthesia**
  A. **There is no accurate measure of the overall risk of anesthesia.**
    1. Recent data suggest that anesthesia may contribute to death in about 1 per 10,000 anesthetics. These estimates are speculative because control of the conditions is impossible.
    2. Preventable mortality related to anesthesia in healthy patients (American Society of Anesthesiologists classes 1 and 2) may be on the order of 1 in 100,000. Higher-risk patients undergoing increasingly complex surgical interventions are more likely to be affected by adverse events.
    3. Many other patients suffer serious and costly nonfatal injuries such as permanent neurologic damage.
    4. Although anesthesiology is recognized as a leading specialty in patient safety and adverse outcomes have been markedly reduced, the risks of anesthesia remain substantial. Previous successful efforts to promote safety and reduce preventable deaths and injuries must be maintained and strengthened.
  B. **Accidents leading to injury are primarily caused by system failures, but human error is a strong contributor to most preventable adverse outcomes.**
    1. At least half of adverse events could have been prevented and may have resulted from deviations from accepted anesthesia practices.
    2. There is rarely a single cause for an accident. Most accidents evolve from one or more trigger events or system failures. System failures are breakdowns in the checks and balances required for the safe operation of the system. The accepted approach to accident prevention now focuses on flaws in the system rather than on flaws in the operator.
    3. Near mishaps are much more prevalent than the events that result in injury. These "near-miss" events can be used as indicators of the overall safety of the system.
    4. Adverse outcomes usually can be attributed to one or more of the following direct or indirect causes: hypovolemia, hypoxia, hypotension, hypoventilation, airway obstruction, drug overdose, aspiration, inadequate preparation, inadequate supervision, miscommunication, or poor crisis management.
  C. **Vigilance and attention to detail are essential for a safely conducted anesthetic.** Vigilance allows the anesthetist to remain aware of surrounding events and signals while performing other tasks. Attention to detail allows the anesthetist to actively focus on an issue (such as accurately labeling a syringe) in the midst of concurrent extensive sensory input. Coordinating different cognitive levels (thinking versus doing) and managing many problems simultaneously are essential parts of dynamic decision making.

D. **Serious mishaps typically involve a lapse in vigilance in combination with errors in knowledge, judgment, or skill.** These combinations may be triggered by the interactions of the patient, the equipment, the anesthetist, the surgeon, and the environment. These factors can combine to obscure the prompt detection or the appropriate correction of a problem. Disorderly personal routines, disorganized workspace ergonomics, and faulty or intermittent charting can contribute to accidents.

II. **General safety strategies**

A. **Prepare a preoperative plan.** Construct a sound anesthesia plan (including prioritizing goals and contingencies for crisis); become familiar with the procedure, equipment, and anesthetic technique; prepare the patient; prepare the workspace (including ergonomic considerations of maneuverability, unobstructed visual field, access to patient and machine); perform a complete checkout of the anesthesia workstation, monitors, and other devices; check backup equipment; label all medications; after reviewing the anesthesia plan obtain any extra medications or equipment that may be needed. Know the location of emergency supplies and equipment.

B. **Develop situational awareness.** Use a systematic approach to scanning the machine, monitors, patient, surgical field, and surroundings. Arrange equipment and appropriate monitors in a way that facilitates this. Constantly assess the "big picture" and construct differential diagnoses to explain the observed events as well as "mental maps" of the different possible interventions. If one vital sign is anomalous, quickly assess the others while repeating the measurement and observing what is happening on the surgical field.

C. **Enhance teamwork; communicate.** Teamwork enhances safety and may be essential for preventing or recovering from a critical situation. A healthy team has mutual collegial respect; members share tasks, goals, and key information, thus enabling all members to do their jobs well. To enhance teamwork and communication, address surgeons and nurses early in the case by knowing names and establishing eye contact. Make requests and delegate tasks clearly and specifically by name; request verbal confirmation of all assigned tasks (e.g., "Jack, do task X and tell me when task X is completed.") Delegate tasks to those who can best perform them. Never assume that crucial interventions or medications have been given as planned, until they are confirmed.

D. **Compensate for stressors.** Recognize conditions that decrease performance: production pressure, noise, poor lighting, fatigue, boredom, illness, hunger, and interpersonal tension. Attempt to optimize the work environment including simple steps, such as turning on a light. Consider more subtle issues such as recognizing one's own limitations by asking for needed relief when overtired or ill.

E. **Verify observations.** Cross-check observations with redundant systems (e.g., check heart rate with both the electrocardiogram and with pulse oximeter), and assess covarying variables (e.g., look for a concomitant change in heart rate with an increase in blood pressure). When a situation does not make sense, review it with a second person.

F. **Implement compensatory responses.** React to a developing problem by implementing time-buying measures until a more definitive solution is found (e.g., increase the fraction of inspired oxygen when oxygen saturation falls; administer intravenous fluids or vasopressors when hypotension occurs). However, do not let the compensatory responses provide the only repair to the problem. Search out any correctable primary cause and treat it appropriately.

G. **Prepare for crisis.** Be prepared for critical events. Actively plan for contingencies, and be prepared to revise the plan. **Calling for help is an appropriate response when confronted with potentially overwhelming circumstances.** Learn to call for help early because it may not be available immediately. Review, practice, and use accepted protocols for emergencies and resuscitation (e.g., advanced cardiac life support, malignant hyperthermia protocols).

H. **Recognize and address production pressures** including **time and economic constraints. These sometimes conflict with** adequate preoperative evaluation, preparation, and monitoring as well as causing pressure to do a case even when there are medical reasons to cancel. If you are uncertain about proceeding with the case or believe it is unsafe to anesthetize the patient, address concerns explicitly to your colleagues. Pressure to put efficiency and output ahead of safety has caused catastrophic accidents in various industries. Patient safety must remain the highest priority, despite overt or covert pressures and incentives on personnel to emphasize production.

I. **Learn from close calls.** An event that nearly results in an adverse outcome should be used to improve future performance under similar circumstances. Every mistake is an opportunity to learn and improve. Report such events via your department's quality assurance mechanism.

III. **Crucial errors to know and avoid**
Following is a partial list of important pitfalls to avoid. This list was compiled from clinician experiences, quality assurance analysis, and theoretical mechanisms described in the literature. Many of these errors may be quickly lethal or result in significant morbidity. While systems factors (discussed above) often promote errors or compound their effects, the errors listed here can arise simply from lack of knowledge of a particular pitfall and therefore are worth specifically knowing about. An expanded list, with significantly more extensive explanations, diagrams, and tips for prevention and treatment, can be found on the website of the Massachusetts General Hospital's Department of Anesthesia and Critical Care (www.etherdome.org under "Patient Care").

A. **Airway errors**
1. A **Passy-Muir valve** left on a tracheostomy when inflating the cuff to deliver positive pressure ventilation causes **repeated inflation of the patient's lungs with no mechanism for exhalation.**
2. **If the backup O_2 tank is left on** after the machine check is performed, it may delay detection of a pipeline failure until the backup O_2 cylinder is also empty.
3. **Insufficient preoxygenation** can lead to significant **desaturation if intubation becomes difficult.**
4. **Accidental extubation during a prone surgery** can cause extreme difficulty in reestablishing an airway.
5. **Extubation of a patient** (accidentally) **during transport** can cause loss of airway control.
6. **Insufficient O_2 in the tank** during **transport** can cause severe desaturation.

B. Medication errors

1. **Administration of undiluted dilantin by rapid intravenous infusion** can cause refractory hypotension, arrhythmias, and death.

2. **Administration of undiluted potassium by rapid intravenous infusion** can cause ventricular fibrillation and cardiac arrest.

3. **Neostigmine given without an antimuscarinic drug (e.g., glycopyrrolate)** can cause **asystole**, severe bradycardia and atrioventricular block and can be fatal.

4. **Succinylcholine** can cause severe **hyperkalemia and dysrhythmias,** may trigger **malignant hyperthermia, and may be fatal** given in situations where it is contraindicated.

5. **Medications** to which a patient is **allergic** can cause **anaphylaxis.**

6. **Administering the wrong blood** (clerical error) can cause an **incompatibility reaction** that can be fatal.

C. Procedure errors

1. Unrecognized **iatrogenic tension pneumothorax** can cause **rapid cardiovascular collapse.**

2. Inadvertent **intravascular injection of local anesthetics** during a nerve block can cause **neurologic** and **cardiac toxicity,** which can be fatal (especially with bupivacaine).

3. **Avoidable epidural hematomas** may develop when spinal or epidural anesthetics are performed in **patients who have coagulopathies.**

4. **Air embolisms** may occur during the placement or removal of **central venous catheters** and may cause significant hemodynamic instability.

5. **Air embolisms** may occur in **pressurized intravenous systems** that contain **air in the intravenous bag or unprimed intravenous tubing.**

6. **Limb necrosis** can develop if the tourniquet used for intravenous placement or blood draw is left on the anesthetized patient for a prolonged period.

7. **Intracranial pressure may be increased** if a **ventriculostomy drain** is connected to a **pressurized bag of heparin-treated saline** (in a patient who likely already has a high intracranial pressure).

IV. Quality assurance

Quality assurance programs take many different forms but must include a spectrum of activities aimed at maintaining and improving the quality of care and minimizing the risk of injury from anesthesia.

A. Documentation. A quality assurance incident report is completed for any unusual occurrence, unforeseen outcome, patient injury, or near miss, especially if follow-up action may be required to prevent recurrence. The report should include the relevant facts and avoid judgmental statements. Incidents are reviewed by the departmental quality assurance committee, which receives additional information from those involved in the event and may suggest compensatory mechanisms as systematic factors are identified. Cases with special educational value should be presented at departmental case conferences. There should be an ongoing analysis and feedback of adverse events (actual and near-miss events) to identify and assess system problems and developing patterns. (See section V.C. for further details.)

B. **Standards and guidelines.** Anesthesiologists should be aware of their institution's safety policies and procedures. These should include those for monitoring, response to an adverse event, hand-off checklist, resuscitation protocols, perioperative testing, and any special procedures or practices for the use of drugs, equipment, and supplies. (See section V below and www.asahq.org for national standards and practice guidelines.)

C. **Safety training.** Anesthesia providers should obtain training in safety to learn and maintain basic skills. Training should include **basic environmental safety** (fire and evacuation, electrical safety (see Chapter 18), **prevention of cross-infection** (see Chapter 7), and **crisis management skills** (e.g., advanced cardiac life support, advanced trauma life support, pediatric advanced life support, anesthesia crisis resource management, malignant hyperthermia treatment). Simulation techniques should be used wherever practical to allow practice under semirealistic conditions. Special attention should be given to learning generic critical-event management skills, including role clarity (e.g., leadership, task delegation), communication (using names, closing the loop of instructions), resource management (e.g., allocating personnel, time, and equipment), appropriate use of support (e.g., assigning responsibilities, monitoring, and cross-checking information), and global assessment (e.g., avoiding fixation errors, maintaining situational awareness).

D. Safety is influenced by an institution's work culture. **A constant commitment to safety, including the presence of redundant systems, continual training, and a dedication to learning from mistakes, are all needed in an organization's culture.**

V. **Standards and protocols**

Three important and illustrative protocols are described here:

A. **The American Society of Anesthesiologists' standards for basic anesthetic monitoring** apply to all anesthesia care, although in emergency circumstances appropriate life support measures take precedence. Under extenuating circumstances, the responsible anesthesiologist may waive some requirements. These standards are not intended for application to the care of the obstetric patient in labor or in the conduct of pain management. All anesthesia providers should be aware of the complete current standards (see Chapter 10 and www.asahq.org), which describe specific provisions and exceptions. The key elements are as follows:

1. **Qualified anesthesia personnel** shall be present in the room throughout the course of all general anesthetics, regional anesthetics, and monitored anesthesia care.

2. **Continually evaluate** the patient's *oxygenation* (via an oxygen analyzer and pulse oximeter), *ventilation* (via clinical signs and capnometry; continual end-tidal carbon dioxide analysis must be used with tracheal intubation; some form of monitoring with an audible alarm must be used during mechanical ventilation), *circulation* (continuous EKG; blood pressure and heart rate at least every 5 min; one or more of the following: palpation of a pulse, auscultation of heart sounds, monitoring of a tracing of intra-arterial pressure, ultrasound peripheral pulse monitoring, pulse plethysmography or oxime-

try), and *temperature* (by any means, when clinically significant changes in body temperature are intended, anticipated, or suspected).

B. **Handoffs and team communication**
1. Periodic breaks should be given to the primary individuals providing anesthesia. **Handoffs** should be avoided, if possible, during short cases and should be used with caution in cases characterized by complexity—i.e., if the anesthesiologist's intuitive sense of anesthetic management cannot be satisfactorily transferred to another person. **The record should indicate the time of the change.**
2. **During a relief handoff, the following information should be clearly presented** before the original anesthesiologist leaves the room. See Figure 8.1 for an example of a handoff checklist.

Handoff Checklist

Prior clinical details:
[ ] Patient name/age, surgery, attending surgeon, diagnosis, HPI
[ ] Team members/introductions
[ ] Allergies (and reactions)
[ ] Baseline status (functional status, mentation, ability to cooperate)
[ ] Weight
[ ] PMH/PSH
[ ] Medications (and pertinent past meds, e.g., steroids, anticoagulants)
[ ] Pertinent labs/studies

Intraoperative (management, anticipated plans):
[ ] Airway assessment, management, difficulties? ventilator settings
[ ] Anesthetics/narcotics/pressors/relaxant/antiernetic (meds due/planned? concentrations of prepared meds?)
[ ] Antibiotics (given? next due?)
[ ] Current vitals and trends
[ ] Fluid status (fluids given, urine, EBL, available blood products, ongoing plans)
[ ] Lines
[ ] Current labs, planned labs (to be drawn)
[ ] Progress of surgery
[ ] Ancillary equipment (e.g., tourniquet, laser)
[ ] Any concerns/issues? (e.g., patient status, lines, machines, equipment, surgery)
[ ] Plan to extubate?
[ ] Anticipate need for monitoring/equipment during transport?
[ ] Postop destination? (bed called for?)
[ ] Postop concerns (e.g., analgesia plan, need for consults, UO)
[ ] Any questions from relieving anesthetist?

Figure 8.1.   Handoff checklist. This is an example of a tool to guide the transfer of patient care intraoperatively, from one anesthetist to another. HPI = History of Present Illness; PMH = Past Medical History; PSH = Past Surgical History; EBL = Estimated Blood Loss; UO = Urine Output.

a. **Prior clinical details.** The patient's diagnosis, surgery, allergies, past medical and surgical history, relevant medications, and any pertinent normal or abnormal laboratory values or studies.

b. **Intraoperative management.** Status of surgery, airway assessment and management techniques, anesthetic plan and current status, current vital signs with an explanation for any apparent abnormalities or trends, intravenous access and monitoring, blood loss and volume status assessment (including status of blood bank sample plus blood product repletion and availability), anticipated need for additional medications (e.g., narcotics, muscle relaxation or reversal, antiemetics), and disposition, including location for recovery as well as anticipated need for continued support or monitoring on transport (e.g., inotropic agents, prolonged intubation).

3. **Communication with surgeons.** Concerns about a patient's ability to tolerate elective surgery/anesthesia and the need for further diagnosis or treatment, to optimize intraoperative management, should be addressed with the primary surgical team. The responsible surgeons should also be informed early of possible postoperative anesthetic complications that may affect postoperative care.

4. **Communication with other physicians,** including recovery room anesthesiologists, should be initiated as deemed appropriate. This is in addition to the standard detailed reports given to nursing staff. The communication should be a brief **alert** as to why the physician should be aware of the patient, including pertinent history and intraoperative management (e.g., patient with difficult airway).

C. **Guidelines for action after an adverse anesthesia event.** The following guidelines for action should be used when a patient has died, or has been injured, from causes suspected to be related to anesthesia management:

1. **The objectives** are to limit patient injury from a specific adverse event associated with anesthesia and to ensure that the causes of the event are identified so that a recurrence can be prevented. The activities aim at ensuring care of the patient, preventing loss or alteration of equipment or supplies related to the event, documenting information, informing appropriate personnel, and providing necessary guidance and support to caregivers.

2. **The guidelines** dictate the responsibilities for the primary anesthesiologist, the incident supervisor (preferably someone other than the primary anesthesiologist involved in the event), the equipment manager, and the follow-up supervisor.

3. **The anesthesiologist** involved in an adverse event should do the following:

a. Provide for continuing care of the patient.

b. Notify the anesthesia operating room administrator as soon as possible. If a resident or certified registered nurse anesthetist was involved in the event, (s)he should notify the attending staff.

c. Not discard supplies or tamper with equipment.

  d. Document events in the patient record (including the serial number of the anesthesia machine).

  e. Not alter the record.

  f. Stay involved with the follow-up care.

  g. Contact consultants as needed.

  h. Submit a follow-up report to the department quality assurance committee.

  i. Document continuing care in the patient's record.

SUGGESTED READING

American Society of Anesthesiologists (www.asahq.org/publicationsServices.htm), accessed January 30, 2006.

Anesthesia Patient Safety Foundation (www.apsf.org) accessed January 30, 2006.

Beckmann U, Runciman WB. The role of incident reporting in continuous quality improvement in the intensive care setting. *Anaesth Intensive Care* 1996;24: 311–313.

Bognar SM. *Human error in medicine.* Hillsdale, NJ: Lawrence Erlbaum, 1994.

Cooper JB, Gaba DM. A strategy for preventing anesthesia accidents. *Int Anesthesiol Clin* 1989;27:148–152.

Cooper JB, Newbower RS, Kitz RJ. An analysis of major errors and equipment failures in anesthesia management: considerations for prevention and detection. *Anesthesiology* 1984;60:34–42.

Gaba DM. Anaesthesiology as a model for patient safety in health care. *BMJ* 2000;320:785–788. Available at: www.bmj.com/cgi/content/full/320/7237/785.

Gaba DM, Fish K, Howard S. *Anesthesia crisis management.* New York: Churchill Livingstone, 1994.

Goldhaber-Fiebert SN, Torri A. Crucial Errors in Anesthesia to Know and Avoid. Internal Anesthesia Department Materials at Massachusetts General Hospital. Personal Communication. Dec. 2005. Available at : www.etherdome.org under patient care.

Howard SK, Gaba DM, Fish KJ, et al. Anesthesia crisis resource management training: teaching anesthesiologists to handle critical incidents. *Aviat Space Environ Med* 1992;63:763–770.

Institute for Safe Medication Practice (www.ISMP.org), accessed January 30, 2006.

Keats AS. Anesthesia mortality in perspective. *Anesth Analg* 1990;71:113–119.

Kohn LT, Corrigan JM, Donaldson MS, eds. *To err is human: building a safer healthcare system.* Washington, DC: National Academy Press, 1999.

Leape LL. Error in medicine. *JAMA* 1994;272:1851–1857.

Morrell RC, Eichhorn JH. *Patient safety in anesthetic practice.* New York: Churchill Livingstone, 1997.

National Patient Safety Foundation (www.npsf.org), accessed January 30, 2006

Rall M, Gaba DM. Human performance in patient safety. In: *Miller's Anesthesia,* Miller RD, ed. New York: Elsevier Churchill Livingstone, 2005;3021–3072.

9

The Anesthesia Machine

Greg Ginsburg and Jane C. Ballantyne

I. **Overview.** The basic function of the anesthesia machine is to pre-
    pare a gas mixture of precisely known and variable composition for
    delivery to the patient. The machine provides a controlled flow of oxy-
    gen, nitrous oxide, air, and anesthetic vapors. These are delivered to a
    breathing system, which provides a means to deliver positive pressure
    ventilation and to control alveolar carbon dioxide by minimizing re-
    breathing and/or by absorbing carbon dioxide. A mechanical ventilator
    is connected to the breathing system, freeing the anesthetist's hands
    for other tasks. Various monitors are used to survey the functioning of
    the system, to detect equipment failures, and to provide information
    about the patient.

II. **The gas delivery system** (Figure 9.1)

A. **Gas supplies**

1. **Piped gases.** Wall outlets supply oxygen, nitrous oxide, and
    air at a pressure of 50 to 55 pounds/in^2 (psi). These outlets
    and the supply hoses to the machine are diameter indexed
    and color-coded.

2. **Cylinders**

    a. **A full cylinder (size E) of oxygen** has a pressure of 2,000
        to 2,200 psi and contains the equivalent of 660 L of
        gas at atmospheric pressure and room temperature. The
        oxygen cylinder pressure decreases in direct proportion
        to the amount of oxygen in the cylinder.

    b. **A full cylinder (size E) of nitrous oxide** has a pressure
        of 745 psi and contains the equivalent of 1,500 L of
        gas at atmospheric pressure and room temperature. The
        nitrous oxide in the full cylinder is mostly in the liquid
        phase; the cylinder pressure does not decrease until the
        liquid content is exhausted, at which time one-fourth of
        the total volume of gas remains.

    c. **Air cylinders** are present on some machines. A full cylin-
        der (size E) has a pressure of 1,800 psi and contains the
        equivalent of 630 L at atmospheric pressure and room
        temperature.

    d. **Pressure regulators** reduce the high pressure from the
        cylinders to about 45 psi (just below pipeline pressure)
        so that, when cylinder gases are used, adjustments at the
        rotameter are not needed to compensate for the chang-
        ing pressure that occurs as the cylinders empty. If both
        cylinders and pipelines are connected and open, gas flows
        preferentially from the pipeline because its pressure is
        slightly higher than the regulated cylinder pressure. The
        regulators divide the machine into high-pressure (prox-
        imal to the regulator) and low-pressure (distal to the
        regulator) systems.

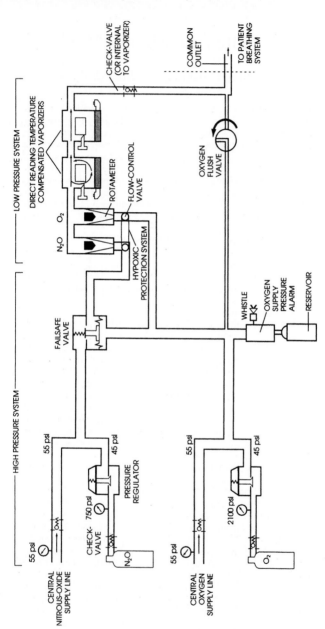

Figure 9.1. Schematic of an anesthesia machine. There are many variations in design depending on vintage and manufacturer.

B. **Flow control valves and flowmeters** control and measure gas flows.

1. **A needle valve** controls the flow of each gas. As a safety feature, the oxygen control knob is fluted and protrudes more than the nitrous oxide and air controls. Gas pressures are reduced from 45 to 55 psi (high pressure) to near atmospheric pressure (low pressure) by the needle valves.

2. **Flowmeters.** Each flowmeter is a calibrated tapered glass tube in which a bobbin or ball floats to indicate the flow of gas. The oxygen flowmeter is always placed downstream so that a leak will be less likely to result in delivery of a hypoxic gas mixture.

C. **Vaporizers.** Anesthesia machines are outfitted with one or more temperature-compensated flow-over vaporizers calibrated to deliver a specific concentration of anesthetic measured as percent by volume. These vaporizers operate on the principle that a small proportion of the total gas mixture delivered to them is diverted into a vaporizing chamber, where it becomes fully saturated with anesthetic before it is added back to the main flow. The concentration of anesthetic delivered by the vaporizer is therefore proportional to the amount of gas passing through the vaporizing chamber, which is controlled primarily by the vaporizer dial. Because saturated vapor pressure varies with temperature, a secondary mechanism alters the amount of gas diverted through the chamber to compensate for temperature changes. The vaporizers are calibrated for a specific anesthetic and have pin-indexed filling adapters to prevent inadvertent mixing of anesthetics. The vaporizing chamber is enclosed in a metal case to enhance heat transfer and to compensate for the heat lost from cooling as the anesthetic evaporates. The desflurane vaporizer is heated and pressurized to compensate for the anesthetic's relatively high vapor pressure and the extreme cooling that occurs when high concentrations are vaporized.

D. The **common gas outlet** is the port where gases exit the machine; it is connected to the breathing system via the fresh gas hose.

E. **Oxygen flush valve.** One hundred percent oxygen at 45 to 55 psi comes directly from the high-pressure system to the common gas outlet. Oxygen flow can be as high as 40 to 60 L/min.

III. **Breathing systems.** The circle system is most commonly used. The T-piece systems (Mapleson D and F) are used in infants because of low resistance and small dead space.

A. **The circle system.** The circle system incorporates a carbon dioxide absorber and prevents rebreathing of exhaled carbon dioxide. The system allows low fresh gas flows that conserve use of expensive inhalation anesthetics and maintain higher humidity and temperature within the breathing circuit. The circle consists of an absorber, two one-way valves, a Y-piece adapter, a reservoir bag, and an adjustable pressure limiting (APL) "pop off" valve (Figure 9.2).

1. The **carbon dioxide absorber.** Sodalime ($CaOH_2$ + NaOH + KOH + silica) or Baralyme ($Ba[OH]_2$ + $Ca[OH]_2$) contained in the absorber combines with carbon dioxide, forming $CaCO_2$ and liberating heat and moisture (H_2O). A pH-sensitive dye changes to blue-violet, indicating exhaustion of the absorbing capacity. The top canister should be changed

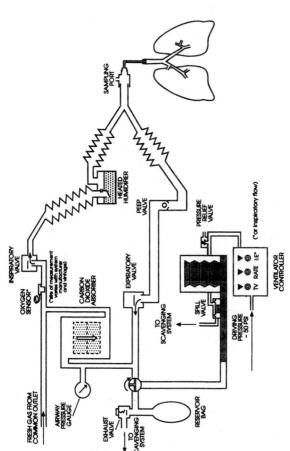

Figure 9.2. Representative circle breathing system with ventilator. The airway pressure gauge may sense on the patient side of the inspiratory valve. The positive end-expiratory pressure (PEEP) valve may be integral to the ventilator. Other variations are possible depending on the manufacturer.

when 25% to 50% of the pellets have changed color, although a second canister provides a safety margin.

2. Two **one-way valves** (inspiratory and expiratory) ensure that exhaled gas is not rebreathed without passing through the carbon dioxide absorber.

3. The **Y-piece adapter** is used to connect the inspiratory and expiratory sides of the system to the patient.

4. The **reservoir bag and APL valve** are located on the expiratory limb. The reservoir bag accumulates gas between inspirations. It is used to visualize spontaneous ventilation and to assist ventilation manually. Typically a 3-L reservoir bag is used for adult patients; smaller bags may be appropriate for pediatric patients. The APL valve is used to control the pressure in the breathing system and allows excess gas to escape. The valve can be adjusted from fully open (for spontaneous ventilation, minimal peak pressure 1 to 3 cm H_2O) to fully closed (maximum pressure 75 cm H_2O or greater). Dangerously high pressures that can produce barotrauma and hemodynamic compromise may occur if the valve is left unattended in the fully or partially closed position.

B. **The T-piece systems.** The T-piece systems are single-limbed rebreathing systems. Because there is no CO_2 absorber, rebreathing of CO_2 is inevitable unless a fresh gas flow at least equal to the patient's peak flow is used. Inspired CO_2 concentration is controlled by the fresh gas flow and/or by varying the minute ventilation. Mapleson classified all possible configurations of single-limbed rebreathing systems (the T-pieces included) according to the relative position of patient, fresh gas flow, reservoir bag, and valve. The Mapleson D and F systems are used most frequently and are both T-piece systems. All the T-piece systems require high fresh gas flows (at least two to three times minute ventilation) to prevent rebreathing during spontaneous ventilation. Capnography is useful to verify sufficient washout of carbon dioxide.

1. The **Mapleson D** circuit is a semiclosed system with a reservoir bag and APL valve at the machine end with fresh gas entering at the patient end (Figure 9.3).

2. The **Bain** circuit is a coaxial version of the Mapleson D. The fresh gas delivery tube is a small-diameter uncorrugated tube that runs inside the corrugated wide-diameter expiratory limb. Inspired gases are warmed and the system appears simpler, but there is a risk of hypoxia if leaks develop, so the circuit should always be carefully checked for leaks before use.

3. The **Mapleson F** circuit (Jackson-Rees modification of the Ayres T-piece or Mapleson E) is particularly useful in neonates and small infants. It consists simply of an open-ended reservoir bag and a defined length of corrugated breathing tube, with fresh gas entering the system at the patient end. Manual ventilation of small patients is accomplished well with this system because the anesthetist can adjust the filling of the open-ended reservoir bag with his or her hand, making the bag a sensitive indicator of lung compliance. The system also allows the anesthetist to be close to the infant while manually ventilating. The advantages of this system have been reduced by the introduction of scavenging systems

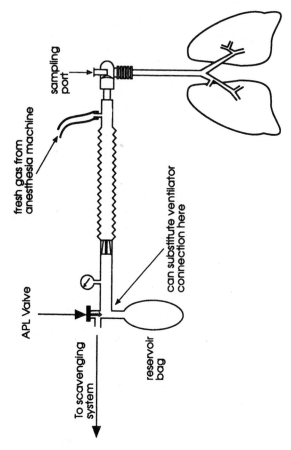

Figure 9.3. Schematic of a Mapleson D breathing system. In the Bain modification, the fresh gas flows through a tube that runs through the corrugated tubing.

that increase its weight and by improvements in alternative systems (e.g., low-compliance breathing tubes and improvements in mechanical ventilators).

IV. Anesthesia ventilators

A. Conventional anesthesia machines are fitted with a mechanical ventilator that uses a **collapsible bellows within a closed chamber.** The bellows is compressed intermittently when oxygen or air is directed into the chamber, thereby pressurizing it. The ventilators are time-cycled flow (as opposed to pressure) generators, controlled both mechanically and electronically, and pneumatically driven (requiring 10 to 20 L of driving gas per minute). Ventilator controls vary among makes and models. Some ventilators require setting of minute ventilation, rate, and inspiratory/expiratory (I/E) ratio to produce the desired tidal volume; other ventilators allow direct adjustment of tidal volume, with I/E ratio dependent on the inspiratory flow rate, which is set independently. A portion of the fresh gas flow delivered by the machine adds to the set tidal volume during the inhalation phase. For example, an increase in total fresh gas flow from 3 to 6 L/min will increase delivered minute ventilation by an additional 1 L/min at an I/E ratio of 1:2 or by 1.5 L/min at an I/E ratio of 1:1 (more inspiratory time in the latter). Although gas-driven ventilators can be safely driven with either oxygen or air, most often oxygen is chosen and is supplied by pipeline. Whether cylinder gases are used to drive the ventilator in the event of pipeline failure is usually determined by the user. If the machine is set up to drive the ventilator using cylinder oxygen, mechanical ventilation should be discontinued in the event of pipeline failure to conserve oxygen supplies.

B. **Flow generators** deliver a set tidal volume regardless of changes in patients' compliance (unlike pressure generators) but will not compensate for system leaks and may produce barotrauma because high pressures can be generated. They reliably deliver the preset tidal volume (even in the presence of a small leak). The risk of barotrauma is minimal because most patients presenting to the operating room have healthy normally compliant lungs.

C. For infants and patients with diseased lungs, maintaining preset tidal volumes may produce unacceptably high airway pressures and increased risk of barotrauma. **Pressure generators** are more appropriate in these situations, because airway pressure is controlled and barotrauma risk is minimized.

D. The lack of flexibility of many anesthesia machine ventilators severely limits their use in the setting of abnormal lung mechanics. In these situations, the use of manual ventilation or a critical care ventilator may be preferred. Relatively new anesthesia machines feature versatile **microprocessor-controlled ventilators,** which allow for sophisticated manipulation and monitoring of airway pressures (e.g., variable positive end-expiratory pressure [PEEP]) and flow rates. These ventilators incorporate a piston rather than a bellows and are also notable for more consistent delivery of set tidal volumes independent of fresh gas flow rates. As is the case with ICU ventilators, newer anesthesia machines are capable of multiple modes (such as pressure control, pressure support, synchronized mandatory, and inverse ratio ventilation), thereby enabling the anesthetist to optimize ventilation, oxygenation, hemodynamics, and weaning.

V. **Safety features**

A. An **audible oxygen alarm** is fitted in the oxygen supply line of the high-pressure system. It consists of a pressure regulator and a reed or whistle that will sound when the pressure in the supply line is greater than 0 and less than about 25 psi.

B. A pressure-operated **"fail safe" valve** in the high-pressure system of the nitrous oxide supply line opens only when oxygen pressure in the high-pressure system is above 25 psi. If the oxygen pressure falls below that, nitrous oxide will cease to flow. Because both the audible oxygen alarm and the fail-safe valve respond specifically to low pressure in the oxygen supply line of the high-pressure system, neither protects against the delivery of a hypoxic mixture downstream in the low-pressure system (e.g., if the oxygen flow control valve is accidentally shut off).

C. **Oxygen ratio control.** All new anesthetic machines are fitted with a device to control the proportion of oxygen delivered. This may take the form of a mechanical link between the oxygen and nitrous oxide flow control knobs that will not allow a fraction of inspired oxygen (FIO_2) of <25% to be set. Alternatively, some machines incorporate an oxygen ratio monitor that sounds an alarm if a low FIO_2 is set.

D. **Pressure alarms** are incorporated into all anesthesia machines, but different manufacturers use different pressure alarm systems.

1. A **low-pressure alarm** is triggered by a period of no pressure in the system or by a sustained pressure drop below atmospheric pressure. Low pressure may be caused by a disconnection or large leak in the system. Negative pressure usually indicates a scavenging system malfunction or that the patient is inhaling against an obstruction.

2. A **high-pressure alarm** may have a variable or a preset (e.g., 65 cm H_2O) limit. A high-pressure alarm may indicate obstruction in the tubing or endotracheal tube or a change in pulmonary compliance (e.g., bronchospasm or pneumothorax).

3. A **continuing pressure alarm** alerts the user in the event of high pressure being sustained for more than a few seconds. A blocked or closed pop-off valve, a malfunctioning ventilator pressure relief valve, or an obstruction in the scavenging system could create this condition.

VI. **Scavenging.** A scavenging system channels waste gases away from the operating room to a location outside the hospital building or a location where the gases can be discharged safely (e.g., to a nonrecirculating exhaust ventilating system). The ambient concentration of anesthetic gases in the operating room should not exceed 25 parts per million (ppm) for nitrous oxide and 2 ppm for halogenated agents. Specific anesthetic gas-scavenging systems should be used routinely. These systems consist of a collecting system, a transfer system, a receiving system, and a disposal system.

A. The **collecting system** delivers waste gases to the transfer system and operates from the APL valve and from the expiratory valve of the ventilator. In addition, waste gases may be collected from the gas analyzers.

B. The **transfer system** consists of tubing that connects the collecting and receiving systems.

C. The **receiving system** ensures that neither positive nor negative pressure builds at the patient end of the system. The system may be open or closed. An open system consists of a reservoir canister opened to atmosphere at one end. Suction usually is applied to the canister, exhausting the waste gas. A closed system consists of a reservoir bag with positive and negative pressure relief valves to maintain the pressure in the bag within an acceptable range.

D. The **disposal system** may be passive or active, although passive systems are inadequate for modern hospitals. A passive system consists of wide-bore tubing that carries gases directly to the exterior or into the exhaust ventilation ducts. Active systems can be powered by vacuum systems, fans, pumps, or Venturi systems.

VII. Gas analysis. Several methods are used to monitor concentrations of O_2, CO_2, and anesthetic gases in the breathing system. The oxygen analyzer is the most important monitor for detecting a hypoxic gas mixture. Capnometry, the measurement of CO_2, has many uses, including monitoring the adequacy of ventilation and detecting breathing system faults. Breath-to-breath monitoring of anesthetic concentrations provides tracking of anesthetic uptake and distribution. Most gas analyzers incorporate alarms. Among the techniques for measurement are the following:

A. **Mass spectrometry** can provide rapid response measurement of the concentration of any gas, but the spectrometer itself is very large and must be housed in a central location where it can serve a number of operating rooms. A sample of gas is withdrawn through a side port in the breathing system near the Y piece and carried through a nylon catheter to the central mass spectrometer. The sample is ionized in an electron beam. The resulting fragments are accelerated through a high-voltage field and then subjected to a deflecting magnetic field. The specific fragments are detected on collectors, and the relative concentration of each agent is determined. Calibration is performed automatically at the central system. By a switching system, the mass spectrometer can sample from as many as 32 locations. The time between measurements in each room may be one or several minutes depending on the number of rooms "on line." A "stat" sample may be requested.

B. **Infrared analysis** uses spectrophotometry and Beer's law to provide continuous measurement of the concentration of gas or anesthetic in a gas mixture. Gases that have two or more different atoms in the molecule absorb infrared radiation; thus, infrared analysis can be used to measure concentrations of CO_2, N_2O, and halogenated anesthetics but not O_2. Typically, some gas is withdrawn from the breathing system at a steady rate (50 to 300 mL/min) and passed into a small measurement chamber in the instrument. Pulses of infrared energy at a wavelength that is absorbed only by the gas of interest are beamed through the gas, and the difference in energy absorbed is used to determine the gas concentration. In some capnographs, a miniaturized measurement chamber and sensor are placed in the breathing system. In most infrared instruments, only one preselected volatile anesthetic can be measured at a time.

C. **Oxygen analyzers.** Continuous measurements of oxygen concentrations in a mixture of gases can be provided by mass spectrometry; polarographic, galvanic or fuel cell analysis; or paramagnetic analysis.

1. **Polarographic oxygen analyzers.** The analyzer sensor is placed in the inspiratory limb of the circuit. The sensor consists of an anode and a cathode in an electrolyte solution with a polarizing voltage. Oxygen diffuses through a semipermeable membrane into the electrolyte solution, after which a current flows dependent on the uptake of oxygen at the cathode and thus on the partial pressure of oxygen. Sensors have a limited life span; replacement cells are needed periodically. The sensor should be placed in the upright position to avoid accumulation of moisture and may require occasional removal and drying.

2. **Galvanic or fuel cell analyzers** are similar to polarographic cell analyzers except that different anode, cathode, and electrolyte materials are used and no polarizing voltage is applied. This cell is similar to a battery that consumes oxygen.

3. **Paramagnetic analyzers.** These analyzers are based on the principle that oxygen is paramagnetic and therefore attracted to a magnetic field, whereas most other gases are weakly diamagnetic and therefore repelled from a magnetic field. Modern miniaturized paramagnetic analyzers incorporate a rapidly oscillating magnetic chamber and are capable of breath-to-breath analysis. They are often combined with another gas analysis technique in an anesthetic agent monitor.

VIII. **Accessories**

A. A **backup means of positive-pressure ventilation** (self-inflating bag) should be available for any anesthetic procedure.

B. A **humidifier** may be used and is indicated especially for infants and small children and during high-flow anesthesia. Two types generally are used during anesthesia: water bath and condenser humidifiers. Water bath humidifiers are associated with a risk of overheating (with consequent injury to the patient) and with risk of infection. Condenser humidifiers increase the resistance of the breathing system but are simpler to use than water bath humidifiers. High resistance makes them unsuitable for use with small children.

C. A **PEEP valve** can be connected to the expiratory limb of the breathing system. Many new machines have built-in PEEP capability.

D. A **flashlight** should be available in case of power failure.

E. **Computerized information management systems,** including electronic anesthetic records, are increasingly replacing written medical and anesthetic records. Advantages may include enhanced documentation including automated perioperative patient data collection, accessible databases that facilitate quality improvement and resource utilization, enhanced billing accuracy and completeness, and efficient compliance with various regulatory and accreditation requirements.

IX. **Next-generation anesthesia machines.** The conventional anesthesia machine works well and meets almost all needs. Machine-related morbidity and mortality is usually attributable to human misuse (e.g., unrecognized breathing circuit disconnection) rather than to true equipment failure. Conventional machines are at the end of their evolutionary cycle, however, and production of a new generation of machines has begun. **Next-generation anesthesia machines** present many challenges to anesthetists in terms of their increased complexity, changed layout and function, and integration of new technologies. Notable advantages of some newer machines include the following:

A. **Electronic interfaces** that facilitate more versatile and precise measurement and manipulation of gas concentrations, airway pressures, and ventilation (controlled and assisted).

B. **More-numerous and adaptable alarms.**

C. **Fewer external connections,** possibly reducing the incidence of disconnections, misconnections, kinking, and other mishaps.

D. **Automated machine self-checkout,** which likely enhances the detection rate of malfunctions while also freeing the anesthetist to perform other tasks.

E. **Enhanced data collection** to facilitate integration with computerized information management systems.

X. **Anesthesia machine checkout recommendations.** This checkout, or a reasonable equivalent, should be conducted before administering anesthesia. These recommendations are valid only for an anesthesia system that conforms to current and relevant standards and includes an ascending bellows ventilator and at least the following monitors: capnograph, pulse oximeter, oxygen analyzer, respiratory volume monitor (spirometer), and breathing system pressure monitor with high-and low-pressure alarms. This is a guideline that users are encouraged to modify to accommodate differences in equipment design and variations in local clinical practice. Such local modifications should have appropriate peer review. Users should refer to the operator's manual for manufacturer's specific procedures and precautions, especially the manufacturer's low-pressure leak test (see section X.C.2). **Note:** If an anesthesia provider uses the same machine in successive cases, the steps denoted by an asterisk (*) below do not need to be repeated or may be abbreviated after the initial checkout.

A. **Emergency ventilation equipment. Verify that backup ventilation equipment is available and functioning.***

B. **High-pressure system**
1. **Check oxygen cylinder supply.***
   a. Open oxygen cylinder and verify that it is at least half full (about 1,000 psi).
   b. Close cylinder.
2. **Check central pipeline supplies.*** Check that hoses are connected properly and pipeline gauges read about 50 psi.

C. **Low-pressure system**
1. **Check initial status of low pressure system.***
   a. Close flow control valves and turn vaporizers off.
   b. Check fill level and tighten vaporizers' filler caps.
2. **Perform leak check of machine low-pressure system.***
   a. Verify that the machine master switch and flow control valves are "OFF."
   b. Attach suction bulb to common (fresh) gas outlet.
   c. Squeeze bulb repeatedly until it is fully collapsed.
   d. Verify that bulb stays fully collapsed for at least 10 seconds.
   e. Open one vaporizer at a time and repeat "c" and "d" as above.
   f. Remove suction bulb and reconnect fresh gas hose.

3. **Turn on machine master switch and all other necessary electrical equipment.***
4. **Test flowmeters.***
   a. Adjust flow of all gases through their full range, checking for smooth operation of floats and undamaged flow tubes.
   b. Attempt to create a hypoxic O_2/N_2O mixture and verify correct changes in flow and/or alarm.

D. **Scavenging system. Adjust and check scavenging system.***
   1. Ensure proper connections between the scavenging system and both APL (pop-off) valve and ventilator relief valve.
   2. Adjust waste gas vacuum (if necessary).
   3. Fully open APL valve and occlude Y-piece.
   4. With minimum O_2 flow, allow scavenger reservoir bag to collapse completely and verify that absorber pressure gauge reads nearly 0.
   5. With the O_2 flush activated, allow the scavenger reservoir bag to distend fully and then verify that the absorber pressure gauge reads less than 10 cm H_2O.

E. **Breathing system**
   1. **Calibrate O_2 monitor.**
      a. Expose sensor to room air and verify monitor reads 21%.
      b. Verify that low O_2 alarm is enabled and functioning.
      c. Reinstall sensor in circuit and flush breathing system with O_2.
      d. Verify that monitor now reads greater than 90%.
   2. **Check initial status of breathing system.**
      a. Set selector switch to "bag" mode.
      b. Check that breathing circuit is complete, undamaged, and unobstructed.
      c. Verify that CO_2 absorbent is adequate.
      d. Install breathing circuit accessory equipment (e.g., humidifier, PEEP valve) to be used during the case.
   3. **Perform leak check of the breathing system.**
      a. Set all gas flows to 0 (or minimum).
      b. Close APL (pop-off) valve and occlude Y-piece.
      c. Pressurize breathing system to 30 cm H_2O with O_2 flush.
      d. Ensure that pressure remains fixed for at least 10 seconds.
      e. Open APL (pop-off) valve and ensure that pressure decreases.

F. **Manual and automatic ventilation systems. Test ventilation systems and unidirectional valves.**
   1. Place a second breathing bag on the Y-piece.
   2. Set appropriate ventilator parameters for next patient.
   3. Switch to automatic ventilation (Ventilator) mode.
   4. Fill bellows and breathing bag with O_2 flush and then turn ventilator "ON."
   5. Set O_2 flow to minimum and other gas flows to 0.
   6. Verify that during inspiration bellows delivers appropriate tidal volume and that during expiration bellows fills completely.
   7. Set fresh gas flow to about 5 L/min.

8. Verify that the ventilator bellows and simulated lungs fill and empty appropriately without sustained pressure at end expiration.
9. Check for proper action of unidirectional valves.
10. Test breathing circuit accessories to ensure proper function.
11. Turn ventilator "OFF" and switch to manual ventilation mode.
12. Ventilate manually and ensure inflation and deflation of artificial lungs and appropriate feel of system resistance and compliance.
13. Remove second breathing bag from Y-piece.

G. **Monitors. Check, calibrate, and/or set alarm limits of all monitors.**

H. **Final position. Check final status of the machine.**
   1. Vaporizers off.
   2. APL valve open.
   3. Selector switch to "Bag."
   4. All flowmeters to 0.
   5. Patient suction level adequate.
   6. Breathing system ready to use.

SUGGESTED READING

Dorsch JA, Dorsch SE, eds. *Understanding anesthesia equipment*, 4th ed. Philadelphia: Lippincott Williams & Wilkins, 1999.

Ehrenwerth J, Eisencraft JB. *Anesthesia equipment*, 2nd ed. St. Louis: Mosby Year Book, 2001.

Olympio MA. Modern anesthesia machines offer new safety features. *Anesthesia Patient Safety Foundation Newsletter* 2003;18:17–32.

10

Monitoring

Arthur J. Tokarczyk and Warren S. Sandberg

I. **Standard monitoring.** In addition to the continual presence of the anesthetist, standard monitoring is applied to maintain appropriate vital organ functioning during patient care. It was approved by ASA House of Delegates on October 21, 1996, and last amended October 25, 2005.

A. **Standard monitoring for general anesthesia** involves oxygenation (oxygen analyzer, pulse oximetry), ventilation (capnography, minute ventilation), circulation (electrocardiogram [ECG], arterial blood pressure, perfusion assessment), and temperature, if necessary.

B. **Standard monitoring for monitored anesthesia care and regional anesthesia** involves oxygenation (pulse oximetry), ventilation (respiratory rate), circulation (ECG, blood pressure, perfusion assessment), and temperature, if necessary.

C. **Additional monitoring** may be added, such as invasive arterial and venous pressure monitoring, echocardiography, neuromuscular blockade monitoring, and central nervous system monitoring.

II. **Cardiovascular system.** The circulatory system is responsible for oxygen delivery to and removal of waste products from the organs, and this must be maintained during anesthesia.

A. **Circulation**

1. **Flow to organs** is directly related to pressure gradient and inversely related to vascular resistance. So even if pressure is high, flow may be reduced in the face of elevated resistance.

2. **Pressure gradient** can be estimated by the difference between mean arterial pressure (MAP) and venous pressure, or, for the cerebral circulation in the case of increased intracerebral pressure (ICP), the difference between MAP and ICP.

3. **Signs and symptoms of perfusion abnormalities**

a. Central nervous system: mental status changes, neurologic deficits.

b. Cardiovascular system: chest pain, shortness of breath, ECG abnormalities, wall motion abnormalities on echocardiogram.

c. Renal: decreased urine output, elevated blood urea nitrogen and creatinine, decreased fractional excretion of sodium.

d. Gastrointestinal: abdominal pain, decreased bowel sounds, hematochezia.

e. Peripheral: cool limbs, poor capillary refill, diminished pulses.

B. **ECG.** The ECG monitors the conduction of electrical impulses through the heart. It is used to determine the heart rate and to detect and diagnose dysrhythmia, myocardial ischemia, pacemaker function, and electrolyte abnormalities. The presence of an ECG signal does not guarantee cardiac contraction and output.

1. **Mechanism of monitoring**
   a. **Electrode pads.** ECG electrodes measure a small electrical signal (about 1 mV). This makes the ECG prone to electrical interference from outside sources and requires proper electrode application to clean, dry skin.
   b. **Electrode locations.** To effectively detect dysrhythmias and ischemia, the pads must be placed in consistent locations on the body. Limb leads must be placed on or near their appropriate limbs and the precordial lead (V5) at the fifth intercostal space, anterior axillary line.
   c. **Modes and options**
      (1) Monitors often have several choices for filtering of noise, most commonly called "diagnostic" and "monitor" modes. The monitor mode filters out noise by using a narrowed bandpass (0.5 to 40 Hz), while the diagnostic mode filters less signal and noise by using a wider bandpass (0.05 to 100 Hz). The diagnostic mode should be used when monitoring for ischemia.
      (2) Automatic trending of ST segment changes is often available and useful for monitoring the development of ischemia over time.
2. **Rhythm detection.** The relationship between the P and QRS waves allows for dysrhythmia diagnosis; the P wave is best seen in lead II.
3. **Ischemia detection.** Monitoring leads II and V5 allows for detection of ischemia anywhere in a large area of the myocardium. Lead II monitors the inferior portion of the heart, supplied by the right coronary artery. Lead V5 monitors the bulk of the left ventricle, supplied by the left anterior descending artery. Lead I may be monitored on patients in whom the left circumflex artery is at risk.

C. **Arterial blood pressure.** Arterial blood pressure is used as a surrogate for blood flow. It is composed of resistance and flow. Thus, blood supply to an organ may be low despite adequate blood pressure because of high resistance. Individual organs manifest a degree of autoregulation, which allows for local changes in resistance to maintain a constant blood flow.
   1. **Analysis. Systolic and diastolic blood pressures** are measured by a variety of methods. The pressure created by a contracting heart corresponds to the systolic pressure, while the pressure during relaxation corresponds to the diastolic blood pressure. **Mean arterial blood pressure** is the average arterial blood pressure during systole and diastole. It may be either directly measured or calculated from the systolic and diastolic values.
   2. **Manual blood pressure** directly measures the systolic and diastolic blood pressures by auscultation of Korotkoff sounds. An occlusive cuff is inflated above the systolic blood pressure and is slowly deflated (3 to 5 mm Hg/second) while auscultating for blood flow. The first sound of blood flow corresponds to the systolic blood pressure, while the point at which the sounds diminish gives the diastolic blood pressure.
      a. **Auscultation** involves using a stethoscope to detect Korotkoff sounds.
      b. **Limitations**

(1) Cuff size may give incorrect values; a cuff that is too small may result in falsely high blood pressures, while a cuff that is too large may result in falsely low blood pressures. The cuff width should cover two-thirds of the upper arm or thigh.

(2) Requires active operator participation

(3) Prone to operator error and interpretation

(4) Vasoconstriction and low blood pressure may make sounds difficult to auscultate.

(5) Rapid deflation may give low pressure readings.

c. **Doppler or palpation** uses ultrasound or touch. The systolic pressure correlates to the point at which the first pulse is palpated or Korotkoff sounds are heard. Palpation also may be used to determine approximate systolic blood pressure based on whether the pulse may be palpated at key points: radial artery (80 mm Hg), femoral artery (60 mm Hg), or carotid artery (50 mm Hg). This method provides estimates when the blood pressure is very low.

d. **Limitations**

(1) Cannot determine diastolic blood pressure.

(2) Same limitations as auscultation method.

3. **Automated noninvasive blood pressure** is the most common noninvasive method of measuring blood pressure in the operating room. The blood pressure cuff is inflated initially to a preset point (150 mm Hg or 40 mmHg above prior measurement) and then incrementally decreased while sensing the pressure oscillation in the cuff. This method directly measures the mean arterial blood pressure, which correlates to the point of maximum oscillation amplitude, and the systolic and diastolic pressures are determined by an algorithm. This method allows passive participation by the operator and limits operator interpretation.

a. **Limitations**

(1) Motion artifact may result in erroneous values or may not give any values at all, resulting in a delay in accurate measurements.

(2) Venous congestion and ischemia may result from frequent blood pressure measurements during rapid or large blood pressure fluctuations.

(3) Dysrhythmias may make values difficult to interpret or increase cycle time.

(4) Very low or high blood pressures may not correlate with intra-arterial measurements; noninvasive blood pressure measurement often overestimates low blood pressure (i.e., systolic blood pressure below 80 mm Hg).

4. **Invasive blood pressure monitoring** uses an indwelling arterial catheter coupled through fluid-filled tubing to a pressure transducer. The transducer converts pressure into an electrical signal to be displayed.

a. **Indications**

(1) Need for tight blood pressure control (e.g., induced hyper- or hypotension).

(2) Hemodynamically unstable patient.

(3) Frequent arterial blood sampling.

       (4) Inability to utilize noninvasive blood pressure measurements.

b. Interpretation
- **(1)** Systolic blood pressure is often monitored in situations when high pressure may cause rupture (e.g., aneurysm).
- **(2)** MAP is often monitored for assessing adequate perfusion pressure of vital organs.

c. Materials include appropriately sized arterial catheter and transducer apparatus. Generally, catheter size is 22- to 24-gauge for infants, 20- to 22-gauge for children, and 18- to 20-gauge for adults.
- **(1) Transducer** is connected to fluid-filled tubing and a pressurized bag of saline with or without heparin. The line is continuously flushed at 3 mL/hour to prevent clotting. The signal should have a flat frequency response below 20 Hz to monitor all physiologic heart rates.
- **(2) Tubing** should be rigid and as short as possible, with no kinks or air bubbles.
- **(3) Set-up.** The transducer should be electronically zeroed while open to air and placed at the height of the coronary sinus for most patients. Exceptions include placing the transducer at the level of the head during cerebral aneurysm surgery.
- **(4) Flush apparatus** is available for flushing the catheter of blood after placement. This apparatus includes, in order, a 10-mL syringe with about 7 mL of saline, a stopcock, and a T-connector. This is flushed before arterial cannulation.

5. Procedure: arterial cannulation

a. Locations. The most common site for placement is the radial artery. Other locations include ulnar, brachial, axillary, femoral, and dorsalis pedis arteries. As the distance from the heart increases, the systolic blood pressure increases, mean arterial pressure generally decreases, and the pressure waveform displayed narrows.

b. Direct cannulation technique of the radial artery.
- **(1)** Immobilize the forearm and slightly hyperextend the wrist using a padded arm board or roll (Fig. 10.1) The thumb may be extended to improve the extension of the wrist. Palpate the course of the radial artery medial to the head of the radius. The wrist may be returned to the normal position after the catheter is secured.
- **(2)** The skin is prepped in sterile fashion and a 25- to 27-gauge needle is used to raise a skin wheal with 1% lidocaine with or without bicarbonate. A small skin puncture with a 16-gauge needle may ease catheter insertion.
- **(3)** For the **direct cannulation method,** use an acute angle (see Figure 10.1) for catheter placement. The needle is advanced until the artery is entered and a good flow of blood is observed. The catheter is advanced over the needle without moving the needle.

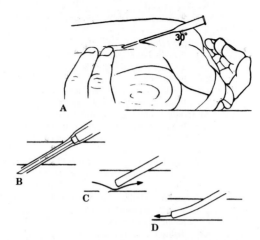

Figure 10.1. Percutaneous radial artery cannulation. A: Direct threading method. B–D: Transfixing method. Positioning of the hand and forearm is the same for both methods.

Proximal pressure is applied to occlude the artery while the needle is removed and flush apparatus is attached.

(4) A sterile arterial guide wire can be used to ease catheter insertion, as in a Seldinger technique.

(5) The T-connector is attached to the transducer tubing and 2 mL of blood is aspirated from the catheter. The line is then flushed with solution to remove residual blood.

(6) Do not flush the line with more than 3 mL as retrograde flow into the cerebral circulation has been demonstrated.

c. **Transfixion technique (also called bloodless technique).** All steps are identical to the direct cannulation method, except for step 3.

(1) The catheter is advanced completely through the artery, often with a flash of blood in the hub of the needle (except for 22- and 24-gauge catheters). The catheter is held in place while the needle is removed and the flush apparatus is firmly connected to the catheter. The catheter is lowered almost parallel to the skin and slowly retracted until blood pulsates freely into the flush apparatus. The catheter is then advanced into the vessel using a twisting motion. The catheter is then aspirated and flushed with solution to clear it of blood, and the stopcock is turned to "off." A sterile guidewire can be used if catheter insertion is difficult.

d. **Considerations for placement**

(1) Femoral and axillary artery cannulation is best performed with an 18- or 20-gauge catheter to cannulate

the vessel and then inserting a longer 6-inch, 18-gauge catheter via the Seldinger technique.

(2) The **modified Allen test** may be used to assess the relative patency and contribution of the radial and ulnar arteries to the blood supply to the hand. The results do not correlate well with outcomes, though, and the test is often omitted.

(3) Blood pressure and pulses should be assessed in both right and left sides; if disparity exists, the catheter should be placed on the side with the higher pressure.

(4) Prior cannulation may result in thrombosis and proximal pulsation should be assessed before placement. Distal pulsation may simply indicate collateral flow.

e. **Complications** may necessitate using an alternative means of blood pressure measurement.

(1) Dampened waveforms may result from arterial obstruction, catheter occlusion or clot, kinking of the pressure tubing, air in the tubing, loss of flush pressure in tubing, or transducer failure. Catheter patency should be assessed with aspiration and flushing. If the problem persists, the catheter may be replaced over a wire or with a new insertion.

(2) Rare complications include arterial thrombosis, ischemia, infection, and fistula or aneurysm formation. The catheter should be removed and the indication for invasive monitoring reassessed. The opposite side should be considered for new placement, and the ipsilateral ulnar artery should not be cannulated in the event of radial artery complications.

D. **Central venous pressure (CVP) and cardiac output**

1. **CVP** is measured by coupling the intravascular space to a pressure transducer using fluid-filled tubing. Pressure is monitored at the level of the vena cava or the right atrium. The transducer apparatus (see section II.C.4.c.) is placed at the level of the coronary sinus.

a. **Indications**

(1) Measurement of the right heart filling pressures to assess intravascular volume and right heart function.

(2) Drug administration to the central circulation.

(3) Intravenous access for patients with poor peripheral access.

(4) Indicator injection for cardiac output determination (e.g., green dye cardiac output).

(5) Access for insertion of pulmonary artery catheter.

b. **Waveform.** The CVP tracing contains three positive deflections—the **a, c,** and **v** waves—and two negative slopes—the **x** and **y descents** (Fig. 10.2). The waves correspond to atrial contraction, isovolemic ventricular contraction including tricuspid bulging, and right atrial filling, respectively. The x descent corresponds to atrial relaxation and systolic collapse, and the y descent corresponds to early ventricular filling and diastolic collapse.

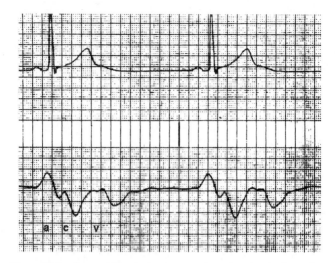

Figure 10.2. A normal central venous pressure tracing is shown in the bottom half of the figure with its corresponding electrocardiogram in the top half. Waves a, c, and v on the venous pressure tracing are labeled. The *x* descent occurs between waves c and v; the *y* descent occurs after the v wave. (From Kaplan JA. *Cardiac anesthesia*, 2nd ed. Philadelphia: WB Saunders, 1987:186, with permission.)

    c. **Analysis**
        (1) **Range.** The CVP is read between the a and c waves at end-expiration, thus minimizing the interaction of respiration. **The CVP is normally 2 to 6 mm Hg.**
        (2) **Decreases in CVP** indicate an increase in cardiac performance, decreased venous return, or a decrease in intravascular volume (mean systemic pressure). When a CVP decrease is associated with an increase in blood pressure, without changes to the systemic vascular resistance, the CVP has fallen because of increased cardiac performance. If blood pressure is decreased, then decreased CVP is due to decreased intravascular volume or venous return.
        (3) **Increases in CVP** indicate either a decrease in cardiac performance, increased venous return, or an increase in volume (mean systemic pressure). When this increase is associated with increased blood pressure, without changes to the systemic vascular resistance, the cause of increased CVP is an increase in volume or venous return. With an associated decrease in blood pressure, the increased CVP is due to decreased cardiac performance.
    d. **Pathology and CVP**
        (1) **Cannon a waves** are due to the atrium contracting against a closed tricuspid valve, as during atrioventricular dissociation.

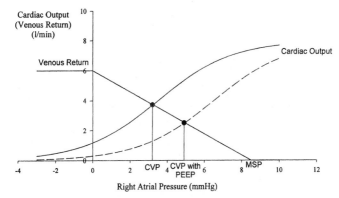

Figure 10.3. Effect of positive end-expiratory pressure (PEEP) on the venous return/cardiac output curves. PEEP has the effect of shifting the Starling curve to the right by a degree equal to the transmitted extracardiac pressure. At high levels of PEEP (>15 cm H_2O), the curve can be depressed secondary to increased right ventricular afterload. The central venous pressure measured is consequently higher. MSP, mean systemic pressure.

(2) **Large v waves** are due regurgitant flow during ventricular contraction, as with tricuspid regurgitation.

e. **Positive pressure ventilation** will affect both the cardiac output and venous return, and this relationship dictates the effect of positive end-expiratory pressure (PEEP) on CVP (Fig. 10.3). According to the Starling rule, the transmural pressure, which is the difference between atrial pressure and extracardiac pressure, correlates with cardiac output. At low levels of PEEP, the CVP increases with increased PEEP. At high levels of PEEP (over about 15 cm H_2O), CVP increases as the cardiac output is depressed because of impaired right ventricular output.

2. **Procedure: CVP**

a. **Locations.** The central venous catheter essentially can be placed wherever access to a central vein is possible. Common locations include internal jugular vein, subclavian vein, external jugular vein, axillary vein, cephalic vein, and femoral vein.

b. **Materials** include a pressure bag, fluid-filled tubing, and a transducer. The transducer is placed at the level of the coronary sinus.

(1) **Multiple lumen catheters** are directly inserted and are available with one to four lumens to provide access for multiple drugs, pressure monitoring, and blood sampling.

(2) An **introducer catheter** is a large-bore catheter with a septum valve. A special multiple lumen catheter or a pulmonary artery catheter is then placed through the introducer.

(3) **Ultrasound imaging** can be used to help identify the anatomy, assist catheter insertion, and verify placement. Ultrasound systems specifically designed for catheter placement (e.g., SiteRite, Dynamax Corporation, Pittsburgh, PA) have a small probe to ease manipulation.

c. **Complications**

(1) **Dysrhythmias,** caused by the guide wire or pulmonary artery catheter (PAC) irritating the endocardium, are temporary and resolve with withdrawal of the catheter or wire.

(2) **Arterial puncture** is a complication that can occur at any point of catheter placement and can cause significant vessel damage if the dilator or catheter is placed into the artery. Before dilation, intravenous position should be verified by color, blood gas, or pressure measurement through the finder needle, thin-walled needle, or 18-gauge catheter. Furthermore, the guide wire should not feel tethered with dilator placement, as this may signify venous damage or puncture. If an artery is punctured before dilatation, the needle should be removed and pressure applied for at least 5 min (10 min in the case of coagulopathy) and a new site chosen. If the catheter is placed in the artery, it should remain in place and a vascular surgeon should be consulted.

(3) **Pneumothorax, hemothorax, hydrothorax, chylothorax, or pericardial tamponade** may become evident with vital sign changes. They are in part ruled out with chest radiography. The risk of pneumothorax is highest with subclavian vein insertion.

(4) **Infection and air embolism** may occur at any time before removal of the catheter. The risk of infection is higher with femoral venous placement. To reduce the chance of air embolism upon catheter removal, the site is occluded with the patient performing a Valsalva maneuver. The Trendelenberg position helps to prevent air entrainment at neck and subclavian sites.

d. For the **internal jugular Seldinger technique,** the **right side** is preferred because the vessels run a straighter course to the right atrium (Fig. 10.4).

(1) **Position and preparation.** Patient is supine or in the Trendelenberg position with the head extended and turned toward the left side. An oxygen mask is placed, and the neck is prepped in sterile fashion. The site is widely surrounded with a fluid-impervious sterile drape.

(2) **Landmarks** include the suprasternal notch, clavicle, lateral border of sternocleidomastoid (SCM) muscle, and angle of the mandible. For insertion, locate the midpoint between the mastoid process and the sternal attachment of the SCM.

(3) **Placement** via the middle approach is performed between the clavicular and sternal heads of the SCM, while the posterior approach is approximately 1 cm

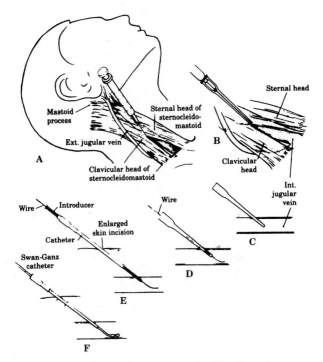

Figure 10.4. Cannulation of the right internal jugular vein (Seldinger technique). See text for details.

superior to the external jugular vein at the lateral border of the clavicular head of the SCM.

(4) Lidocaine (1%) is used to infiltrate the soft tissues, while avoiding the carotid artery. The carotid artery is palpated and gently retracted medially, taking care not to apply so much pressure as to compress the vein. The patient may be asked to perform a Valsalva maneuver during insertion to increase the size of the vein.

(5) While aspirating, a finder needle is inserted at a 45° angle to the skin and advanced toward the ipsilateral nipple until venous blood is aspirated. If the vessel is not encountered, the needle is withdrawn slowly while observing for venous flow and may be redirected laterally.

(6) Once the vein is located, the finder needle is removed and a thin-wall needle or a catheter over needle is inserted at the same angle as the finder needle.

(7) The syringe is removed and a guide wire is passed through the needle or catheter. During insertion, the wire should pass easily. The needle or catheter

is then removed, and the site should be enlarged laterally with a scalpel.

(8) With countertraction, a rigid dilator is advanced over the wire with gentle twisting; the guide wire should still be easily mobile, indicating preserved intravascular position.

(9) The dilator is removed while maintaining the guide wire, and a central catheter or introducer is inserted over the wire. Alternatively, an introducer and dilator are inserted simultaneously. The wire is removed, the ports are aspirated and flushed, and the catheter is secured to the skin.

(10) A chest radiograph is required to confirm the position and exclude complications, such as pneumothorax. The tip of the catheter should be at the subclavian vein (SVC) and right atrial junction and should not encounter the wall of the SVC at a right angle.

e. The **SCV** may be easily accessed as the vessel passes under the clavicle at the midclavicular line. It is one of the most common central venous line locations. Although the artery is not compressible in case of puncture, coagulopathy is not a contraindication to placement. The SCV is often preferred for patient comfort, and the left SCV is often chosen in the case of PAC placement.

(1) **Position and preparation** is the same as in section II.D.2.b. A roll may be placed between shoulder blades to facilitate positioning.

(2) **Landmarks** include the clavicle, suprasternal notch, and lateral border of the SCM as it inserts onto the clavicle.

(3) **Placement** is similar to that described in section II.D.2.b. Lidocaine is infiltrated around the insertion site, medial to the midclavicular line. The thin-walled needle is placed at this insertion site and aimed at the suprasternal notch. It is used to identify the clavicle, and the tip is then "walked" posteriorly under the clavicle. The bevel of the thin-walled needle is directed vertically up toward the ceiling with initial insertion but then turned 90° caudad to ease guide wire insertion. Total length of the catheter should not be greater than 16 to 17 cm, as this may place the tip in the right atrium.

f. **Femoral vein** is one of the most easily accessible central veins and using it does not carry a risk of pneumothorax. Limitations include hip immobility and limited utility during cardiopulmonary resuscitation.

(1) **Position and preparation** are done with the patient supine and the leg slightly abducted.

(2) **Landmarks** include the femoral artery, inguinal ligament, anterior superior iliac spine (ASIS), and pubic tubercle. The femoral vein is immediately medial to the femoral artery. If the artery is not palpable, it is reliably located one-third of the distance from the pubic tubercle to the ASIS. In either case, the

insertion point is just inferior to the inguinal ligament, 1 to 2 cm medial to the artery.

(3) **Placement** uses the Seldinger technique. Lidocaine
(1%) is infiltrated at the insertion point, and the
needle is advanced cephalad at a 45° angle from the
skin. If the guide wire does not pass easily beyond
the needle, the needle may be brought more parallel
to the skin to ease wire threading.

g. **External jugular vein** is cannulated similarly to an internal
jugular vein placement described in section II.D.2.b. It
runs obliquely across the SCM, along a line running from
the angle of the mandible to the midpoint of the clavicle.
Occlusive pressure at the inferior portion of the vein near
the clavicle may ease cannulation. Because the vessel bends
to join the SCV, threading of a guide wire may be difficult
and should not be forced. For this reason, internal jugular
cannulation may be easier for central catheter placement.

h. **Basilic vein** may be used to access the central circulation
with a long catheter. Passing the guide wire into the SCV
may be difficult but may be facilitated by abducting the
ipsilateral arm and turning the head toward the side of
insertion.

3. **Pulmonary artery catheterization and pulmonary artery
occlusion pressures.** The PAC gives information about ventricular function and vascular volume by measuring CVP, pulmonary artery pressure (PAP), pulmonary artery occlusion
pressure (PAOP), mixed-venous sampling, and cardiac output.

a. **Mechanism.** The PAC is inserted through a central venous
introducer catheter. It passes through the vena cava, right
atrium, and right ventricle and into the pulmonary artery.
By coupling the intravascular space to a transducer with
fluid-filled tubing, the PAC is able to measure the pressure
at each of the locations mentioned above. Inflating the
balloon at the tip of the catheter allows measurement of
PAOP, or "wedge" pressure, reflecting the left atrial pressure and left ventricular preload. To minimize the effect
of alveolar pressure on PAOP, the tip should rest in West
zone III, where pulmonary venous pressure is greater than
alveolar pressure. Fortunately, the tip usually ends up in
this location.

b. **Indications**

(1) Unexplained hypotension.

(2) Access for cardiac pacing.

(3) Surgical procedures with significant physiologic
changes (e.g., open aortic aneurysm repair, lung or
liver transplant).

(4) Acute myocardial infarction with shock.

(5) The PAC should be used only if the potential benefit of diagnosis or guidance in treatment outweighs
the risks of complications. The PAC should be discontinued once active measurement is no longer
necessary.

c. **PA and PAOP**

(1) **Waveform.** The PAP waveform is similar in shape
to the systemic arterial waveform. Because of the

location, the waveform is smaller and precedes the systemic waveform. With the balloon inflated, the PAC will measure the PAOP recording, which is similar to the CVP waveform, with a and v waves. This waveform approximates the left atrial pressures and is slightly delayed because of the interposed lung.

(2) **Range.** The **normal PAP is 15 to 30 mm Hg systolic and 5 to 12 mm Hg diastolic.** The **normal range for PAOP is 5 to 12 mm Hg.** At end expiration, this approximates the left atrial pressure and correlates with the left ventricular end diastolic volume.

d. **PAOP analysis** is used to assess the left heart performance. A basic model of left heart function is given by the relationship between the end-systolic pressure volume curve and diastolic pressure volume curve. Because the left ventricular end diastolic pressure, which correlates with the left ventricular end diastolic volume, is known, the following deductions are possible (Fig. 10.5).

(1) **Increase in PAOP** can be due to an increase in end-diastolic volume, decrease in compliance, or both.

(2) **Decrease in PAOP** can be due to a decrease in end-diastolic volume, increase in compliance, or both.

e. **Pathology and PAOP**

(1) **Large a waves** may be due to either left ventricular hypertrophy (LVH) or atrioventricular dissociation. LVH will decrease the compliance of the left ventricle and will elevate the left ventricular end diastolic pressure (LVEDP). Thus, the PAOP should be measured at the peak of the a wave. During atrioventricular dissociation, pressure should be measured before the a wave.

(2) **Large v waves** are the result of mitral regurgitation.

(3) **Right heart dilatation** can cause shifting of the interventricular septum into the left ventricle, effectively decreasing the left ventricular end diastolic compliance. Thus, LVEDP will be elevated.

(4) **Pulmonary embolism** will cause an elevation of the PAP without a concomitant elevation of the PAOP.

f. **Materials/catheter types.** Most catheters are available with or without bonded heparin. Types of PACs include the following:

(1) **Venous infusion** (VIP, VIP+) catheters provide extra ports for infusion and sampling.

(2) **Paceports** allow placement of cardiac pacing wires.

(3) **Continuous cardiac output** catheters perform frequent automated determinations of cardiac output by using frequent low-heat pulses to obtain a thermodilution curve; the values are usually an average over time.

(4) **Oximetric** catheters monitor mixed venous O_2 saturation.

(5) **Right ventricular ejection fraction** catheters use a rapid response thermistor to calculate the right

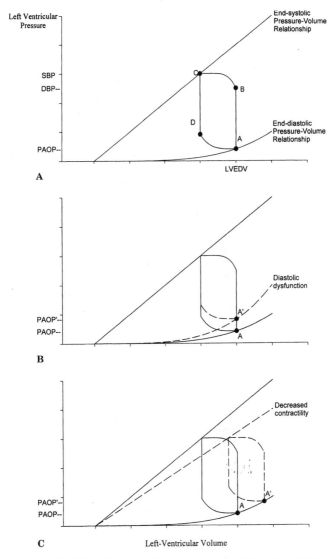

Figure 10.5. Left ventricular pressure–volume relationships. (A) The cardiac cycle (A-B-C-D-A) is limited by the end-systolic pressure–volume relationship (describing the contractility) and the end-diastolic pressure–volume relationship. The pulmonary artery occlusion pressure (PAOP) approximates the left ventricular end-diastolic pressure. An increase in PAOP may be ascribed to decreased diastolic compliance (B), an increase in left ventricular end-diastolic volume (LVEDV) (C), or a combination of both. An increase in LVEDV often results from decreased contractility in the setting of a properly performing right ventricle (C). SBP, systolic blood pressure; DBP, diastolic blood pressure.

ventricular ejection fraction in addition to cardiac output.

4. **Cardiac output**
    a. **Mechanism.** Cardiac output is most commonly determined with either thermodilution or dye dilution. A known quantity of tracer (cold saline or dye) is injected into the central circulation, and the concentration of the tracer is plotted as a function of time as it is pumped through the circulation. An algorithm is then used to correlate this with cardiac output/index.
    b. **Methods of measurement**
        (1) **Thermodilution** is performed with only a PAC to measure blood flow. Typically, 10 mL of cold (room temperature or less) saline or 5% dextrose in water is injected into the CVP port over 4 seconds and the change in temperature is monitored at the thermistor located at the tip of the catheter within the main pulmonary artery. The area under the bell-shaped temperature-time curve is inversely proportional to the blood flow and correlates with the cardiac output in the absence of intracardiac shunting. Injectate spillage, very slow injection, or use of the wrong catheter constant produces errors in measured cardiac output.
        (2) **Dye dilution** is commonly done with a central venous catheter and an arterial line. This method uses a known volume and concentration of a nontoxic dye injected into the central circulation, and the concentration over time is measured from the arterial circulation. Again, the area under the curve is inversely proportional to the cardiac output. The tracer agent is usually indocyanine green, but other agents include lithium chloride and radioisotopes.
    c. **Physiologic interpretation**
        (1) The typical range of cardiac output is 4 to 8 L/min, while the cardiac index is 2.4 to 4.0 L/min/m^2.
        (2) **Respiration** will affect the cardiac output. During spontaneous breathing, the negative intrathoracic pressure generated by inspiration will increase venous return and left ventricular transmural pressure. During positive pressure ventilation, positive intrathoracic pressure during inspiration will decrease venous return and left ventricular transmural pressure. Thus, cardiac output should be measured at a consistent point in the respiratory cycle, usually end-expiration.
        (3) **Pathology and cardiac output**
            (a) **Tricuspid regurgitation** tends to underestimate the cardiac output/cardiac index by prolonging and increasing the area under the cardiac output curve, although values may be erroneously high as well.
            (b) **Intracardiac shunting** will produce erroneous cardiac output measurements.

5. Procedure: pulmonary artery catheter

   a. Locations and prep are similar to that of the central venous catheter described in section II.D.2. The PAC is invariably placed through an introducer catheter. The operator typically dons a fresh pair of sterile gloves between the introducer and PAC placement.

   b. Technique. The PAC is prepared and examined as follows:

      (1) Sheath placement is done before balloon examination and placed at 70 cm.

      (2) Balloon examination includes inflating the balloon with 1.5 mL of air. The balloon should be symmetrical and inflate and deflate smoothly.

      (3) All ports are flushed to ensure patency and are attached to calibrated pressure transducers. Raising and lowering the PAC distal end should produce changes on the pressure tracing and serves as a quick test of the system before insertion.

      (4) Placement (Fig. 10.6). The PAC is held so that it follows a natural curve through the heart during passage through the introducer. Once the 20-cm mark is reached, the balloon is inflated with 1.5 mL of air and the CVP waveform is confirmed. As the catheter is advanced, the waveform will change to a right ventricular waveform and then to a pulmonary artery waveform (with an elevated, down-sloping diastolic plateau). The PAC is advanced until a PAOP waveform is seen, and the balloon is then deflated. The waveform should return to a pulmonary artery tracing upon deflation. If it does not, then the PAC should be withdrawn about 5 cm with the balloon deflated, the balloon should be reinflated, and the PAC should be advanced until a PAOP tracing is encountered. The balloon should remain deflated normally.

      (5) Securing the sheath to the introducer proximally and at the 70-cm mark distally ensures the ability to manipulate the PAC aseptically. The introducer and PAC are secured to the patient, and an occlusive dressing is applied.

   c. Distances. From the right internal jugular vein, each location appears "on the tens." The right atrium is reached at 20 cm, the right ventricle is reached at 30 cm, the pulmonary artery is reached at 40 cm, and the PAOP should be at 50 cm. For subclavian vein placement, subtract 5 cm from these distances; for femoral vein placement, add 20 cm to these distances.

   d. During PAC insertion, difficulty in passing the catheter into the right ventricle and pulmonary artery may be encountered because of balloon malfunction, valvular lesions, a low-flow state, or a dilated right ventricle. The monitoring equipment should be rechecked for calibration and scale. Inflating the balloon with a full 1.5 mL of air, slow PAC advancement, and large inspirations by

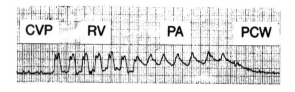

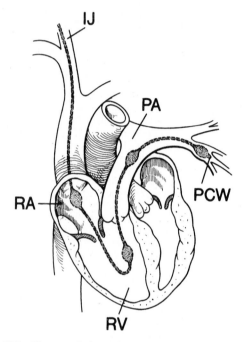

Figure 10.6. Characteristic pressure waves seen during insertion of a pulmonary artery catheter. CVP, central venous pressure; IJ, internal jugular; RA, right atrium; RV, right ventricle; PA, pulmonary artery; PCW, pulmonary capillary wedge.

the patient to augment venous return may be helpful. The PAC may have to be withdrawn to a depth of 20 to 30 cm, rotated slightly, and readvanced.

e. **Complications**

(1) **Dysrhythmias** are possible because of direct stimulation of the atrium or ventricle in 50% to 70% of placements. They are usually transient and resolve spontaneously or with withdrawal of the PAC. Complete heart block and ventricular tachycardia are possible (up to 0.3% of placements) and should be treated appropriately.

(2) **Right bundle-branch block** is a specific risk in patients with either a left bundle-branch block or a

first-degree heart block, as this may result in complete heart block. In this event, the PAC should be withdrawn and temporary pacing initiated.

(3) **Pulmonary artery rupture or infarction** is possible from overinflation or prolonged inflation of the balloon or from direct pressure by the PAC. Thus, the balloon should be slowly inflated, and volume to achieve PAOP should be monitored. Furthermore, the PAP should be monitored by default; if a persistent PAOP appears, the catheter should be pulled back immediately and repositioned.

(4) **Pacemakers** do not contraindicate PAC placement, although fluoroscopic guidance should be used if the pacemaker is less than 6 weeks old.

(5) **Balloon rupture** may occur with overinflation with more than the recommended 1.5 mL.

(6) **Valve damage, catheter knotting, thrombus formation, and infection** can occur with PACs.

6. **Echocardiography (echo)**

   a. **Mechanism.** Echocardiography is performed with ultrasonic waves to create a two-dimensional image of the heart and surrounding structures. This may be done from a transthoracic or transesophageal approach, depending on the targeted structures, patient compliance, and conditions during placement. It provides independent assessments of the same parameters that a PAC measures, but it also reveals cardiac valve function, ventricular contractility, diastolic function, and intracardiac structures.

   b. **Indications**

      (1) **Hypotension** of unknown cause.
      (2) **Uninterpretable PAC values.**
      (3) **Suspected intracardiac masses or vegetations.**
      (4) **Valvular abnormalities.**
      (5) **Shunts.**
      (6) **Air embolism.**
      (7) **Pericardial disease.**
      (8) **Thoracic aneurysm/dissection.**

   c. **Methods**

      (1) **Transthoracic echocardiogram** can be performed with the patient awake and provides good visualization of right heart structures and qualitative estimates of contractile performance, although visualization of the left heart is limited and may not be allowed by the surgical location.

      (2) **Transesophageal echocardiogram** requires that the patient be topically, locally, or generally anesthetized, but it may be performed intraoperatively and allows superior visualization of the left heart.

III. **Respiratory system.** The respiratory system is responsible for oxygen uptake and carbon dioxide removal and provides a conduit for delivery of anesthetic agents.

   A. **Mandatory respiratory monitors** during general anesthesia include pulse oximetry, capnography, a fraction of inspired oxygen analyzer, and a disconnect alarm. Direct visualization of the chest and a precordial or esophageal stethoscope may provide additional information. During regional anesthesia, respiration may be monitored with direct visualization, oximetry, and capnography.

B. **Oxygenation** is most easily measured by **pulse oximetry.** Other methods include qualitative assessment of skin color, transcutaneous oximetry, and arterial blood bas sampling.

1. **Method.** Oxygenated and deoxygenated hemoglobin absorb light differently at most wavelengths, including 660 and 960 nm, the wavelengths examined by most devices. The Beer-Lambert law allows the concentration of each species to be calculated from the absorption of light at those wavelengths. The ratio of absorption is processed to give the oxygen saturation of hemoglobin. The sensor has at least two light-emitting diodes (960 and 660 nm) and a light detector. This may be applied to fingers, toes, earlobes, tongue, or, with a special probe, the nose.

2. **Interpretation.** Normal range in a healthy adult is 96% to 99%, while values above 88% may be acceptable in patients with lung disease. A high pulse oximeter reading (SpO_2) generally indicates that oxygen is available in the lungs, taken up in the blood, and delivered to distal tissues. A low SpO_2 may be due to a problem along the above pathway or to an error in monitoring.

3. **Limitations.**

   a. Oximetry may be a late reporter of inadequate gas exchange.

   b. **Carboxyhemoglogin** absorbs light similarly to oxygenated hemoglobin at 660 nm and will provide falsely elevated readings, although it does not contribute to oxygenation.

   c. **Methemoglobin** absorbs light at both 660 and 940 nm, resulting in a saturation of 85%, which does not correlate with the true saturation. Methemoglobinemia may often be treated with methylene blue.

   d. **Methylene blue, indocyanine green, indigo carmine,** and **isosulfan blue** injections transiently result in falsely low saturation readings.

   e. SpO_2 tends to be falsely overestimated at low saturations (below 80%).

   f. Low perfusion, motion, and nail polish may cause SpO_2 measurements to be uninterpretable or unreliable.

C. **Ventilation** is assessed by end-tidal carbon dioxide measurements (i.e., capnography) and spirometry. Capnometry and capnography are often used as synonyms, as both analyze and record carbon dioxide, with the latter including a waveform. Capnography not only evaluates respiration but also confirms of endotracheal intubation and is diagnostic of pathologic conditions.

1. **Method.** The measurement of carbon dioxide is often based on infrared light absorption to determine concentration. Carbon dioxide may be measured either at the breathing circuit (mainstream capnograph) or via aspiration of gas samples by the capnograph (sidestream capnograph). Mainstream capnographs often cause traction on the endotracheal tube and can cause burns by radiant heat, while sidestream capnographs have a measurement delay based on sample volumes and may result in significant leaks from sampling. Sidestream capnography

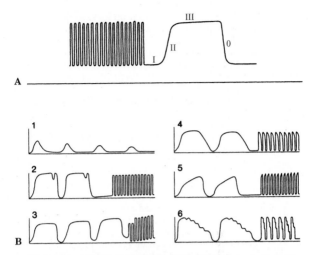

Figure 10.7. A: Normal capnograph. I, dead space expiration; II, mixed dead space and alveolar gas expiration; III, alveolar gas expiration and plateau; 0, inspiration. Phase IV is an upswing that occurs at the end of phase III. B: Capnographs that may be seen in practice. 1, rapidly extinguishing uncharacteristic waveform, compatible with esophageal intubation; 2, regular dips in end-expiratory plateau, seen in underventilated lungs or in patients recovering from neuromuscular blockade; 3, upward shift in baseline and plateau, seen with rebreathing of carbon dioxide, miscalibration, and so forth; 4, restrictive pulmonary disease; 5, obstructive pulmonary disease; 6, cardiogenic oscillations.

may also be used on a nonintubated patient to give a qualitative assessment of respiration.

2.   **Waveform.** The normal end-tidal carbon dioxide ($Petco_2$) waveform (Fig. 10.7) contains the expiratory portion (phases I, II, III, and occasionally IV) and inspiratory portion (phase 0). Two angles, the alpha angle (between phase II and III) and the beta angle (between phase III and 0), also aide in interpretation (see Fig. 10.7).

a.   **Phase 0** is the inspiratory segment.

b.   **Phase I** is the carbon dioxide-free gas that is not involved in gas exchange (dead space).

c.   **Phase II** is the rapid upswing and includes both alveolar gas and dead space gas.

d.   **Phase III** is a plateau that involves alveolar gas and has a small positive slope. $Petco_2$ is measured at the end of phase III.

e.   **Phase IV** is a terminal upswing seen in obese and pregnant patients with reduced thoracic compliance.

f.   **Alpha angle** is between phases II and II and is related to the ventilation:perfusion matching of the lung. The **beta angle** is between phases III and 0 and usually is about 90°, and it may be used to assess rebreathing.

3. **Range and analysis**
    a. Normally, $Petco_2$ is 2 to 5 mm Hg lower than arterial CO_2 pressure, so the typical range for end-tidal carbon dioxide during general anesthesia is 30 to 40 mm Hg.
    b. Due to swallowed gas, **esophageal intubation** may result in carbon dioxide return similar to that of endotracheal intubation, except that $Petco_2$ diminishes to zero with a few breaths.
    c. **An early sign of malignant hyperthermia** is a rapidly rising end-tidal carbon dioxide, especially if it is unresponsive to hyperventilation.
    d. Shock/low perfusion, embolism, auto-PEEP, airway obstruction, and system leaks will result in diminishing end-tidal carbon dioxide.
    e. Carbon dioxide absorption during laparoscopic procedures, reperfusion after releasing an arterial clamp or tourniquet, and absorbent exhaustion or channeling will result in rising end-tidal carbon dioxide.
    f. Widening of the beta angle with an elevation of both phase 0/I and III is a sign of **inspiratory valve failure.**
    g. Elevation of both phase 0/I and phase III is a sign of **expiratory valve failure** or **absorbent malfunction.**

IV. **Central nervous system (level of consciousness) monitoring**
    A. **Bispectral index (BIS)** (Aspect Medical Systems, Newton, MA) and related devices assess central nervous system depression during general anesthesia. This makes available an additional monitor independent of blood pressure and heart rate to assess hypnosis. It is based on the surface electroencephalogram (EEG), which predictably changes in amplitude and frequency as the depth of anesthesia increases.
        1. **Mechanism.** The BIS monitor uses a sensor to transmit EEG signals from the patient to a digital signal converter, which digitizes the signal and sends it to the monitor for processing and analysis.
            a. The BIS reading is a processed numeric value that correlates with the level of hypnosis. It is derived from the preceding 15 to 30 seconds of EEG measurements. The range is 0 (flat line EEG) to 100 (awake).
            b. The **signal quality index** indicates the quality of the EEG signal and is primarily based on impedance and artifact.
            c. The **electromyograph indicator** displays power from muscles in the frequency range of 70 to 110 Hz. The range is 30 to 55 dB.
            d. The **EEG display** presents a filtered EEG waveform.
            e. **Suppression ratio** displays the percentage that an isoelectric (flat line) condition exists over the prior 63 seconds. The range is 0% to 100%.
        2. **Indications.** Level-of-consciousness monitoring is helpful for assessing depth of anesthesia and effectively may reduce the incidence of unplanned intraoperative recall. Specific indications include the following:
            a. Challenging emergence, such as during neurologic procedures or prolonged neuromuscular blockade.

    b. Reducing excessive administration of hypnotic agent, as in the case of hemodynamic instability or to speed recovery.

    c. During total intravenous anesthetic.

    d. Closed-loop anesthesia, in which BIS directly guides administration of the hypnotic agent. This is not available in the United States at this time because of its investigational nature.

3. BIS interpretation

    a. Recall of words or pictures is depressed at BIS values of 70 to 75. Explicit recall is significantly diminished as BIS decreases below 70, and a BIS of 40 to 60 correlates with general anesthesia.

    b. Increasing concentrations of hypnotic agents predictably lower BIS. The response of BIS to hypnotic agents increases with age.

    c. BIS is not affected by opioids, so the target BIS needs to be selected based on anesthetic technique. Thus, in the absence of opioids or analgesics, BIS should be 25 to 35; with the use of opioid or analgesic supplementation, BIS can be 45 to 60.

4. Complications. BIS may be inaccurate because of artifacts from different sources.

    a. Excessive muscle activity may elevate BIS. This is treated with paralysis.

    b. Seizure and "abnormal brain" rarely result in erroneous BIS values due to atypical EEG patterns or anatomy.

    c. Specific hypnotic agents have different effects on BIS. The response of BIS to nitrous oxide is not linear and may be unreliable. Ketamine has little effect on BIS, even with clinically effective doses, but may blunt the response to stimulation in the presence of other agents. Etomidate is associated with increased muscle activity upon induction and thus may falsely elevate BIS.

    d. External electrical or mechanical interference may make BIS unreliable.

5. Materials. The required materials, connected in series, are the BIS monitor, monitor interface cable, digital signal converter, patient interface cable, and sensor. The sensor is applied to either side of the patient's forehead according to the included diagram. The sensor should not be located between the surgical site and the electrocautery skin electrode.

B. Other methods of awareness monitoring are **entropy monitoring,** using a Datex-Ohmeda spectral entropy algorithm, and **midlatency auditory evoked potentials,** both of which correlate well with anesthetic agent effect on awareness.

V. Temperature monitoring

  A. Mechanism. Temperature may be measured intermittently or continuously. The limitation of more external methods of temperature determination is that they may not reflect changes in the core body temperature, especially in the presence of vasoconstriction.

  B. Indications

    1. Need to control temperature during induced hypothermia and rewarming (e.g., during cardiopulmonary bypass or vascular neurosurgery).

2. **Infants and small children** are prone to thermal lability due to their high surface area to volume ratio.

3. **Adults subjected to large evaporative losses or low ambient temperatures** (as occur with exposed body cavity, large volume transfusion of unwarmed fluids, or burns) are prone to hypothermia.

4. **Febrile patients** need to be monitored because of the risk of hyper- or hypothermia.

5. Patients with **autonomic dysfunction** are unable to autoregulate their body temperature.

6. **Malignant hyperthermia** is always a possible complication, and temperature monitoring should always be available.

C. **Monitoring sites**

1. **Skin temperature,** as measured on the forehead, is normally 3°F to 4°F below core temperature, and this gradient may increase with further cooling.

2. **The axilla** is a common site for noninvasive temperature determination and is usually 1°F below body temperature. The probe needs be placed at the axillary artery with the arm adducted.

3. **Tympanic membrane temperature** correlates well with core temperature by measuring near the eardrum. Intervening cerumen may enlarge the gradient with respect to core temperature.

4. **Rectal temperature** changes lag behind those of core body temperature. This phenomenon is often noted during rewarming after hypothermia and indicates the slower peripheral, or "shell," rewarming. The risk of rectal perforation is a rare complication.

5. **Nasopharyngeal temperature,** measured at the posterior nasopharynx, reflects the brain temperature. This measurement is performed by measuring the distance from the external meatus of the ear to the external nare and inserting the temperature probe to that distance. This method may be associated with epistaxis in coagulopathic or pregnant patients or may result in skin necrosis if the probe is allowed to press on the nare during longer procedures. This method is discouraged in patients with head trauma or cerebrospinal fluid rhinorrhea.

6. **Esophageal temperature** monitoring reflects the core temperature well. The probe should be located at the lower third of the esophagus and rarely may be misplaced in the airway.

7. **Blood temperature** measurements may be obtained with the thermistor of a PAC.

VI. **Neuromuscular blockade monitoring (see Chapter 12)**

SUGGESTED READING

Jacobsohn E, Chorn R, O'Connor M. The role of the vasculature in regulating venous return and cardiac output: historical and graphical approach. *Can J Anaesth* 1997;44:849–867.

Kodali BS. *Capnography. A comprehensive educational website,* May 2005. Harvard Medical School. 30 September 2005 <http://www.capnography.com>

Lake CL. *Clinical monitoring: practical applications for anesthesia & critical care,* 1st ed. Philadelphia: WB Saunders, 2001.

Mark JB. *Atlas of cardiovascular monitoring.* New York: Churchill Livingstone, 1998.

Pagel PS, Grossman W, Haering JM, et al. Left ventricular diastolic function in the normal and diseased heart (pt 1). *Anesthesiology* 1993;79:836–854.

Pagel PS, Grossman W, Haering JM, et al. Left ventricular diastolic function in the normal and diseased heart (pt 2). *Anesthesiology* 1993;79:1104–1120.

Perret C, Tagan D, Feihl F, et al. *The pulmonary artery catheter in critical care.* Oxford: Blackwell Science, 1996.

Sagawa K, Maughan L, Suga H, et al. *Cardiac contraction and the pressure-volume relationship.* Oxford: Oxford University Press, 1988.

11

Intravenous and Inhalation Anesthetics

Owais Saifee and Ken Solt

I. **Pharmacology of intravenous (IV) anesthetics.** IV anesthetics are commonly used for induction of general anesthesia, maintenance of general anesthesia, and sedation during local or regional anesthesia. The rapid onset and offset of these drugs are due to their physical translocation in and out of the brain. After a bolus IV injection, fat-soluble drugs like propofol, thiopental, and etomidate rapidly distribute into highly perfused tissues like brain and heart, causing an extremely rapid onset of effect. Plasma concentrations decrease rapidly as the drugs continue to be distributed into muscle and fat. When plasma concentrations have decreased sufficiently, these drugs rapidly **redistribute** out of the brain, and their effects are terminated. Active drug remains in the body, so clearance still needs to occur, typically by hepatic **metabolism** and renal **elimination. Elimination half-time** is defined as the time required for the plasma concentration of drug to decrease by 50% during the terminal (elimination) phase of clearance. **Context-sensitive half-time (CSHT)** (Fig. 11.1) is defined as the time for a 50% decrease in the central compartment drug concentration after an infusion of specified duration.

A. **Propofol** (2,6-diisopropylphenol) is used for induction or maintenance of general anesthesia as well as for conscious sedation. It is prepared as a 1% isotonic oil-in-water emulsion, which contains egg lecithin, glycerol, and soybean oil. Bacterial growth is inhibited by either ethylenediaminetetraacetic acid or sulfite, depending on the manufacturer.

1. **Mode of action:** Increases activity at inhibitory γ-aminobutyric acid (GABA) synapses. Inhibition of glutamate (*N*-methyl-D-aspartate [NMDA]) receptors may play a role.

2. **Pharmacokinetics**

   a. Hepatic (and some extrahepatic) metabolism to inactive metabolites.

   b. The CSHT of propofol (see Fig. 11.1) is 15 min after a 2-hour infusion.

3. **Pharmacodynamics**

   a. **Central nervous system (CNS)**

      (1) Induction doses rapidly produce unconsciousness (30 to 45 seconds), followed by rapid reawakening due to redistribution. Low doses produce sedation.

      (2) Weak analgesic effects at hypnotic concentrations. The plasma EC_{50} (concentration for an effect to occur in 50% of individuals) is 3.3 μg/mL for unconsciousness and >12 μg/mL for suppression of movement.

      (3) Raises seizure threshold more than methohexital. Decreases intracranial pressure (ICP) but also cerebral perfusion pressure. High doses cause isoelectric electroencephalogram.

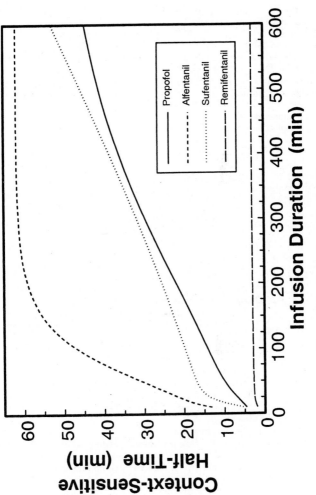

Figure 11.1. Context-sensitive half-time.

Table 11.1. Dosages of commonly used IV anesthetics

Drug	Dose		
	Induction (mg/kg)	Maintenance (μg/kg/min)	Sedation (titrate to effect)
Propofol IV	2.0–2.5	100–150	25–75 μg/kg/min
Thiopental IV	3–5		
Midazolam IV	0.1–0.4	0.5–1.5	0.5–1.0 mg
Midazolam IM			0.07–0.1 mg/kg
Ketamine IV	0.5–2	15–90	0.1–0.8 mg/kg
Ketamine IM	5–10		2–4 mg/kg
Etomidate IV	0.2–0.4	10	5–8 μg/kg/min[a]
Dexmedetomidine IV			0.2–0.7 μg/kg/hour[b]

[a] For brief periods.
[b] After loading dose of 1 μg/kg over 10 minutes.

     b. Cardiovascular system
       (1) Dose-dependent decrease in preload and afterload and depression of contractility leading to decreases in arterial pressure and cardiac output.
       (2) Heart rate is minimally affected, and baroreceptor reflex is blunted.
     c. Respiratory system
       (1) Produces a dose-dependent decrease in respiratory rate and tidal volume.
       (2) Ventilatory response to hypercarbia is diminished.
4. Dosage and administration: Table 11.1.
     a. Titrate with reduced incremental doses in elderly or hemodynamically compromised patients or if administered with other anesthetics.
     b. May be diluted, if necessary, only in 5% dextrose in water to a minimum concentration of 0.2%.
     c. Propofol emulsion supports bacterial growth; prepare drug under sterile conditions, label with date and time, and discard unused opened propofol after 6 hours to prevent inadvertent bacterial contamination.
5. Other effects
     a. Venous irritation
       (1) May cause pain during IV administration in as many as 50% to 75% of patients.
       (2) Pain may be reduced by administering IV in a large vein or by adding lidocaine to the solution. Alternatively, lidocaine (0.5 mg/kg) may be given IV 1 to 2 min before the propofol with a tourniquet proximal to the IV site. Many treatments have been investigated for this problem, but none has been proven more effective than lidocaine.
     b. Postoperative nausea and vomiting occurs less frequently after a propofol-based anesthetic compared with other techniques, and subhypnotic doses have antiemetic effects.

       c. **Lipid disorders.** Propofol is a lipid emulsion and should be used cautiously in patients with disorders of lipid metabolism (e.g., hyperlipidemia, pancreatitis).

       d. **Myoclonus** can occur after induction doses of propofol in the absence of concomitant muscle relaxation.

       e. **Propofol infusion syndrome** is a rare and often fatal disorder that occurs in critically ill patients (usually children) subjected to prolonged, high-dose propofol infusions. Typical features include rhabdomyolysis, metabolic acidosis, cardiac failure, and renal failure.

B. **Barbiturates** for anesthesia include thiopental and methohexital. These medications, like propofol, rapidly produce unconsciousness (30 to 45 seconds), followed by rapid reawakening due to redistribution. Barbiturates are very alkaline (pH >10) and are usually prepared as dilute solutions (1.0% to 2.5%) for IV administration.

    1. **Mode of action:** Barbiturates occupy receptors adjacent to GABA receptors in the CNS and augment the inhibitory tone of GABA.

    2. **Pharmacokinetics**

       a. Hepatic metabolism. Methohexital (half-life = 4 hours) has a much higher clearance than thiopental (half-life = 12 hours). Thiopental is metabolized to pentobarbital, an active metabolite with a longer half-life.

       b. Multiple doses or a prolonged infusion may produce prolonged sedation or unconsciousness. The CSHT of thiopental is long, even after short infusions.

    3. **Pharmacodynamics**

       a. **CNS**

          (1) Produce unconsciousness (thiopental EC_{50} = 15.6 μg/mL) and suppress responses to pain at much higher concentrations. Thiopental can cause hyperalgesia at subhypnotic concentrations (clinical relevance uncertain).

          (2) Produce a dose-dependent cerebral vasoconstriction and decrease in cerebral metabolism which decrease cerebral blood flow and intracranial pressure.

          (3) At high doses, thiopental will produce an isoelectric electroencephalogram, but methohexital can produce seizure activity.

       b. **Cardiovascular system**

          (1) Cause venodilation and depress myocardial contractility, so arterial blood pressure and cardiac output decrease in a dose-dependent manner, especially in patients who are preload dependent.

          (2) May increase heart rate. Very little effect on baroreceptor reflexes.

       c. **Respiratory system**

          (1) Produce a dose-dependent decrease in respiratory rate and tidal volume. Apnea may result for 30 to 90 seconds after an induction dose.

          (2) Laryngeal reflexes more active than with propofol. Incidence of laryngospasm is higher.

    4. **Dosage and administration:** See Table 11.1.

       a. Reduce doses in sick, elderly, or hypovolemic patients.

5. **Adverse effects**
   a. **Allergy.** True allergies are unusual. Thiopental occasionally causes anaphylactoid reactions (hives, facial edema, hypotension).
   b. **Porphyria**
      (1) **Absolutely contraindicated** in patients with acute intermittent porphyria, variegate porphyria, and hereditary coproporphyria.
      (2) Barbiturates induce porphyrin synthetic enzymes like δ-aminolevulinic acid synthetase; patients with porphyria may accumulate toxic heme precursors and suffer an acute attack.
   c. **Venous irritation and tissue damage**
      (1) May cause pain at the site of administration because of venous irritation.
      (2) Subcutaneous infiltration or intra-arterial administration of thiopental (but not methohexital) may cause severe pain, tissue damage, arterial spasm, and necrosis. If intra-arterial administration occurs, heparin treatment, vasodilators, and/or regional sympathetic blockade may be helpful in treatment.
   d. **Myoclonus, twitching, and hiccoughing** are often associated with the administration of methohexital.
C. **Benzodiazepines** include midazolam, diazepam, and lorazepam. They are often used for sedation and amnesia or as adjuncts to general anesthesia. Midazolam is prepared in a water-soluble form at pH 3.5, while diazepam and lorazepam are dissolved in propylene glycol and polyethylene glycol, respectively.
   1. **Mode of action:** Enhance the inhibitory tone of GABA receptors.
   2. **Pharmacokinetics**
      a. After IV administration, the onset of CNS effects occurs in 2 to 3 minutes for midazolam and diazepam (slightly longer for lorazepam). All have effects terminated by redistribution, so the durations of a single dose of diazepam and midazolam are similar. The effects of lorazepam are somewhat more prolonged.
      b. All three drugs are metabolized in the liver. Elimination half-lives for midazolam, lorazepam, and diazepam are approximately 2, 11, and 20 hours, respectively. The active metabolites of diazepam last longer than the parent drug and accumulate with repeated dosing. Hydroxymidazolam can accumulate and cause sedation in patients with renal failure.
      c. Diazepam clearance is reduced in the elderly, but this is less of a problem with midazolam and lorazepam. Obese patients may require higher initial doses of benzodiazepines, but clearance is not markedly different.
   3. **Pharmacodynamics**
      a. **CNS**
         (1) Produce amnestic, anticonvulsant, anxiolytic, muscle-relaxant, and sedative-hypnotic effects in a dose-dependent manner. Amnesia may last only 1 hour after a single premedicant dose of midazolam. Sedation may sometimes be prolonged.

        (2) Do not produce significant analgesia.
        (3) Reduce cerebral blood flow and metabolic rate.
   b. **Cardiovascular system**
        (1) Produce a mild systemic vasodilation and reduction in cardiac output. Heart rate is usually unchanged.
        (2) Hemodynamic changes may be pronounced in hypovolemic patients or in those with little cardiovascular reserve if rapidly administered in a large dose or if administered with an opioid.
   c. **Respiratory system**
        (1) Produce a mild dose-dependent decrease in respiratory rate and tidal volume.
        (2) Respiratory depression may be pronounced if administered with an opioid, in patients with pulmonary disease, or in debilitated patients.
  4. **Dosage and administration:** See Table 11.1 for midalozam.
   a. Incremental IV doses of diazepam (2.5 mg) or lorazepam (0.25 mg) may be used for sedation. Appropriate oral doses are 5 to 10 mg of diazepam or 2 to 4 mg of lorazepam.
  5. **Adverse effects**
   a. **Drug interactions.** Administration of a benzodiazepine to a patient receiving the anticonvulsant valproate may precipitate a psychotic episode.
   b. **Pregnancy and labor**
        (1) May be associated with birth defects (cleft lip and palate) when administered during the first trimester.
        (2) Cross the placenta and may lead to a depressed neonate.
   c. **Superficial thrombophlebitis and injection pain** may be produced by the vehicles in diazepam and lorazepam.
  6. **Flumazenil** is a competitive antagonist for benzodiazepine receptors in the CNS.
   a. Reversal of benzodiazepine-induced sedative effects occurs within 2 min; peak effects occur at approximately 10 min. Flumazenil does not completely antagonize the respiratory depressant effects of benzodiazepines.
   b. Flumazenil is shorter acting than the benzodiazepines it is used to antagonize. Repeated administration may be necessary because of its short duration of action.
   c. Metabolized to inactive metabolites in the liver.
   d. **Dose:** 0.3 mg IV every 30 to 60 seconds (to a maximum dose of 5 mg).
   e. Flumazenil is **contraindicated** in patients with tricyclic antidepressant overdose and in those receiving benzodiazepines for control of seizures or elevated intracranial pressure. Use cautiously in patients who have had long-term treatment with benzodiazepines because acute withdrawal may be precipitated.
D. **Ketamine** is a congener of phencyclidine. It is a sedative-hypnotic agent with powerful analgesic properties. Usually used as an induction agent.
  1. **Mode of action:** Not well defined but includes antagonism at the NMDA receptor.

2. **Pharmacokinetics**
   a. Produces unconsciousness in 30 to 60 seconds after an IV induction dose. Effects are terminated by redistribution in 15 to 20 min. After intramuscular (IM) administration, the onset of CNS effects is delayed for approximately 5 min, with peak effect at approximately 15 min.
   b. Metabolized rapidly in the liver to multiple metabolites, some of which have modest activity. Elimination half-life = 2 to 3 hours.
   c. Repeated bolus doses or an infusion results in accumulation.

3. **Pharmacodynamics**
   a. **CNS**
      (1) Produces a "dissociative" state accompanied by amnesia and analgesia. Analgesia occurs at much lower concentrations than hypnosis, so analgesic effects persist after awakening.
      (2) Increases cerebral blood flow (CBF), metabolic rate, and intracranial pressure. CBF response to hyperventilation is not blocked.
   b. **Cardiovascular system**
      (1) Increases heart rate as well as systemic and pulmonary artery blood pressures by causing centrally mediated release of endogenous catecholamines.
      (2) Often used to induce general anesthesia in hemodynamically compromised patients, particularly those for whom heart rate, preload and afterload, should remain high.
      (3) May act as a direct myocardial depressant if administered to patients with maximal sympathetic nervous system stimulation or in those with autonomic blockade.
   c. **Respiratory system**
      (1) Usually depresses respiratory rate and tidal volume only mildly and has minimal effect on CO_2 response.
      (2) Alleviates bronchospasm by a sympathomimetic effect.
      (3) Laryngeal protective reflexes are relatively well-maintained, but aspiration can still occur.

4. **Dosage and administration:** See Table 11.1.
   a. Ketamine may be especially useful for IM induction in patients in whom IV access is not available (e.g., children). Ketamine is water soluble and may be administered either IV or IM.
   b. A concentrated 10% solution is available for IM use only.

5. **Adverse effects**
   a. **Oral secretions** are markedly stimulated by ketamine. Coadministration of an antisialagogue (e.g., glycopyrrolate) may be helpful.
   b. **Emotional disturbance.** Administration of ketamine may cause restlessness and agitation during emergence; hallucinations and unpleasant dreams may occur postoperatively. Risk factors for these adverse effects include increased age, female gender, and dosages greater than 2 mg/kg. The

incidence (up to 30%) may be greatly reduced with coadministration of a benzodiazepine (e.g., midazolam) or propofol. Children seem to be less troubled than adults by the hallucinations. Alternatives to ketamine should be considered in patients with psychiatric disorders.

c. **Muscle tone.** May lead to random myoclonic movements, especially in response to stimulation. Muscle tone is often increased.

d. **Increases intracranial pressure** and is relatively contraindicated in patients with head trauma or intracranial hypertension.

e. **Ocular effects.** May lead to mydriasis, nystagmus, diplopia, blepharospasm, and increased intraocular pressure; alternatives should be considered during ophthalmologic surgery.

f. **Anesthetic depth may be difficult to assess.** Common signs of anesthetic depth (e.g., respiratory rate, blood pressure, heart rate, eye signs) are less reliable when ketamine is used.

E. **Etomidate** is an imidazole-containing hypnotic unrelated to other anesthetics. It is supplied in a solution containing 35% propylene glycol. It is most commonly used as an IV induction agent for general anesthesia.

1. **Mode of action:** Augments the inhibitory tone of GABA in the CNS.

2. **Pharmacokinetics**

   a. Very high clearance in the liver and by circulating esterases to inactive metabolites.

   b. Times to loss of consciousness and awakening after an induction dose are similar to those of propofol. Effects of a bolus dose are terminated by redistribution.

3. **Pharmacodynamics**

   a. **CNS**

      (1) No analgesic properties, so it is often supplemented with opioids.

      (2) Cerebral blood flow, metabolism, and ICP decrease while cerebral perfusion pressure is usually maintained.

   b. **Cardiovascular system.** Produces minimal changes in heart rate, blood pressure, and cardiac output. Does not affect sympathetic tone or baroreceptor function and will not effectively suppress hemodynamic responses to pain. Etomidate is often chosen to induce general anesthesia in hemodynamically compromised patients.

   c. **Respiratory system.** Produces a dose-dependent decrease in respiratory rate and tidal volume; transient apnea may occur. The respiratory depressant effects of etomidate appear to be less than those of propofol or the barbiturates.

4. **Dosage and administration:** See Table 11.1.

5. **Adverse effects**

   a. **Myoclonus** may occur after administration, particularly in response to stimulation.

   b. **Nausea and vomiting** occur more frequently in the postoperative period than with other anesthetic agents.

   c. **Venous irritation and superficial thrombophlebitis** may be caused by the propylene glycol vehicle.

Minimized by administration into a free-flowing IV carrier infusion.

  d. **Adrenal suppression.** A single dose suppresses adrenal steroid synthesis for up to 24 hours (probably an effect of little clinical significance). Repeated doses or infusions are not recommended because of the risk of significant adrenal suppression.

F. **Dexmedetomidine** is a sedative agent with analgesic properties. It is used as an adjunct to general and regional anesthesia and for sedation in the ICU.

 1. **Mode of action:** Selective $\alpha 2$ adrenoceptor agonist. **Clonidine** is a less selective $\alpha 2$ agonist with similar sedating and analgesic properties.

 2. **Pharmacokinetics**

  a. Undergoes rapid redistribution after IV administration. Elimination half-time is approximately 2 hours.

  b. Metabolized extensively in the liver.

 3. **Pharmacodynamics**

  a. **CNS**

   (1) Elicits a sedated but arousable state with features similar to natural sleep.

   (2) Potentiates CNS effects of propofol, volatile anesthetics, benzodiazepines, and opioids.

  b. **Cardiovascular system**

   (1) Decrease blood pressure and heart rate, although transient hypertension may occur after an IV bolus.

   (2) Baroreflex is well preserved.

  c. **Respiratory system:** Minimal respiratory depression, although it may add to respiratory depressant effects of other anesthetics.

  d. **Endocrine system:** May decrease adrenal response to adrenocorticotropic hormone after prolonged infusions, although clinical significance is unclear.

 4. **Dosage and administration:** See Table 11.1.

  a. Decreased dosage should be considered in patients with significant hepatic dysfunction. Because the activity of dexmedetomidine metabolites has not been studied, decreased dosage may be prudent for patients with severe renal dysfunction.

  b. Indicated only for infusions lasting <24 hours.

G. **Opioids.** Morphine, meperidine, hydromorphone, fentanyl, sufentanil, alfentanil, and remifentanil are the opioids commonly used in general anesthesia. Their primary effect is analgesia, and therefore they are used to supplement other agents during induction or maintenance of general anesthesia. In high doses, opioids are occasionally used as the sole anesthetic (e.g., cardiac surgery). Opioids differ in their potency, pharmacokinetics, and side effects.

 1. **Mode of action:** Opioids bind at specific receptors in the brain, spinal cord, and on peripheral neurons. The opioids listed above are all relatively selective for μ opioid receptors.

 2. **Pharmacokinetics**

  a. Pharmacokinetic data are presented in Table 11.2, and the CSHTs for alfentanil, sufentanil, and remifentanil are shown in Figure 11.1.

Table 11.2. Dose, time to peak effect, and duration of analgesia for intravenous opioid agonists and agonist-antagonists[a]

Opioid	Dose (mg)[b]	Peak (min)	Duration (h)[c]
Morphine	10	30–60	3–4
Meperidine	80	5–7	2–3
Hydromorphone	1.5	15–30	2–3
Oxymorphone	1.0	15–30	3–4
Methadone	10	15–30	3–4
Fentanyl	0.1	3–5	0.5–1
Sufentanil	0.01	3–5	0.5–1
Alfentanil	0.75	1.5–2	0.2–0.3
Remifentanil	0.1	1.5–2	0.1–0.2
Pentazocine	60	15–30	2–3
Butorphanol	2	15–30	2–3
Nalbuphine	10	15–30	3–4
Buprenorphine	0.3	<30	5–6

[a] Data for fentanyl derivatives are derived from intraoperative studies; the remainder from postoperative pain studies.
[b] Approximately equianalgesic doses (see text).
[c] Average duration of first single dose.

    b. Elimination is primarily by the liver and depends on hepatic blood flow. Remifentanil is metabolized by circulating and skeletal muscle esterases. Morphine and meperidine have important active metabolites; hydromorphone and the fentanyl derivatives do not. The metabolites are primarily excreted in the urine.

    c. After IV administration, onset of action is within minutes for the fentanyl derivatives; hydromorphone and morphine may take 20 to 30 minutes for peak effect. Termination of effect for all except remifentanil is by redistribution.

3. Pharmacodynamics

    a. CNS

        (1) Produce sedation and analgesia in a dose-dependent manner; euphoria is common. Very large doses may produce amnesia and loss of consciousness, but opioids are not reliable hypnotics.

        (2) Reduce the minimum alveolar concentration (MAC) of volatile and gaseous anesthetic agents, and reduce the requirements for IV sedative-hypnotic drugs.

        (3) Decrease CBF and metabolic rate. Meperidine, in repeated doses, may produce CNS excitation and seizures, secondary to the accumulation of normeperidine.

    b. Cardiovascular system

        (1) All except meperidine produce minimal changes in cardiac contractility. Opioids do not block low- or high-pressure baroreceptor responses.

        (2) Systemic vascular resistance (SVR) usually is moderately reduced because of reduced medullary sympathetic outflow. Bolus doses of meperidine or morphine may reduce SVR because of histamine release.

(3) Produce bradycardia in a dose-dependent manner by stimulation of the central vagal nuclei. Meperidine has a weak atropine-like effect and does not cause bradycardia.

(4) The relative hemodynamic stability offered by opioids often leads to their use in sedation or anesthesia for hemodynamically compromised or critically ill patients.

c. **Respiratory system**

(1) Produce respiratory depression in a dose-dependent manner. Initially, respiratory rate decreases; with larger doses, tidal volume decreases. Effect is accentuated in the presence of sedatives, other respiratory depressants, or preexisting pulmonary disease.

(2) Decrease ventilatory response to hypercapnia and hypoxia. Effects are markedly increased if the patient falls asleep.

(3) Opioids decrease the cough reflex in a dose-dependent manner. Higher doses suppress tracheal and bronchial foreign body reflexes, so endotracheal tubes and mechanical ventilation are better tolerated.

d. **Pupil size** is decreased (miosis) by stimulation of the Edinger-Westphal nucleus of the oculomotor nerve.

e. **Muscle rigidity** may occur after opioid administration, especially in the chest, abdomen, and upper airway, resulting in the inability to ventilate the patient. The incidence increases with drug potency, dose, rate of administration, and presence of nitrous oxide. This rigidity may be reversed by administering neuromuscular relaxants or opioid antagonists. Rigidity is less likely after pretreatment with a sedative dose of a benzodiazepine or propofol.

f. **Gastrointestinal system**

(1) Produce a decrease in gastric emptying and intestinal secretions. Colonic tone and sphincter tone increase, and propulsive contractions decrease.

(2) Increase biliary pressure and may produce biliary colic; spasm of the sphincter of Oddi can prevent cannulation of the common duct. The incidence is lower with the agonist-antagonist opioids.

g. **Nausea and vomiting** can occur because of direct stimulation of the chemoreceptor trigger zone. Nausea is more likely if the patient is moving.

h. **Urinary retention** may occur because of increased tone in the vesical sphincter and inhibition of the detrusor (voiding) reflex. May also decrease awareness of the need to urinate.

i. **Allergic reactions** are rare, although anaphylactoid (histamine) reactions are seen with morphine and meperidine.

j. **Drug interactions.** Administration of meperidine to a patient who has received a monoamine oxidase inhibitor may result in delirium or hyperthermia and may be fatal.

4. **Dosage and administration.** Opioids are usually administered IV, either by bolus or infusion. Appropriate dosages are presented in Table 11.2. Clinical dosing must be individualized and based on the patient's underlying condition and clinical response. Larger doses may be required in patients chronically receiving opioids.

5. **Naloxone** is a pure opioid antagonist used to reverse unanticipated or undesired opioid-induced effects such as respiratory or CNS depression.

   a. **Mode of action.** Naloxone is a competitive antagonist at opioid receptors in the brain and spinal cord.

   b. **Pharmacokinetics**
      (1) Peak effects are seen within 1 to 2 min; a significant decrease in its clinical effects occurs after 30 min because of redistribution.
      (2) Metabolized in the liver.

   c. **Pharmacodynamics**
      (1) Reverses the pharmacologic effects of opioids such as CNS and respiratory depression.
      (2) Crosses the placenta; administration to the parturient before delivery will decrease opioid-induced respiratory depression in the neonate.

   d. **Dosage and administration:** Perioperative respiratory depression in an adult can be treated with 0.04 mg IV every 2 to 3 min as needed.

   e. **Adverse effects**
      (1) **Pain.** May lead to the abrupt onset of pain as opioid analgesia is reversed. This may be accompanied by sudden hemodynamic changes (e.g., hypertension, tachycardia).
      (2) **Cardiac arrest.** Naloxone administration has, in rare cases, precipitated pulmonary edema and cardiac arrest.
      (3) Repeated administration may be necessary because of its short duration of action.

II. **Pharmacology of inhalation anesthetics.** Inhalation anesthetics are usually administered for maintenance of general anesthesia but also can be used for induction, especially in pediatric patients. General properties of inhalation anesthetics are presented in Table 11.3. Dosages of inhalation anesthetics are expressed as **MAC**, the **minimum alveolar concentration** at one atmosphere at which 50% of patients do not move in response to a surgical stimulus.

A. **Mode of action**
   1. **Nitrous oxide.** Produces general anesthesia through interaction with cellular membranes of the CNS; exact mechanisms are not clear.
   2. **Volatile anesthetics.** Exact mechanisms are unknown. Various ion channels in the CNS (including GABA, glycine, and NMDA receptors) have been shown to be sensitive to inhalation anesthetics and may play a role.

B. **Pharmacokinetics**
   1. Nitrous oxide
      a. Uptake and elimination of nitrous oxide are relatively rapid compared with other inhaled anesthetics, primarily as a result of its low blood-gas partition coefficient (0.47).

Table 11.3. Properties of inhalation anesthetics

Anesthetic	Vapor Pressure (mm Hg, 20°C)	Partition Coefficients Blood Gas[a] (37°C)	Partition Coefficients Brain-blood (37°C)	MAC (% with O_2 only)
Halothane	243	2.3	2.0	0.74
Enflurane	175	1.8	1.4	1.68
Isoflurane	239	1.4	1.6	1.15
Desflurane	664	0.42	1.3	6.0
Sevoflurane	157	0.69	1.7	2.05
Nitrous oxide	39,000	0.47	1.1	104

MAC, minimum alveolar concentration that inhibits movement in response to a skin incision in 50% of patients.
[a] The blood-gas partition coefficient is inversely related to the rate of induction.

    b. Nitrous oxide is eliminated via exhalation.
    c. Significant biotransformation has not been demonstrated.
  2. Volatile anesthetics
    a. Determinants of speed of onset and offset. The alveolar anesthetic concentration (F_A) may differ significantly from the inspired anesthetic concentration (F_I). The rate of rise of the ratio of these two concentrations (F_A/F_I) determines the speed of induction of general anesthesia (Fig. 11.2). Two opposing processes, anesthetic delivery to and uptake from alveoli, determine the F_A/F_I at a given time. Determinants of uptake include the following:
      (1) Blood-gas partition coefficient. A lower solubility in blood will lead to lower uptake of anesthetic into the bloodstream, thereby increasing the rate of rise of F_A/F_I. The solubility of halogenated volatile anesthetics in blood is increased somewhat with hypothermia and hyperlipidemia.
      (2) Inspired anesthetic concentration, which is influenced by circuit size, fresh gas inflow rate, and absorption of volatile anesthetic by circuit components.
      (3) Alveolar ventilation. Increased minute ventilation, without alteration of other processes that affect anesthetic delivery or uptake, increases F_A/F_I. This effect is more pronounced with the more blood-soluble agents.
      (4) Concentration effect. As F_I increases, the rate of rise of F_A/F_I also increases. For a gas with a high F_I like nitrous oxide, a large amount is taken up into blood, but this causes a large loss of total gas volume. The remaining nitrous oxide is thus "concentrated," and addition of more anesthetic with the next breath will increase the concentration further. The uptake of a large gas volume also creates a void that draws more fresh gas into the alveoli, thereby increasing F_A and augmenting the inspired tidal volume. The concentration effect explains why the rate of rise of F_A/F_I is

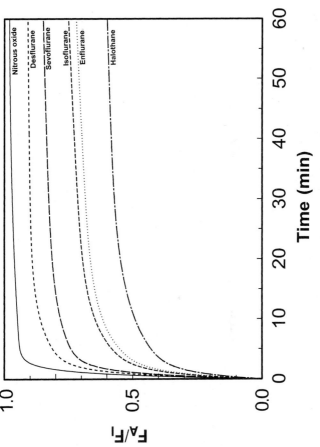

Figure 11.2. Ratio of alveolar to inspired gas concentration (F_A/F_I) as a function of time at constant cardiac output and minute ventilation.

faster for nitrous oxide than for desflurane (see Fig. 11.2), even though the blood-gas partition coefficient for desflurane is smaller.

(5) **The second gas effect.** This is a direct outcome of the concentration effect. When nitrous oxide and a potent inhalation anesthetic are administered together, the uptake of nitrous oxide concentrates the "second" gas (e.g., isoflurane) and increases the input of additional second gas into alveoli via augmentation of inspired volume.

(6) **Cardiac output.** An increase in cardiac output (and therefore pulmonary blood flow) will increase anesthetic uptake and thus decrease the rate of rise in F_A/F_I. A decrease in cardiac output will have the opposite effect. This effect of cardiac output is more pronounced with nonrebreathing circuits or highly soluble anesthetics and is most prominent early in the course of anesthetic administration.

(7) **Gradient between alveolar and venous blood.** Uptake of anesthetic in blood will decrease as the anesthetic partial pressure gradient between the alveoli and blood decreases. This gradient is particularly large early in the course of anesthetic administration.

b. **Distribution in tissues.** The partial pressure of an inhalation anesthetic in arterial blood usually approximates its alveolar pressure. The arterial partial pressure may be significantly less, however, when marked ventilation-perfusion abnormalities (e.g., shunt) are present, especially with less-soluble anesthetics (e.g., nitrous oxide). The rate of equilibration of anesthetic partial pressure between blood and a particular organ system depends on the following factors:

(1) **Tissue blood flow.** Equilibration occurs more rapidly in tissues receiving increased perfusion. The most highly perfused organ systems receive approximately 75% of cardiac output; these organs include the brain, kidney, heart, liver, and endocrine glands and are referred to as the vessel-rich group. The remainder of the cardiac output perfuses predominantly muscle and fat.

(2) **Tissue solubility.** For a given arterial anesthetic partial pressure, anesthetic agents with high tissue solubility are slower to equilibrate. Solubilities of anesthetic agents differ among tissues. Blood-brain partition coefficients of inhalation agents are shown in Table 11.3.

(3) **Gradient between arterial blood and tissue.** Until equilibration is reached between the anesthetic partial pressure in the blood and a particular tissue, a gradient exists that leads to uptake of anesthetic by the tissue. The rate of uptake will decrease as the gradient decreases.

c. **Elimination**

(1) **Exhalation.** This is the predominant route of elimination. After discontinuation, an anesthetic's tissue and alveolar partial pressures decrease by reversing

the processes that occurred when the anesthetic was introduced.

(2) **Metabolism.** Volatile anesthetics may undergo different degrees of hepatic metabolism (halothane, 15%; enflurane, 2% to 5%; sevoflurane, 1.5%; isoflurane, <0.2%; desflurane, <0.2%). When anesthetizing concentrations of an agent are present, metabolism probably has little effect on the alveolar concentration because of saturation of hepatic enzymes. After discontinuation of the anesthetic, metabolism may contribute to the decrease in the alveolar concentration; however, the effect is not clinically significant.

(3) **Anesthetic loss.** Inhalation anesthetics may be lost both percutaneously and through visceral membranes, although such losses are probably negligible.

C. **Pharmacodynamics**

1. **Nitrous oxide**

   a. **CNS**

      (1) Produces analgesia.

      (2) Concentrations greater than 60% may produce amnesia, although not reliably.

      (3) Because of its high MAC (104%), it is usually combined with other anesthetics to attain surgical anesthesia.

   b. **Cardiovascular system**

      (1) Mild myocardial depressant and a mild sympathetic nervous system stimulant.

      (2) Heart rate and blood pressure are usually unchanged.

      (3) May increase pulmonary vascular resistance in adults.

   c. **Respiratory system.** Nitrous oxide is a mild respiratory depressant, although less so than the volatile anesthetics.

2. **Volatile anesthetics**

   a. **CNS**

      (1) Produce unconsciousness and amnesia at relatively low inspired concentrations (25% MAC).

      (2) Produce a dose-dependent generalized CNS depression and depression of electroencephalographic activity up to and including burst suppression.

      (3) Produce decreased amplitude and increased latency of somatosensory evoked potentials.

      (4) Increase CBF (halothane > enflurane > isoflurane, desflurane, or sevoflurane).

      (5) Decrease cerebral metabolic rate (isoflurane, desflurane, or sevoflurane > enflurane > halothane).

      (6) Uncouple autoregulation of CBF; decreased cerebral metabolic rate does not lead to decreased CBF.

   b. **Cardiovascular system**

      (1) Produce dose-dependent myocardial depression (halothane > enflurane > isoflurane (desflurane or sevoflurane) and systemic vasodilation (isoflurane > desflurane or sevoflurane > enflurane > halothane).

      (2) Heart rate tends to be unchanged, although desflurane has been associated with sympathetic stimulation, tachycardia, and hypertension at induction or when the inspired concentration is abruptly

increased. Isoflurane administration may lead to similar effects but to a lesser degree than desflurane.

    (3) Sensitize the myocardium to the arrhythmogenic effects of catecholamines (halothane > enflurane > isoflurane or desflurane > sevoflurane), which is of particular concern during infiltration of epinephrine-containing solutions or administration of sympathomimetic agents. With halothane, subcutaneous infiltration with epinephrine should not exceed 2 μg/kg/20 minutes. In a subgroup of patients with coronary artery disease, isoflurane may redirect coronary flow away from ischemic areas; the clinical significance of this is not clear (see Chapter 23).

  c. **Respiratory system**

    (1) Produce dose-dependent respiratory depression with a decrease in tidal volume, an increase in respiratory rate, and an increase in arterial CO_2 pressure.

    (2) Produce airway irritation (desflurane > isoflurane > enflurane > halothane > sevoflurane) and, during light levels of anesthesia, may precipitate coughing, laryngospasm, or bronchospasm, particularly in patients who smoke or have asthma. The lower pungency of sevoflurane and halothane may make them more suitable as inhalation induction agents.

    (3) Equipotent doses of volatile agents possess similar bronchodilator effects, with the exception of desflurane, which has mild bronchoconstricting activity.

  d. **Muscular system**

    (1) Produce a dose-dependent decrease in muscle tone, often enhancing surgical conditions.

    (2) May precipitate malignant hyperthermia in a susceptible patient (see Chapter 18).

  e. **Liver.** May cause a decrease in hepatic perfusion (halothane > enflurane > isoflurane, desflurane, or sevoflurane). Rarely, a patient may develop hepatitis secondary to exposure to a volatile agent, most notably halothane ("halothane hepatitis") (see Chapter 5).

  f. **Renal system.** Decrease renal blood flow through either a decrease in mean arterial blood pressure or an increase in renal vascular resistance.

D. **Problems related to specific agents**

  1. **Nitrous oxide**

    a. **Expansion of closed gas spaces.** The predominant constituent in closed gas-containing spaces in the body is nitrogen. Because nitrous oxide is 31 times more soluble in blood than nitrogen, closed air spaces will expand as the amount of nitrous oxide diffusing into these spaces is greater than the amount of nitrogen diffusing out. Spaces containing air such as a pneumothorax, occluded middle ear, bowel lumen, or pneumocephalus will markedly enlarge if nitrous oxide is administered. Nitrous oxide will diffuse into the cuff of an endotracheal tube and may increase pressure within the cuff; this pressure should be assessed intermittently and, if necessary, adjusted.

    b. **Diffusion hypoxia.** After discontinuation of nitrous oxide, its rapid diffusion from the blood into the lung may lead to a low partial pressure of oxygen in the alveoli, resulting in hypoxia and hypoxemia if supplemental oxygen is not administered.

    c. **Inhibition of tetrahydrofolate synthesis.** N_2O inactivates methionine synthetase, a vitamin B_{12}-dependent enzyme necessary for the synthesis of DNA. Nitrous oxide should be used with caution in pregnant patients and those deficient in vitamin B_{12}.

2. **Desflurane** can be degraded to carbon monoxide in carbon dioxide absorbents (especially Baralyme). This is most likely to occur when the absorbent is new or dry from the passage of large volumes of dry gas; a few cases of clinically significant carbon monoxide poisoning have been reported.

3. **Sevoflurane** can be degraded in CO_2 absorbents (especially Baralyme) to fluoromethyl-2,2,-difluoro-1-vinyl ether (Compound A), which has been shown to produce renal toxicity in animal models. Compound A concentrations increase at low fresh gas rates. So far, there has been no evidence of consistent renal toxicity with sevoflurane usage in humans.

4. **Enflurane** can produce electroencephalographic epileptiform activity at high inspired concentrations (>2%).

SUGGESTED READING

Campagna JA, Miller KW, Forman SA. Mechanisms of actions of inhaled anesthetics. *N Engl J Med* 2003;348:2110–2124.

Eger EI. Uptake and distribution. In: Miller RD, ed. *Anesthesia*, 6th ed. New York: Churchill Livingstone, 2005;131–153.

Kennedy, SK. Pharmacology of intravenous anesthetic agents. In: Longnecker DE, Tinker JH, Morgan GE Jr, eds. *Principles and practice of anesthesiology*, 2nd ed. Philadelphia: Mosby-Year Book, 1998;1211–1232.

Rosow CE, Dershwitz M. Pharmacology of opioid analgetic agents. In: Longnecker DE, Tinker JH, Morgan GE Jr, eds. *Principles and practice of anesthesiology*, 2nd ed. Philadelphia: Mosby-Year Book, 1998;1233–1259.

12

Neuromuscular Blockade

Jaianand S. Sethee and Peter F. Dunn

The principal pharmacologic effect of neuromuscular blocking drugs (NMBDs) is to interrupt transmission of synaptic signaling at the neuromuscular junction (NMJ) by antagonism of the nicotinic acetylcholine receptor (AChR).

I. **Anatomy and physiology of the NMJ**

   A. **The NMJ** comprises portions of three cell types: motor neuron, muscle fiber, and Schwann cell. It is a chemical synapse located in the peripheral nervous system that is composed of **the neuronal presynaptic terminal,** where **acetylcholine** (ACh) is stored and released, and the postsynaptic muscle cell (**motor endplate**), where high densities of the AChR reside. In the nerve terminal, ACh is stored for eventual release in specialized organelles known as **synaptic vesicles.** These vesicles are found in high concentrations in the regions of the nerve terminal that lie in direct apposition to areas of muscle membrane with high concentrations of AChRs. On the folds of the postsynaptic muscle membrane, AChRs are found in densities as high as $10,000/\mu m^2$ at the synapse and fall to concentrations as low as 10 to $100/\mu m^2$ at extrajunctional regions of the muscle cell (Fig. 12.1).

   B. In response to an action potential in the nerve, **voltage dependent N-type calcium channels,** which are also highly concentrated in close proximity to synaptic vesicles, open and cause a rapid influx of calcium into the nerve terminal. These calcium transients, lasting approximately 0.5 milliseconds, elevate calcium concentrations intracellularly to approximately 100 μM and induce fusion of synaptic vesicles with the plasma membrane and release of the stored ACh. The ACh then diffuses across the synaptic cleft where two molecules of ACh bind simultaneously to a single AChR.

   C. Junctional AChRs are composed of five subunits (α, α, β, δ, and ϵ). Of these, the α subunits constitute the binding sites for ACh. When two molecules of ACh are bound, the AChR undergoes a conformational change, "activation," that allows influx of Na^+ and Ca^{2+} into the muscle cell, depolarizing the membrane, and allowing contraction. As the membrane becomes depolarized, Na^+ and Ca^{2+} cease to enter and K^+ begins to move out, beginning the process of repolarization. At this point, the AChR is "inactivated." The amount of ACh released and the number of postsynaptic AChRs is much greater than that actually needed to induce contraction. This is termed the "safety factor" for neuromuscular transmission and plays a crucial role in certain pathologic conditions.

   D. After triggering depolarization, the ACh diffuses into the synaptic cleft where it is broken down by **acetylcholinesterase** (AchE) into choline and acetyl CoA. These molecules are then recycled to synthesize new ACh for use in synaptic vesicles and synaptic

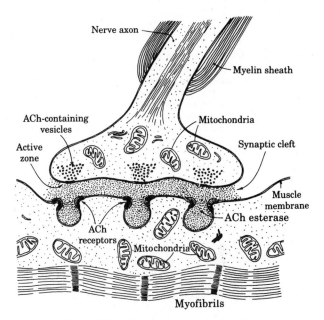

Figure 12.1. The neuromuscular junction.

transmission. Inactivated AChRs are now returned to their "resting" state, able to be activated once more.

II. General pharmacology of the NMJ

The precise apposition of a motor nerve terminal and the muscle membrane make the NMJ a very efficient specialized structure. AChR and AChE are the primary targets of most NMBDs used in clinical anesthesia.

A. **Cholinergic receptors** are categorized as **nicotinic** and **muscarinic** by their responses to the alkaloids nicotine and muscarine, respectively. There are two broad classes of nicotinic cholinergic receptors, muscular (N_M) and neuronal (N_N). N_M receptors are found at the NMJ, whereas N_N are in autonomic ganglia and the central nervous system (CNS). The various classes of muscarinic receptor are found in autonomic ganglia, at end-organ sites of parasympathetic innervation, and in the CNS. All these cholinergic receptors have different subunit composition and are affected differently by various agonists and antagonists. Nonspecific cholinergic agonists (e.g., reversal agents) can affect all of them, however.

B. There are well-described **signaling systems** that regulate the distribution and density of AChR at the NMJ. Conditions that affect AChR distribution are quite common clinically. For example, with burns, trauma, or disuse, the density of postsynaptic junctional AChRs decreases, whereas extrajunctional densities increase.

C. **All NMBDs are antagonists of the AChR.** Each is designated **depolarizing** or **nondepolarizing** based on whether it induces a depolarization of the muscle membrane after binding to the receptor. The agents differ substantially in their onset, duration of blockade, metabolism, side effects, and interactions with other drugs.

D. **Succinylcholine** (SCh) is currently the only available depolarizing NMBD. Nondepolarizing NMBDs are often divided by chemical class: **aminosteroid derivatives** (e.g., pancuronium, vecuronium, and rocuronium) and **benzylisoquinolines** (e.g., *d*-tubocurarine, cisatracurium, and mivacurium). The NMBDs also are commonly classified by duration of effect: ultrashort (SCh), short (mivacurium), intermediate (vecuronium, rocuronium, cisatracurium), and long (pancuronium, *d*-tubocurarine).

III. Neuromuscular blockade

A. **Depolarizing blockade** occurs when a drug mimics the action of the neurotransmitter ACh. SCh, like ACh, binds and activates the AChR, which leads to depolarization of the endplate and adjacent muscle membrane. Because SCh is not degraded as quickly as ACh, persistent endplate depolarization inhibits the inward flow of sodium ions, and there is inexcitability of the perijunctional muscle membrane. The inability to further activate sodium channels explains how muscle relaxation can occur in the presence of an endplate potential sufficient to trigger an action potential.

1. **Depolarizing blockade** (Fig. 12.2) is characterized by the following:
   a. Muscle fasciculation followed by relaxation.

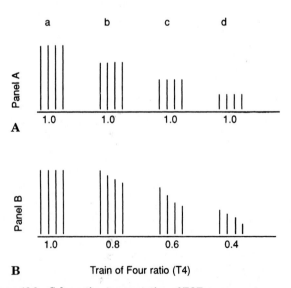

Figure 12.2. Schematic representation of TOF responses to a depolarizing (A) and a nondepolarizing (B) relaxant, showing the control response before the relaxant (*a*) and afterward (*b, c, d*). Note no fade with the depolarizing relaxant and progressive fade with the nondepolarizing relaxant.

b. Absence of fade after tetanic or train-of-four (TOF) stimulation (see section IV).

c. Absence of posttetanic potentiation (PTP). (See section IVC.)

d. Potentiation of the block by anticholinesterases.

e. Antagonism of the block by nondepolarizing relaxants.

2. Depolarizing blockade from SCh ends when the molecule diffuses away from the receptor and is broken down to choline and succinic acid in the plasma. SCh is hydrolyzed by **plasma cholinesterase** (also called butyrylcholinesterase or pseudocholinesterase) to choline and succinic acid. This enzyme is not the same as AChE and is not found in the synaptic cleft. Inhibitors of AchE tend to affect both enzymes, however.

3. **Side effects** of SCh are related to its transient agonist effects at both the nicotinic and muscarinic AChRs.

   a. **Myalgias** are common postoperatively, especially in the muscles of the abdomen, back, and neck and may occur secondary to muscle fasciculations. They occur more frequently in women and in young ambulatory patients after minor surgical procedures. The incidence of myalgias is reduced by administering a small dose of a nondepolarizing relaxant (e.g., 1 mg of cisatracurium intravenously [IV] or 3 mg of rocuronium IV) 3 min before SCh administration. When pretreating for a rapid sequence induction, the subsequent dose of SCh is increased to 1.5 mg/kg IV. Awake patients pretreated with a nondepolarizing relaxant may experience diplopia, weakness, or dyspnea. Pretreatment with lidocaine, propofol, benzodiazepines, Mg^{2+}, vitamin C, and combinations have been tried but their effectiveness remains unproven. No technique can completely eliminate myalgias.

   b. **Arrhythmias. Ganglionic stimulation** will often increase heart rate and blood pressure in adults. **SCh** may produce sinus bradycardia, junctional rhythm, and sinus arrest in children after the first dose and in adults receiving a second dose within a short dose interval (i.e., 5 minutes). Pretreatment with atropine (0.4 mg IV) immediately before SCh blocks this bradycardia.

   c. SCh normally causes serum K^+ to increase 0.5 to 1.0 mEq/L but dangerous **hyperkalemia** and cardiovascular collapse have occurred in patients with burns, upper and lower motor neuron disease, and injuries. This effect is due to up-regulation of extrajunctional ACh receptors. In burned patients, the period of greatest risk is from 2 weeks to 6 months after the burn has been sustained; however, it is advisable to avoid SCh in burned patients after the first 24 hours and for 2 years from the injury. Patients with renal failure may safely receive SCh if they are not currently hyperkalemic or acidemic.

   d. **A transient increase in intraocular pressure** occurs after an intubating dose of SCh presumably due to fascicular contractions of the extraocular muscles. The use of SCh in open eye injuries is still possible (see Chapter 25, section I.C.1.a for a full discussion).

e. **Increased intragastric pressure** results from fasciculation of abdominal muscles. The pressure increase averages 15 to 20 mm Hg in an adult but does not occur to a significant extent in infants and children.

f. SCh produces a mild brief **increase in cerebral blood flow and intracranial pressure** (see Chapter 24, section II.C).

g. A history of **malignant hyperthermia** is an absolute contraindication to the use of SCh. Malignant hyperthermia may be triggered in susceptible patients. Failure of the masseter muscle to relax or generalized myotonia after SCh should alert one to this possibility (see Chapter 18, section XVII).

h. **Pretreatment with nondepolarizing NMBDs** may block visible fasciculations but is not uniformly effective in attenuating the above-mentioned side effects.

i. **Phase II block** is most likely to occur after repeated or continuous administration of SCh. Phase II block may occur with dosages of 2 to 5 mg/kg IV in conjunction with inhalation anesthetics and 8 to 12 mg/kg with nitrous oxide-opioid anesthesia. Phase II blockade has some of the characteristics of a nondepolarizing block:

(1) Fade after tetanic or TOF stimulation. (See section IV.C.)

(2) Tachyphylaxis (increasing dose requirement).

(3) Partial or complete reversal with anticholinesterases.

j. **Prolonged blockade** may be caused by low levels of plasma cholinesterase, drug-induced inhibition of cholinesterase activity, or a genetically atypical enzyme.

(1) **Decreased plasma cholinesterase levels** are seen in the last trimester of pregnancy, liver disease, starvation, carcinomas, hypothyroidism, burn patients, shock, uremia, cardiac failure, and after therapeutic radiation.

(2) **Inhibition of plasma cholinesterase** occurs with the use of organophosphate compounds (e.g., insecticides, echothiophate eye drops) and other drugs that inhibit AChE (e.g., neostigmine, pyridostigmine, donepezil, rivastigmine). Plasma cholinesterase levels are not usually altered after hemodialysis.

(3) **Heterozygous atypical plasma cholinesterase** occurs in 4% of the general population, whereas the incidence of **homozygous atypical cholinesterase** enzyme is about 0.04% (1 in 2,800 patients). Homozygous atypical patients have prolonged neuromuscular blockade and respiratory insufficiency for 2 to 3 hours after SCh administration. The **dibucaine number** is a laboratory assay used to characterize plasma cholinesterase abnormality. Normal plasma cholinesterase is 80% inhibited in vitro by the local anesthetic dibucaine (dibucaine number 80), whereas the homozygous atypical plasma cholinesterase is only 20% inhibited (dibucaine number 20). A range of dibucaine numbers from

30 to 65 occurs in heterozygotes. Less commonly, individuals sensitive to SCh may have a fluoride-resistant enzyme (with a normal dibucaine number but a low fluoride number) or a silent gene with complete absence of plasma cholinesterase (dibucaine number 0) and no esterase activity.

B. **Nondepolarizing blockade** is most commonly due to reversible competitive antagonism of ACh at the α subunits of the AChR.

1. **Other mechanisms** can be involved under the following circumstances:

a. **Noncompetitive blockade** around the extracellular entrance of the channel may be produced by high concentrations of nondepolarizing relaxants and by some antibiotics, quinidine, tricyclic antidepressants, and naloxone.

b. **Desensitization** can be produced by long duration of exposure of the AChR to an agonist, resulting in a conformational change in the receptor. This may be the mechanism of phase II block from SCh.

c. **Interference** with presynaptic ACh mobilization. The commonly used nondepolarizing NMBDs probably inhibit ACh release by binding to cholinergic autoreceptors on the presynaptic terminal.

d. **Interference** with presynaptic Ca^{2+} influx. Aminoglycoside antibiotics are thought to inhibit ACh release presynaptically by competing with Ca^{2+}. Ca^{2+} channel blockers potentiate neuromuscular blockade as well, although the precise mechanisms have not been defined.

2. **Nondepolarizing blockade** (Figs. 12.2 and 12.3) is characterized by the following:

a. Absence of fasciculations.

b. Fade during tetanic and TOF stimulation. (See section IV.)

c. PTP. (See section IVC3.)

d. Antagonism of depolarizing block; reversible by anticholinesterases.

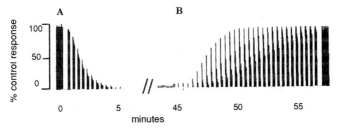

Figure 12.3. A: Electromyographic response to repeated TOF stimulation after injection of a nondepolarizing agent. Each vertical bar is composed of four individual twitch responses. Fade of TOF response eventually leaves only one twitch (approximately 90% block). B: Reversal of the blockade by neostigmine and atropine given 45 min later shows a progressive recovery of the TOF response and reduction in fade with a TOF ratio of 0.9.

Table 12.1. Comparative clinical pharmacology of relaxants[a,b]

	ED_{95}[c] (mg/kg IV)	Intubating Dose (mg/kg IV)[d]	Time to Intubation (min)[e]	Time to 25% Recovery (min)[f]	Elimination
Depolarizing drug					
Succinylcholine	0.25	1	1	5–20	Hydrolysis by plasma cholinesterase.
Nondepolarizing drug					
Atracurium	0.25	0.4–0.5	2–3	25–30	Ester hydrolysis and Hoffman elimination
Cisatracurium	0.05	0.15–0.2	2–2.5	50–60	Hoffman elimination
d-tubocurarine	0.51	0.5–0.6	3–5	80–100	70% renal, 15%–20% biliary secretion
Gallamine	3.0	3.0–4.0	3–5	80–120	100% renal
Metocurine	0.28	0.3–0.4	3–5	80–100	80%–100% renal
Mivacurium	0.09	0.15–0.25	1.5–2.0	16–20	Hydrolysis by plasma cholinesterase
Pancuronium	0.07	0.08–1.0	3–5	80–100	70%–80% renal, 15%–20% biliary excretion and hepatic
Rocuronium	0.3	0.6–1.2	1–1.5	40–150	Primarily excreted by liver
Vecuronium	0.06	0.1–0.12	2–3	25–30	10%–20% renal, 80% biliary excretion and hepatic

Synergistic combinations

Pancuronium and d-tubocurarine	0.02 + 0.15	3–5	40–60
Pancuronium and metocurine	0.02 + 0.07	3–6	40–60

[a] All doses were determined under balanced (nitrous oxide-opioid) technique.

[b] There is a large variability in the response to all relaxants, especially at the extremes of age and with profound illness. Therefore, all patients should be monitored as described in the text.

[c] An ED_{95} dose of a relaxant gives adequate surgical relaxation with nitrous oxide-opioid anesthesia.

[d] These are customary intubating doses and not all equipotent. All relaxants are potentiated by potent inhalational anesthetics, including newer agents such as desflurane and sevoflurane.

[e] These times reflect the use of customary intubating doses and may be altered very substantially by very light or very deep anesthesia. For rapid sequence induction with nondepolarizing agents, onset time can be reduced by using a "priming dose" 3–5 min before the full dose. No nondepolarizing relaxant has as rapid an onset as succinylcholine.

[f] Maintenance doses to be given when the twitch height reaches 25% of control are generally 20%–25% of the initial dose.

    e. Potentiation of block by other nondepolarizing NMBDs and other anesthetic agents.

  3. **Synergistic blockade** may result when aminosteroid NMBDs (pancuronium, vecuronium, or rocuronium) are combined with benzylisoquinolines (mivacurium, atracurium, or cisatracurium). The combined effects of agents with similar chemical structure, such as mivacurium and atracurium, are additive.

  4. **The clinical pharmacology** of the commonly used nondepolarizing NMBDs is outlined in Table 12.1.

  5. **Cisatracurium** is 1 of 10 stereoisomers that constitute atracurium. It is two to three times as potent as atracurium. High molar potency results in a relatively slow onset time. Unlike atracurium, it does not produce histamine release or hemodynamic effects after rapid injection of doses as high as eight times its 95% effective dose (ED_{95}). In usual doses, intubating conditions are achieved in 3 to 5 minutes. The drug is cleared primarily by spontaneous, nonenzymatic Hoffman degradation (into laudanosine metabolites), so its duration of action is largely independent of renal or hepatic function.

  6. **Rocuronium** is an analog of vecuronium that has lower potency. Low potency (large intubating dose) results in a fast onset time. At a dose of 0.6 mg/kg, good to excellent intubating conditions occur by 60 seconds. Increasing the dose to 1.2 mg/kg (four times the ED_{95}) shortens the time even more but significantly prolongs the duration of action. Rocuronium's duration of action can be highly variable among patients. It is often chosen when rapid sequence induction is necessary and SCh is contraindicated.

  7. **Mivacurium** is a short-acting nondepolarizing NMBD that is rapidly hydrolyzed by plasma cholinesterase. The onset time is similar to that of *cis*-atracurium, although this may be improved by dividing a 0.25-mg/kg intubating dose and administering 0.10 mg/kg just before the induction agent. It should be used with caution in patients with known atypical plasma cholinesterase activity or in those given cholinesterase inhibitors. Histamine release can occur with higher doses. In the event that mivacurium must be antagonized with an anticholinesterase, edrophonium may be preferred to neostigmine because it has much less effect on plasma cholinesterase activity.

  8. The **cardiovascular side effects** of nondepolarizing NMBDs are summarized in Table 12.2. Hypotension caused by histamine release (e.g., with atracurium or mivacurium) can be reduced or prevented if the drug is administered over 30 seconds.

C. **Clinical choice of NMBD**

  1. **Many factors** must be considered simultaneously when selecting a NMBD: the urgency for tracheal intubation, the duration of the procedure, coexisting medical conditions that may affect the NMJ, and side effects and metabolism of the drug. For example, SCh is a good choice for rapid intubation of the trachea, but rocuronium may be a better choice in a burned patient. Pancuronium can produce a tachycardia that is undesirable in patients with severe ischemic heart disease but may be appropriate in pediatric patients.

  2. **Cost-effectiveness** is also a consideration in the choice of drug, and some have suggested that the additional expense

Table 12.2. Cardiovascular side effects of relaxants

Drugs	Histamine Release[a]	Ganglionic Effects	Vagolytic Activity	Sympathetic Stimulation
Atracurium	+	0	0	0
Cisatracurium	0	0	0	0
Doxacurium	0	0	0	0
d-Tubocurarine	+ + +	−	0	0
Gallamine	0	0	+ + +	+
Metocurine	+	0	0	0
Mivacurium	+	0	0	0
Pancuronium	0	0	+ +	+ +
Pipecuronium	0	0	±	0
Rocuronium	0	0	0	0
Succinylcholine	±	+	0	0
Vecuronium	0	0	0	0

[a] Histamine release is dose and rate dependent, and, therefore, less pronounced if drugs are given slowly.

of newer short-acting NMBDs is not justified in longer cases. A large Danish study (Berg et al., 1997) compared pancuronium with vecuronium and atracurium. Despite the use of intraoperative neuromuscular monitoring, pancuronium-treated patients had a significantly higher incidence of postoperative residual blockade and pulmonary complications. The cost of any drug-induced morbidity should be a part of assessing cost-effectiveness.

IV. **Monitoring neuromuscular function**
   A. There are several reasons to monitor neuromuscular function under anesthesia:
      1. To facilitate timing of intubation.
      2. To provide an objective measurement of relaxation during surgery and degree of recovery before extubation.
      3. To titrate dosage according to patient response.
      4. To monitor for the development of phase II block.
      5. To permit early recognition of patients with abnormal plasma cholinesterase activity.
   B. **Peripheral nerve stimulators** use various patterns of stimulation: single-twitch, tetanus, TOF, and double-burst stimulation as well as the "posttetanic count." The **adductor pollicis response to ulnar nerve stimulation** at the wrist is most often used, because it is easily accessible, and results are not confused with direct muscle activation. Cutaneous electrodes are placed at the wrist over the ulnar nerve and attached to a battery-driven pulse generator, which delivers a graded impulse of electrical current at a specified frequency. For maximal twitch response, the negative pole (active) should be placed distally over the ulnar nerve at the wrist. Evoked muscle tension can be estimated by feeling for thumb adduction or measured by using a force transducer attached to the thumb. After the administration of a muscle relaxant, the developed tension and twitch height decrease with the onset of neuromuscular blockade. If the ulnar nerve is unavailable, other sites may be used

Table 12.3. Clinical assessment of blockade

Twitch Response	Clinical Correlate
95% suppression of single twitch at 0.15–0.1 Hz	Adequate intubating conditions
90% suppression of single twitch; train-of-four count of one twitch	Surgical relaxation with nitrous oxide-opioid anesthesia
75% suppression of single twitch; train-of-four count of three twitches	Adequate relaxation with inhalation agents
25% suppression of single twitch	Decreased vital capacity
Train-of-four ratio >0.75; sustained tetanus at 50 Hz for 5 s	Head lift for 5 s; vital capacity = 15–20 mL/kg; inspiratory force = –25 cm H_2O; effective cough
Train-of-four ratio >0.9	Sit up unassisted; intact carotid body response to hypoxemia; normal pharyngeal function
Train-of-four ratio = 1.0	Normal expiratory flow rate, vital capacity, and inspiratory force. Diplopia resolves

(e.g., facial, posterior tibial, peroneal, or lateral popliteal nerves). It is difficult to estimate twitch strength accurately by palpation, so significant residual muscular blockade may be missed by all these techniques.

C. The twitch response to various patterns of stimulation has been correlated with clinical endpoints, and these data are summarized in Table 12.3.

1. **Single twitch** is a supramaximal stimulus, typically lasting 0.2 milliseconds at a frequency of 0.1 Hz (one impulse every 10 seconds). The height of the muscle twitch (its amplitude for a given load and peak tension) is determined as a percent of control. A supramaximal stimulus ensures recruitment of all muscle fibers, and a short duration prevents repetitive nerve firing. The stimulus frequency is important because it affects twitch height and degree of fade. Single twitch is not a sensitive measure of onset or recovery from blockade because 75% of receptors must be blocked before twitch height begins to decrease and 75% may still be blocked when it returns to control height.

2. **Tetanic stimulus** frequencies vary from 50 to 200 Hz. All NMBDs reduce twitch height, but with nondepolarizing block and phase II block tetanic fade is also demonstrated. This occurs when NMBDs bind to presynaptic receptors and decrease mobilization of ACh during high-frequency stimulation. A tetanic stimulus at 50 Hz for 5 seconds is clinically useful,

because a sustained tension at this frequency corresponds to that achieved with maximum voluntary effort. However, tetanic stimuli are painful and can speed recovery in the stimulated muscle, thus misleading the observer with respect to the degree of recovery in important respiratory and upper airway muscles.

3. **Posttetanic single twitch** is measured by single-twitch stimulation 6 to 10 seconds after a tetanic stimulus. An increase in this twitch is called **PTP**. This transient reversal is due to partial increased mobilization and synthesis of ACh during and after tetanic stimulation. Both nondepolarizing and phase II blockade will cause PTP, but depolarizing blockade will not. Repeated tetanic stimuli can change contractile function and may occasionally cause an artifactual PTP.

4. **The TOF** is four supramaximal stimuli at a frequency of 2 Hz, repeated at intervals of at least 10 seconds. Responses at this frequency show fade during partial curarization. During nondepolarizing neuromuscular blockade, elimination of the fourth response corresponds to 75% depression of a single twitch. Disappearance of the third, second, and first responses correspond to 80%, 90%, and 100% depression of a single twitch, respectively. The ratio of the height of the fourth to the first twitch (TOF ratio) correlates with the degree of clinical recovery. A TOF ratio of 0.75 correlates with some indices of clinical recovery (see Table 12.3). Studies have demonstrated that functional impairment of the muscles of the upper airway may exist up to TOF ratios as high as 0.9, with an increased risk of regurgitation and aspiration. NMBDs may also impair the carotid body hypoxic response, even at a TOF ratio of 0.7. In addition, several studies suggest that experienced clinicians often overestimate TOF ratios and are unable to detect fade when the TOF ratio is greater than 0.4. Nevertheless, TOF is a very useful method for clinical monitoring, because it does not require a control measurement, it is not as painful as tetanic stimulation (may be performed in an awake patient to identify residual block), and it does not induce changes in subsequent recovery. It is a good measure in the range of blockade required for surgical relaxation (75% to 90%) and is useful in assessing recovery from blockade. It is not helpful in quantifying the degree of depolarizing blockade because no fade will be evident. However, TOF monitoring may be used to detect fade, signifying the onset of phase II blockade during continuous or repeated administration of SCh.

5. **Posttetanic count** is used to quantify *deep* levels of nondepolarizing block. A 50-Hz tetanic stimulus is given for 5 seconds, followed 3 seconds later by repeated single stimuli at 1.0 Hz. The number of responses detectable predicts the time for spontaneous recovery.

6. **Double-burst stimulation** uses a burst of two or three tetanic stimuli at 50 Hz followed 750 ms later by a second burst. A decrease in the second response indicates residual curarization. It has been suggested that fade in response to double-burst stimulation is more easily detected than fade in response to TOF stimulation.

  D.   Recording instruments are the only objective means to accurately
       quantify muscle contraction in response to nerve stimulation.
       Mechanomyography converts the force of muscle contraction into
       an electric signal and is considered the gold standard. Electromyog-
       raphy measures the electrical activity of the muscle action potential.
       Acceleromyography measures acceleration of muscle contraction via
       a force transducer and is the only monitor commercially available
       for clinical use. Acoustic myography is a relatively new modal-
       ity that measures low-frequency sounds generated by muscular
       contraction.

V. **Reversal of neuromuscular blockade**

  A.   **Recovery from SCh-induced depolarizing blockade** usually oc-
       curs in 10 to 15 min. Patients with atypical or inhibited plasma
       cholinesterase will have a greatly prolonged duration of blockade.
       Reversal of phase II blockade occurs spontaneously within 10 to
       15 min in approximately 50% of patients. The remaining patients
       have prolonged responses. It is advisable to allow these patients
       to recover spontaneously for 20 to 25 minutes, and then reversal
       with an anticholinesterase may be attempted if there is no further
       improvement in twitch height. Earlier reversal could worsen the
       block.

  B.   **Nondepolarizing block** spontaneously recovers when the drugs
       diffuse from their sites of action. Reversal can be accelerated by ad-
       ministering agents that inhibit AChE (anticholinesterases), thereby
       increasing the ACh available to compete for binding sites.

  C.   **AChEs.** The three principal drugs are **edrophonium, neostigmine,**
       and **pyridostigmine.** Table 12.4 summarizes the clinical pharma-
       cology of these three relaxant antagonists. Because they work by
       increasing ACh, all have nicotinic and muscarinic effects. Saliva-
       tion, bradycardia, tearing, miosis, and bronchoconstriction can be
       minimized by administering an antimuscarinic drug (e.g., atropine
       or glycopyrrolate) with the anticholinesterase. Some data suggest
       that higher doses of neostigmine (>2.5 mg) increase the incidence
       of postoperative nausea and vomiting. However, the potential harm
       associated with lack of reversal outweighs the risk of side effects.

  D.   **Time to adequate reversal** is related to the degree of spontaneous
       recovery, so it will take longer to reverse a deeper block. Reversal may
       be more difficult with the use of long-acting NMBDs, high total
       doses, and large amounts of inhalation anesthetics. Other factors
       that may prolong the blockade include hypothermia, antibiotics
       (particularly aminoglycosides, clindamycin, and uridopenicillins),
       electrolyte disturbances (hypokalemia, hypocalcemia, and hyper-
       magnesemia), and acid-base disturbances (alkalosis prolongs block-
       ade, acidosis impairs reversal). If residual weakness is present after
       attempted reversal, the endotracheal tube should be left in place
       to provide adequate ventilation and airway protection. Reversal
       should not be attempted unless at least one response to TOF stim-
       ulation is present. Attempts to reverse a deep or resistant block with
       excessive doses of neostigmine may increase the degree of residual
       weakness.

  E.   **Evidence of neuromuscular recovery** should include a TOF ra-
       tio greater than 0.75, maintenance of a patent airway without
       assistance, adequate ventilation and oxygenation, sustained grip
       strength, the ability to sustain head lift or movement of an extrem-
       ity without fade, and the absence of discoordinated muscle activity.

Table 12.4. Clinical pharmacology of reversal drugs

Drugs	Dosage	Time to Peak Antagonism (min)	Duration of Antagonism (min)	Excretion Pattern[a]	Dosage of Atropine Required[b] (μg/kg)
Edrophonium	0.05–1.0 mg/kg	1	40–65	70% renal 30% hepatic	7–10
Neostigmine	0.03–0.06 mg/kg up to 5 mg	7	55–75	50% renal 50% hepatic	15–30
Pyridostigmine	0.25 mg/kg	10–13	80–130	75% renal 25% hepatic	15–20

[a]The increased duration during renal failure exceeds the increased durations of pancuronium and curare and so there is no "recurarization."
[b]Dosage of glycopyrrolate = $\frac{1}{2}$ dosage of atropine. The onset time of atropine is much faster than that of glycopyrrolate, and it peaks in a little over a minute compared with 4–5 min for glycopyrrolate. Therefore, glycopyrrolate is a good choice with pyridostigmine, which has a longer time to peak antagonism. However, glycopyrrolate should be given at least 3 min before edrophonium. There appears to be less tachycardia, fewer arrhythmias, and a greater secretory drying effect with glycopyrrolate.

These may be sufficient for a patient emerging from major surgery or remaining in the hospital overnight. However, an outpatient may not tolerate residual diplopia, inability to sit up unassisted, fatigue, or malaise. For these patients, more stringent criteria (TOF ratio >0.9, ability to clench down on an oral airway and prevent its withdrawal) may be more appropriate.

VI. **Disorders that influence the response to NMBDs**
Certain illnesses, both those confined to the NMJ and those affecting more general systems, dramatically affect the use and safety of NMBDs. Generally, transmission at the NMJ is abnormal in these disorders and there are ultrastructural and biochemical changes in motor nerves, muscle, or both.

A. **Burns and immobilization**

1. **Thermal injury** affects fluid and electrolyte regulation, cardiovascular and pulmonary function, drug metabolism, and musculoskeletal structure and function.

2. **Burn patients and many immobilized patients** (such as those found in intensive care unit [ICU] settings) have a greatly exaggerated response to depolarizing agents and a decreased responsiveness to nondepolarizing agents. Burn patients exhibit ultrastructural and biochemical alterations in both muscle cells and neuromuscular contacts. Administration of SCh can cause dramatic, and sometimes fatal, hyperkalemia. These effects can be seen for greater than 1 year after the initial thermal insult. Similar problems have been reported in patients who have sustained major crush injuries or large areas of devitalized tissue.

B. **Critical illness**

1. **The prevalence of neuromuscular dysfunction in critical illness** is exceedingly high. The frequency of diagnosis ranges from 30% to 70% and the incidence approaches 76% with more sensitive electrophysiologic tests.

2. **Myopathy of critical illness** is the name given the collective group of disorders that can cause weakness in ICU patients. The underlying pathology is quite heterogeneous, ranging from pure neuropathies and myopathies to mixed neuromuscular-transmission disorders. Sepsis and multiorgan system failure are commonly associated with myopathy of critical illness.

3. **Weakness** is the common manifestation of all these disorders. In critically ill patients, such weakness can cause ventilator dependence and increased morbidity and mortality. Other signs and symptoms that may be present include altered deep tendon reflexes, increased creatine kinase levels, and electrophysiologic alterations in nerve, muscle, or both.

4. **Corticosteroids, NMBDs, and certain antibiotics** can contribute to or precipitate weakness in ICU patients. One subtype of myopathy of critical illness, acute necrotizing myopathy, has been linked to the repeated administration of NMBDs, often in conjunction with high doses of corticosteroids. These patients exhibit profound weakness, elevated serum creatine kinase levels, and sparing of sensory-nerve action potentials. Limiting steroid and NMBD use in critically ill patients is advisable.

C. **Myasthenia gravis (MG)**
1. **MG** is an autoimmune disease with a prevalence of 1 in 20,000 in the general population. It is most common in young adult women.
2. **The loss of AChR at motor endplates** in MG is induced by antireceptor antibodies that increase the degradation of junctional and extrajunctional receptors. The antibodies are detectable in the serum of 90% of MG patients, but antibody titers correlate poorly with clinical signs.
3. MG often presents with the gradual onset of **pharyngeal or ocular weakness.** All muscle groups may be affected. The hallmark of MG is weakness that becomes worse with exercise.
4. The diagnosis is supported by the clinical history and confirmed by transiently improved muscle strength after 10 mg of IV edrophonium (the **Tensilon test**), by characteristic electromyographic findings, and most specifically by the presence of anti-AChR antibodies in the patient's serum.
5. **Treatment** includes anticholinesterases (e.g., pyridostigmine), corticosteroids, immunosuppressive drugs such as azathioprine and cyclophosphamide, plasmapheresis, and thymectomy. Remission of the disease is common after thymectomy.
6. Special attention needs to be given to MG patients receiving either regional or general anesthetics.
   a. **The use of neuraxial regional anesthesia** is associated with skeletal muscle relaxation and some degree of diaphragmatic weakness. This normal effect of regional anesthesia often unmasks underlying weakness that may have been only partially treated by cholinesterase inhibitors. These patients, therefore, may suffer from profound respiratory weakness even when not challenged with neuromuscular blocking agents. They need careful respiratory monitoring throughout anesthesia and recovery.
   b. **Anticholinesterase therapy** should not be discontinued before surgery.
   c. These patients are often resistant to depolarizing agents, although clearance of SCh is inhibited by pyridostigmine. They are also extremely sensitive to nondepolarizing agents. Both longer-acting agents such as pancuronium and shorter-acting agents such as cisatracurium have been associated with prolonged blockade, refractoriness to reversal agents, and profound postoperative weakness. NMBDs are best avoided, if possible.
   d. **Monitoring of the degree of neuromuscular blockade is strongly advised,** although complete recovery of the TOF does not ensure recovery of either the muscles of the upper airway or of ventilation.
   e. **Surgery and anesthesia may exacerbate the underlying illness.** Postoperative ventilation may be required even after minor surgical procedures.
D. **Muscular dystrophies** are a heterogeneous group of inherited muscle disorders characterized by a progressive loss of skeletal muscle function. **Duchenne muscular dystrophy** is the most common and the most severe of the disorders. The gene responsible encodes

a membrane-associated protein known as dystrophin that is critical for the stability of the muscular membrane. The disorder is X-linked recessive and clinically evident in males. The clinical course is characterized by painless degeneration and atrophy of skeletal muscle, which manifests as weakness by the age of 5 years. By the preteen years, the patient often is confined to a wheelchair, and death usually occurs by the mid-20s secondary to congestive heart failure.

1. **Serum creatine kinase levels** are elevated and track the progression of muscular degeneration. By the late stages of the disease, creatine kinase levels are near normal because of significant loss of muscle mass.

2. Cardiac (progressive systolic dysfunction and ventricular thinning) and smooth muscle (gastrointestinal hypomotility with delayed gastric emptying) are affected to various degrees.

3. Although the diaphragm is spared, accessory muscle weakness produces a restrictive pattern on pulmonary function testing. Because coughing is impaired, pneumonia is a frequent complication.

4. **SCh** can cause massive rhabdomyolysis, hyperkalemia, and death. Studies involving nondepolarizing NMBDs exhibit variable results. Because the intensity and duration of drug effect is hard to predict, short-acting agents may be preferable. **Volatile inhalational agents,** particularly halothane, can have exaggerated myocardial depressant effects. **Malignant hyperthermia** occurs with increased frequency, but there are no good predictive tests for which patients are at risk. The delayed gastric emptying and ineffective cough place these patients at greater risk for regurgitation and aspiration. Postoperatively, these patients require aggressive pulmonary physiotherapy to ensure adequate secretion clearance. Opioids, which may further depress deep breathing and coughing, should be used cautiously.

E. **The myotonic syndromes** are a group of disorders characterized by a defect in skeletal muscle relaxation and persistent contraction of skeletal muscles after stimulation. The persistent contraction is a consequence of ineffective calcium removal from the cytoplasm to the sarcoplasmic reticulum. **Myotonic dystrophy** is the most common syndrome in this group of disorders.

1. Myotonic dystrophy patients have progressive involvement and deterioration of skeletal, cardiac, and smooth muscle throughout the body, with weakened respiratory effort, a restrictive pattern on pulmonary function testing, and diminished gastrointestinal motility. Other symptoms include cataracts, cardiac conduction abnormalities, baldness, and mental retardation.

2. Regional anesthesia, neuromuscular blocking agents, and increasing depth of general anesthesia do not relieve myotonic muscle rigidity. Pregnancy exacerbates this condition, and cesarean section is often indicated because of uterine muscle dysfunction. These patients are exquisitely sensitive to the respiratory depressant effects of opioids, benzodiazepines, and inhalational agents. Neuraxial opiates that have minimal effect on respiratory function in normal persons can have a

substantial effect in these patients. Like patients with Duchenne muscular dystrophy, these patients have frequent cardiac arrhythmias and are at increased risk for cardiac arrest during general anesthesia.

SUGGESTED READING

Ali HH, Savarese JJ. Monitoring of neuromuscular function. *Anesthesiology* 1976;45:216–249.

Baraka A. Onset of neuromuscular block in myasthenic patients. *Br J Anaesth* 1992;69:227–228.

Baraka A, Taha S, Yazbeck V, et al. Vecuronium block in the myasthenic patient. Influence of anticholinesterase therapy. *Anaesthesia* 1993;48:588–590.

Belmont MR, Lien CA, Quessy S, et al. The clinical neuromuscular pharmacology of 51W89 in patients receiving nitrous oxide/opioid/barbiturate anesthesia. *Anesthesiology* 1995;82:1139–1145.

Berg H, Roed J, Viby-Mogensen J, et al. Residual neuromuscular block is a risk factor for postoperative pulmonary complications. A prospective, randomised, and blinded study of postoperative pulmonary complications after atracurium, vecuronium and pancuronium. *Acta Anaesthesiol Scand* 1997;41:1095–1103.

Chiu JW, White PF. The pharmacoeconomics of neuromuscular blocking drugs. *Anesth Analg* 2000;90:S19–S23.

Eriksson LI. The effects of residual neuromuscular blockade and volatile anesthetics on the control of ventilation. *Anesth Analg* 1999;89:243–251.

Eriksson LI, Sundman E, Olsson R, et al. Functional assessment of the pharynx at rest and during swallowing in partially paralyzed humans. *Anesthesiology* 1997;87:1035–1043.

Ibebunjo C, Martyn JA. Fiber atrophy, but not changes in acetylcholine receptor expression, contributes to the muscle dysfunction after immobilization. *Crit Care Med* 1999;27:275–285.

Kim C, Fuke N, Martyn JA. Burn injury to rat increases nicotinic acetylcholine receptors in the diaphragm. *Anesthesiology* 1988;68:401–406.

Kopman AF, Yee SY, Neuman GG. Relationship of the train-of-four fade ratio to clinical signs and symptoms of residual paralysis in awake volunteers. *Anesthesiology* 1997;86:765–771.

Lin RC, Scheller RH. Mechanisms of synaptic vesicle exocytosis. *Annu Rev Cell Dev Biol* 2000;16:19–49.

Martyn JA, Richtsfeld M. Succinylcholine-induced Hyperkalemia in Acquired Pathologic States. *Anesthesiology* 2006;104:158–169.

Martyn JA, Vincent A. A new twist to myopathy of critical illness. *Anesthesiology* 1999;91:337–339.

Murphy GS, Szokol JW. Monitoring neuromuscular blockade. *Int Anesthesiol Clin* 2004;42(2):25–40.

Murphy GS, Szokol JW, et al. Residual paralysis at the time of tracheal extubation. *Anesth Analg* 2005;100:1840–1845.

Pino RM. Neuromuscular blocker studies of critically ill patients. *Intensive Care Med* 2002;28:1695–1697.

13

Airway Evaluation and Management

Matthew W. Zeleznik and Peter F. Dunn

I. **Applied anatomy**
   A. **The pharynx** is divided into the nasopharynx, the oropharynx, and the laryngopharynx.
      1. The **nasopharynx** consists of the nasal passages, including the septum, turbinates, and adenoids.
      2. The **oropharynx** consists of the oral cavity, including the dentition and tongue.
      3. The epiglottis separates the **laryngopharynx** into the larynx (leading to the trachea) and the **hypopharynx** (leading to the esophagus).
   B. **The larynx**
      1. The **larynx,** located at the level of the fourth to the sixth cervical vertebrae, originates at the laryngeal inlet and ends at the inferior border of the cricoid cartilage. It consists of nine cartilages, three unpaired (thyroid, cricoid, and epiglottis) and three paired (corniculates, cuneiforms, arytenoids); ligaments; and muscles.
      2. The **cricoid cartilage** (C5-6), located just inferior to the **thyroid cartilage,** is the only complete cartilaginous ring in the respiratory tree.
      3. The **cricothyroid membrane** connects the thyroid and cricoid cartilages and measures 0.9 × 3.0 cm in adults. The membrane is superficial, thin, and devoid of major vessels in the midline, making it an important site for emergent surgical airway access (see cricothyroidotomy below).
      4. **The laryngeal muscles** can be divided into two groups: muscles that open and close the glottis (lateral cricoarytenoid [adduction], posterior cricoarytenoid [abduction], transverse arytenoid) and muscles that control the tension of the vocal ligaments (cricothyroid, vocalis, and thyroarytenoid).
      5. **Innervation**
         a. **Sensory.** The **glossopharyngeal nerve** (cranial nerve IX) provides sensory innervation to the posterior one-third of the tongue, the oropharynx from its junction with the nasopharynx, including the pharyngeal surfaces of the soft palate, epiglottis, and the fauces, to the junction of the pharynx and esophagus. The **internal branch of the superior laryngeal nerve,** a branch of the vagus nerve (cranial nerve X), provides sensory innervation to the mucosa from the epiglottis to and including the vocal cords. The sensory fibers of the **inferior laryngeal nerve,** a branch of the recurrent laryngeal nerve (also a branch of the vagus nerve), provides sensory innervation to the mucosa of the subglottic larynx and trachea.

b. **Motor.** The external branch of the **superior laryngeal nerve** provides motor innervation to the cricothyroid muscle. Activation of this muscle results in tensing of the vocal cords. The motor fibers of the **inferior laryngeal nerve** provide motor innervation to all other intrinsic muscles of the larynx. **Bilateral injury to the inferior laryngeal nerves** (e.g., via injury to the recurrent laryngeal nerves) can produce unopposed activation of the cricothyroideus, leading to tensing of the vocal cords and airway closure.

C. The **glottis** is composed of the vocal folds (true and "false" cords) and the rima glottidis.

1. The **rima glottidis** describes the aperture between the true vocal cords.

2. The **glottis** represents the narrowest point in the adult airway (more than 8 years of age), whereas the cricoid cartilage represents the narrowest point in the infant airway (birth to 1 year of age).

D. **The lower airway** extends from the subglottic larynx to the bronchi.

1. The subglottic larynx extends from the vocal folds to the inferior border of the cricoid cartilage (C-6).

2. The **trachea** is a fibromuscular tube that is 10 to 12 cm long with a diameter of approximately 20 mm in adults. It extends from the cricoid cartilage to the carina. The trachea is supported by 16 to 20 U-shaped cartilages, with the open end facing posteriorly. Noting the posterior absence of cartilaginous rings provides anterior-posterior orientation during fiberoptic exam of the tracheobronchial tree.

3. The trachea bifurcates into the right and left main stem bronchi at the carina. The right main stem bronchus is approximately 2.5 cm long with a take-off angle of approximately 25°. The left main stem bronchus is approximately 5 cm long with a take-off angle of approximately 45°.

II. **Evaluation**

A. **History.** A history of difficult airway management in the past may be the best predictor of a challenging airway. If old medical records are available, prior anesthetic records should be reviewed for the ease of intubation and ventilation (number of intubation attempts, ability to mask ventilate, type of laryngoscope blade used, use of stylet, or any other modifications of technique). Particular importance should also be placed on diseases that may affect the airway. Specific symptoms related to airway compromise should be sought, including hoarseness, stridor, wheezing, dysphagia, dyspnea, and positional airway obstruction.

1. **Arthritis or cervical disk disease** may decrease neck mobility. Cervical spine instability and limitation of mandibular motion are common in rheumatoid arthritis; the temporomandibular and cricoarytenoid joints may also be involved. Aggressive neck manipulation in these patients may lead to atlantoaxial subluxation and spinal cord injury. The risk of atlantoaxial subluxation is highest in patients with severe hand deformities and skin nodules.

2. **Infections** of the floor of the mouth, salivary glands, tonsils, or pharynx may cause pain, edema, and trismus with limited mouth opening.

3. **Tumors** may obstruct the airway or cause extrinsic compression and tracheal deviation.

4. **Morbidly obese** individuals may have a history of obstructive sleep apnea from hypertrophied tonsils and adenoids as well as a short neck or increased soft tissue at the neck and upper airway.

5. **Trauma** may be associated with airway injuries, cervical spine injury, basilar skull fracture, or intracranial injury.

6. **Previous surgery, radiation, or burns** may produce scarring, contractures, and limited tissue mobility (also see Chapter 32).

7. **Acromegaly** may cause mandibular hypertrophy and overgrowth and enlargement of the tongue and epiglottis. The glottic opening may be narrowed because of enlargement of the vocal cords.

8. **Scleroderma** may produce skin tightness and decrease mandibular motion and narrow the oral aperture.

9. **Trisomy 21 patients** may have atlantoaxial instability and macroglossia.

10. **Dwarfism** may be associated with atlantoaxial instability and potentially difficult airway management because of mandibular hypoplasia (micrognathia).

11. **Other congenital anomalies** may complicate airway management, particularly patients with craniofacial abnormalities such as Pierre-Robin syndrome, Treacher-Collins syndrome, or Goldenhar syndrome.

B. **Physical examination**

1. **Specific findings** that may indicate a difficult airway include the following:
   a. Inability to open the mouth.
   b. Poor cervical spine mobility.
   c. Receding chin (micrognathia).
   d. Large tongue (macroglossia).
   e. Prominent incisors.
   f. Short muscular neck.
   g. Morbid obesity.

2. **Injuries** to the face, neck, or chest must be evaluated to assess their contribution to airway compromise.

3. **Head and neck examination**
   a. **Nose.** The patency of the nares or the presence of a deviated septum should be determined by occluding one nostril at a time and assessing ease of ventilation through the other nostril. This is especially important should nasotracheal intubation be required.
   b. **Mouth.** Identify macroglossia and conditions that reduce mouth opening (e.g., facial scars or contractures, temporomandibular joint disease). **Poor dentition** may increase the risk of tooth injury or loss during airway manipulation. Loose teeth should be identified preoperatively and protected or removed before initiation of airway management.

c. Neck

   (1) If the **thyromental distance** (the distance from the lower border of the mandible to the thyroid notch with the neck fully extended) is less than 6 cm (three to four finger breadths), there may be difficulty visualizing the glottis. The mobility of laryngeal structures should be assessed, and the trachea should be palpable in the midline above the sternal notch. Look for scars from previous neck surgery, an enlarged thyroid, and other paratracheal masses.

   (2) **Cervical spine mobility.** Patients should be able to touch their chin to their chest and extend their neck posteriorly. Lateral rotation should not produce pain or paresthesia.

   (3) The presence of a healed or patent **tracheostomy** stoma may be a clue to subglottic stenosis or prior complications with airway management. Smaller diameter endotracheal tubes (ETTs) should be available for these patients.

4. The **Mallampati classification** to predict difficult intubation is based on the finding that visualization of the glottis is impaired when the base of the tongue is disproportionately large. Assessment is made with the patient sitting upright, with the head in the neutral position, the mouth open as wide as possible, and the tongue protruded maximally. The modified classification includes the following four categories (Fig. 13.1):

   a. **Class I.** Faucial pillars, soft palate, and uvula are visible.

   b. **Class II.** Faucial pillars and soft palate may be seen, but the uvula is masked by the base of the tongue.

   c. **Class III.** Only soft palate is visible. Intubation is predicted to be difficult.

   d. **Class IV.** Soft palate is not visible. Intubation is predicted to be difficult.

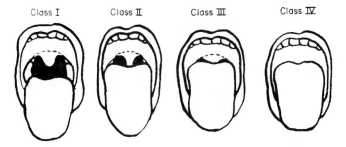

Figure 13.1. Mallampati classification of the oropharyngeal structures as modified by Samsoon and Young, as defined in a patient sitting upright with mouth maximally opened and tongue protruded without phonation. (From Samsoon GLT, Young JRB. Difficult tracheal intubation, a retrospective study. *Anaesthesia* **1987;42:487–490, with permission.)**

C. **Special studies.** In most patients, a careful history and physical examination will be all that is needed to evaluate an airway. Useful adjuncts may include the following:

1. **Laryngoscopy** (direct, indirect, or fiberoptic) will provide information about the hypopharynx, laryngeal inlet, and vocal cord function. It can be performed in a conscious patient with topical anesthesia or nerve blocks.

2. **Chest or cervical radiographs** may reveal tracheal deviation or narrowing and bony deformities in the neck. Cervical spine films are particularly important in trauma cases and should be performed whenever there is an injury above the clavicle or serious multiple traumatic injuries. Lateral cervical spine films may be useful in the rheumatoid patient to assess for atlantoaxial subluxation.

3. **Tracheal tomograms or computed tomography** can delineate masses obstructing the airway.

4. **Pulmonary function tests** and flow volume loops can help determine the degree and site of airway obstruction (see Chapter 3).

5. **Baseline arterial blood gas tensions** can indicate the functional consequences of airway abnormalities and alert the clinician to patients who are chronically hypoxemic or hypercarbic.

III. **Mask airway**

A. **Indications**

1. To provide inhalation anesthesia in patients not at risk for regurgitation of gastric contents.

2. To preoxygenate (denitrogenate) a patient before endotracheal intubation.

3. To assist or control ventilation as part of initial resuscitation.

B. **Technique** involves placing a face mask and maintaining a patent airway.

1. **The mask** should fit snugly around the bridge of the nose, cheeks, and mouth. Clear plastic masks allow for observation of the lips (for color) and mouth (for secretions or vomitus).

2. **Mask placement.** The mask is held in the left hand so that the little finger is at the angle of the mandible, the third and fourth fingers are along the mandible, and the index finger and thumb are placed on the mask. The right hand is available to control the reservoir bag. Two hands may be required to maintain a good mask fit, necessitating an assistant to control the bag. Head straps may be used to assist mask fit.

3. **Edentulous patients** may present a problem when attempting to achieve an adequate seal with the face mask because of decreased distance between the mandible and the maxilla. An oral airway will often correct this problem, and the cheeks may be compressed against the mask to decrease leaks. Two hands may be required to do this. Alternatively, dentures may be left in place during mask ventilation.

4. **Airway obstruction** during spontaneous ventilation may be recognized by a "rocking" motion of the chest and abdomen, and stridor may be heard if the obstruction is partial. Respiratory excursions in the reservoir bag will be decreased or absent. Peak airway pressures will be increased when positive pressure ventilation is attempted.

5. **Airway patency** may be restored by the following:
    a. Neck extension.
    b. Jaw thrust, by placing the fingers under the angles of the mandible and lifting forward.
    c. Turning the head to one side.
    d. Insertion of an oral airway. An airway may not be well tolerated if the gag reflex is intact. Complications from use of oral airways include vomiting, laryngospasm, and dental trauma. The wrong size oral airway may worsen obstruction. If the oral airway is too short, it may compress the tongue; if it is too long, it may lie against the epiglottis.
    e. A nasal airway helps maintain upper airway patency in a patient with minimal to moderate obstruction and is reasonably tolerated by awake or sedated patients. Nasal airways can cause epistaxis and should be avoided in patients who are coagulopathic.
C. **Difficult mask ventilation** may be anticipated in patients who are obese or edentulous and in those who have beards, cervical arthritis, or a history of snoring. Appropriate oral and nasal airways and laryngeal mask airways (LMAs) should be available.
D. **Complications.** The mask may cause pressure injuries to soft tissues around the mouth, mandible, eyes, or nose. Loss of the airway may produce laryngospasm or vomiting. Mask ventilation does not protect the airway from aspiration of gastric contents. **Laryngospasm,** a tonic contraction of the laryngeal and pharyngeal muscles, causes airway obstruction that may be relieved by jaw thrust and the application of constant positive airway pressure. If this fails, a small dose of succinylcholine (20 mg intravenously or intramuscularly in the adult) may be required.

IV. **LMAs**
A. The LMA Classic is a reusable airway management device that can be used as an alternative to both mask ventilation and endotracheal intubation in appropriate patients. The LMA also plays an important role in management of the difficult airway. When inserted appropriately, the LMA lies with its tip resting over the upper esophageal sphincter, cuff sides lying over the pyriform fossae, and cuff upper border resting against the base of the tongue. Such positioning allows for effective ventilation with minimal inflation of the stomach.
    1. **Indications**
        a. As an alternative to mask ventilation or endotracheal intubation for airway management. The LMA is not a replacement for endotracheal intubation when endotracheal intubation is indicated.
        b. In the management of a known or unexpected difficult airway.
        c. In airway management during the resuscitation of an unconscious patient.
    2. **Contraindications**
        a. Patients at risk of aspiration of gastric contents (emergency use is an exception).
        b. Patients with decreased respiratory system compliance, because the low-pressure seal of the LMA cuff will leak at high inspiratory pressures and gastric insufflation may occur. Peak inspiratory pressures should be maintained at

Table 13.1. Laryngeal mask airway (LMA) sizes

Patient Age/Size	LMA Size	Cuff Volume	ETT Size (ID)
Neonates/infants to 5 kg	1	Up to 4 mL	3.5 mm
Infants, 5–10 kg	1.5	Up to 7 mL	4.0 mm
Infants/children, 10–20 kg	2.0	Up to 10 mL	4.5 mm
Children, 20–30 kg	2.5	Up to 14 mL	5.0 mm
Children, 30 kg to small adults	3.0	Up to 20 mL	6.0 cuffed
Average adults	4.0	Up to 30 mL	6.0 cuffed
Large adults	5.0	Up to 40 mL	7.0 cuffed

ETT, endotracheal tube; ID, inner diameter.

    less than 20 cm H_2O to minimize cuff leaks and gastric insufflation.

    c. Patients in whom long-term mechanical ventilatory support is anticipated or required.

    d. Patients with intact upper airway reflexes, because insertion can precipitate laryngospasm.

3. Use

    a. LMAs are available in a variety of pediatric and adult sizes (see Table 13.1). Using the proper size maximizes the probability of appropriate cuff fit. Maneuvers for appropriate insertion of the LMA are shown in Figure 13.2.

    b. Ensure correct cuff deflation and lubrication. Lubrication of the LMA inner surface should be avoided because any lubricant dripping into the larynx can precipitate laryngospasm.

    c. Follow usual preoxygenation and monitoring requirements.

    d. Ensure an adequate level of anesthesia and suppression of upper airway reflexes.

    e. Position the patient's head appropriately. The "sniffing" position (slight flexion of the lower cervical spine with extension of C1-2) used to optimize endotracheal intubation also typically provides the best positioning for LMA insertion.

    f. Insert the LMA (see Fig. 13.2). A soft bite block can be used to protect against a patient biting down on the LMA tube.

    g. Inflate cuff (see Table 13.1). Typically, one sees a smooth ovoid expansion of the tissues above the thyroid cartilage with adequate inflation of the appropriately positioned LMA.

    h. Ensure adequate ventilation.

    i. Connect to anesthetic circuit. The LMA can be secured with tape, if necessary.

    j. **LMA removal.** The LMA generally is well tolerated by a patient emerging from general anesthesia as long as the

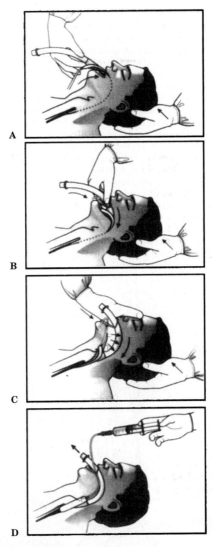

Figure 13.2. A: With the head extended and the neck flexed, carefully flatten the laryngeal mask airway (LMA) tip against the hard palate. B: With the index finger, push the LMA in a cranial direction following the contours of the hard and soft palate. C: Maintaining pressure with the finger on the tube in the cranial direction, advance the mask until definite resistance is felt at the base of the hypopharynx. D: Inflation without holding the tube allows the mask to seat itself optimally. (From Brain AIJ, Denman WY, Goudsouzian NG. *Laryngeal mask airway instructional manual.* Berkshire, UK: Brain Medical Ltd., 1996:21–25.)

cuff is not overinflated (cuff pressure less than 60 cm H_2O). The LMA can be removed by deflating the cuff once the patient has emerged from general anesthesia and has return of upper airway reflexes.

  k. The LMA is a suitable airway for some patients having procedures in the prone position. If this technique is chosen, patients can position themselves on the operating table before induction. After induction of anesthesia, the LMA can be inserted with the patient's head turned to the side and resting on a pillow or blankets.

  4. Adverse effects. The most common adverse effect is sore throat, with an estimated incidence of 10%, and is most often related to overinflation of the LMA cuff. The primary major adverse effect is aspiration, which has been estimated to occur at a comparable incidence as with mask or endotracheal anesthesia.

B. The LMA Fastrach (intubating LMA) includes a curved stainless steel tube (13 mm inner diameter [ID]) covered with silicone, a 15-mm end connector, a handle, cuff, and an epiglottic lifting bar (Fig. 13.3). The tube is of sufficient diameter to accept a cuffed 8-mm ID ETT and is short enough to ensure that the ETT cuff will rest beyond the vocal cords. The primary differences between

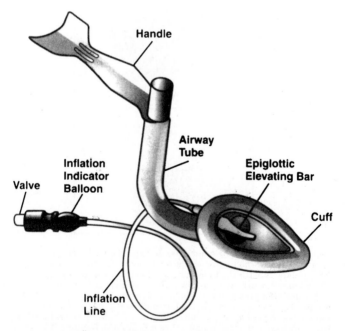

Figure 13.3. Features of the laryngeal mask airway Fastrach. (From Brain AIJ, Verghese C. *LMA-Fastrach instruction manual*. San Diego: *LMA* North America, Inc., 1998.)

the LMA Classic and the LMA Fastrach are the steel tube, handle, and epiglottic lifting bar.

1. The LMA Fastrach is inserted similarly to the LMA Classic. Once inserted, it can be used with the cuff inflated as the sole airway device. It can also be used as a conduit for fiberoptic or blind intubation.

2. For intubation, a special ETT with a blunt bullnose tip (the Euromedical ILM ETT) can be used to minimize soft tissue damage. If attempting blind intubation, the tube should be lubricated and gently inserted into the LMA tube. At 15 cm, the ETT tip will lie at the epiglottic lifting bar. The ETT should be gently pushed into the trachea while grasping the LMA handle for support. The Fastrach handle should not be used as a lever during intubation. Once the intubation is deemed successful, the tube position should be verified and the cuff inflated and ETT secured (see section V).

3. **After intubation,** the LMA Fastrach can either be left in place or removed leaving the ETT in place. If the LMA Fastrach is left in place, the LMA cuff should be deflated. If the LMA Fastrach is removed, the LMA cuff should be deflated and the LMA gently removed by manipulating the handle while using an ETT stabilizer to keep the ETT in place. The ETT stabilizer can be removed once the LMA has cleared the patient's mouth and the ETT stabilized with the operator's other hand or by an assistant.

C. The LMA Proseal has two design features that may offer advantages over the standard LMA during positive pressure ventilation. First, improved airway seal pressures are achieved with lower mucosal pressure. Second, the LMA Proseal allows for separation of the respiratory and gastrointestinal tracts by the integration of a drainage tube that may vent esophageal gases or facilitate the passage of an orogastric tube for decompression of the stomach. In addition, the absence of bars or an epiglottic elevator in the bowl of the LMA Proseal allows for unimpeded fiberoptic bronchoscopy.

V. **Endotracheal intubation**
   A. **Orotracheal intubation**
      1. **Indications.** Endotracheal intubation is required to provide a patent airway when patients are at risk for aspiration, when airway maintenance by mask is difficult, and for prolonged controlled ventilation. Intubation also may be required for specific surgical procedures (e.g., head/neck, intrathoracic, or intra-abdominal procedures).
      2. **Technique.** Intubation is usually performed with a laryngoscope. The Macintosh and Miller blades are most commonly used.
         a. The **Macintosh blade** is curved, and the tip is inserted into the vallecula (the space between the base of the tongue and the pharyngeal surface of the epiglottis) (Fig. 13.4A). It provides a good view of the oro- and hypopharynx, thus allowing more room for passage of the ETT with decreased epiglottic trauma. Size ranges are designated as no. 1 through 4, with most adults requiring a Macintosh no. 3 blade.
         b. The **Miller blade** is straight, and it is passed so that the tip lies beneath the laryngeal surface of the epiglottis

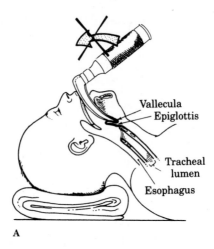

Vallecula
Epiglottis

Tracheal
lumen

Esophagus

A

Straight Blade Placement

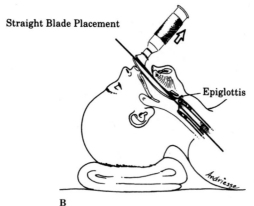

Epiglottis

B

Curved Blade Placement

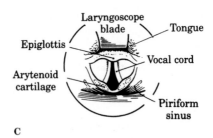

Laryngoscope
blade — Tongue

Epiglottis

Vocal cord

Arytenoid
cartilage

Piriform
sinus

C

Figure 13.4. Anatomic relations for laryngoscopy and endotracheal intubation.

(Fig. 13.4B). The epiglottis then is lifted to expose the vocal cords. The Miller blade provides excellent exposure of the glottic opening but provides a smaller passageway through the oro- and hypopharynx. Sizes are designated as no. 0 through 4, with most adults requiring a Miller no. 2 or 3 blade.

c. Many specially modified laryngoscopes (e.g., Bullard, Upsher, Wu) and laryngoscope blades (e.g., McCoy, Siker) are available that may facilitate endotracheal intubation under difficult or unusual conditions. Facility with the use of these devices should first be gained under elective conditions.

d. The patient should be positioned in the so-called **sniffing position,** with the occiput elevated by pads or folded blankets and the neck extended. On average, this improves the laryngoscopic view, although intubation and mouth opening may be facilitated in some patients by simple neck extension. Neck flexion may make it more difficult to open the mouth.

e. The laryngoscope is held in the left hand near the junction between the handle and blade. After propping the mouth open with a scissoring motion of the right thumb and index finger, the laryngoscope is inserted into the right side of the patient's mouth while sweeping the tongue to the left. The lips should not be pinched by the blade and the teeth should be avoided. The blade is then advanced toward the midline until the epiglottis comes into view. The tongue and pharyngeal soft tissues are then lifted to expose the glottic opening. The laryngoscope should be used to lift (see Fig. 13.4B) rather than act as a lever (see Fig. 13.4A) to prevent damage to the maxillary incisors or gingiva.

f. An appropriate ETT size depends on the patient's age, body habitus, and type of surgery. A 7.0-mm ETT is used for most women and an 8.0-mm ETT is used for most men. The ETT is held in the right hand as one would hold a pencil and advanced through the oral cavity from the right corner of the mouth and then through the vocal cords. The anatomic view for visualization with a Macintosh laryngoscope is shown in Figure 13.4C. If visualization of the glottic opening is incomplete, it may be necessary to use the epiglottis as a landmark, passing the ETT immediately beneath it and into the trachea. External pressure on the cricoid and/or thyroid cartilage may aid in visualization. The proximal end of the ETT cuff is placed just below the vocal cords, and the markings on the tube are noted in relation to the patient's incisors (or lips). The cuff is inflated just to the point of obtaining a seal in the presence of 20 to 30 cm H_2O positive airway pressure.

g. **Proper placement of the ETT** can be verified by the detection of carbon dioxide in end-tidal or mixed expiratory gas as well as inspection and auscultation of the stomach and both lung fields during positive pressure ventilation. If breath sounds are heard on one side of the thorax only, an endobronchial intubation should be suspected and the ETT should be withdrawn until breath sounds are heard bilaterally. Listening for breath sounds high in each axilla may decrease the chances of being misled by transmitted breath sounds from the opposite lung. No single verification technique is foolproof, and the consequences of misdiagnosis may be disastrous. Additional confirmatory techniques, such as use of an esophageal bulb detector, bronchoscopy, and radiography, may be necessary. A high index of suspicion of an esophageal intubation should be maintained until adequate oxygenation and ventilation are ensured.

    h. The ETT should be fastened securely with tape, preferably to taut skin overlying bony structures.

  3. Complications of orotracheal intubation include injury of the lips or tongue, teeth, pharynx, or tracheal mucosa. There may rarely be avulsion of arytenoid cartilages or damage to vocal cords or trachea.

B. Nasotracheal intubation

  1. Indications. Nasotracheal intubation may be required in patients undergoing an intraoral procedure. Compared with oral ETTs, the maximal diameter that can be accommodated is usually smaller, and, accordingly, resistance to breathing may be higher. The nasotracheal route is now rarely used for long-term intubation because of increased airway resistance and the increased risk of sinusitis.

  2. Contraindications. Basilar skull fractures, especially of the ethmoid bone, nasal fractures, epistaxis, nasal polyps, coagulopathy, and planned systemic anticoagulation and/or thrombolysis (i.e., the patient with acute myocardial infarction), are relative contraindications to nasal intubation.

  3. Technique. Topical anesthesia and vasoconstriction of the nasal mucosa may be achieved by applying a mixture of 3% lidocaine and 0.25% phenylephrine, using cotton-tipped pledgets. If both nares are patent, the right naris is preferred because this will direct the bevel of most ETTs toward the flat nasal septum, reducing damage to the turbinates. The inferior turbinates can interfere with passage and limit the size of the ETT. Usually, a 6.0- to 6.5-mm ETT is used for women and a 7.0- to 7.5-mm ETT is used for men. After it passes through the naris into the pharynx, the tube is advanced through the glottic opening. Intubation may be performed blindly, under direct vision with a laryngoscope or fiberoptic bronchoscope, or assisted by Magill forceps.

  4. Complications are similar to those described for orotracheal intubation (see section V.A.3). Additionally, epistaxis, submucosal dissection, and dislodgement of enlarged tonsils and adenoids may occur. Compared with orotracheal intubation, the nasotracheal route has been associated with an increased incidence of sinusitis and bacteremia.

C. Fiberoptic intubation. The flexible fiberoptic laryngoscope consists of glass fibers that are bound together to provide a flexible unit for the transmission of light and images. The fiberoptic bundle is fragile, and excessive bending can damage the fibers. Working channels are usually present that can be used to administer topical anesthetics and provide suction or oxygen. The visual field often becomes limited as the fiberoptic bronchoscope nears the glottic opening. Secretions, blood, or fogging of the lens may obscure the view. Immersing the tip of the fiberoptic scope in warm water helps to prevent fogging.

1. **Standard equipment** for oral or nasal fiberoptic intubation includes an oral bite block or Ovassapian airway, topical anesthetics and vasoconstrictors, suction, and a sterile fiberoptic scope with a light source.

2. **Indications**

   a. The flexible fiberoptic laryngoscope or bronchoscope can be used in both awake and anesthetized patients to evaluate and intubate their airways. It can be used for both nasal and oral endotracheal intubation and should be used as a first option in an anticipated difficult airway rather than as a "last resort."

   b. Initial fiberoptic intubation is recommended for patients with known or suspected cervical spine pathology, head and neck tumors, morbid obesity, or a history of difficult ventilation or intubation.

3. **Technique.** An ETT is placed over a lubricated fiberoptic scope, suction or oxygen tubing is attached to the working port, and the control lever is grasped with one hand while the scope is advanced or maneuvered with the other hand. An oral Ovassapian airway is helpful and well tolerated for oral laryngoscopy. It is important to keep the fiberoptic scope in the midline to prevent entering the piriform fossa. The tip of the scope is positioned anteriorly when in the hypopharynx and advanced toward the epiglottis. If mucous or secretions impair the view, the scope should be retracted or removed to clean the tip and then reinserted in the midline. As the scope slides beneath the epiglottis, the vocal cords will be seen. The scope is advanced with the tip in a neutral position until tracheal rings are noted. If topical anesthesia is adequate, the patient will tolerate this without coughing. The scope is stabilized within the trachea, and the ETT is advanced over it and into the trachea. If there is resistance to passage, the ETT may need to be turned 90° counterclockwise to avoid the anterior commissure and permit passage through the vocal cords.

D. **Alternative intubation techniques**

   1. **The gum elastic bougie,** a 60 cm long, 15 French semirigid device with a slight J angle at its distal tip, exemplifies the various types of hollow and solid introducers that may facilitate passage of the ETT into the trachea when direct laryngoscopy is difficult. During direct laryngoscopy, the bougie is advanced under the epiglottis and its angled end is directed anteriorly toward the glottic opening. If the bougie is inserted into the trachea, the tracheal rings will be felt as a characteristic "clicking" sensation. The ETT is then advanced over the bougie and proper placement is confirmed as described above (section V.A.2.g). The bougie may also be used as an ETT exchanger.

   2. The **light wand** consists of a malleable lighted stylet over which an oral ETT can be passed blindly into the trachea. To insert, the operating room lights are dimmed, and the light

wand and ETT are advanced following the curve of the tongue. A glow noted in the lateral neck indicates that the tip of the ETT lies in the piriform fossa. If the tip enters the esophagus, there is a marked diminution in the light's brightness. When the tip is correctly positioned in the trachea, a glow is noted in the anterior neck. At this point, the ETT is slid off the stylet and into the trachea.

3. **Retrograde tracheal intubation** can be performed when previously described techniques have been unsuccessful. It is performed in a conscious patient who is ventilating with a stable airway. For this technique, the cricothyroid membrane is identified and punctured in the midline with an 18-gauge intravenous (IV) catheter. An 80-cm, 0.025-inch guidewire is introduced and directed cephalad. A laryngoscope is used to visualize and retrieve the wire. An ETT is passed over the wire, which serves as a guide through the vocal cords.

VI. **The difficult airway and emergency airway techniques**

A. **Difficult airway.** The 2003 revision of the American Society of Anesthesiologists (ASA) algorithm for managing difficult airways is shown in Figure 13.5. Familiarity with this algorithm is crucial for the anesthesiologist. Since its adoption in 1993, the number of death or brain death claims associated with airway-related events during induction of anesthesia has decreased significantly.

1. The difficult airway can be divided into the recognized difficult airway and the unrecognized difficult airway; the latter presents the greater challenge for the anesthesiologist.

2. The ASA defines **a difficult airway** as failure to intubate with conventional laryngoscopy after three attempts and/or failure to intubate with conventional laryngoscopy for more than 10 min. Others have suggested that a more appropriate definition of a difficult airway would be that of failure to intubate with conventional laryngoscopy after an optimal/best attempt. This optimal/best attempt is defined as an attempt with a reasonably experienced laryngoscopist, no significant resistive muscle tone, use of optimal sniffing position, use of external laryngeal manipulation, change of laryngoscope blade type a single time, and change of laryngoscope blade length a single time.

3. The use of **regional anesthesia** as a way to avoid the known or anticipated difficult airway deserves special mention. Although the difficult airway algorithm advocates considering regional anesthesia, it must be kept in mind that the regional block can fail, or the patient may require rapid conversion to a general anesthetic for other reasons. Regional anesthesia generally should not be elected for a patient with a known difficult airway if the surgery cannot be terminated rapidly (in case of failed or inadequate block) or access to the patient's airway is compromised.

4. The **LMA** (Classic and Fastrach) is a prominent airway option throughout the 2003 ASA difficult airway algorithm:

a. **Nonemergency**

(1) An airway in patients who can be mask ventilated after general anesthesia is induced but cannot be intubated. It is also an alternative if awake intubation has failed (but only when general anesthesia

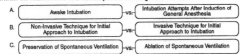

DIFFICULT AIRWAY ALGORITHM

1. Assess the likelihood and clinical impact of basic management problems:
   A. Difficult Ventilation
   B. Difficult Intubation
   C. Difficulty with Patient Cooperation or Consent
   D. Difficult Tracheostomy

2. Actively pursue opportunities to deliver supplemental oxygen throughout the process of difficult airway management

3. Consider the relative merits and feasibility of basic management choices:

A. [Awake Intubation] vs. [Intubation Attempts After Induction of General Anesthesia]

B. [Non-Invasive Technique for Initial Approach to Intubation] vs. [Invasive Technique for Initial Approach to Intubation]

C. [Preservation of Spontaneous Ventilation] vs. [Ablation of Spontaneous Ventilation]

4. Develop primary and alternative strategies:

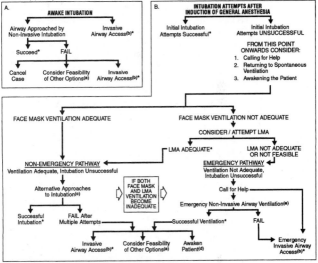

* Confirm ventilation, tracheal intubation, or LMA placement with exhaled CO_2

a. Other options include (but are not limited to): surgery utilizing face mask or LMA anesthesia, local anesthesia infiltration or regional nerve blockade. Pursuit of these options usually implies that mask ventilation will not be problematic. Therefore, these options may be of limited value if this step in the algorithm has been reached via the Emergency Pathway.

b. Invasive airway access includes surgical or percutaneous tracheostomy or cricothyrotomy.

c. Alternative non-invasive approaches to difficult intubation include (but are not limited to): use of different laryngoscope blades, LMA as an intubation conduit (with or without fiberoptic guidance), fiberoptic intubation, intubating stylet or tube changer, light wand, retrograde intubation, and blind oral or nasal intubation.

d. Consider re-preparation of the patient for awake intubation or canceling surgery.

e. Options for emergency non-invasive airway ventilation include (but are not limited to): rigid bronchoscope, esophageal-tracheal combitube ventilation, or transtracheal jet ventilation.

Figure 13.5. American Society of Anesthesiologists difficult airway algorithm. (From ASA: Practice guidelines for management of the difficult airway: an updated report by the American Society of Anesthesiologists Task Force on Management of the Difficult Airway. *Anesthesiology* **2003;98:1269–1277.)**

and mask ventilation are not considered problematic).

(2) A conduit for intubation in patients who can be mask ventilated but cannot be intubated with conventional laryngoscopy.

b. Emergency

(1) An airway in patients who cannot be intubated and cannot be ventilated. The Combitube and transtracheal jet ventilation are other options here.

(2) A conduit for intubation in patients who cannot be intubated and cannot be ventilated (when a supraglottic airway is insufficient and intubation per se is needed).

B. Emergency airway techniques

1. **Percutaneous needle cricothyroidotomy** involves placing a 14-gauge IV catheter or 7.5 French introducer through the cricothyroid membrane into the trachea. Oxygen can be administered by connecting the breathing circuit to a 3-mm ID ETT adapter inserted directly into the IV catheter or to a 7.5-mm ID ETT adapter inserted into a 3-mL syringe barrel and connected to the IV catheter.

   a. Oxygenation, but not ventilation, can be achieved by administering oxygen through the catheter at flow rates of 10 to 12 L/min. This is a temporary maneuver and is absolutely contraindicated in cases of complete upper airway obstruction, because severe barotrauma may result.

   b. Some ventilation may be achieved by pressing the oxygen flush valve for 1 second and allowing for passive exhalation over 2 to 3 seconds.

   c. Once in place, the catheter must be carefully and firmly held in position to **avoid dislodgment,** which can be life threatening.

   d. Complications include barotrauma, pneumothorax, subcutaneous emphysema of the neck and anterior chest, loss of the airway, and death. Furthermore, the airway is not "protected," and aspiration is a possibility.

2. **Rigid bronchoscopy** may be necessary to support an airway partially obstructed by a foreign body, traumatic disruption, stenosis, or mediastinal mass. General anesthesia will usually be required for insertion. It is important to have a range of bronchoscope sizes available (including pediatric sizes). An inhalation induction with spontaneous ventilation is most commonly used (see Chapter 21).

3. **Cricothyroidotomy** is a rapid effective method for relieving severe upper airway obstruction. With the neck extended, a small incision is made in the cricothyroid membrane in the midline. The handle of a scalpel or a Kelley forceps is used to separate the tissues while a tracheostomy tube or ETT is inserted percutaneously.

4. **Tracheostomy** may be performed under local anesthesia before the induction of general anesthesia for a patient with a particularly difficult airway.

   a. Technique. After careful dissection of vessels, nerves, and the thyroid isthmus, a tracheal incision is made, usually between the third and fourth cartilaginous rings.

Percutaneous dilational tracheostomy, using commercially available techniques and a modified Seldinger technique, may also be performed.

    b. **Complications** include hemorrhage, false passage, and pneumothorax.

VII. Special considerations

A. Rapid sequence induction

1. **Indications.** Patients at risk for aspiration include those who have recently eaten (full stomach), pregnant patients, and those with bowel obstruction, morbid obesity, or symptomatic reflux.

2. **Technique**

    a. **Equipment** necessary for a rapid sequence induction should include the following:

       (1) Functioning tonsil-tip (Yankauer) suction.

       (2) Several different laryngoscope blades (Macintosh and Miller).

       (3) Several styletted ETTs, including one that is a size smaller than normal.

       (4) An assistant who can apply cricoid pressure effectively.

    b. The patient is **preoxygenated** using high flow rates of 100% oxygen for 3 to 5 min (denitrogenation). Four vital capacity breaths of 100% oxygen achieve nearly the same results when time is of the essence.

    c. **The neck is extended** so the trachea is directly anterior to the esophagus. After IV administration of an induction agent (e.g., thiopental, propofol, or ketamine), followed immediately by succinylcholine (1 to 1.5 mg/kg IV), an assistant places firm downward digital pressure on the cricoid cartilage, effectively compressing and occluding the esophagus (**Sellick maneuver**). This maneuver reduces the risk of passive regurgitation of gastric contents into the pharynx and may bring the vocal cords into better view by displacing them posteriorly. It should not be used if the patient is actively vomiting, because high pressures could injure the esophagus.

    d. There should be no attempt to ventilate the patient by mask. Intubation can usually be performed within 30 to 60 seconds. Cricoid pressure is maintained until successful endotracheal intubation is verified.

    e. If intubation attempts are unsuccessful, cricoid pressure should be maintained continuously during subsequent intubation maneuvers and while mask ventilation is in progress.

B. Awake intubation

1. **Indications.** Awake oral or nasal intubation should be considered when there is:

    a. A difficult intubation anticipated in a patient at risk for aspiration.

    b. Uncertainty about the ability to ventilate or intubate after induction of general anesthesia (e.g., morbidly obese patients).

    c. A need to assess neurologic function after intubation or positioning for surgery.

2. **Technique**
   a. To perform an awake intubation, a 4% lidocaine gargle, followed by a lidocaine spray or nebulizer, is used to decrease upper airway sensation.
      (1) **Superior laryngeal nerve block** may be used to anesthetize supraglottic structures. A 25-gauge needle is directed anterior to the greater cornu of the hyoid bone and inserted in the thyrohyoid membrane. After negative aspiration, 2 mL of 2% lidocaine is injected on each side.
      (2) **Translaryngeal injection of local anesthetic** can anesthetize the glottis and upper trachea. A 25-gauge needle is inserted through the cricothyroid membrane in the midline. After aspiration of air to confirm placement within the tracheal lumen, 2 mL of 2% lidocaine is injected, and the needle is withdrawn. The patient will cough when local anesthetic is injected, aiding in anesthetic spread. This block may increase the risk for aspiration in a patient with a full stomach.
   b. **Awake oral laryngoscopy** often allows one to assess the airway. Sedatives such as midazolam, propofol, and fentanyl may be used in addition to the nerve blocks described above.
   c. **Awake (blind) nasal intubation** may be performed after adequate topical anesthesia and regional airway blocks.
      (1) Incremental doses of sedatives are useful adjuncts.
      (2) A well-lubricated ETT is passed into the nasopharynx with gentle pressure.
      (3) Deep resonant breath sounds may be noted as the tube is advanced toward the glottis. An exaggerated sniffing position may be useful. The ETT is usually passed into the trachea during inspiration.
      (4) Successful intubation is noted when the patient is unable to phonate, breath sounds and humidification within the ETT are noted with ventilation, and carbon dioxide is noted on the capnograph.
3. **Complications** are as described in section V.B.4.
C. **ETT changes.** Occasionally, ETT cuff leaks or partial obstruction of the ETT necessitates changing an ETT in a patient with a difficult airway.
   1. The oropharynx is suctioned and the patient is ventilated with 100% oxygen.
   2. A **tracheal tube changer** is a specialized stylet that is placed through the ETT and into the distal trachea. The old ETT is slid off the changer, and a new ETT is passed over the changer into the trachea.
   3. A **fiberoptic bronchoscope** can also be used for reintubation. An ETT is placed over the bronchoscope, the tip of which is passed into the trachea alongside the existing tube. The cuff of the existing ETT is deflated, the bronchoscope is advanced, and tracheal rings are noted to confirm position. The existing ETT is removed (a tracheal tube changer may be left in its place) and the new one is advanced as described in section V.C.

SUGGESTED READING

Adnet F, Baillard C, Borron SW, et al. Randomized study comparing the "sniffing position" with simple head extension for laryngoscopic view in elective surgery patients. *Anesthesiology* 2001;95:836–841.

ASA: Practice guidelines for management of the difficult airway: an updated report by the American Society of Anesthesiologists Task Force on Management of the Difficult Airway. *Anesthesiology* 2003;98:1269–1277.

Brain AIJ, Verghese C, Strube PJ. The LMA 'Proseal' – a laryngeal mask with an oesophageal vent. *Br J Anaesthesia* 2000;84:650–654.

Cormack RS, Lehane J. Difficult tracheal intubation in obstetrics. *Anaesthesia* 1984;39:1105–1111.

Ferson DZ, Rosenblatt WH, Johansen MJ, et al. Use of the intubating LMA-Fastrach in 254 patients with difficult-to-manage airways. *Anesthesiology* 2001;95:1175–1181.

Hurford WE. Nasotracheal intubation. *Respir Care* 1999;44:643–649.

Langeron O, Masso E, Huraux C, et al. Prediction of difficult mask ventilation. *Anesthesiology* 2000;92:1229–1236.

Peterson GN, Domino KB, Caplan RA, Posner KL, et al. Management of the difficult airway: a closed claims analysis. *Anesthesiology* 2005;103:33–39.

Samsoon GLT, Young JRB. Difficult tracheal intubation: a retrospective study. *Anaesthesia* 1987;42:490–497.

Scmitt H, Buchfelder M, Radespil-Troger M, et al. Difficult intubation in acromegalic patients. *Anesthesiology* 2000;93:110–114.

Sellick B. Cricoid pressure to control regurgitation of stomach contents during induction of anesthesia. *Lancet* 1961;2:404–406.

14

Administration of General Anesthesia

Stuart A. Forman and Roy P. H. Yang

The **primary goals** of general anesthesia are to maintain the health and safety of the patient while providing amnesia, hypnosis (lack of awareness), analgesia, and optimal surgical conditions (e.g., immobility). **Secondary goals** may vary, depending on the patient's medical condition, the surgical procedure, and the surgical setting (e.g., outpatient surgical unit versus inpatient operating room [OR]; see Chapters 31 and 32). Perioperative planning involves the integration of pre-, intra-, and postoperative care. Flexibility is an essential component in this planning; multiple approaches to induction, maintenance, and emergence should be considered. Furthermore, intraoperative changes in the surgical procedure or the patient's condition may occur, requiring modification of anesthetic goals and plans.

I. **Preoperative preparation.** The anesthetist assumes responsibility for the patient when the preoperative medication is administered. An anesthetist or other responsible physician should accompany an unstable patient during transport to the OR.

   A. **Preoperative evaluations** may be performed minutes to weeks before administration of the anesthetic and sometimes not by the anesthetist of record. The administering anesthetist performs an airway examination and checks for interim changes in the patient's condition, medications, laboratory data, and consultant notes. Time of last oral intake is confirmed, the anesthetic plan is reviewed with the patient, and proper informed consent for administration of anesthesia is obtained from either the patient or his/her legal proxy.

   B. **Intravascular volume.** Patients may arrive in the OR with intravascular volume deficits or dehydration due to prolonged lack of oral intake, severe inflammatory illness, hemorrhage, fever, vomiting, or diuretic use. Currently available isotonic bowel preparations may not directly induce water loss but can decrease absorption of fluids ingested before surgery. The patient's volume status is evaluated either clinically or with appropriate monitors. If a **fluid deficit** is present, the patient should be adequately hydrated before the induction of anesthesia. The fluid deficit for fasting adults is estimated at 60 mL/hour plus 1 mL/kg/hour for each kilogram greater than 20 kg (maintenance fluids). In general, at least half of this deficit is corrected before induction; the remainder may be corrected intraoperatively. The type and amount of fluids given may be modified in the presence of systemic diseases (see Chapters 2 to 6) or when specific types of surgery are planned (see Chapters 21 to 26).

   C. **Intravenous (IV) access.** The size and number of IV catheters placed varies with the procedure, anticipated blood loss, and the need for continuous drug infusions. At least one 14- or 16-gauge catheter is indicated when rapid fluid or blood infusion is anticipated. When continuous drug infusions are to be delivered concurrently with rapid fluid infusion, an additional IV catheter often is dedicated for this purpose. Some medications used for cardiovascular support (e.g., norepinephrine) are best delivered via a central venous catheter.

D. **Preoperative medications**

1. **Anxiety.** The preoperative period is one of great anxiety, especially for patients who have not had a prior interview with an anesthetist. Anxiety may be managed effectively with calm reassurance and expression of interest in the patient's well-being. When deemed appropriate, a benzodiazepine (e.g., diazepam, midazolam) with or without a small dose of an opioid (e.g., fentanyl, morphine) may be administered. Oral diazepam or lorazepam may be given with a small amount of water 30 to 60 min before the procedure. Patients complaining of pain on arrival in the OR may be given opioids in incremental amounts to alleviate symptoms. Dosages are based on the patient's age, medical condition, and anticipated time of discharge (see Chapters 1 and 11). Appropriate monitoring should be used and resuscitative equipment should be available.

2. **Drugs to neutralize gastric acid and decrease gastric volume** are used when the patient is at increased risk of aspiration of gastric contents (i.e., recent meal, trauma, bowel obstruction, pregnancy, history of gastric surgery, increased intra-abdominal pressure, or history of active reflux; see Chapter 1).

E. **Monitoring.** Standard monitoring (see Chapter 10) is established before the induction of anesthesia. Invasive monitors (e.g., arterial catheter, central venous line, pulmonary artery catheter) should be placed before induction of anesthesia when indicated by the patient's medical condition and potential anesthetic effects (e.g., an arterial line for a patient at risk for cerebral ischemia). Invasive monitors may be placed after induction of anesthesia when indicated primarily by the surgical procedure (e.g., a central line for a patient undergoing elective aortic surgery).

F. **Trauma and cardiac, thoracic, aortic, and intracranial surgery** pose significant risks to the patient that prolong the need for close monitoring and highly skilled care (see Chapters 21 to 24). If necessary, intensive care unit (ICU) bed availability must be confirmed before elective cases and planned for during emergency surgery.

II. **Induction of anesthesia** produces an unconscious patient with depressed reflexes who is entirely dependent on the anesthetist for maintenance of homeostatic mechanisms and safety.

A. **The environment** in the OR should be warm, with minimal noise, and with all attention focused on the patient.

B. **The patient's position** for induction is usually supine, with extremities resting comfortably on padded surfaces in a neutral anatomic position. The head should rest comfortably on a firm support, which is raised in a "sniff" position (see Chapter 13). Routine preinduction administration of oxygen minimizes the risk of hypoxia developing during induction of anesthesia. High-flow (8 to 10 L/min) oxygen should be delivered via a face mask placed gently on the patient's face. The patient can be instructed to take deep breaths and exhale fully to speed the exchange of oxygen.

C. **Induction techniques.** The choice of induction technique is guided by the patient's medical condition, anticipated airway management (i.e., risk of aspiration, difficult intubation, or compromised airway), and patient preference.

1. **IV induction** begins with administration of a potent short-acting hypnotic drug (specific agents and doses are given in Chapter 11). After loss of consciousness, inhalation or additional IV agents are administered to maintain anesthesia. The patient may continue to breathe spontaneously or with assistance.

2. **An induction using only inhalational anesthetics** may be used to maintain spontaneous ventilation when there is a compromised airway or to defer the placement of an IV catheter (e.g., in pediatric patients). After preoxygenation, inhalational anesthetics are added at a low concentration (0.5 times minimum alveolar concentration [MAC]) and then increased every three to four breaths until the depth of anesthesia is adequate for IV placement or airway manipulation. Alternatively, a "single vital capacity breath" inhalation induction can be achieved with a high concentration of a less pungent agent like halothane or sevoflurane. Physiological signs should be closely observed to assess anesthetic depth (Table 14.1).

3. Intramuscular injection of ketamine, oral transmucosal fentanyl, and oral midazolam are agents and routes more commonly used in uncooperative patients and young children (see Chapters 11 and 29).

D. **Airway management** (see Chapter 13). The patency of the patient's airway is critically important during induction of anesthesia. Patients with difficult or unstable airways may require endotracheal intubation before the induction of anesthesia. The anesthetized patient's airway may be managed with a face mask, oral or nasopharyngeal airway, cuffed oropharyngeal airway, laryngeal mask airway (LMA), or endotracheal tube (ETT). If tracheal intubation is planned, a muscle relaxant may be given to facilitate laryngoscopy and intubation, but the ability to ventilate the patient via face mask should be assessed before muscle relaxant administration. An exception to this rule is the "rapid sequence induction" for patients at risk for pulmonary aspiration (see Chapter 13).

E. **Laryngoscopy** and **intubation** may cause profound sympathetic responses such as hypertension and tachycardia; these can be attenuated by the prior administration of additional hypnotics, volatile anesthetics, opioids, or β-adrenergic blockers.

F. **Positioning for surgery** usually occurs after the induction of general anesthesia. Patients at risk for neurologic injury during positioning may undergo awake intubation and then be assisted into their surgical position before induction of anesthesia. Movement of a supine anesthetized patient into a different position may cause hypotension because of the lack of intact compensatory hemodynamic reflexes. Positioning should occur at a controlled pace with frequent assessments of the patient's cardiovascular status and with close attention to the patient's airway and ventilation. The anesthetist should ensure that the patient's head and limbs are protected and sufficiently padded to prevent compressive ischemia or neurologic damage. Hyperextension or overrotation of the patient's neck and joints must be avoided.

III. **Maintenance** begins when the patient is sufficiently anesthetized to block awareness and movements in response to surgery. Vigilance on

Table 14.1. Stages of general anesthesia

Stage I: Amnesia	This period begins with induction of anesthesia and continues to loss of consciousness. The threshold of pain perception is lowered during stage I.
Stage II: Delirium	This period characterized by uninhibited excitation and potentially injurious responses to noxious stimuli, including vomiting, laryngospasm, hypertension, tachycardia, and uncontrolled movement. The pupils are often dilated, gaze may be divergent, respiration is frequently irregular, and breath holding is common. Desirable induction drugs accelerate transition through this stage.
Stage III: Surgical anesthesia	In this target depth for anesthesia, the gaze is central, pupils are constricted, and respirations are regular. Anesthesia is considered sufficient when painful stimulation does not elicit somatic reflexes or deleterious autonomic responses (e.g., hypertension, tachycardia).
Stage IV: Overdosage	Commonly described as "too deep," this stage is marked by shallow or absent respirations, dilated and nonreactive pupils, and hypotension that may progress to circulatory failure. Anesthesia should be lightened immediately.

The "stages" or planes of anesthesia were defined by Guedel after careful observation of patient responses during induction with diethyl ether. Induction with modern anesthetic agents is sufficiently rapid that these descriptions of individual stages are often not applicable or appreciated. However, modification of these categories still provides useful terminology to describe progression from the awake to the anesthetized state.

the part of the anesthetist is required to maintain homeostasis (vital signs, acid-base balance, temperature, coagulation, and volume status) and regulate anesthetic depth.

A. **Ensuring lack of awareness and amnesia** are implicit goals of a general anesthetic. **Intraoperative awareness** with recall is estimated to occur in 0.1% to 0.2% of general anesthetics and is more frequent in certain high-risk surgical populations (e.g., trauma, cardiac surgery, obstetrics, difficult airway). Factors that increase the risk of awareness include the use of muscle relaxants with "light" anesthesia techniques such as nitrous oxide–opioid relaxant. Alcoholism or long-term use of sedatives and/or opioids may increase a patient's dosage requirements for general anesthetics. Preoperative discussion with the patient before obtaining consent is recommended when risk factors for awareness during general anesthesia are present. **Depth of anesthesia** should be continuously assessed from induction through emergence. Changes in the intensity of surgical stimulation may cause rapid changes in anesthetic depth, which should be anticipated. Responses suggesting inadequate anesthetic depth are nonspecific and unreliable. These may be somatic (movement, coughing, changes of respiratory pattern) or autonomic (tachycardia, hypertension, mydriasis, sweating, or tearing). Purposeful movements in response to surgical stimulation or voice command are evidence of "perceptive awareness" but can occur without recall. These should be attenuated by first ensuring adequate hypnosis and analgesia and then, if indicated, by the administration of muscle relaxants. In paralyzed patients, changes in physiologic signs (see Table 14.1) can indicate inadequate anesthesia, but these are unreliable. Awareness can occur without any autonomic signs and sympathetic activation may be caused by stimuli other than awareness or pain (e.g., hypoxia, hypercarbia, hypovolemia, caval compression, adrenal manipulation). Furthermore, autonomic responses are modified by IV analgesics, regional anesthesia, antihypertensives, and other drugs. Intraoperative monitors that analyze features of the cortical electroencephalogram and auditory evoked potentials have been shown to help predict the hypnotic state under many, but not all, types of general anesthesia. The use of electroencephalogram bispectral index monitoring to guide anesthesia has been shown to reduce the incidence of awareness with recall in high-risk patients.

B. **Methods**
1. **The use of volatile agents** with minimal opioid use usually permits spontaneous ventilation. The concentration of the volatile anesthetic is titrated to patient movement (if muscle relaxants are not used), blood pressure (which decreases with increasing depth), and ventilation. Nitrous oxide, if used, is adjusted to ensure adequate oxygenation. High concentrations of nitrous oxide are contraindicated in patients with closed air-filled compartments (e.g., pneumothorax, pneumocephalus, bowel obstruction, intravitreal bubbles in eye surgery). Nitrous oxide has the potential to exacerbate hematologic or neurologic diseases in patients with vitamin B12 or folate deficiency or methionine synthase abnormalities.
2. **In a nitrous oxide–opioid relaxant technique,** an inspired gas mixture of 65% to 70% nitrous oxide is combined with IV opioids, which are titrated to the patient's heart rate and blood pressure in response to surgical stimulation. Ventilation is controlled during the procedure to prevent hypoventilation because of the combination of muscle relaxants and opioids. An estimate of the total opioid requirement should be calculated and large doses should be avoided near the end of surgery to prevent delayed emergence and hypoventilation. Depending on the nitrous oxide concentration, patient's age, and physical status, awareness during surgery may be a concern requiring additional amnestic or hypnotic agents.
3. **IV anesthesia** uses the continuous infusion or repeated boluses of a short-acting hypnotic drug (e.g., propofol) with or without opioids (e.g., remifentanil) and a muscle relaxant. This technique allows for a rapid emergence, and it is particularly useful when ventilation is frequently interrupted (e.g.,

bronchoscopy, laser airway surgery) or when it is desirable to avoid drugs that can trigger malignant hyperthermia.

4. **Combinations** of the above methods are often used. A low concentration of a volatile anesthetic (0.3 to 0.5 × MAC) may be added to a nitrous oxide–opioid relaxant technique to decrease the possibility of awareness. Nitrous oxide is frequently used in conjunction with IV anesthetics. Continuous ketamine infusions at analgesic doses can be used with other inhaled or IV anesthetics to reduce the need for intra- and postoperative opioids. Multiple anesthetics reduce the need for and the potential toxicity of large doses of single anesthetic agents. However, adverse medication reactions and interactions increase with the number of anesthetics administered.

5. **General anesthesia can be combined with a regional anesthetic technique** (i.e., peripheral or neuraxial nerve block). The required dose of general anesthesia is significantly reduced with blockade of painful surgical stimulation but still needs to be sufficient to ensure lack of awareness when muscle relaxants are used.

C. **Ventilation** of the patient during general anesthesia may be spontaneous, assisted, or controlled.

1. **Spontaneous or assisted ventilation** may help assess the depth of anesthesia by observing the respiratory rate and pattern. A patient may breathe spontaneously with or without assistance, via a mask, LMA, or ETT. Intraoperatively, respiratory function may be significantly compromised because of the patient's medical condition, positioning, external pressure on the thorax and abdomen, surgical maneuvers (e.g., peritoneal insufflation, open chest, surgical packing), and medications (e.g., opioids). Most inhaled and IV anesthetic agents depress respiration in a dose-dependent manner, with a moderate rise in arterial partial pressure of carbon dioxide.

2. **Controlled ventilation.** Although a mask or LMA may be used, an ETT and mechanical ventilator are generally used if ventilation is to be controlled for a significant period of time. Initial ventilator settings in healthy patients usually consist of a tidal volume of 10 to 12 mL/kg and a respiratory rate of 8 to 10 breaths/min. Lower tidal volumes (6 to 7 mL/kg) and the addition of positive end-expiratory pressure (PEEP) reduce the likelihood of barotrauma in patients with pulmonary pathology (see Chapter 36). Peak inspiratory pressure (PIP) should be noted. High airway pressure (>25 to 30 cm H_2O in nonobese patients) or changes of PIP must be investigated immediately and may signal a breathing circuit problem, ETT obstruction or movement, altered lung compliance or resistance, change in muscle relaxation, or surgical compression.

3. **Assessment of ventilation.** Adequate ventilation is confirmed by continual observation of the patient, auscultation of breath sounds, inspection of the anesthesia machine (e.g., reservoir breathing bag, ventilator bellows, airway pressures and gas flows), and patient monitors (e.g., capnograph, pulse oximeter). Arterial blood gas measurement and adjustments in the patient's ventilation may be required intraoperatively. If

gas exchange is inadequate, manual controlled ventilation, increased inspired oxygen concentrations, PEEP, or special ventilator modes (sometimes requiring a stand-alone ventilator) may be used (see Chapter 36) while the source of the problem is sought and treated.

D. IV fluids

1. **Intraoperative IV fluid requirements**

   a. **Maintenance fluid requirements** as described in section I.B. should be continued intraoperatively. In some instances (e.g., extremity surgery with tourniquet use), this may be the major component of the fluid requirement.

   b. **"Third space losses"** are caused by tissue edema from surgical trauma, whereas **"insensible losses"** are cause by evaporation from the airways and surgical wounds. These losses are difficult to assess and may be substantial (up to 20 mL/kg/hour) depending on the site and extent of surgery. The rate of evaporative loss is increased in febrile patients.

   c. **Blood losses may be difficult to estimate.** The amount present in the suction canisters should be monitored, taking into consideration the presence of other fluids (e.g., irrigation, ascites). Used surgical sponges should be checked and may be weighed to improve estimates of blood loss. Blood lost on the surgical field (e.g., surgical drapes) and on the floor should be estimated. If blood loss is substantial, serial monitoring of hematocrits is warranted.

2. **IV fluids** are administered to correct preoperative deficits and intraoperative losses.

   a. **Crystalloid solutions** are used to replace maintenance fluid requirements, evaporative losses, and third space losses. The IV solution should be a balanced salt solution that is approximately isotonic (e.g., lactated Ringer's). Other IV solutions may be indicated for patients with specific metabolic conditions (e.g., added glucose for diabetic patients receiving insulin, reduced sodium in diabetes insipidus, or increased sodium in syndrome of inappropriate secretion of antidiuretic hormone). Blood loss may be replaced with balanced salt solution, administered in a 3:1 ratio of volume to estimated blood loss. With continued blood loss, this ratio will increase.

   b. **Colloid solutions** (e.g., 5% albumin, 6% hydroxyethyl starch) may be used to replace blood loss or restore intravascular volume. To replace blood loss, colloid solutions should be administered in an approximately 1:1 ratio of volume to estimated blood loss (see Chapter 34).

   c. **Blood transfusion** is discussed in Chapter 34.

3. **Assessment.** Trends in heart rate, blood pressure, and urine output may serve as guides to intravascular volume status and adequacy of replacement therapy. Measurement of central venous pressure, pulmonary artery occlusion pressure, right and left end-diastolic volumes (using transesophageal echocardiography), and cardiac output provide additional data to guide fluid administration when intraoperative losses are large or when cardiopulmonary disease mandates strict control of the patient's central pressures. Hematocrit, platelet count, fibrinogen concentration, prothrombin time, and partial

thromboplastin time are used to assess the adequacy of blood product therapy.

IV. **Emergence from general anesthesia.** During this period, the patient makes the transition from an unconscious state to an awake state with intact protective reflexes.

    A. **Goals.** Patients should be awake and responsive, with full muscle strength and adequate pain control. Full recovery of airway reflexes and muscle function minimizes the risk of airway obstruction or pulmonary aspiration upon extubation and facilitates immediate neurologic assessment. In patients with cardiovascular disease, hemodynamics should be controlled.

    B. **Technique.** Surgical stimulation diminishes as the procedure nears completion and anesthetic depth is reduced, enabling rapid emergence. Residual muscle relaxation is reversed, and the patient may start to breathe spontaneously. Analgesic requirements should be estimated and addressed before awakening.

    C. **Environment.** The OR should be warmed, blankets placed on the patient, and noise and conversation minimized.

    D. **Positioning.** The patient is usually returned to the supine position before extubation. The patient may be extubated in a lateral or prone position if the anesthetist is confident that the airway can be maintained and protected. A method for quickly returning the patient to the supine position must be available.

    E. **Mask ventilation.** A patient who has received mask ventilation should continue to breathe 100% oxygen by mask during emergence. A period of light anesthesia (stage II; see Table 14.1) often occurs before the patient regains consciousness. Stimulation (especially of the airway) during this period may precipitate vomiting or laryngospasm and is best avoided. The patient can be moved when fully awake, following verbal commands, breathing spontaneously, and oxygenating adequately.

    F. **Extubation.** Removal of the ETT from the trachea of an intubated patient is a critical moment. Patients with respiratory failure, hypothermia, impaired sensorium, marked hemodynamic instability, or whose airway may be significantly jeopardized (e.g., extensive oral surgery or possible glottic edema after neck surgery or prolonged head-down positioning) may remain intubated postoperatively until these conditions have improved.

        1. **Awake extubation.** Extubation of the airway usually occurs after the patient fully regains protective reflexes. Awake extubation is indicated in patients at risk of aspiration of gastric contents, patients who have difficult airways, and patients who have just undergone tracheal or maxillofacial surgery.

            a. **Criteria.** Before extubation, the patient should be awake and hemodynamically stable. The patient should have regained full muscle strength (see Chapter 12), be able to follow simple verbal commands (e.g., lift head), and breathe spontaneously with acceptable oxygenation and ventilation.

            b. **Technique.** The presence of an ETT may be irritating to patients emerging from anesthesia. Lidocaine (0.5 to 1.0 mg/kg IV) can be given to suppress coughing but may prolong emergence. The patient breathes 100% oxygen, and the oropharynx is suctioned. Mild positive airway pressure (20 cm H_2O) is applied via the ETT, the ETT cuff is deflated, and the tube is removed. Oxygen (100%) administration is continued by face mask. The anesthetist's attention should remain focused on the patient until the patient's ability to ventilate, oxygenate, and protect the airway is confirmed. The extubated patient may become unconscious again and lose protective airway reflexes when stimulation decreases.

   c. **Removal of the ETT over a flexible stylette** (e.g., ETT exchanger, jet stylette, fiberoptic bronchoscope) can be performed when the patency of the patient's airway is uncertain or reintubation may be difficult. The airway is first anesthetized with lidocaine at 0.3 to 0.5 mg/kg administered via the ETT and the patient is allowed to breathe spontaneously. A lubricated ETT exchanger is passed into the trachea through the ETT, the ETT cuff is deflated, and the ETT removed, leaving the exchange device in place until the anesthetist is certain that the patient's airway is stable. If airway obstruction develops, oxygen can be insufflated via the hollow exchange device or an ETT can be inserted over the device, which acts as a guide.

2. **Deep extubation.** Stimulation of airway reflexes by the ETT during emergence can be avoided by extubating the trachea while the patient is still deeply anesthetized (stage III). This reduces the risk of laryngospasm and bronchospasm, making it a useful technique for severely asthmatic patients. It also avoids coughing and straining that may be undesirable after middle-ear surgery, open-eye procedures, and abdominal or inguinal herniorrhaphy.

   a. **Criteria.** Contraindications to deep extubation are noted above (section IV.F.1.). Anesthetic depth must be sufficient to avoid responses to airway stimulation. Anesthesia may be deepened with a short-acting IV anesthetic or ventilation with a high concentration of a volatile agent.

   b. **Technique.** All necessary airway equipment and medications should be readily available for replacement of the ETT. Surgical positioning must allow unrestricted access to the head for airway management. The oropharynx should be suctioned, the ETT cuff deflated, and, if there is no response to cuff deflation, the ETT is removed. Inhalation anesthesia is continued by mask and emergence is managed as described above (section IV.F.).

G. **Agitation.** Severe agitation is occasionally seen on emergence from general anesthesia. Physiologic causes (e.g., hypoxia, hypercarbia, airway obstruction, or a full bladder) must be excluded. Pain, a common reason for agitation, may be treated with cautious titration of opioids (e.g., fentanyl, 0.025 mg IV, or meperidine, 25-mg IV increments) if vital signs and oxygenation are reassuring.

H. **Delayed awakening.** On occasion, a patient will not awaken promptly after the administration of general anesthesia. Ventilatory support and airway protection should be continued, and specific etiologies should be investigated (see Chapter 35).

V. **Transport.** The anesthetist should accompany the patient from the OR to the postanesthesia care unit (PACU) or ICU. Monitoring of blood pressure, hemoglobin saturation, and electrocardiogram is continued

Table 14.2.   Postoperative assessment for awareness during general anesthesia

The Modified Brice Interview[a]

1) What is the last thing you remember before going to sleep?
2) What is the first thing you remember after waking up?
3) Do you remember anything between going to sleep and waking up?
4) Did you dream during your procedure?
5) What was the worst thing about your operation?

[a]These questions are a modification of the interview approach first reported by D.D. Brice et al. *British Journal of Anaesthesia* 1970;42:535–541. Responses to this type of postoperative interview have been reported to vary depending on the interval after surgery and the setting (hospital versus home).

during transport to an ICU but generally is not needed for transport of stable patients to the PACU. Supplemental oxygen should be available, and the patient's airway, ventilation, and overall condition should be continually observed. Placing the patient in the lateral position may help to prevent aspiration and upper airway obstruction. Medications and airway equipment should be available during transport if the patient is unstable or if transport is over a significant distance. Upon transfer of responsibility for patient care in the PACU or ICU, the anesthetist should provide a concise but thorough summary of the patient's past medical history, intraoperative course, postoperative condition, and current therapy.

VI. Postoperative visit. A postoperative evaluation of the patient should be performed by the anesthetist within 24 to 48 hours of surgery and documented in the patient's medical record. The visit should include a review of the medical record, examination of the patient, and discussion of the patient's perioperative experience. Specific complications such as nausea, sore throat, dental injury, nerve injury, ocular injury, altered pulmonary function, or change in mental status should be sought. Questions to elicit evidence of awareness during the general anesthetic (Table 14.2) should be asked. Responses along with an evaluation and plan, if needed, should be recorded in the patient's chart. Complications that require further therapy or consultations should be actively managed and the patient's course should be followed until these issues are resolved.

SUGGESTED READING

Ghoneim MM. Awareness during anesthesia. *Anesthesiology* 2000;92:597–602.

Myles PS, et al. Bispectral index monitoring to prevent awareness during anaesthesia: The B-Aware Randomised Controlled Trial. *Lancet* 2004;363:1757–1763.

Sebel PS, et al. The incidence of awareness during anesthesia: a multicenter United States study. *Anesth Analg* 2004;99:833–839.

Stanski DR, Shafer SL. Monitoring depth of anesthesia. In: Miller RD, ed. *Anesthesia*, 5th/6th ed. Philadelphia: Churchill Livingstone, 2005:1227–1264.

Willenkin RL, Polk SL. Management of general anesthesia. In: Miller RD, ed. *Anesthesia*, 4th ed. New York: Churchill Livingstone, 1994:1045–1056.

15

Local Anesthetics

Ping Jin and Jeannie C. Min

I. **General principles**
   A. **Chemistry.** Local anesthetics are weak bases whose structure consists of an aromatic moiety connected to a substituted amine through an ester or amide linkage. The pK_a values of local anesthetics are near physiologic pH; thus, in vivo, both charged and uncharged forms are present. The degree of ionization is important because the uncharged form is more lipophilic and able to gain access to the axon. The clinical differences between the ester and amide local anesthetics involve their potential for producing adverse effects and the mechanisms by which they are metabolized.
   1. **Esters.** Procaine, cocaine, chloroprocaine, and tetracaine. The ester linkage is cleaved by plasma cholinesterase. The half-life of esters in the circulation is very short (about 1 minute). The degradation product of ester metabolism is *p*-aminobenzoic acid.
   2. **Amides.** Lidocaine, mepivacaine, bupivacaine, etidocaine, and ropivacaine. The amide linkage is cleaved through initial *N*-dealkylation followed by hydrolysis, which occurs primarily in the liver. Patients with severe hepatic disease may be more susceptible to adverse reactions from amide local anesthetics. The elimination half-life for amide local anesthetics is 2 to 3 hours.
   B. **Mechanism of action**
   1. **Local anesthetics block nerve conduction** by impairing propagation of the action potential in axons. They have no effect on the resting or threshold potentials but decrease the rate of rise of the action potential so that the threshold potential is not reached.
   2. **Local anesthetics interact directly with specific receptors** on the Na^+ channel, inhibiting Na^+ ion influx. The anesthetic molecule must traverse the cell membrane through passive nonionic diffusion in the uncharged state and then bind to the sodium channel in the charged state. In addition, recent data suggest that local anesthetics may also act on K^+ and Ca^{2+} channels.
   3. **Physiochemical properties** of the local anesthetics affect neural blockade.
      a. **Lipid solubility** determines potency, as more lipophilic local anesthetic agents more easily cross nerve membranes.
      b. Agents with a high degree of **protein binding** will have a prolonged duration of effect.
      c. **pK_a** determines the speed of onset of neural blockade. pK_a is the pH at which 50% of the local anesthetic is in the uncharged form. Agents with a lower pK_a value will have a faster onset because a greater fraction of these weak bases

Table 15.1. Classification of nerve fibers

Fiber Type	Myelin	Diameter (μm)	Function
A-α	++	6–22	Motor efferent, proprioception afferent
A-β	++	6–22	Motor efferent, proprioception afferent
A-γ	++	3–6	Muscle spindle efferent
A-δ	++	1–4	Pain, temperature, touch afferent
B	+	<3	Preganglionic autonomic
C	−	0.3–1.3	Pain, temperature, touch afferent, postganglionic autonomic

will exist in the uncharged form at pH 7.4 and thus will more readily diffuse across nerve membranes.

  d. **Higher pH of the drug solution** will speed onset by increasing the proportion of molecules in the uncharged form.

4. **Differential blockade of nerve fibers**

  a. **Peripheral nerves** are classified according to size and function (Table 15.1). Traditionally, thin nerve fibers were believed to be more easily blocked than thick ones; however, the opposite susceptibility has been found. Myelinated fibers are more readily blocked than unmyelinated ones, as myelinated fibers need to be blocked only at the nodes of Ranvier.

  b. **Differential blockade** of pain, temperature sensation, and motor function can occur and is a reflection of the variable sensitivities of different nerve fibers to local anesthetics. This may be due to different ion channel compositions of the nerve fibers and their arrangement within the peripheral nerve. Dilute solutions of local anesthetics cannot be relied upon to produce differential blockade in a reproducible manner.

5. **Sequence of clinical anesthesia.** Neural blockade of peripheral nerves usually progresses in the following order:

  a. Sympathetic block with peripheral vasodilatation and skin temperature elevation.

  b. Loss of pain and temperature sensation.

  c. Loss of proprioception.

  d. Loss of touch and pressure sensation.

  e. Motor paralysis.

6. **Pathophysiologic factors**

  a. **A decrease in cardiac output** reduces the plasma and tissue clearance of local anesthetics, increasing plasma concentration and the potential for toxicity.

  b. **Severe hepatic disease** may prolong the duration of action of amino amides.

  c. **Renal disease** has minimal effect.

Table 15.2. Clinical uses of local anesthetics

Anesthetics	Onset	Duration	Toxicity	Maximal Recommended dose (mg)[a]	Applications/Comments
Esters					
Procaine (Novocaine)	Rapid	Short	Low	400 (600)	Local infiltration Spinal anesthesia (very short duration)
Chloroprocaine (Nescaine)	Very rapid	Short	Very low	800 (1000)	Local blocks Epidural anesthesia Rapid hydrolysis in plasma
Tetracaine (Pontocaine)	Slow	Long	High	100 (200)	Spinal anesthesia Nerve blocks Motor and sensory blockade of similar duration and intensity
Amides					
Lidocaine (Xylocaine)	Rapid	Intermediate	Moderate	300 (500)	Most frequently used local anesthetic All types of local and regional anesthesia Neurotoxicity especially after subarachnoid administration (see text)
Mepivacaine (Carbocaine)	Moderate	Intermediate	Moderate	300 (500)	Local infiltration Nerve blocks Epidural anesthesia
Benzocaine	Rapid	Intermediate	Moderate		High lipophilicity, used for topical anesthesia, risk of methemoglobinemia

Bupivacaine (Marcaine, Sensorcaine)	Slow	Long	High	175 (225)	Sensory greater than motor blockade* All types of local and regional anesthesia requiring long duration
Etidocaine (Duranest)	Rapid	Long	Moderate	300 (400)	Nerve blocks Epidural anesthesia Motor greater than sensory blockade
Ropivacaine	Slow	Long	Moderate	200 (n/a)	Epidural anesthesia Sensory greater than motor blockade[b] Less cardiac toxicity than bupivacaine

[a]Maximal recommended dose for a major nerve block; epinephrine-containing solution in parenthesis. Maximal dose may be less after intercostal or intratracheal block due to rapid absorption from these sites.
[b]Sensory versus motor blockade dependent on concentration.

    d. Patients with **reduced cholinesterase activity** (newborns and pregnant patients) and patients with **atypical cholinesterase** may have an increased potential for toxicity from ester-type anesthetics.

    e. **Fetal acidosis** may result in greater transplacental transfer and trapping of local anesthetics from mother to fetus and thus may have an increased potential for fetal toxicity.

    f. Conditions such as **sepsis, malignancy, and cardiac ischemia** can increase the concentration of the binding protein α_1-acid glycoprotein, and this may decrease the plasma concentration of free local anesthetics.

C. Commercial preparations

    1. Commercially available solutions of local anesthetics are supplied as **hydrochloride salts** to increase solubility in water. These solutions are usually acidic to enhance the formation of the water-soluble ionized form. Plain solutions usually are adjusted to pH 6. Those containing epinephrine are adjusted to pH 4 because of the lability of catecholamine molecules at alkaline pH.

    2. **Antimicrobial preservatives** (paraben derivatives) are added to multidose vials. Only preservative-free solutions should be used in spinal, epidural, or caudal anesthesia to prevent potentially neurotoxic effects.

    3. **Antioxidants** (sodium metabisulfite, sodium ethylenediaminetetraacetic acid [EDTA]) may be added to slow breakdown of local anesthetics.

II. Clinical uses of local anesthetics. The choice of local anesthetic must take into consideration the duration of surgery, regional technique used, surgical requirements, the potential for local or systemic toxicity, and any metabolic constraints (Tables 15.2 and 15.3).

A. Combinations of local anesthetics

    1. Chloroprocaine–bupivacaine, lidocaine–bupivacaine, and mepivacaine–bupivacaine mixtures are reported to have a rapid onset and long duration. The systemic toxicity appears to be additive. The clinical benefit of local anesthetic combinations is unproven.

    2. **Eutectic mixture of local anesthetics (EMLA)** cream is a mixture of 2.5% lidocaine and 2.5% prilocaine for use as a topical skin anesthetic.

B. Epinephrine

    1. **Epinephrine** may be added to local anesthetics for the following reasons:

        a. To prolong the duration of anesthesia. This varies with the specific agent and its concentration as well as the type of regional block.

        b. To decrease systemic toxicity by decreasing the rate of absorption of anesthetic into the circulation, thus minimizing peak blood levels of local anesthetics.

        c. To increase intensity of the block by a direct α agonist effect on antinociceptive neurons in the spinal cord.

        d. To provide local vasoconstriction and decrease surgical bleeding.

        e. To assist in the detection of intravascular injections (see Chapter 16).

Table 15.3. Local anesthetic agents

Anesthetic Technique	Anesthetic	Concen-tration (%)	Dura-tion (hours)[a]	Usual Dose (mL; 70-kg patient)
Peripheral nerve block	Lidocaine	1–2	1.5–3.0	20–40
	Mepivacaine	1–2	3–5	20–40
	Bupivacaine	0.25–0.5	6–12	30–40
	Etidocaine	1.0–1.5	6–12	20–40
	Ropivacaine	0.5	5–8	30–40
Epidural and caudal	Chloroprocaine	2–3	0.25–0.5	15–20
	Lidocaine	1–2	0.5–1.0	15–20
	Mepivacaine	1–2	0.75–1.0	15–20
	Bupivacaine	0.25–0.75	1.5–3.0	20–30
	Etidocaine	0.5–1.5	1.5–3.0	20–30
	Ropivacaine	0.5–1.0	2–5	15–30
Local infiltration	Procaine	0.5–1.0	0.25–0.5	1–60
	Lidocaine	0.5–1.0	0.5–2.0	1–50
	Mepivacaine	0.5–1.0	0.25–2.0	1–50
	Bupivacaine	0.25–0.5	2–4	1–45
	Ropivacaine	0.5	2–6	1–40
Spinal	Lidocaine (hyperbaric)	1.5–2.0	1–1.5	2–3
	Bupivacaine (hyperbaric)	0.75	2–4	2–3
	Bupivacaine (isobaric)	0.5	2–4	2–4
	Tetracaine (hyperbaric)	0.5–1.0	2–4	1–2
	Tetracaine (isobaric)	0.5–1.0	3–5	1–2
	Tetracaine (hypobaric)	0.1	3–5	3–6

[a] Adding epinephrine to local anesthetic solution prolongs the analgesia duration of lidocaine, mepivacaine, and tetracaine. However, the analgesia duration of bupivacaine and ropivacaine is not significantly affected by epinephrine, partly because of the vasoconstriction produced by these agents.

2. **Adding epinephrine** (1:200,000 solution) to plain solutions of local anesthetics just before administration permits the use of a solution with a high pH, which speeds onset of the block. A 1:200,000 dilution is achieved by adding 0.1 mL of 1:1,000 epinephrine (with a tuberculin syringe) to 20 mL of local anesthetic solution.

3. The **maximum dose of epinephrine** probably should not exceed 10 μg/kg in pediatric patients and 200 to 250 μg in adults.

4. Epinephrine should not be used in peripheral nerve blocks in areas with poor collateral blood flow (e.g., digits, penis, toes) or in intravenous regional techniques. Caution is advised in

patients with severe coronary artery disease, arrhythmias, uncontrolled hypertension, hyperthyroidism, and uteroplacental insufficiency.

C. Phenylephrine has been used like epinephrine, but no particular advantages have been demonstrated; 1 to 2 mg of phenylephrine can be added to solutions of local anesthetics to prolong spinal anesthesia.

D. Opioids such as fentanyl and hydromorphone have been used together with local anesthetics in spinal/epidural anesthesia with improved analgesia.

E. Sodium bicarbonate added to local anesthetic solutions raises the pH and increases the concentration of nonionized free base. The increased percentage of uncharged drug will increase the rate of diffusion and speed the onset of neural blockade. Typically, 1 mEq of sodium bicarbonate is added to each 10 mL of lidocaine or mepivacaine; only 0.1 mEq of sodium bicarbonate may be added to each 10 mL of bupivacaine to avoid precipitation. Carbonated local anesthetics (e.g., lidocaine carbonate) are thought to augment neural block by lowering intraneural pH and promoting formation of the active (charged) species.

F. Meperidine has local anesthetic properties, and it has been used as the sole anesthetic agent in spinal anesthesia for cesarean section. There is no proven advantage to using the drug this way.

III. Toxicity

A. Allergic reactions. True allergic reactions to local anesthetics are uncommon. It is important to differentiate them from common nonallergic responses such as vasovagal episodes and responses to intravascular injection of local anesthetic and/or epinephrine.

1. **Ester-type local anesthetics** may cause allergic reactions from the metabolite p-aminobenzoic acid. These anesthetics also may produce allergic reactions in persons sensitive to sulfa drugs (e.g., sulfonamides or thiazide diuretics).

2. **Amide-type local anesthetics** are essentially devoid of allergic potential. Multidose vials of anesthetic solutions containing **methylparaben** as the preservative may produce an allergic reaction in patients sensitive to p-aminobenzoic acid.

3. **Local hypersensitivity reactions** may produce local erythema, urticaria, edema, or dermatitis.

4. **Systemic hypersensitivity reactions** are rare and can present with generalized erythema, urticaria, edema, bronchoconstriction, hypotension, and cardiovascular collapse.

5. **Treatment** is supportive (see Chapter 18).

B. Local toxicity

1. **Tissue toxicity** is rare.

2. **Transient radicular irritation (TRI) or transient neurologic symptoms (TNS)** may occur after subarachnoid injection of local anesthetics. These are usually manifested as pain or dysesthesia in the buttocks or legs. The primary risk factors for the development of TRI/TNS are lidocaine spinals in ambulatory patients undergoing procedures in the lithotomy position or knee arthroscopy. Bupivacaine is associated with virtually no incidence of TRI/TNS. **When a patient complains of signs of TRI/TNS,** treatment may begin once other possible etiologies (hematoma, abscess) have been eliminated. Nonsteroidal antiflammatory drugs, opioids, transcutaneous electrical nerve

stimulation (TENS), physical therapy, and trigger point injections may relieve symptoms.

3. Reports of sensory and motor deficits after intrathecal chloroprocaine solutions containing the antioxidant sodium bisulfite resulted in a change in its formulation. EDTA has replaced bisulfite. Nevertheless, intense back pain has been reported after administration of large volumes of solution. The back pain is thought to be caused by spasms of the paraspinal muscles due to the calcium binding properties of EDTA.

C. Systemic toxicity usually results from intravascular injection or overdose.

1. Intravascular injection most commonly occurs during nerve blockade in areas with large blood vessels (e.g., axillary or vertebral artery and epidural vein). This can be minimized by the following:

a. Aspiration before injection.

b. Use of epinephrine-containing solutions for test doses.

c. Use of small incremental volumes in establishing the block.

d. Use of proper technique during intravenous regional anesthesia (see Chapter 17).

2. Central nervous system (CNS) toxicity

a. Clinical features of CNS toxicity include metallic taste, light-headedness, tinnitus, visual disturbances, and numbness of the tongue and lips. These may progress to muscle twitching, loss of consciousness, grand mal seizures, and coma.

b. CNS toxicity is exacerbated by hypercarbia, hypoxia, and acidosis.

c. Treatment. At the first sign of toxicity, injection of local anesthetic should be discontinued and oxygen administered. If seizure activity interferes with ventilation or is prolonged, anticonvulsant treatment is indicated with midazolam (1 to 2 mg) or thiopental (50 to 200 mg in the adult). Succinylcholine can be given to facilitate intubation.

3. Cardiovascular toxicity. The cardiovascular system is more resistant than the CNS to toxic effects, but cardiovascular toxicity may be severe and difficult to treat.

a. Clinical features. Cardiovascular toxicity produces decreased ventricular contractility, refractory cardiac arrhythmias, and loss of peripheral vasomotor tone, which may lead to cardiovascular collapse. Cocaine is the only local anesthetic that causes vasoconstriction at all doses.

b. The **intravascular injection of bupivacaine or etidocaine** may produce cardiovascular collapse, which is often refractory to therapy because of the high degree of tissue binding by these agents. Hypercarbia, acidosis, and hypoxia enhance the negative inotropic and chronotropic effects of these drugs. Ropivacaine, similar to bupivacaine in potency and duration of action, has less cardiac toxicity because it dissociates more rapidly from sodium channels.

c. Treatment

(1) Oxygen must be administered and circulation supported with volume replacement and vasopressors, including intoropes, as necessary. Advanced cardiac life support may be necessary (see Chapter 37).

(2) **Ventricular tachycardia** should be treated by electrical cardioversion. Local anesthetic-induced cardiac arrhythmias are difficult to treat but usually subside over time if the patient's hemodynamics can be maintained.

(3) **Amiodarone** may be more effective than lidocaine for ventricular arrhythmias associated with intravascular injections of bupivacaine, and large doses of epinephrine may be necessary for successful resuscitation.

(4) **Prolonged cardiopulmonary resuscitation** may be required until the cardiotoxic effects subside with drug redistribution.

D. **Other adverse effects** include **Horner syndrome,** which can result from blockade of B fibers in the T1–4 nerve roots, and **methemoglobinemia,** which can follow administration of benzocaine and large amounts of EMLA cream. Methylene blue (1 to 2 mg/kg over 5 minutes) can be administered intravenously to convert methemoglobin to reduced hemoglobin.

SUGGESTED READING

Berde CB, Strichartz GR. Local anesthetics. In: Miller RE, ed. *Anesthesia*, 5th ed. New York: Churchill Livingstone, 2000:491–522.

Cousins MJ, Bridenbaugh PO. *Neural blockade in clinical anesthesia and management of pain*, 3rd ed. Philadelphia: Lippincott-Raven, 1998.

Kindler CH, Yost CS. Two-pore domain potassium channels: new site of local anesthetic action and toxicity. *Reg Anesth Pain Med* 2005;30(3):260–274.

Milliigan KR. Recent advances in local anesthetics for spinal anaesthesia. *Eur J Anaesthesiol* 2004;21(11):837–847.

Reiz S, Nath S. Cardiotoxicity of local anaesthetic agents. *Br J Anaesth* 1986;58:736–746.

Weinberg L. Current concepts in resuscitation of patients with local anesthetic cardiac toxicity. *Reg Anesth Pain Med* 2002;27(6):568–575.

Spinal, Epidural, and Caudal Anesthesia

Takefumi Nishida and May Pian-Smith

I. **General considerations**
   A. **Preoperative assessment** of the patient for regional anesthesia is similar to that for general anesthesia. The details of the procedure to be performed, including its anticipated length, patient position, and a complete review of any coexisting diseases, should be taken into account in determining the appropriateness of a regional technique.
   B. **The area where the block is to be administered should be examined** for potential difficulties or pathology. Pre-existing neurological abnormalities should be well documented and the presence of kyphoscoliosis determined.
   C. **A history of abnormal bleeding** and a review of the patient's medications may indicate a need for additional coagulation studies.
   D. Patients should be given a **detailed explanation** of the planned procedure, with risks and benefits. They should be reassured that additional sedation and anesthesia can be given during the operation and that general anesthesia is an option if the block fails or the operation becomes more prolonged or extensive than originally thought. In some instances, it is planned from the onset to have a combination of regional and general anesthesia.
   E. As with general anesthesia, patients should receive appropriate monitoring (see Chapter 10) and have an intravenous (IV) line in place. Oxygen, equipment for intubation and positive-pressure ventilation, and drugs to provide hemodynamic support should be available.

II. **Segmental level required for surgery**
   A. A knowledge of the sensory, motor, and autonomic distribution of spinal nerves will help the anesthetist determine the correct segmental level required for a particular operation and anticipate the potential physiologic effects of producing a block to that level. Figure 16.1 illustrates the dermatomal distribution of the spinal nerves.
   B. **Afferent autonomic nerves** innervate visceral sensation and viscerosomatic reflexes at spinal segmental levels much higher than would be predicted from skin dermatomes.
   C. **Minimal suggested levels** for common surgical procedures are listed in Table 16.1.

III. **Contraindications to neuraxial anesthesia**
   A. **Absolute**
      1. Patient refusal.
      2. Localized infection at skin puncture site.
      3. Generalized sepsis (e.g., septicemia, bacteremia).

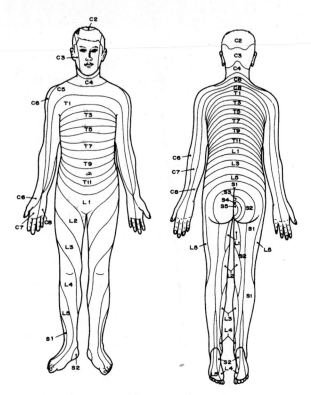

Figure 16.1.   Skin dermatomes corresponding to respective sensory innervation by spinal nerves.

Table 16.1.   Suggested minimum cutaneous levels for spinal anesthesia

Operative Site	Level
Lower extremities	T-12
Hip	T-10
Vagina, uterus	T-10
Bladder, prostate	T-10
Lower extremities with tourniquet	T-8
Testis, ovaries	T-8
Lower intraabdominal	T-6
Other intraabdominal	T-4

      4. Coagulopathy

      5. Increased intracranial pressure.

  B. Relative

      1. Localized infection peripheral to regional technique site.

      2. Hypovolemia.

      3. Central nervous system disease.

      4. Chronic back pain.

IV. Spinal anesthesia involves administering local anesthetic into the subarachnoid space.

  A. Anatomy

      1. The **spinal canal** extends from the foramen magnum to the sacral hiatus. The boundaries of the bony canal are the vertebral body anteriorly, the pedicles laterally, and the spinous processes and laminae posteriorly (Fig. 16.2).

      2. Three **interlaminar ligaments** bind the vertebral processes together:

        a. Superficially, the **supraspinous ligament** connects the apices of the spinous processes.

        b. The **interspinous ligament** connects the spinous processes on their horizontal surface.

        c. The **ligamentum flavum** connects the caudal edge of the vertebrae above to the cephalad edge of the lamina below. This ligament is composed of elastic fibers and is usually recognized by its increased resistance to passage of a needle.

      3. The **spinal cord** extends the length of the vertebral canal during fetal life, ends at about L-3 at birth, and moves progressively cephalad to reach the adult position near L-1 by

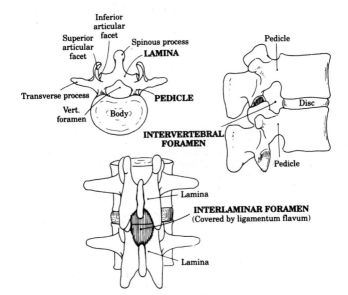

Figure 16.2.   Vertebral anatomy.

2 years of age. The conus medullaris, lumbar, sacral, and coccygeal nerve roots branch out distally to form the cauda equina. Spinal needles are placed in this area of the canal (below L-2), because the mobility of the nerves reduces the danger of trauma from the needle.

4. The spinal cord is invested in three **meninges**:
   a. The **pia mater**.
   b. The **dura mater**, which is a tough fibrous sheath running longitudinally the length of the spinal cord and is tethered caudally at S-2.
   c. The **arachnoid**, which lies between the pia and dura mater.

5. The **subarachnoid space** lies between the pia mater and the arachnoid and extends from the attachment of the dura at S-2 to the cerebral ventricles above. The space contains the spinal cord, nerves, cerebrospinal fluid (CSF), and blood vessels that supply the cord.

6. **CSF** is a clear colorless fluid that fills the subarachnoid space. The total volume of CSF is 100 to 150 mL, whereas the volume in the spinal subarachnoid space is 25 to 35 mL. CSF is continuously formed at a rate of 450 mL/day by secretion or ultrafiltration of plasma from the choroid arterial plexuses located in the lateral, third, and fourth ventricles. CSF is reabsorbed into the bloodstream through the arachnoid villi and granulations that protrude through dura to lie in contact with the endothelium of the cerebral venous sinuses.

B. **Physiological changes.**
   1. **Neural blockade.** Smaller C fibers conveying autonomic impulses are more easily blocked than the larger sensory and motor fibers. As a result, the level of autonomic blockade extends above the level of the sensory blockade by two to three segments. This phenomenon is termed differential blockade. Similarly, fibers conveying sensation are more easily blocked than the larger motor fibers so that sensory blockade will extend above the level of motor blockade.

   2. **Cardiovascular. Hypotension** is directly proportional to the degree of **sympathetic blockade** produced. Sympathetic blockade results in dilatation of arteries and venous capacitance vessels, leading to decreased systemic vascular resistance and decreased venous return. If the block is below T-4, increased baroreceptor activity produces an increase in activity to the cardiac sympathetic fibers and vasoconstriction of the upper extremities. Blockade above T-4 interrupts cardiac sympathetic fibers, leading to bradycardia, decreased cardiac output, and a further decrease in blood pressure. These changes are more marked in patients who are hypovolemic, are elderly, or have obstruction to venous return (e.g., pregnancy). Risk factors for bradycardia after spinal anesthesia include baseline bradycardia, American Society of Anesthesiologists status 1, use of beta blockers, age less than 50, and sensory level above T-6.

   3. **Respiratory.** Low spinal anesthesia has no effect on ventilation. With ascending height of the block into the thoracic area, there is progressive ascending intercostal muscle paralysis. This has little effect on ventilation in the supine

surgical patient who still has diaphragmatic function mediated by the phrenic nerve. Ventilation in patients with poor respiratory reserve, such as the morbidly obese, however, may be profoundly impaired. Paralysis of both intercostal and abdominal muscles decreases the efficiency of coughing, which may be important in patients with chronic obstructive pulmonary disease. Usually a spinal level of T-4 does not result in impaired ventilation, but respiratory compromise may happen in patients with limited respiratory reserve or higher spinal levels.

4. **Visceral effects**

   a. **Bladder.** Physiological changes: Sacral blockade (S-2 to S-4) results in an atonic bladder that can retain large volumes of urine. Blockade of sympathetic efferents (T-5 to L-1) results in an increase in sphincter tone, producing retention.

   b. **Intestine.** Sympathetic blockade (T-5 to L-1) produced by spinal anesthesia leads to contraction of the small and large intestine because of a predominance of parasympathetic tone.

5. **Neuroendocrine.** Peridural block to T-5 inhibits part of the neural component of the stress response through its blockade of sympathetic afferents to the adrenal medulla and blockade of sympathetic and somatic pathways mediating pain. Other components of the stress response and central release of humoral factors are unaffected. Vagal afferent fibers from the upper abdominal viscera are not blocked and can stimulate release of hypothalamic and pituitary hormones, such as antidiuretic hormone and adrenocorticotropic hormone. Glucose tolerance and insulin release are normal.

6. **Thermoregulation.** Hypothermia may occur due to several mechanisms. Redistribution of the central heat to the periphery occurs. Core temperature may drop even though surface temperature is preserved. Thermoregulation is lost during spinal anesthesia. Patients may feel warm despite a decrease in their temperatures. Shivering is often seen. There is loss of the vasoconstriction protective mechanism to preserve heat below the level of sympathectomy. If severe hypothermia occurs, patients should be warmed with hot blankets or other warming devices.

7. **Central nervous system effects.** Spinal anesthesia may have direct effects to suppress the consciousness, probably secondary to decreased afferent stimulation of the reticular activating system. During spinal or epidural anesthesia, requirements of sedative agents may be decreased.

C. **Technique**

1. **Spinal needle.** Newer needles such as the **Sprotte** and **Whitacre** feature a pencil-point design with a lateral opening. These needles may reduce the incidence of postdural puncture headache (to <1%) compared with traditional "cutting tip" needles by splitting rather than cutting dural fibers during insertion. Needles that are 24 and 25 gauge are easily bent and are often inserted through a 19-gauge introducer needle. The 22-gauge **Quincke** needle is more rigid and is more easily directed and inserted. It can be useful in older patients

in whom access may be more difficult and the incidence of postdural puncture headache is low.

2. **Patient position.** The lateral decubitus, prone, and sitting positions can be used for administration of spinal anesthesia

   a. In the **lateral position,** the patient is placed with the affected side up if a hypobaric or isobaric technique is to be used and with the affected side down if a hyperbaric technique is to be used. The spine is horizontal and parallel to the edge of the table. The knees are drawn up toward the chest and the chin is flexed downward onto the chest to obtain maximal flexion of the spine.

   b. The **sitting position** is useful for low spinal blocks required in certain gynecologic and urologic procedures and is commonly used in obese patients to assist in identification of the midline. It is used in conjunction with hyperbaric anesthetics. The head and shoulders are flexed downward onto the trunk with the arms resting on a Mayo stand. An assistant should be available to stabilize the patient, and the patient should not be oversedated.

   c. The **prone position** is used in conjunction with hypobaric or isobaric anesthetics for procedures on the rectum, perineum, and anus. A prone jackknife position can be used for administration of spinal anesthesia and the subsequent surgery.

3. **Procedure**

   a. The L2-3, L3-4, or L4-5 interspaces are commonly used for spinal anesthesia. The L-3 to L-4 interspace or the spinous process of L-4 is aligned with the upper borders of the superior iliac crests.

   b. Disinfect a large area of skin with an appropriate antiseptic solution. Care must be taken to avoid contamination of the spinal kit with antiseptic solution, which is potentially neurotoxic.

   c. Check the stylet for correct fit within the needle.

   d. Raise a skin wheal with 1% lidocaine and a 25-gauge needle at the spinal puncture site.

   e. **Approaches**

      (1) **Midline.** Place the spinal needle (or introducer) through the skin wheal and into the interspinous ligament. The needle should be in the same plane as the spinous processes and angulated slightly cephalad toward the interlaminar space (Fig. 16.3).

      (2) **Paramedian.** This approach is useful in patients who cannot adequately flex their back because of pain or whose interspinous ligaments may be ossified. Place the spinal needle 1.5 cm lateral and slightly caudad (~1 cm) to the center of the selected interspace. Aim the needle medially and slightly cephalad, passing lateral to the supraspinous ligament. If the lamina is contacted, redirect the needle and walk the tip off the lamina in a medial and cephalad direction.

      (3) **Needle placement.** Always keep the stylet in place when advancing the needle so that the needle's

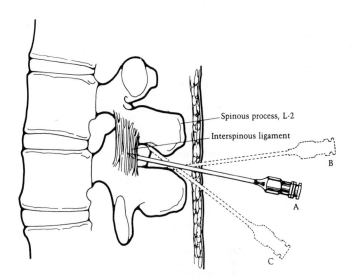

Figure 16.3. Spinal needle insertion, lateral view. For the classic midline approach, the needle is introduced in the middle of the interspace and advanced with a slight cephalad angulation. If correctly angled (A), it will enter the interspinous ligament, ligamentum flavum, and epidural space. If bone is contacted, it may be the inferior spinous process (B), and cephalad redirection will identify the correct path. If angling cephalad causes contact with bone again at a shallower depth (C), it is probably the superior spinous process. If bone is encountered at the same depth after several attempts at redirection (not shown), the needle is most likely on the lamina lateral to the interspace, and the position of the true midline should be reassessed. (From Mulroy MF. *Regional anesthesia: an illustrated procedural guide*, 2nd ed. Boston: Little, Brown and Company, 1996:79, with permission.)

lumen does not become plugged with tissue. If paresthesias occur during placement, immediately withdraw the needle. Allow the paresthesia to pass and reposition the needle before proceeding again. Advance the needle until increased resistance is felt as it passes through the ligamentum flavum. As the needle is advanced beyond this ligament, a sudden loss of resistance will occur as the needle "pops" through the dura.

(4) Remove the stylet and confirm correct placement by noting free flow of CSF into the hub of the needle. Rotate the needle in 90° increments if necessary to confirm or reestablish good flow of CSF.

(5) **Administration of anesthetic:** Connect the syringe containing the predetermined dose of local anesthetic to the needle. Gently aspirate CSF into the syringe, which produces birefringence within dextrose-containing solutions and confirms free

flow. Inject the drug slowly. Repeat aspiration of CSF at the end of the injection confirms that the needle point is still within the subarachnoid space. Remove the needle and place the patient gently into the desired position.

f. **Closely monitor** (every 60 to 90 seconds) blood pressure, pulse, and respiratory function for 10 to 15 min. Determine the ascending anesthetic level by noting the response to a gentle pinprick or an alcohol swab. Stabilization of the local anesthetic level takes approximately 20 min.

g. **Continuous spinal anesthesia** allows small aliquots of drug to be injected repeatedly to produce the desired level of sensory blockade. With this technique, a high or rapid sympathetic block can be avoided (of particular concern in the compromised patient). The duration of anesthesia can be extended for longer surgical procedures by repeated administration of drug through a spinal needle. [This technique is frequently used in orthopedics by administering a dose of the drug through the spinal needle, waiting several minutes, and then adding additional drug. It has been described as a "layering technique." A spinal catheter can also be used for longer cases. A 20-gauge catheter is inserted through a 17-gauge epidural needle. The catheter is advanced 2 to 4 cm into the subarachnoid space. Stimulation of nerve roots during catheter insertion necessitates repositioning of the catheter. **Neurotoxicity** from hyperbaric glucose-containing local anesthetic solutions injected through microbore spinal catheters (26 to 32 gauge) has been reported and may be due to the development of very high concentrations of local anesthetic around the nerves of the cauda equina. The use of such small-bore catheters is not recommended.

D. **Determinants of level of spinal blockade** (Table 16.2)

1. **CSF volume.** Clinical correlation between lumbosacral CSF volume and spinal anesthesia with hyperbaric lidocaine and isobaric bupivacaine is excellent. There are no good predictors of lumbosacral CSF volume, but weight has some correlations.

2. **Drug dose.** The anesthetic level varies directly with the dose of the agent used.

3. **Drug volume.** The greater the volume of the injected drug, the further the drug will spread within the CSF. This is especially applicable to hyperbaric solutions.

4. **Turbulence of CSF.** Turbulence created within the CSF during or after injection will increase spread of the drug and the level obtained. Turbulence is created by rapid injection, barbotage (the repeated aspiration and reinjection of small amounts of CSF mixed with drug), coughing, and excessive patient movement.

5. **Baricity of local anesthetic solution.** Local anesthetic solutions can be described as hyperbaric, hypobaric, or isobaric in relation to the specific gravity of CSF (1.004 to 1.007 g/mL).

Table 16.2. Factors affecting subarachnoid local anesthetic injections

Determinants of spread
   Major factors
      Baricity of solution
      Position of patients (except isobaric solution)
      Dose and volume of drug injected (except isobaric)
   Minor factors
      Level of injection
      Speed of injection/barbotage
      Size of needle
      Physical status of patients
      Intra-abdominal pressure
Determinants of duration
   Drug used
   Dose injected
   Presence of vasoconstrictors
   Total spread of blockade

Adapted from Wildsmith JAW, Rocco AG. Current concepts in spinal anesthesia. *Reg Anesth* 1985;10:119, with permission.

     a. Hyperbaric solutions are typically prepared by mixing the drug with dextrose. They flow by gravity to the most dependent parts of the CSF column (Table 16.3).

     b. Hypobaric solutions are prepared by mixing the drug with sterile water. They slowly rise to the highest part of the CSF column.

     c. Isobaric solutions may have the advantage of a predictable spread through the CSF that is less dependent on patient position. Increasing the dose of an isobaric anesthetic has more of an effect on the duration of anesthesia than on the dermatomal spread. Patient positioning can be altered to limit or increase the spread of these mixtures.

  6. Increased intra-abdominal pressure. Pregnancy, obesity, ascites, and abdominal tumors increase pressure within the inferior vena cava. This pressure increases blood volume within the epidural venous plexus, concomitantly reducing the

Table 16.3. Drugs and dosages for hyperbaric spinal anesthesia

Drug	Level (mg)[a]			Duration (min)
	T-10	T-8	T-6	
Tetracaine	10	12	14	90–120
Bupivacaine	7.5	9.0	10.5	90–120
Lidocaine	50	60	70	30–90

[a] Doses are based on a 66-inch patient. An additional 2 mg of tetracaine, 10 mg of lidocaine, or 1.5 mg of bupivacaine should be added or subtracted for each 6 inches in height above or below 66 inches.

volume of CSF within the vertebral column, which permits greater spread of injected local anesthetic. In obese patients, this effect is potentiated by increased fat within the epidural space.

7. **Spinal curvatures.** Lumbar lordosis and thoracic kyphosis influence the spread of hyperbaric solutions. Drug injected above the L-3 level while the patient is in the lateral position will spread cephalad and will be limited by the thoracic curvature at T-4 (Fig. 16.4).

E. **Determinants of duration of spinal blockade**

1. **Drugs and dose.** A characteristic duration is specific for each drug (see Chapter 15). The addition of opioids to the injected solution can modify the character of the block (see also Chapter 38). **Hydrophilic opioids** (e.g., morphine) offer analgesia that is slow in onset and long in duration. Delayed respiratory depression may occur. If hydrophilic opioids are given intrathecally, patients should be closely observed at least 24 hours. **Lipophilic opioids** (e.g., fentanyl) have less risk of delayed respiratory depression. Onset is fast and duration is moderate.

2. **Vasoconstrictors.** The addition of epinephrine, 0.2 mg (0.2 mL of 1:1,000), or phenylephrine, 2 to 5 mg, can prolong the duration of some spinal anesthetics by up to 50%. This effect has not been definitively demonstrated for bupivacaine, although there is evidence that epinephrine prolongs the analgesic effects of low-dose bupivacaine and fentanyl combinations used for labor analgesia.

F. **Complications**

1. **Neurologic.** Nerve injury is infrequent but can be a serious problem. Several types of nerve injury may occur.

   a. Direct nerve injury related to needle or catheter placement. Pain during insertion of the catheter or injection of the drug is a warning sign for potential nerve injury resulting from needle or catheter placement and requires repositioning of the needle or catheter. **Transient paresthesias,** which can occur during placement of neuraxial blocks, are often without any long-term sequelae.

   b. **Transient neurologic syndrome is a** spontaneous severe radicular pain that is evident after resolution of the spinal anesthetic and may last for 2 to 7 days. The incidence is highest with lidocaine administration but has also been observed with tetracaine, bupivacaine, and mepivacaine. Obesity, outpatient surgery, and lithotomy position are additional risk factors.

   c. Separately, there is an incidence of **back pain** following spinal anesthesia that may be related to the relaxation of the ligaments that occurs with the anesthesia. There is a similar incidence of back pain following general anesthesia, again likely related to the effects of anesthetic agents and muscle relaxants on the structures of the back.

   d. **Bloody tap.** Puncture of an epidural vein during needle insertion may result in either blood or a mixture of blood and CSF emerging from the spinal needle. If the fluid does not rapidly clear, the needle should be withdrawn and reinserted.

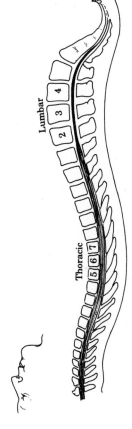

Figure 16.4. Spinal column curvatures that influence the spread of anesthetic solutions.

e. **Spinal hematoma.** Overall incidence is around 1/150,000. The signs and symptoms of severe back pain and persistent neurologic deficit usually present within 48 hours. Risk is higher among patients who are coagulopathic or anticoagulated. Bloody taps are not generally thought to cause a spinal hematoma in patients with normal coagulation. A bloody tap may be a risk factor for spinal hematoma in patients who undergo subsequent anticoagulation, but there are no data to support the mandatory cancelation of a case under these circumstances. Instead, we advocate direct communication with the surgeon and that a specific risk-benefit decision about proceeding be made on an individual basis. **Close postoperative monitoring** for signs consistent with hematoma is warranted. Diagnosis is usually made with magnetic resonance imaging (MRI), and treatment is via emergent hematoma evacuation. Because catheter removal as well as needle placement may cause spinal hematoma, anesthesiologists need to check a patient's coagulation status and use of anticoagulants not only at the time of needle placement but also at the time of catheter removal. The approach to the use of anticoagulants, antiplatelet agents, and nonsteroidal anti-inflammatory drugs at Massachusetts General Hospital is listed in Table 16.4.

f. **Postdural puncture headache** usually develops within 3 days; 70% of headaches resolve within 7 days, 90% within 6 months. The classic "spinal headache" is frontal and occipital in distribution; less frequently, the temporal area is affected. The headache is exacerbated by upright posture and relieved by lying down. Other manifestations include visual disturbances or hearing impairment. Younger age and female gender are risk factors. The incidence may be reduced by using smaller needles and noncutting needles (e.g., pencil-point needles). Initial treatments of symptoms include rehydration, maintenance of supine position, pain medication including opioids, and caffeine. Maintenance of supine position as a prevention is neither proven nor recommended. Caffeine exerts its effect by vasoconstriction of cerebral vessels. The recommended dose of caffeine is 300 to 500 mg orally or IV. One cup of coffee contains 50 to 100 mg of caffeine. If initial therapy fails and severe symptoms persist more than 24 hours, an **epidural blood patch** can be done. Epidural needle insertion is done at the level of presumed dural puncture. Blood is drawn in a sterile fashion and injected into the epidural space. The typical blood volume is 20 to 30 mL, or less if the patient complains of back discomfort during injection. The success rate ranges from 65% to 98%. A second blood patch can be tried with a success rate about the same as the first attempt. The use of a prophylactic epidural blood patch before onset of headache symptoms is of doubtful benefit and not recommended.

Table 16.4. Anticoagulation and epidural anesthesia/analgesia guidelines

Drug (generic)	Common Tradenames	Time Interval for Placement of Catheter after Last Dose	Time Interval for Removal of Catheter after Postop Dose	Time Interval to Restart Med after Catheter Is Removed
Abciximab	Reopro	48 hours	48 hours	12 hours
Argatroban		There are no specific recommendations at the present time. Would recommend waiting at least 6 hours to place or manipulate an epidural catheter in a patient who has been given argatroban (may use in operating room like IV heparin).		
Cilostazol[a]	Pletal[a]	48 hours	48 hours	1 hour
Clopidogrel[b]	Plavix	7 days	Within 24 hours	24 hours
Eptifibatide	Integrilin	8 hours	8 hours	4 hours
Fondaparinux[c]	Arixtra	4 days	4 days	2 hours
Heparin subcutaneously	Heparin	No significant risk		
Heparin IV	Heparin	2–4 hours, PTT <35	2–4 hours, PTT <35	1 hour
Dalteparin[d]	Fragmin (any dose)	24 hours	24 hours	2 hours
LMWH (low dose)	Lovenox (<60 mg qd)	12 hours	12 hours	2 hours
Enoxaparin[d]	Innohep			
Tinzaparin[d]				

continued

Table 16.4. (*Continued*)

Drug (generic)	Common Tradenames	Time Interval for Placement of Catheter after Last Dose	Time Interval for Removal of Catheter after Postop Dose	Time Interval to Restart Med after Catheter Is Removed
LMWH (high dose) Enoxaparin[d] Tinzaparin[d]	bid dosing = high-dose Lovenox Innohep	>24 hours	Catheter SHOULD be removed before first dose; if not, wait >24 hours	2 hours
NSAID, asa	Celebrex, Motrin, Naprosyn, Vioxx etc.	No significant risk		
Thrombolytics: streptokinase, alteplase (tpa)	Streptase activase	10 days	10 days	10 days
Ticlopidine	Ticlid	14 days	14 days	24 hours
Tirofiban	Aggrastat	8 hours	8 hours	4 hours
Warfarin	Coumadin	3–5 days, INR <1.3	Check INR if treatment >24 hours, INR <1.5	Same day

PTT, partial thromboplastin time; NSAID, nonsteroidal anti-inflammatory drug.

[a] If pletal is the only anticoagulant given, then an epidural catheter placement is most likely safe. If pletal is combined with other anticoagulant medicines, epidural catheter placement should be delayed for at least 48 hours.

[b] Clopidogrel (Plavix) has a 24- to 48-hour window to remove an epidural catheter once the medication is given. If it has been more than 48 hours since dosing of clopidogrel, you must wait 7 days.

[c] Fondaparinux should not be given if regional anesthesia is anticipated or has been used. If, however, fondaparinux is given, we suggest the above guidelines.

[d] Low-molecular-weight heparin: single daily dosing may be started 6 to 8 hours postoperatively. Twice daily dosing should be started at least 24 hours postoperatively. Epidural catheters should be removed before initiation of therapy.

2. **Cardiovascular**
   a. **Hypotension.** The incidence of hypotension may be reduced by IV administration of 500 to 1,000 mL of Ringer lactate solution before performing the block. Patients with decreased cardiac function require care in administering large volumes of IV fluid, because translocation of fluid from the peripheral to the central circulation during recession of the block and return of systemic vascular tone could produce volume overload and pulmonary edema. Treatment of hypotension includes increasing venous return and treating severe bradycardia. Trendelenberg position, fluid administration, or the use of vasopressors, such as ephedrine (5 to 10 mg IV bolus) or phenylephrine (40 to 100 μg IV bolus, 10 to 150 μg/min IV infusion) may be necessary. Oxygen should be available.
   b. **Bradycardia.** Bradycardia can be treated with atropine (0.4 to 0.8 mg IV) or glycopyrrolate (0.2 to 0.4 mg). If bradycardia is severe and accompanied by hypotension, ephedrine or epinephrine may be used.
3. **Respiratory**
   a. **Dyspnea** is a common complaint with high spinal levels. It is caused by proprioceptive blockade of afferent fibers from abdominal and chest wall muscles. Reassuring the patient may be all that is required, although adequate ventilation must be ensured.
   b. **Apnea** can be caused by reduced medullary blood flow accompanying severe hypotension or from direct blockade of C-3 to C-5 ("total spinal"), inhibiting phrenic nerve output. Immediate ventilatory support is required.
4. **Visceral**
   a. **Urinary retention.** The mechanism of urinary retention is described in section IV.B.4.a. Urinary retention may outlast the sensory and motor blockade. This effect may be problematic, particularly if the patient has pre-existing urinary obstructive symptoms or if large volumes of IV fluids have been administered during surgery. A urinary catheter should be placed if anesthesia or analgesia is maintained for a prolonged period.
   b. **Nausea and vomiting** are usually caused by hypotension or unopposed vagal stimulation. Treatment involves restoring blood pressure, administering oxygen, and IV atropine.
5. **Infection** after spinal anesthesia is exceedingly rare. Nevertheless, meningitis, arachnoiditis, and epidural abscess can occur. Possible etiologies include chemical contamination and viral or bacterial infection. Consultation and prompt diagnosis and treatment are essential.

V. **Epidural anesthesia** is achieved by introducing local anesthetics into the epidural space.
   A. **Anatomy.** The epidural space extends from the base of the skull to the sacrococcygeal membrane. Posteriorly, it is bounded by the ligamentum flavum, the anterior surfaces of the laminae, and the articular processes. Anteriorly, it is bounded by the posterior longitudinal ligament covering the vertebral bodies and

intervertebral discs. Laterally, it is bounded by intervertebral foramina and the pedicles. It has direct communications with the paravertebral space. It contains fat and lymphatic tissue as well as epidural veins, which are most prominent in the lateral aspects of the space. The veins have no valves and directly communicate with the intracranial veins. The veins also communicate with the thoracic and abdominal veins through the intervertebral foramina and with the pelvic veins through the sacral venous plexus. The epidural space is widest in the midline and tapers off laterally. In the lumbar region, it is 5 to 6 mm wide in the midline; in the midthoracic region, the space is 3 to 5 mm wide.

B. **Physiology**

1. **Neural blockade.** Local anesthetic placed in the epidural space acts directly on the spinal nerve roots located in the lateral part of the space. These nerve roots are covered by the dural sheath, and local anesthetic gains access to the CSF by uptake through the dura. The onset of the block is slower than with spinal anesthesia, and the intensity of the sensory and motor block is less. Anesthesia develops in a segmental manner, and selective blockade can be achieved.

2. **Cardiovascular.** Physiological changes from sympathetic blockade are similar to those described for spinal anesthesia (see section IV.B.2), but usually hemodynamic change is slower. Large doses of local anesthetic may be absorbed or inadvertently injected into the systemic circulation and depress the myocardium. Epinephrine used to prolong the duration of the local anesthetics may also be absorbed or injected into the systemic circulation, producing tachycardia and hypertension.

3. **Respiratory.** Physiological changes are similar to those described for spinal anesthesia. When we use postoperative epidural analgesia with dilute local anesthetics after major abdominal, upper abdominal, or thoracic surgery, the reduction in functional residual capacity and impairment of diaphragm function are minimized, which improves overall pulmonary outcome. With epidural anesthesia, the incidence of postoperative hypoxemia can be decreased by reducing the dose and effects of systemic opioids.

4. **Coagulation.** Epidural anesthesia has been reported to reduce venous thrombosis and subsequent pulmonary embolism. Proposed mechanisms include increased pelvic blood flow, decreased sympathetic response to surgery, and earlier mobility. Epidural anesthesia may reduce intraoperative blood loss during hip, pelvic, and lower abdominal surgery.

5. **Gastrointestinal.** Epidural anesthesia can be administered for patients undergoing bowel resection with anastomosis. As with spinal anesthesia, the predominance of the parasympathetic system may cause contraction of the bowel. Early return of bowel function with use of epidural anesthesia and analgesia may be due to lower systemic narcotic levels.

6. Other physiologic changes seen are similar to those described for spinal anesthesia (see section IV.B).

C. **Technique**

1. **Epidural needles.** Most commonly, the 17-gauge **Tuohy** or **Weiss** needle is used for identification of the epidural space.

These needles are styleted, have a blunt leading edge with a lateral opening, and have a thin wall to allow passage of a 20-gauge catheter.

2. **Patient position.** Patients can be positioned for epidural anesthesia in either the sitting or the lateral position. The same considerations apply as for spinal anesthesia (see section IV.C.2).

3. **Approaches.** Whether from a midline or paramedian approach, the needle should enter the epidural space in the midline, because the space is widest here and there is a decreased risk of puncturing epidural veins, spinal arteries, or spinal nerve roots, all of which lie predominantly in the lateral aspects of the epidural space. Palpation of landmarks, skin preparation, and draping are as described for spinal anesthesia (see section IV.C.3) (Fig. 16.5).

   a. **Lumbar.** Use a long 25-gauge needle for superficial and deep infiltration of local anesthetic into the supraspinous and interspinous ligaments. This needle also assists in defining the direction in which the epidural needle should be inserted. A skin puncture can be made with a 15-gauge needle to facilitate epidural needle passage. Advance the epidural needle through the supraspinous and interspinous ligaments in a slightly cephalad direction,

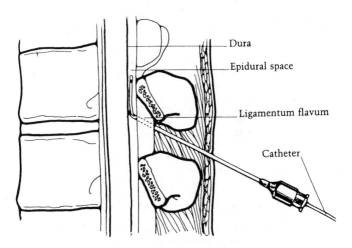

Figure 16.5. Insertion of an epidural catheter. The needle is secured by resting one hand on the back and grasping the hub firmly (not shown) while the other hand inserts the catheter into the hub and gently advances it beyond the tip of the needle. The bevel is usually directed cephalad, which produces the most reliable insertion; caudad orientation may allow the catheter to exit one of the intervertebral foramina. Ideally, the catheter is advanced 3 to 4 cm beyond the needle tip; further placement increases the potential for lateral misdirection or foraminal exit. (From Mulroy MF. *Regional anesthesia: an illustrated procedural guide*. Boston: Little, Brown and Company, 1996:109, with permission.)

until it comes to lie within the "rubbery" ligamentum flavum.

- **(1) Loss of resistance techniques.** Remove the stylet and attach a glass or plastic loss-of-resistance syringe containing approximately 3 mL of air or saline to the needle hub. Apply constant pressure to the plunger of the syringe while slowly advancing the needle. When the bevel enters the epidural space, there is a marked "loss of resistance" to plunger displacement. Alternatively, an "intermittent" technique can be used, where the change in resistance is tested repeatedly in between small careful advances of the epidural needle. When air is used for loss of resistance, the amount of air injection should be minimized. Patchy block, pneumocephalus, and air embolism have been reported with loss of resistance with the air technique.

- **(2)** The **hanging drop technique** relies on the principle that a drop of fluid placed on the hub of the epidural needle (once the ligamentum flavum has been entered) will retract into the needle as the tip of the needle is advanced into the epidural space. This negative pressure is provided by "tenting" of the dura by the needle tip but may be altered by transmitted changes in intra-abdominal and intrathoracic pressure (e.g., pregnancy, obesity). Drop retraction occurs only about 80% of the time, so if a change in compliance is felt while advancing through the ligamentum flavum, it should be checked by "loss of resistance."

b. Thoracic epidural anesthesia provides upper abdominal and thoracic anesthesia with a smaller dose of local anesthetic. Postoperative analgesia can be produced without lower extremity blockade. Although the technique is the same as for lumbar placement, the thoracic vertebral spinous processes are much more sharply angulated downward so that the tip of the superior spinous process overlies the lamina of the vertebra below, and the epidural needle should be directed in a more acute cephalad direction. In addition, there is a risk of producing trauma to the underlying spinal cord if dural puncture occurs. Occasionally, a paramedian approach is necessary.

c. Technique for catheter placement. An epidural catheter permits repeated injections of local anesthetic for prolonged procedures and provides a route for postoperative analgesia.

- **(1)** Thread a 20-gauge radiopaque catheter with 1-cm graduations through the epidural needle. If the catheter contains a wire stylet, the stylet should first be withdrawn 1 to 2 cm before insertion of the catheter to decrease the incidence of paresthesia and dural or venous puncture. Polyvinyl chloride catheters are relatively stiff and resist kinking but can be associated with dural and venous puncture. Teflon catheters are very soft and flexible but may be more likely to kink and occlude. Newer catheters of nylon, polyamide, and polyvinyl offer compromises between flexibility and rigidity. Wire-reinforced soft catheters do not kink and are much less prone to slipping out. When multipore catheters are used, the distance from the catheter tip to the most proximal lateral hole should be noted to ensure that all injected medication reaches the epidural space.

(2) Advance slowly the catheter ~5 cm into the epidural space. The patient may experience an abrupt paresthesia, which is usually transient. If it is sustained, the catheter must be repositioned. If the catheter must be withdrawn, the catheter and needle should be removed together to avoid shearing the catheter tip.

(3) Measure the distance from the surface of the patient's back to a mark on the catheter.

(4) Carefully withdraw the needle over the catheter and remeasure the distance from the patient's back to the mark on the catheter. If the catheter was advanced, withdraw it, leaving 4 to 5 cm within the epidural space.

d. Administer a **test dose** of local anesthetic agent through the needle if a single-dose technique is used or through the catheter for continuous techniques. A test dose usually consists of 3 mL of 2% lidocaine with 1:200,000 epinephrine. This should have little effect in the epidural space. If the solution has been injected into the CSF, a spinal block will occur rapidly. If the solution has been injected into an epidural vein, a 20% to 30% increase in heart rate may be seen. Other symptoms of an intravascular injection include perioral numbness, a metallic taste, tinnitus, and palpitations. A corresponding increase in blood pressure and heart rate usually can be seen.

e. **Injection of anesthetic.** Administer the anesthetic solution in 3- to 5-mL increments every 3 to 5 min until the total dose has been given. Aspirate the catheter or needle, checking for the appearance of blood or CSF, before each injection.

D. **Determinants of the level of epidural blockade**

1. **Volume of local anesthetic.** A maximum dose of 1.6 mL of local anesthetic per segment has been suggested for the induction of epidural blockade. This maximum can be exceeded if dilute mixtures of medications are used, as for postoperative or labor analgesia.

2. **Age.** The volume of local anesthetic should be reduced by approximately 50% in the elderly and in neonates. Stenosis of intervertebral foramina in the elderly reduces the lateral paravertebral spread of injected drug, allowing for more cephalad spread.

3. **Pregnancy.** A 30% reduction in dose is expected in pregnant women. Hormonal effects during pregnancy render nerves more sensitive to the effects of local anesthetic, and inferior vena cava compression increases blood volume within the epidural venous plexus, reducing the potential volume of the epidural space.

4. **Speed of injection.** Rapid injection of drug into the epidural space may produce a less reliable block than a slow steady injection at approximately 0.5 mL/second. Very rapid injection of large volumes of drug has the potentially hazardous effect of increasing pressure within the epidural space. Such a rise in pressure can produce headache, increased intracranial pressure, and possibly spinal cord ischemia by decreasing spinal cord blood flow.

5. **Position.** The position of the patient has a slight effect on the level of epidural blockade. Patients sitting upright have greater caudad spread of blockade; patients in the lateral position have a higher level of block on the dependent side.

6. **Spread of epidural blockade.** Onset of blockade occurs first and is most dense at the level of injection. Spread of the block usually occurs faster in a cephalad than in a caudad direction. This is likely because of the relative difference in size between the large lower lumbar and sacral nerve roots compared with the smaller thoracic nerve roots. There is often anesthetic sparing of the L-5 to S-1 nerve roots because of their large size.

E. **Determinants of onset and duration of epidural blockade**

1. **Selection of drug** (see Chapter 15).

2. **Addition of epinephrine.** Epinephrine, added at a concentration of 1:200,000, decreases the systemic uptake and plasma levels of local anesthetic and prolongs its duration of action (see Chapter 15).

3. **Addition of opioid.** The addition of fentanyl, 50 to 100 μg, to the local anesthetic solution speeds the onset, increases the level, prolongs the duration, and improves the quality of the block. Fentanyl is thought to produce this effect by having a selective action at the substantia gelatinosa of the dorsal horn of the spinal cord to modulate pain transmission. This action appears to be synergistic with the actions of the local anesthetics.

4. **pH adjustment of solution.** The addition of sodium bicarbonate to the local anesthetic solution in a ratio of 1 mL of 8.4% sodium bicarbonate to each 10 mL of lidocaine (0.1 mL for each 10 mL of bupivacaine) decreases the onset time for blockade. It is thought that this effect is due to an increased amount of local anesthetic base, which increases the rate at which nonionized drug crosses axonal membranes.

F. **Complications**

1. **Dural puncture** occurs in about 1% of epidural catheter placements. If dural puncture occurs during attempted epidural catheter insertion, the chance of postdural puncture headache is higher than with spinal anesthesia. Several management options are available. A conversion to spinal anesthesia can be made by injecting an appropriate amount of anesthetic into the CSF. Continuous spinal anesthesia can be performed by inserting an epidural catheter into the subarachnoid space through the epidural needle. If epidural anesthesia is required (e.g., for postoperative analgesia),

the catheter can be repositioned at a different interspace so that the tip of the epidural catheter lies well away from the site of dural puncture. The possibility of spinal anesthesia occurring with injection of the epidural catheter should be considered.

2. **Bloody tap.** If a bloody tap occurs during epidural needle placement, some practitioners advocate for epidural placement at a different interspace. Advantages include minimizing confounding effects of visualized blood on determination of correct catheter placement and potentially decreasing amounts of systemically absorbed local anesthetic that may be falsely interpreted as a positive "test dose." In patients with normal coagulation function, such bloody taps rarely lead to serious sequelae (e.g., epidural hematoma). Bloody epidural taps may be risk factors for epidural hematoma in patients who undergo subsequent anticoagulation, but there are no data to support the mandatory cancelation of a case under these circumstances. Instead, we advocate direct communication with the surgeon and that a specific risk-benefit decision about proceeding be made on an individual basis. Close postoperative monitoring for signs consistent with hematoma is warranted.

3. **Catheter complications**
   a. **Inability to thread the epidural catheter** is relatively common. This problem can occur if the epidural needle is inserted into the lateral aspect of the epidural space rather than the midline or if the bevel of the needle is at too acute an angle to the epidural space for the catheter to emerge. It can also occur if the bevel of the needle is only partially through the ligamentum flavum when loss of resistance is found. In the latter case, slight (1 mm) advancement of the needle into the epidural space may facilitate catheter insertion.
   b. **The catheter can be inserted into an epidural vein.** Blood cannot always be aspirated back through the catheter. This may be noticed only when an initial test dose with epinephrine is administered, and tachycardia is noted. The catheter should be withdrawn until blood can no longer be aspirated, flushed with saline, and then retested. Withdrawal of the catheter more than 1 to 2 cm should prompt removal and reinsertion.
   c. **Catheters can break off or become knotted** within the epidural space. In the absence of infection, a retained catheter is no more reactive than a surgical suture. The patient should be informed of the problem and reassured. The complications of surgical exploration and removal of an asymptomatic catheter are greater than conservative management.
   d. **Cannulation of the subdural space.** The subdural space is a potential space between the dural and arachnoid membranes and may be entered with a needle or with a catheter. CSF is not aspirated but the effects of the local anesthetic are quite different from usual epidural anesthesia and often quite variable. In the absence of myelography, it is a diagnosis of exclusion. It can result

in dissociation of blocked modalities (e.g., full sensory anesthesia without motor block or motor block with minimal sensory block). It should be suspected whenever an epidural dose produces a more extensive spread than expected. Subdural catheters should be removed and an epidural catheter should be placed.

4. **Unintentional subarachnoid injection.** The injection of a large volume of local anesthetic into the subarachnoid space can produce total spinal anesthesia. Treatment is similar to that described for spinal complications (see section IV.F).

5. **Intravascular injection** of local anesthetic into an epidural vein causes central nervous system and cardiovascular toxicity and may result in convulsions and cardiopulmonary arrest. Resistant ventricular fibrillation with IV bupivacaine 0.75% has been described. Cardiopulmonary bypass is an option if ventricular fibrillation or cardiac arrest is resistant to pharmacological therapy (see Chapters 15 and 37).

6. **Local anesthetic overdose.** Systemic local anesthetic toxicity may occur due to the relatively large amounts of drug required for anesthesia. Inadvertent intravascular injection is the most common cause of local anesthetic overdose. Vasoconstrictors such as epinephrine decrease the incidences of toxicity by decreasing the rate of absorption of the local anesthetic. Therapy is geared toward support of compromised functions.

7. **Direct spinal cord injury** is more likely if the epidural injection is above L-2. The onset of a unilateral paresthesia during needle insertion suggests lateral entry into the epidural space. Further injection or insertion of a catheter at this point may produce trauma to a nerve root. Small feeder arteries to the anterior spinal artery also run in this area as they pass through the intervertebral foramen. Trauma to these arteries potentially may result in anterior spinal cord ischemia or an epidural hematoma. Placement of epidural catheters after the induction of general anesthesia negates the ability to appreciate symptoms of paresthesia and is done only when such potential risk is deemed necessary. Pediatric patients frequently have catheters placed after induction of general anesthesia, often at the caudal level.

8. **Postdural puncture headache.** If the dura is punctured with a 17-gauge epidural needle, there is a greater than 75% chance of a young patient developing a postdural puncture headache. Management is the same as that described under spinal anesthesia (see section IV.F.1.f.).

9. **Epidural abscess** is an extremely rare complication of epidural anesthesia. The source of infection usually is from hematogenous spread to the epidural space from an infection in another area. Infection can also arise from contamination during insertion, contamination of an indwelling catheter used for postoperative pain relief, or a cutaneous infection at the insertion site. The patient presents with fever, severe back pain, and localized back tenderness. Progression to nerve root pain and paralysis can occur. Initial laboratory investigations include a leukocytosis and a lumbar puncture suggestive of

a parameningeal infection. Definitive diagnosis is by MRI. Treatment includes antibiotics and sometimes urgent decompression laminectomy. Rapid diagnosis and treatment are associated with good neurological recovery. Epidural catheter dressings should be inspected daily for signs of leakage and inflammation.

10. **Epidural hematoma** is an extremely rare complication of epidural anesthesia. Trauma to epidural veins in the presence of a coagulopathy may result in a large epidural hematoma. The patient can present severe back pain and persistent neurological deficit after epidural anesthesia. Diagnosis is confirmed by MRI. Decompression laminectomy is required to preserve neurological function.

VI. **Combined spinal-epidural anesthesia**
  A. Spinal anesthesia offers the benefits of rapid onset. Placement of an epidural catheter at the same time offers the advantage of prolonged anesthesia and analgesia for longer procedures or postoperative pain management. This technique often is used in the labor and delivery setting (see Chapter 30).
  B. **Technique.** Prepare the patient as for epidural placement (see section V.C). After placing the epidural needle in the epidural space, advance a long spinal needle (Sprotte 24-gauge × 120 mm or Whitacre 25 gauge) through the epidural needle until the characteristic pop of dural penetration occurs. At this point, withdraw the stylet from the spinal needle and confirm free flow of CSF. Inject medication into the subarachnoid space and withdraw the spinal needle. Thread an epidural catheter through the epidural needle in the standard fashion. If epidural anesthesia is used subsequently, a test dose is required.

VII. **Caudal anesthesia** is obtained by placing local anesthetic into the epidural space in the sacral region.
  A. **Anatomy.** The caudal space is an extension of the epidural space. The sacral hiatus is formed by the failure of the laminae of S-5 to fuse. The hiatus is bounded laterally by the sacral cornua, which are the inferior articulating processes of S-5. The **sacrococcygeal membrane** is a thin layer of fibrous tissue that covers the sacral hiatus. The caudal canal contains the sacral nerves, the sacral venous plexus, the filum terminale, and the dural sac, which usually ends at the lower border of S-2. In neonates, the dural sac may extend to S-4.
  B. **Physiology.** The physiology of caudal anesthesia is similar to that described for epidural anesthesia (see section V.B). It is indicated for surgical and obstetric procedures of the perineal and sacral areas.
  C. **Technique**
    1. Caudal epidural anesthesia is performed with the patient in the lateral, prone, or jackknife position.
    2. Palpate the sacral cornua. If they are difficult to palpate directly, the location of the sacral hiatus in adults can be estimated by measuring 5 cm from the tip of the coccyx in the midline.
    3. Skin preparation and draping are as described for spinal anesthesia (see section IV.C.3).
    4. Raise a skin wheal with 1% lidocaine between the sacral cornua.

5. Insert a 22-gauge spinal needle at an angle of 70° to 80° to the skin. Advance the needle advanced through the sacrococcygeal membrane, which is identified by a characteristic pop. Avoid attempting to thread the needle up the caudal canal, because this increases the likelihood of puncturing an epidural vein (Fig. 16.6).

6. Withdraw the stylet and inspect the hub of the needle for passive CSF or blood flow. The needle can be aspirated as a further check. Reposition the needle if either blood or CSF appears.

7. Administer a test dose of 3 mL of local anesthetic solution with epinephrine (1:200,000), similar to that used for lumbar epidural anesthesia (see section V.C.3.d), observing the patient for signs of subarachnoid or IV injection. Because the caudal canal has a rich epidural venous plexus, IV injections are seen frequently and can occur even though blood cannot be aspirated from the needle.

8. A caudal catheter can be placed in a manner analogous to that for lumbar epidural anesthesia with a 17-gauge Tuohy needle (see section V.C.3.a). The catheter can be used for postoperative analgesia.

9. The level, onset, and duration for caudal anesthesia follow the same principles outlined for epidural anesthesia (see sections V.D and V.E). The extent of caudal block is less predictable than other epidural techniques because of the variability in content and volume of the caudal canal and the amount of local anesthetic solution that leaks out of the sacral foramina. To obtain sacral anesthesia, a volume of 12 to 15 mL should be sufficient.

D. **Complications.** The complications of caudal anesthesia are similar to those of epidural anesthesia (see section V.F).

VIII. **Anticoagulation and neuraxial blockade.** Neuraxial blockade should be avoided in the presence of prophylactic or therapeutic anticoagulation because of the increased risk of epidural hematoma formation. Massachusetts General Hospital guidelines regarding neuraxial anesthesia in anticoagulated patients are listed in Table 16.4.

A. **Oral anticoagulants.** In patients receiving low-dose oral anticoagulants (warfarin), regional techniques may be performed if the thromboprophylaxis was initiated less than 24 hours previously. If epidural or spinal is planned, hold warfarin 3 to 5 days before the operation and the patient's international normalized ratio (INR) should be checked before the operation. An INR less than 1.3 is generally acceptable for many anesthesiologists, but there is no definite cutoff value above which epidurals or spinals are specifically discouraged.

B. **Unfractionated heparin.** Subcutaneous (minidose) heparin prophylaxis is not necessarily a contraindication for the use of neuraxial techniques. Caution should be used in debilitated patients, in whom the action of the drug may be prolonged and in whom neurological monitoring may be difficult. IV heparin should be stopped at least 4 hours before the initiation of neuraxial blockade, and a repeat coagulation profile should be checked if a patient's state of heparinization was excessive before the drug was discontinued. Administration of heparin should be delayed for at least 1 hour after placement. When patients with an indwelling

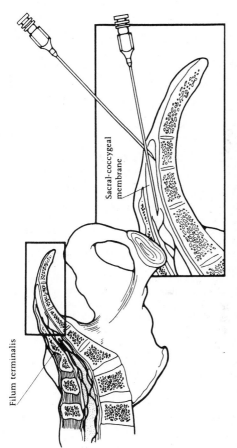

Figure 16.6.   Sacral anatomy, lateral view. A needle directed through the sacral-coccygeal membrane at a 45°-angle will usually "pop" through the ligament and contact the anterior bone of the sacral canal. The needle needs to be rotated so that the bevel does not scrape the periosteum of this layer, and the angle of advancement changed to allow passage directly 2 to 3 cm up the canal without contacting the bone again. This space is generously endowed with blood vessels, and the terminal point of the dural sac extends a variable distance in the sacral canal but usually lies at the S-2 level. (From Mulroy MF. *Regional anesthesia: an illustrated procedural guide.* Boston: Little, Brown and Company, 1996:124, with permission.)

catheter are receiving heparin anticoagulation, IV heparin should be stopped 2 to 4 hours before removal of the catheter and should not be restarted until 1 hour after removal.

C. **Low-molecular-weight heparin** (LMWH). Patients receiving LMWH for thromboembolism prophylaxis have altered coagulation parameters. Spinal or epidural needle placement should not be done for at least 12 hours after the last dose. Patients receiving higher doses of LMWH (enoxaparin 1 mg/kg twice daily) will require longer delays (24 hours). In patients requiring continuing LMWH administration, spinal or epidural catheters should be removed before administration of LMWH. The subsequent administration of LMWH should be delayed for 2 hours after catheter removal.

D. **Antiplatelet drugs.** Patients receiving aspirin or nonsteroidal anti-inflammatory drugs do not appear to be at higher risk for epidural hematoma formation. These drugs could contribute to an increased bleeding risk, however, if they are used concurrently with other anticoagulants. With regard to thienopyridine derivatives (ticlopidine, clopidogrel), the suggested time interval between discontinuation of medication and initiation of neuraxial block is 14 days for ticlopidine and 7 days for clopidogrel. Following platelet GP2b/3a inhibitors, normal platelet function returns in 24 to 48 hours with abciximab and in 4 to 8 hours with eptifibatide, tirofiban.

E. **Fibrinolytic and thrombolytic agents.** Although the plasma half-life of thrombolytic drugs is only hours, it takes several days before thrombolytic effects disappear. Surgery or puncture of noncompressible vessels within 10 days of thrombolytic therapy is contraindicated. There is no definitive guideline regarding the neuraxial anesthesia and thrombolytic therapy. Measurement of the fibrinogen level may be helpful in guiding the decision.

F. **Herbal medication (see Chapter 39).** Herbal medications including garlic, ginkgo, and ginseng are all known to affect coagulation. Currently, there are no specific guidelines for timing the neuraxial block in relationship to herbal medication use. Because it is not known at which doses potential coagulopathies occur, management decisions are often based more on a clinical history of abnormal bleeding. Herbal medications are thought to be more problematic when taken concurrently with other conventional anticoagulant medications.

SUGGESTED READINGS

Aida S, et al. Headache after attempted epidural block: the role of intrathecal air *Anesthesiology* 1998;88:76–81.

Moraca RJ, et al. The role of epidural anesthesia and analgesia in surgical practice. *Ann Surg* 2003;238:663–673.

The Second Consensus Conference on Neuraxial Anesthesia and Anticoagulation. Regional anesthesia in the anticoagulated patient: defining the risks. *Regional Anesth Pain Med* 2003;28:172–197.

Turnbull DK, et al. Post-dural puncture headache: pathogenesis, prevention and treatment. *Br J Anaesth* 2003;91(5):718–729.

Vibeke M, et al. Severe neurological complications after central neuraxial blockades in Sweden 1990–1999. *Anesthesiology* 2004;101:950–959.

Regional Anesthesia

George W. Pasvankas and Deepal S. Sidhu

I. **General considerations**

   A. **Peripheral nerve blockade** can be an excellent alternative to general anesthesia for many surgical procedures and does not significantly disrupt autonomic function. Regional blockade provides optimal surgical conditions while providing prolonged postoperative analgesia. Patient safety, satisfaction, and quicker initial recovery are among the benefits of regional anesthesia.

   B. **The preoperative assessment,** preparation of the patient, and degree of monitoring are the same as for central neuraxial blockade. Patients should follow fasting (nothing by mouth) guidelines whenever possible, and regional anesthesia should not be chosen just to avoid complications of a full stomach or difficult airway. Any neurologic conditions should be documented fully before performance of any block.

   C. **Consent for regional anesthesia** should include a thorough description of the risks, benefits, options, and common side effects. Need for supplemental local anesthesia, sedation, or backup general anesthesia should also be discussed.

   D. **Preoperative medication** may be prescribed as long as the patient remains cooperative and alert. Usually, short-acting agents such as fentanyl and midazolam are adequate.

   E. **All blocks should be performed with strict sterile technique** (i.e., sterile equipment, preparation of the skin with an antiseptic solution). Before inserting any block needle, a skin wheal should be raised with local anesthetic.

II. **Equipment**

   A. **Needles used for nerve blockade**

   1. **A block needle** should be the minimum diameter possible for patient comfort. However, regional block needles often are inserted into deep tissue and therefore need a more rigid shaft. For superficial blocks, such as an axillary block, a 23-gauge needle is suitable. For most peripheral regional blocks, a 22-gauge needle is preferable.

   2. **Short bevel needles** (30° to 45°) are associated with decreased nerve trauma and intravascular injection compared with standard A-bevel needles and therefore have become standard for peripheral nerve blocks. However, some argue that use of smaller, sharp needles may be associated with less damage in the event of a nerve injury because of a "clean cut" of the nerve. Newer needles with a Sprotte or Whitacre tip may be less traumatic.

   3. Upper- and lower-extremity blocks are best performed with a 50- to 150-mm needle. Brachial plexus blocks usually do not require more than a 100-mm needle and can frequently be accomplished, in the case of interscalene block, with a 25- to 50-mm needle.

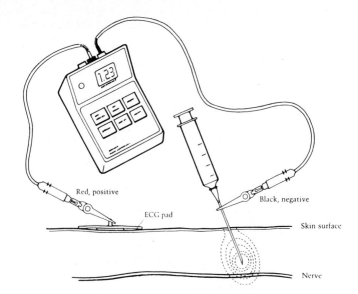

Figure 17.1. **Nerve stimulator attached to regional block needle. The negative (*black*) lead is attached to the exploring needle, whereas the positive (*red*) is connected to a reference electrocardiogram pad used as a "ground." The stimulator is set to deliver 1 to 2 mA of current to detect the nerve. The current is reduced further as the needle approaches the nerve. A current of 0.5 mA will produce motor stimulation when the needle is adjacent to the nerve. (From Mulroy MF. *Regional anesthesia: an illustrated procedural guide*, 2nd ed. Boston: Little, Brown and Company, 1996:65, with permission.)**

   B. **Nerve stimulators** (Fig. 17.1) designed for regional anesthesia deliver a current of 0.1 to 10.0 mA at a frequency of 1 to 2 pulses/second. **Insulated needles** provide the best results.

   C. Many blocks require depositing a large volume of local anesthetic in a single injection. Connecting a large-volume (20 mL) syringe to the block needle with sterile extension tubing will ensure stable needle position during aspiration and injection. For larger volumes of local anesthesia, multiple syringes can be attached with a stopcock.

   D. **Continuous catheter techniques** for nerve blockade are accomplished with commercially available kits.

   E. **Ultrasound equipment** ideally should have the following characteristics:

      1. **High resolution:** Depends on many factors, including the frequency of the ultrasound waves, the density of piezoelectric crystals on the sensing probe, and the processing and display capabilities of the hardware.

      2. **Portability**

      3. **Video and still image recording capabilities:** For review of exam/procedure at a later date, teaching/academic uses, and use in billing/reimbursement.

      4. **Network connection capability**

5. **Probe capabilities:** Different ultrasound frequencies may be utilized using a variable frequency probe. In addition, probes of various shapes, sizes, and frequencies may facilitate imaging of different parts of the body.

6. **Printing capability**

7. **Color Doppler capability:** In peripheral nerve blockade, the primary use is to identify landmark vessels and to distinguish them from nervous tissue when needed.

III. **Nerve localization techniques**

A. **Eliciting a paresthesia** by contacting a nerve with a needle is a time-honored method of nerve localization. However, this may cause patient discomfort and possibly a higher incidence of postanesthetic dysesthesia or neuropathy.

B. **Electrical stimulation** of a mixed nerve produces a motor response without significant pain.

1. Ground the positive lead of the stimulator to the patient and attach the negative terminal of the stimulator to the needle.

2. Set the nerve stimulator to an initial current of 1 to 1.5 mA and move the needle toward the nerve until a motor response in the desired muscle group occurs. Twitches may also arise from local muscle stimulation. Regardless of its origin, if a twitch is uncomfortable the current should be reduced. The needle position and stimulator output should be adjusted to produce the maximum twitch at the lowest current (usually <0.5 mA, although many clinicians accept <0.3 mA as an end point for successful block). This suggests that the needle is close to the nerve and the local anesthetic may be injected.

3. The nerve stimulation technique may be used on patients who are unable to report paresthesias reliably. Patient discomfort and the incidence of postanesthetic neuropathies related to paresthesia may be reduced. However, performing blocks on heavily sedated patients or on those under general anesthesia is not desirable.

C. **The use of ultrasound guidance** for peripheral nerve blockade

1. Frequencies used for medical imaging usually range from 1 to 15 MHz. Using higher frequencies increases the resolution at the expense of penetration (suitable for highly detailed examination of superficial tissues such as breast and thyroid). Conversely, using lower frequencies increases the depth of penetration at the expense of resolution (suitable for examination of deep structures such as the heart, abdominal viscera, and uterus). Most nerve blocks (e.g., supraclavicular, infraclavicular, femoral, sciatic nerve at the popliteal fossa) are done at an intermediate depth and thus are done at intermediate frequencies. Axillary and interscalene blocks, however, are more superficial and are best done at higher frequencies. In obese patients, frequencies may need to be set to favor penetration, particularly for infraclavicular and popliteal fossa blocks.

2. **Performance** of the block relies on three interrelated principles: the insertion point of the needle, the direction of needle advancement, and the end point of the needle tip. Typically, the ultrasound probe is placed where the needle insertion point would be in a conventional block technique. This leaves

two options for needle insertion. The needle may be inserted immediately above or below the midline of the probe and is then advanced perpendicular to the ultrasound beam. Entry point, direction, and end point are somewhat similar to the conventional approach. This permits only a cross-section view of the needle tip as a hyperechoic (white) dot in the image. Alternatively, the needle may be inserted several centimeters away from the probe site and then advanced in the plane of the ultrasound beam. This allows continuous visualization of the length of the needle as a hyperechoic (white) line during advancement. While technically more difficult, this would seem to minimize the likelihood of contacting nerves, blood vessels, pleura, and other vital structures during needle passage.

IV. **General contraindications.** Not all patients are suitable for regional anesthesia. Absolute contraindications to regional anesthesia include lack of patient consent or when nerve blockade would hinder the proposed surgery. Relative contraindications include coagulopathy, infection at the skin entry site, excessive anxiety, mental illness, anatomic distortion, and an unskilled anesthetist. Diseases such as multiple sclerosis, polio, neurologic trauma, and muscular dystrophy may be aggravated by peripheral nerve blockade.

V. **Complications common to all nerve blocks**

   A. **Complications of local anesthetics** include intravascular injection (Fig. 17.2), overdose, and allergic responses. Test doses and

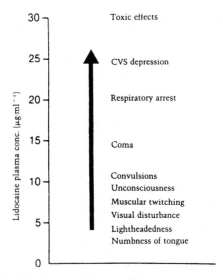

Figure 17.2. Progressive continuum of symptoms of lidocaine local anesthetic toxicity. These symptoms are seen in roughly the same progression and proportion with the other local anesthetics, except that cardiovascular system (CVS) toxicity may be seen with the more potent amino amides at blood levels closer to the convulsion threshold. (From Barash PG, Cullen BF, Stoelting RK, eds. *Clinical anesthesia.* Philadelphia: JB Lippincott, 1988:389, with permission.)

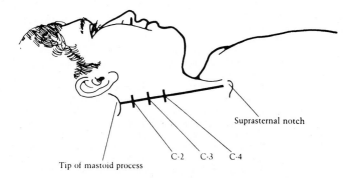

Figure 17.3.   Superficial landmarks for cervical plexus block. A line is drawn from the mastoid process to the prominent tubercle of the sixth cervical vertebra. The transverse processes of the second, third, and fourth cervical vertebrae lie 0.5 cm posterior to this line and at 1.5-cm intervals below the mastoid. (From Mulroy MF. *Regional anesthesia: an illustrated procedural guide*, 2nd ed. Boston: Little, Brown and Company, 1996:235, with permission.)

        intermittent aspiration during injection may help identify intravascular injection. Benzodiazepine premedication increases the seizure threshold and may decrease the central nervous system toxicity of local anesthetics as well as the level of patient anxiety.

B. **Nerve damage** resulting from needle trauma or from painful intraneural injection is a rare complication. This pain can be confused with a paresthesia that is potentiated on injection. If the pain is severe or does not subside after a few milliliters of local anesthetic, the needle should be repositioned.

C. **Hematomas** may result from arterial puncture but usually resolve without residual problems.

VI. **Cervical plexus block for regional anesthesia of the neck**

A. **Anatomy.** The cervical plexus lies in the paravertebral region of the upper four cervical vertebrae (Fig. 17.3). It is formed from the ventral rami of the C-1 to C-4 spinal nerve roots. It is deep to the sternocleidomastoid muscle and anterior to the middle scalene muscle, in continuity with the nerve roots forming the brachial plexus (see section VII.A). The plexus has superficial and deep branches. The **superficial branches** pierce the cervical fascia anteriorly, just posterior to the sternocleidomastoid, and supply the skin of the back of the head, side of the neck, and anterior and lateral shoulder. The **deep branches** supply the muscles and deep structures of the neck and form the phrenic nerve.

B. **Indications. Superficial cervical plexus block** produces only cutaneous anesthesia and is useful for superficial procedures on the neck and shoulder. **Deep cervical plexus block** is a paravertebral block of the C-1 to C-4 nerve roots that form the plexus, anesthetizing both the deep and the superficial branches. Common indications for cervical plexus block are as follows:

1. Cervical lymph node biopsy/excision.

2. Carotid endarterectomy.

3. Thyroid operations.

4. Tracheostomy (when combined with topical airway anesthesia).

C. **Techniques**

1. **For a superficial block,** inject 10 mL of local anesthetic subcutaneously along the posterior border of the sternocleidomastoid.

2. **For a deep block,** position the patient supine with the neck slightly extended and the head turned toward the opposite side. Draw a line connecting the tip of the mastoid process and **Chassaignac tubercle** (the most prominent of the cervical transverse processes, located at C-6, the level of the cricoid cartilage). Draw a second line 1 cm posterior to the first line. The C-2 transverse process can be palpated 1 to 2 cm caudad to the mastoid process, with the C-3 and C-4 processes lying at 1.5-cm intervals along the second line. At each level, insert a 22-gauge 5-cm needle perpendicular to the skin with caudal angulation. Advance the needle 1.5 to 3.0 cm until it contacts the transverse process. After careful aspiration for cerebrospinal fluid or blood, inject 10 mL of local anesthetic solution at each transverse process.

D. **Complications** are possible with deep cervical plexus block because of the close proximity of the needle to neural and vascular structures.

1. **Phrenic nerve block** is the most common complication. This block should be used cautiously in patients with diminished pulmonary reserve. Bilateral deep cervical plexus block will produce bilateral phrenic and recurrent laryngeal nerve blockade and therefore should be avoided.

2. **Subarachnoid injection** resulting in total spinal anesthesia.

3. **Epidural injection** with resultant bilateral cervical epidural anesthesia.

4. **Vertebral artery injection** causing central nervous system toxicity with very small doses of local anesthetic.

5. **Recurrent laryngeal nerve block** causing hoarseness and vocal cord dysfunction.

6. **Cervical sympathetic nerve block** producing Horner syndrome.

VII. **Regional anesthesia of the upper extremity**

A. **Anatomy**

1. Except for some areas of skin over the shoulder and axilla, the upper extremity is innervated by the brachial plexus.

2. The **brachial plexus** is formed from the anterior roots of the spinal nerves from C-5 to C-8 and T-1, with frequent contributions from C-4 and T-2. Each **root** exits posterior to the vertebral artery and travels laterally in the trough of its cervical transverse process, where it is directed toward the first rib and fuses with the other four roots to form the three trunks of the plexus. The roots are sandwiched between the fascial sheaths of the anterior and middle scalene muscles.

3. The **trunks** pass over the first rib through the space between the anterior and middle scalene muscles, in association with the subclavian artery, which shares the same fascial sheath. The roots and trunks have several

branches, innervating the neck, shoulder girdle, and chest wall.

4. As the trunks pass over the first rib and under the clavicle, they reorganize to form the three **cords** of the plexus. The cords descend into the axilla, where each has one major branch, in addition to several minor branches, before becoming a major terminal nerve of the upper extremity. Branches of the lateral and medial cords form the **median nerve.** The lateral cord gives off a branch that forms the **musculocutaneous nerve,** whereas the posterior cord becomes the **axillary and radial nerves.** The medial cord also forms the **ulnar nerve, medial antebrachial,** and **brachial cutaneous nerves.** In the axilla, the median nerve lies lateral to the axillary artery, the radial nerve posterior, and the ulnar nerve medial. The axillary and musculocutaneous nerves exit the sheath high up in the axilla, the musculocutaneous nerve traveling through the substance of the coracobrachialis muscle before becoming subcutaneous below the elbow. The median cutaneous nerves of the arm and forearm are minor branches of the medial cord (Fig. 17.4). The cutaneous peripheral nerve supply of the upper extremity is summarized in Figure 17.5.

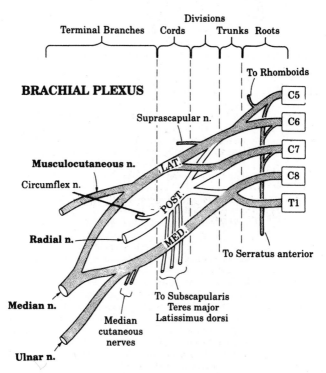

Figure 17.4. Diagram of the brachial plexus and peripheral nerve formation.

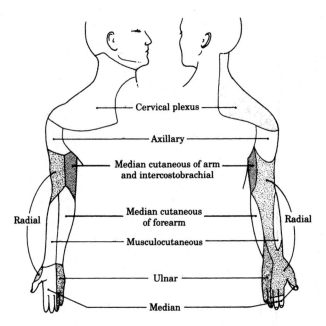

Figure 17.5. Cutaneous peripheral nerve supply of the upper extremity.

5. The **cutaneous and sclerotome distribution of the nerves** of the body is summarized in Figure 17.6. Cutaneous innervation does not necessarily correlate with deep structures; therefore, knowledge of the sclerotomes can be very useful in predicting the ultimate success of any regional technique.

6. **The major motor functions** of the five nerves are as follows:

   a. **Axillary (circumflex nerve):** shoulder abduction (deltoid contraction).

   b. **Musculocutaneous:** elbow flexion (biceps contraction).

   c. **Radial:** elbow (triceps contraction), wrist, and finger extension (extensor carpi radialis longus).

   d. **Median:** wrist and finger flexion (flexor carpi radialis).

   e. **Ulnar:** wrist and finger flexion (flexor carpi ulnaris).

B. **Indications**

1. **Brachial plexus blockade** anesthetizes various areas of the upper extremity, depending on which level of the brachial plexus is blocked. The preferred approach to the plexus depends on the surgical site, the risk of complications, and the experience of the individual anesthetist.

   a. The **interscalene approach** blocks the cervical plexus in addition to the brachial plexus, thereby anesthetizing the skin over the shoulder. The ulnar nerve is frequently spared. This approach is most useful for shoulder and

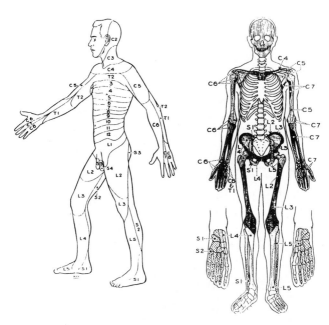

Figure 17.6. A side view of the dermatomes (*left*) and an anterior view of the sclerotomes indicated by the different styles of shading (*right*). (From Haymaker W, Woodhall B. *Peripheral nerve injuries.* Philadelphia: WB Saunders, 1945:20, 41, with permission.)

proximal humerus surgery. It is less useful for forearm and hand operations, unless accompanied by an ulnar nerve block.

b. The **supraclavicular approach** anesthetizes the entire plexus distal to the trunks because of its compact nature at the point of injection and the fact that very few nerves have yet left the plexus.

c. The **infraclavicular approach** provides excellent coverage for surgery distal to the midhumerus.

d. The **axillary approach** is very common. However, because the musculocutaneous and medial cutaneous nerves of the arm exit the sheath more proximally, they are not blocked by this approach, making it unreliable for operations proximal to the elbow.

2. The **intercostobrachial nerve** must be blocked in addition to the plexus for procedures involving the medial arm or using a proximal humeral tourniquet.

3. **Blockade of an individual peripheral nerve** may be useful when limited anesthesia is required or a plexus block is incomplete. The musculocutaneous nerve may be blocked at the axilla or the elbow. Each of the other major terminal nerves may be blocked at either the elbow or the wrist.

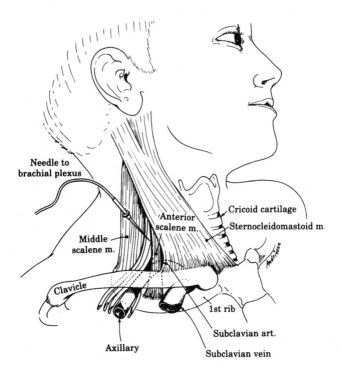

Needle to brachial plexus

Anterior scalene m.

Cricoid cartilage

Sternocleidomastoid m.

Middle scalene m.

Clavicle

1st rib

Axillary

Subclavian art.

Subclavian vein

Figure 17.7. Interscalene approach to brachial plexus block.

C. **Techniques**
   1. **Interscalene** (Fig. 17.7)
      a. Position the patient supine with the head turned slightly away from the side to be blocked.
      b. Identify the lateral border of the sternocleidomastoid by having the patient lift his or her head off the bed. The anterior scalene muscle lies below the posterior edge of the sternocleidomastoid. By rolling your fingers posteriorly over the anterior scalene muscle, you will feel a groove between the anterior and middle scalenes. The intersection of this groove with a transverse plane at the level of the cricoid cartilage is the point at which the needle should enter the skin in a caudal direction. Because the scalenes are accessory muscles of respiration, asking the patient to take slow deep breaths while palpating for the groove may be helpful. The external jugular vein frequently crosses the groove at the level of the C-6 vertebra and may also be a useful landmark.
      c. Advance a 25- to 50-mm needle into the groove at a 45° angle in the caudal direction. Stimulation of the plexus will result in a paresthesia or muscle twitch in the deltoid, biceps, or pectoris major muscles. Paresthesia or twitches

confined to the shoulder may result from suprascapular or cervical plexus stimulation and indicate that the needle is posterior to the plexus. Paresthesia or twitches of the diaphragm (phrenic nerve) indicate that the needle is just anterior to the plexus. Despite being accurately placed in the groove, the needle will sometimes contact the cervical transverse process without stimulating the plexus. If this happens, withdrawing the needle and redirecting it slightly will likely elicit the correct response.

d. A volume of 30 to 40 mL of anesthetic solution should be injected.

e. Applying digital pressure distal to the injection site may facilitate cervical plexus blockade in addition to brachial plexus blockade.

f. **Complications** are identical to those of the cervical plexus block (see section VI.D).

g. **Interscalene block using ultrasound guidance** is performed with the patient supine or semireclined with the arms at the side. The probe (linear or tight curved array) is held over the sternocleidomastoid muscle at the level of the cricoid cartilage (C-6), and the internal carotid artery and internal jugular vein are identified (Fig. 17.8). The probe is moved laterally and the anterior and middle scalene muscles are identified. At this time the roots/trunks will come into view as hypoechoic (dark) nodular structures. They should be centered on the screen, and a needle insertion point should be chosen approximately 2 cm lateral to the probe site. After infiltration with local anesthetic, a 22-gauge 50-mm block needle is inserted and advanced at a 45° angle to the skin, keeping within the plane of the ultrasound image. The middle scalene muscle may or may not be directly traversed. With the former, a distinct increase in resistance followed by a pop will be seen and felt as the needle enters and exits the middle scalene muscle. After aspiration is performed and deemed negative, 15 to 20 mL of local anesthetic solution is deposited between the two scalene muscles and should be visualized in the ultrasound image. Note that motor stimulation is *not* required provided the anatomy and spread of local anesthetic are easily appreciated.

2. The **supraclavicular block** provides anesthesia of the brachial plexus at the level of the nerve trunks and produces reliable anesthesia of the elbow, forearm, and hand. Three approaches will be described; for each, place the patient in the supine position with his or her head turned to the contralateral side. With each of these techniques, it is generally safe to direct the needle laterally, but the medial direction should be avoided to prevent entering the pleural space and producing a pneumothorax.

a. **Parascalene approach.** Palpate the clavicle and lateral border of the sternocleidomastoid muscle. Approximately 1 to 2 cm above the clavicle, identify the interscalene groove as in section VII.C.1.b. Advance a 22-gauge 50-mm needle in an anteroposterior direction.

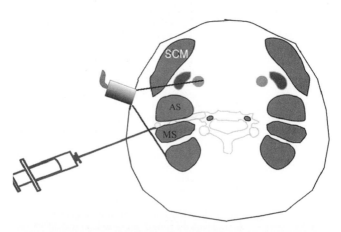

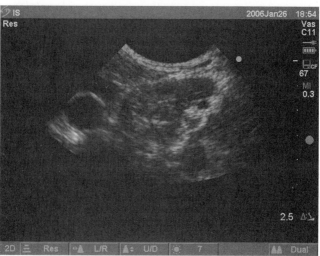

Figure 17.8. Interscalene block using ultrasound guidance. SCM = sternocleidomastoid muscle; AS = anterior scalene muscle; MS = middle scalene muscle.

The plexus can be identified with a nerve stimulator or by the paresthesia technique. If the first rib is contacted, withdraw and redirect the needle in a stepwise fashion. Inject a total of 30 to 40 mL of local anesthetic solution.

b. **Classic supraclavicular approach.** Prepare the patient and identify the interscalene groove as described above. Palpate the pulse of the subclavian artery inferiorly in this space. Advance a 22-gauge 1.5-inch needle directly caudally. The "click" of the needle entering the plexus may be felt, and the plexus may be identified with a nerve

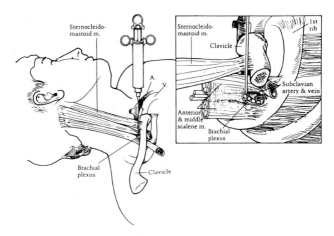

Figure 17.9. The "plumb-bob" approach to the supraclavicular block. The needle is introduced directly posterior to the midpoint of the clavicle. If the nerves are not encountered at the first insertion, the needle is rotated in a caudad direction in very small steps and will encounter the neurovascular bundle before encountering the lung. (From Mulroy MF. *Regional anesthesia: an illustrated procedural guide*, 2nd ed. Boston: Little, Brown and Company, 1996:169, with permission.)

stimulator or by the paresthesia technique. Inject 20 to 30 mL of local anesthetic solution.

  c. **Plumb-bob approach** (Fig. 17.9). Identify the midpoint of the clavicle and advance a 22-gauge 1.5-inch needle in a caudal direction in a plane parallel to that of the head and neck until it contacts the first rib. If a paresthesia or motor response with a nerve stimulator is not elicited, walk the needle in an anterior and then posterior direction across the first rib. Once the plexus has been located, inject 25 to 40 mL of local anesthetic solution.

  d. **Complications** common to each of these approaches include pneumothorax and intravascular injection.

3. **Infraclavicular approach** to the brachial plexus is primarily used for anesthesia of the arm distal to the midhumeral line. It is most useful for medium- to long-duration procedures where prolonged postoperative analgesia would be beneficial (e.g., bone and joint surgery). Soft tissue surgery may be most appropriately accomplished with a **Bier block (see section VII.C.10).**

  a. Position the patient supine with the extremity slightly abducted and the palm upward.

  b. Landmarks to be palpated include the clavicle, coracoid process, and chest wall. After identifying the coracoid process, mark 2 cm inferior and 2 cm medial, making sure this needle insertion mark is superior to the chest wall (between coracoid process and chest wall).

  c. Using a 100-mm insulated needle with a nerve stimulator starting between 1.0 and 1.5 mA, advance the needle in a plumb-bob direction until motor stimulation indicates contact with the cord level of the brachial plexus. If no contact is made, the first redirection should be away from the chest wall.

d. Stimulation of the lateral cord will give flexor carpi radialis stimulation and/or some wrist and finger flexion (median nerve). Stimulation of the posterior cord will produce extension at the elbow and/or wrist (radial nerve). Stimulation of the medial cord produces flexor carpi ulnaris movement with some flexion of the wrist and/or fingers (median and ulnar nerves).

e. Success is seen with motor stimulation below 0.3 mA in any of the three cords; however, some clinicians prefer to take the posterior cord as it is the most central of the three.

f. After aspiration is performed and deemed negative for blood, inject 40 mL of local anesthetic in 3- to 5-mL aliquots.

g. **Complications** include infection, hematoma, pneumothorax, nerve injury, and failed block.

h. **Infraclavicular block using ultrasound guidance** is performed with the patient supine with the arm abducted 90° at the shoulder and the forearm supinated so the palm faces up. The probe (tight curved array is preferable) is positioned in the infraclavicular fossa (at the deltopectoral groove) and the axillary artery is identified and positioned in the center of the screen (Fig. 17.10). A needle insertion site is identified approximately 1 inch superior to the probe and is infiltrated with local anesthetic. A 17- or 18-gauge long block needle is appropriate for placement of a catheter or for use in obese or muscular patients. Smaller 20- or 22-gauge long block needles are appropriate for smaller or thinner patients. The needle is inserted and advanced at a 45° angle to the skin, keeping in the plane of the ultrasound beam, until positioned posterior to the axillary artery (i.e., in the 6 o'clock position). After aspiration is performed and deemed negative for blood, 30 to 40 mL of local anesthetic solution is deposited with a goal of equal distribution on either side of the axillary artery (i.e., between the 6 and 9 o'clock position as well as between the 6 and 3 o'clock position). This may require repositioning after partial injection to achieve spread in both locations. Note that motor stimulation is *not* required provided the anatomy and spread of local anesthetic are easily appreciated.

4. **Axillary approach** (Fig. 17.11)

a. Position the patient supine with the arm abducted 90° at the shoulder, externally rotated and flexed at the elbow.

b. Palpate the axillary artery at its most proximal location in the axilla. If the artery is difficult to palpate, move the patient's hand laterally or reduce the degree of abduction at the shoulder.

c. Advance a 23-gauge needle through the skin just superior to the palpating fingertip, directing the needle

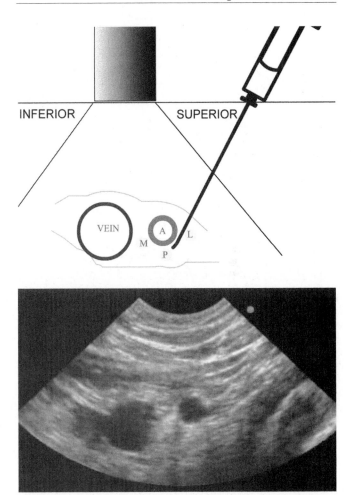

Figure 17.10. Infraclavicular block using ultrasound guidance.
Vein = axillary vein; A = axillary artery; M = medial cord of brachial
plexus; P = posterior cord of brachial plexus; L = lateral cord of
brachial plexus.

> toward the apex of the axilla. Localization of one of
> the nerves of the plexus by either paresthesia or nerve
> stimulation confirms that the needle tip is within the
> plexus sheath; 40 to 50 mL of local anesthetic may be
> injected.
>
> **d.** If the axillary artery is penetrated (see section VII.C.5),
> advance the needle through the posterior wall of the
> artery.
>
> **e.** Frequently, a "pop" will be felt as the sheath is penetrated.
> If this occurs and the needle pulsates in synchrony with

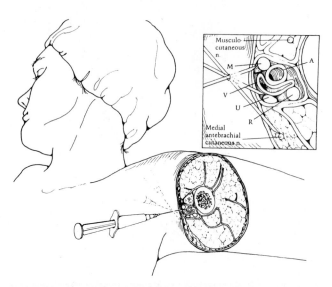

Figure 17.11. Needle position for axillary injection. The median (*M*) and musculocutaneous nerves lie on the superior side of the artery (*A*). The latter usually lies within the body of the coracobrachialis muscle at this point. The ulnar (*U*) nerve lies inferior and the radial (*R*) nerve is inferior and posterior to the artery. These positions may vary with individual patients. The medial antebrachial cutaneous nerve usually lies in the subcutaneous tissues just inferior to the neurovascular bundle and is anesthetized by a subcutaneous wheal along that area, along with the intercostobrachial fibers. (From Mulroy MF. *Regional anesthesia: an illustrated procedural guide*, 2nd ed. Boston: Little, Brown and Company, 1996:172, with permission.)

the pulse, the tip of the needle is located within the sheath and the anesthetic may be injected.

f. While holding distal pressure on the upper arm, redirect the needle so that the tip of the needle is just superior to the artery and perpendicular to the skin in all planes. Advance the needle until the humerus is contacted and then, moving the tip through a 30° arc superiorly, 5 mL of local anesthetic solution can be injected in a fan-wise pattern. This will block the musculocutaneous nerve in the body of coracobrachialis muscle.

g. Intercostobrachial nerve block requires subcutaneous injection of 5 mL of anesthetic, directly inferior to the axillary artery and extending to the inferior border of the axilla.

h. The most common complication specific to the axillary approach is injection of local anesthetic into the axillary artery.

i. Digital pressure may be applied distally to facilitate proximal spread of local anesthetic.

j. Axillary nerve block using ultrasound guidance is performed in the same position as the conventional technique. The probe (tight curved array preferable) is held over the axillary artery on the lateral wall of the axilla and the axillary artery is positioned in the center of the screen (Fig. 17.12). A needle insertion site is chosen 1 to 2 cm superior to the probe, and after infiltration with local anesthetic a 22-gauge 50-mm block needle is inserted and advanced at a 30° angle to the skin. Keeping within the plane of the ultrasound beam, the needle is advanced to the 12 o'clock position above the axillary artery. After aspiration is performed and deemed negative for blood, 10 to 15 mL of local anesthetic solution is deposited. The needle is then withdrawn and positioned at the 6 o'clock position, and once again, after aspiration is performed and deemed negative, 15 to 20 mL of local anesthetic solution is deposited. The goal is 360 degree coverage around the axillary artery and may require further repositioning after partial injection to achieve this spread. The musculocutaneous nerve can be identified as a hyperechoic (white) oval or triangular structure between the coracobrachialis and biceps muscles. Without changing needle entry site, using a more perpendicular trajectory, the needle tip is positioned next to the nerve and 2 to 4 mL of local anesthetic solution is injected. Note that motor stimulation is *not* required provided the anatomy and spread of local anesthetic are easily appreciated.

5. **Axillary transarterial approach**
   a. Prepare the patient as previously described and palpate the axillary artery. Insert a 24-gauge medium bevel at an angle of 30° to the skin and advance it cephalad toward the axillary artery. When blood is aspirated, advance the needle through the posterior wall of the artery until blood can no longer be aspirated. Inject 20 to 40 mL of local anesthetic solution posterior to the artery while aspirating for blood with every 5 mL of anesthetic injected.
   b. Digital pressure may be applied distally to facilitate proximal spread of local anesthetic.
   c. The most common complications with this approach are vascular spasm and hematoma.

6. **Ulnar nerve block**
   a. **Elbow.** Locate the ulnar groove in the medial epicondyle and inject 5 to 10 mL of local anesthetic solution 3 to 5 cm proximal to the groove in a fan-wise pattern.
   b. **Wrist** (Fig. 17.13). The ulnar nerve is just lateral to the flexor carpi ulnaris tendon at the level of the ulnar styloid process. Pierce the deep fascia with the needle oriented perpendicular to the skin, just lateral to the tendon, and inject 3 to 6 mL of solution.

7. **Median nerve block**
   a. **Elbow** (see Fig. 17.13). The median nerve is just medial to the brachial artery. Palpate the artery 1 to 2 cm proximal to the elbow crease and inject 3 to 5 mL of anesthetic just medial to it in a fan-wise pattern.

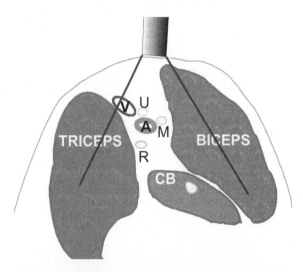

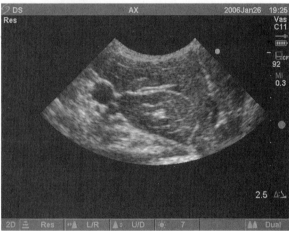

Figure 17.12. Axillary nerve block using ultrasound guidance. V = axillary vein; A = axillary artery; M = median nerve; U = ulnar nerve; R = radial nerve; CB = coracobrachialis muscle.

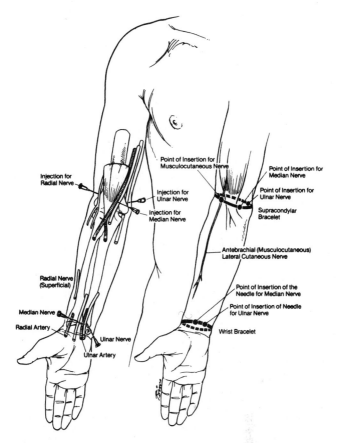

Figure 17.13. Deep anatomy for elbow and wrist block of musculocutaneous, radial, ulnar, and median nerves. (From Raj PP. *Clinical practice of regional anesthesia.* New York: Churchill Livingstone, 1991.)

    b. Wrist (see Fig. 17.13). The median nerve lies between the palmaris longus tendon and the flexor carpi radialis tendon, 2 to 3 cm proximal to the wrist crease. Pierce the deep fascia with the needle oriented perpendicular to the skin close to the lateral border of the palmaris longus and inject 3 to 5 mL of anesthetic.

  8. Radial nerve block

    a. Elbow (see Fig. 17.13). The radial nerve lies lateral to the biceps tendon, medial to the brachioradialis muscle, at the level of the lateral epicondyle of the humerus. Insert the needle 1 to 2 cm lateral to the tendon and advance until it contacts the lateral epicondyle. Inject 3 to 5 mL of anesthetic solution.

b. **Wrist.** The radial nerve divides into its terminal branches in the superficial fascia. Inject 5 to 10 mL of local anesthetic subcutaneously, extending from the radial artery anteriorly to the extensor carpi radialis posteriorly, beginning just proximal to the wrist.

9. **Musculocutaneous nerve block.** The musculocutaneous nerve may be blocked in the axilla, as described in section VII.C.4.f. Its terminal cutaneous component is blocked concomitantly with the radial nerve block at the elbow.

10. **Intravenous (IV) regional anesthesia (Bier block).** IV administration of local anesthetic distal to a tourniquet is a simple way to anesthetize an extremity.

   a. Place a 20- to 22-gauge IV catheter capped off with a heparin-lock device as distally as possible in the extremity. Apply a pneumatic double tourniquet proximally and exsanguinate the extremity by elevating it and wrapping it distally to proximally with an Esmarch bandage.

   b. Both tourniquet cuffs should be checked. Inflate the proximal cuff to 150 mm Hg greater than systolic pressure. Absence of pulses after inflation ensures arterial occlusion. Remove the Esmarch bandage and inject the anesthetic into the previously placed IV catheter. Average drug doses are 50 mL of 0.5% lidocaine for an arm and 100 mL of 0.25% lidocaine for a leg. No vasoconstrictors should be used.

   c. For shorter procedures of the hand, wrist, and distal forearm a single-cuffed tourniquet may be applied proximally on the forearm. Generally 25 to 30 mL of 0.5% lidocaine provides sufficient anesthesia and facilitates early deflation of the tourniquet.

   d. Anesthesia occurs within 5 min of local anesthetic injection. Tourniquet pain generally becomes unbearable after 1 hour and is the limiting factor for the success of this technique. When the patient complains of pain, the distal tourniquet that overlies anesthetized skin should be inflated and the proximal tourniquet released. Some advocate changing cuffs at 45 min, before the onset of pain.

   e. A **toxic reaction to the local anesthetic** is the major complication associated with IV regional anesthesia. It may occur during injection if the tourniquet fails or after tourniquet deflation, particularly with an inflation time of less than 25 min. Careful attention to drug dosage and to the adequacy of vascular occlusion will minimize the risk of a local anesthetic reaction. If the tourniquet is deflated before 25 min, the patient should be observed closely for evidence of toxicity.

VIII. **Regional anesthesia of the lower extremity**

   A. **Anatomy.** There are two major plexuses that innervate the lower extremity: the lumbar plexus and the sacral plexus.

   1. The **lumbar plexus** (Fig. 17.14) is formed within the psoas muscle from the anterior rami of the L-1 to L-4 spinal nerves, with a contribution from the twelfth thoracic nerve. The most cephalad nerves of the plexus are the **iliohypogastric,**

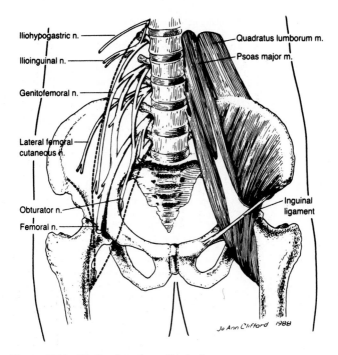

Iliohypogastric n.

Ilioinguinal n.

Genitofemoral n.

Lateral femoral
cutaneous n.

Obturator n.

Femoral n.

Quadratus lumborum m.

Psoas major m.

Inguinal
ligament

Jo Ann Clifford 1988

Figure 17.14.   The lumbar plexus lies in the psoas compartment between the psoas major and quadratus lumborum. (From Miller RD. *Anesthesia*, 3rd ed. New York: Churchill Livingstone, 1991.)

ilioinguinal, and genitofemoral nerves. These nerves pierce the abdominal musculature anteriorly before supplying the skin of the hip and groin. The remainder of the lower abdomen is supplied by intercostal nerves. The three caudal nerves of the lumber plexus are the **lateral femoral cutaneous (LFC), femoral, and obturator nerves.**

a. The **LFC nerve** passes under the lateral end of the inguinal ligament, supplying sensory innervation to the lateral thigh and buttock.

b. The **femoral nerve** passes under the inguinal ligament just lateral to the femoral artery and supplies the muscles and skin of the anterior thigh as well as the knee and hip joints. The **saphenous nerve** is the cutaneous termination of the femoral nerve, supplying the skin of the medial leg and foot. It is the only nerve of the lumbar plexus that innervates the leg below the knee.

c. The **obturator nerve** exits from the pelvis through the obturator canal of the ischium, innervating the adductor muscles of the thigh, the hip and knee joints, and a portion of the skin of the medial thigh.

2. The **sacral plexus** is formed from the anterior rami of the L-4 to L-5 lumbar nerves and the S-1 to S-3 sacral nerves.

The two major nerves of the sacral plexus are the sciatic nerve and the posterior cutaneous nerve of the thigh.

   a. The **posterior cutaneous nerve of the thigh** travels with the sciatic nerve in its proximal extent and supplies the skin of the posterior thigh. Techniques for blocking the sciatic nerve will also block the posterior cutaneous nerve of the thigh.

   b. The **sciatic nerve** passes out of the pelvis through the greater sciatic foramen, becomes superficial at the lower border of the gluteus maximus, descends along the medial aspect of the femur supplying branches to the hamstrings, and becomes superficial again at the popliteal fossa. There it divides into the tibial nerve and the common peroneal nerve.

   (1) The **tibial nerve** travels down the posterior calf and passes under the medial malleolus before dividing into its terminal branches. It supplies the skin of the medial and plantar foot and causes plantar flexion.

   (2) The **common peroneal nerve** winds around the head of the fibula before dividing into the superficial and deep peroneal nerves.

   (a) The **superficial peroneal nerve** is a sensory nerve that passes down the lateral calf, dividing into its terminal branches just medial to the lateral malleolus supplying the anterior foot.

   (b) The **deep peroneal nerve** enters the foot just lateral to the anterior tibial artery, lying at the superior border of the malleolus, in between the anterior tibialis tendon and the extensor hallucis longus tendon. Although primarily a motor nerve causing dorsiflexion of the foot, it also sends a sensory branch to the web space between the first and second toes.

   (3) The **sural nerve** is a sensory nerve formed from branches of the common peroneal and tibial nerves. It passes under the lateral malleolus, supplying the lateral foot.

B. Indications. Anesthetizing the entire lower extremity requires blocking components of both the lumbar and sacral plexuses. Because multiple injections may be required, lower extremity blocks are unpopular with many clinicians. However, they are useful when limited anesthesia is required (making a single injection feasible) or when a regional technique is preferable, but a central neuraxis block is contraindicated. Many of these blocks may be used as adjuncts to general anesthesia to provide postoperative analgesia.

   1. Although **lower abdominal operations** can be performed with combined lumbar plexus block and intercostal nerve blocks, this is rarely done. However, an **ilioinguinal–iliohypogastric block** is a simple and very useful block, providing excellent analgesia for groin operations (e.g., hernia repair).

   2. **Hip operations** require anesthesia of the entire lumbar plexus with the exception of the ilioinguinal and ilioinguinal nerves.

This is most easily accomplished with a lumbar plexus block (psoas block).

3. **Major thigh operations** (e.g., placement of a femoral rod) require anesthesia of the LFC, femoral, obturator, and sciatic nerves. Obturator nerve block may be difficult to perform. Alternatively, these operations may be performed with a combined psoas–sciatic block.

4. **Operations limited to the anterior thigh** may be performed with a combined LFC–femoral block. The nerves may be blocked separately or together with a "3-in-1" block (see section VIII.C.2). Alone, an LFC block gives excellent analgesia for skin graft donor sites. An isolated femoral nerve block is particularly useful for providing postoperative analgesia for femoral shaft fractures or as the sole anesthetic for quadricepsplasty or repair of a patellar fracture.

5. **For tourniquet pain,** a combined LFC–femoral nerve block, in concert with a sciatic block, will usually provide adequate analgesia. This is because the area of skin that the obturator nerve supplies is generally small.

6. **Open operations on the knee** require anesthesia of the LFC, femoral, obturator, and sciatic nerves, which is most easily accomplished with a combined psoas–sciatic block. For knee arthroscopy, combined 3-in-1 and femoral–sciatic nerve blocks provide adequate anesthesia.

7. **Operations distal to the knee** require sciatic block and block of the saphenous component of the femoral nerve. The branches of the sciatic nerve can be blocked with multiple injections at the ankle or with a single injection in the popliteal fossa. The latter is particularly useful when cellulitis is present at the ankle. Ankle block will provide reliable anesthesia for transmetatarsal and toe amputations.

C. **Techniques.** Although paresthesias may be used for nerve localization in the lower extremity, in general, a nerve stimulator is more accurate, and the use of ultrasound can increase the safety and efficacy even further.

1. **Lumbar plexus block (psoas block)**
    a. Local anesthetic deposited into the substance of the psoas muscle will be confined by its fascia and will anesthetize the entire plexus.
    b. Place the patient in the lateral position, hips flexed, with the surgical side uppermost. Insert a 22-gauge 3.5-inch spinal needle perpendicular to the skin at a point 3 cm cephalad to a line connecting the iliac crests and 4 to 5 cm lateral to the midline. If the transverse process of L-4 is contacted, redirect the needle. Localize the plexus by using a nerve stimulator, which will produce a quadriceps muscle twitch. Inject 30 to 40 mL of local anesthetic.
    c. **Epidural blockade** is a complication of this approach, occurring with an incidence of approximately 10%.

2. **3-in-1 block**
    a. The three branches of the lumbar plexus can be blocked with a single injection.
    b. With the patient in the supine position, insert a 2.5- to 3-inch needle just caudad to the inguinal ligament and lateral to the femoral artery. Direct the needle cephalad

at a 45° angle until a quadriceps twitch or paresthesia is elicited. While maintaining distal pressure, which may force the anesthetic more proximally onto lumbar nerve roots, inject 30 to 40 mL of local anesthetic.

c. An alternative approach is the **fascia iliaca compartment block.** It consists of injecting local anesthetic behind the fascia iliaca at the junction of the lateral and middle thirds of the inguinal ligament and forcing it upward by finger compression.

3. **Ilioinguinal–iliohypogastric nerve block.** Insert a 1.5-inch needle perpendicular to the skin and 3 cm medial to the anterior superior iliac spine (ASIS). Contact the ASIS and inject 10 to 15 mL of local anesthetic while withdrawing the needle to the skin.

4. **LFC nerve block** (Fig. 17.15). Insert a 1.5-inch needle 1.5 cm caudad and 1.5 cm medial to the ASIS. Direct the needle in a slightly lateral and cephalad direction, striking the iliac bone medially just below the ASIS, and inject 5 to 10 mL of local anesthetic.

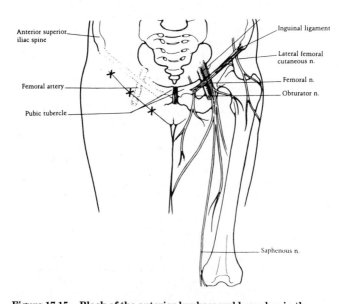

Figure 17.15. Block of the anterior lumbosacral branches in the groin. The lateral femoral cutaneous nerve emerges approximately 2.5 cm medial to the anterior superior iliac spine and is best blocked along that line 2.5 cm caudad to the anterior superior iliac spine. The femoral nerve emerges alongside and slightly posterior to the femoral artery and is again easily approached approximately 2.5 cm below the inguinal ligament. On that same line, the obturator nerve emerges from the obturator canal but is deeper and less reliably located. (From Mulroy MF. *Regional anesthesia: an illustrated procedural guide*, 2nd ed. Boston: Little, Brown and Company, 1996:204, with permission.)

5. **Femoral nerve block** (see Fig. 17.15) is carried out identically to the 3-in-1 block (see section VIII.C.2), except that the needle is directed perpendicular to the skin rather than at a 45° angle. A volume of 15 to 20 mL of local anesthetic suffices.

   a. **Fascia iliaca/femoral nerve block using ultrasound guidance** is performed with the patient supine. The ultrasound probe is placed over the femoral artery at the level of the femoral crease and is moved approximately 1 cm laterally so that the femoral artery is at the lateral edge of the image (Fig. 17.16). Two separate fascial layers can be visualized overlying the iliopsoas muscle: the superficial fascia lata and the deeper fascia iliaca. A needle entry site is chosen approximately 2 cm lateral to the probe and is infiltrated with local anesthetic. A 17- to 22-gauge needle at least 50 mm long is inserted and advanced medially at a 60° angle to the skin. As the needle is advanced, two distinct "pops" are felt and seen (each an initial increase of resistance followed by sudden loss of resistance as the two fascial layers are traversed). At this point, having passed through the fascia lata and the fascia iliaca, the needle tip should lie between the fascia iliaca and the iliopsoas muscle. After aspiration is performed and deemed negative for blood, local anesthetic is injected. Approximately 20 mL is sufficient to block the femoral nerve alone, while approximately 40 mL is required to additionally block the lateral femoral cutaneous and obdurator nerves. Note that it is not necessary for the needle tip to be anywhere near the femoral artery or nerve for the block to be successful. If the needle is in the proper plane, local anesthetic spread is seen mostly in the horizontal direction, easily reaching the femoral and lateral femoral cutaneous nerves.

6. **Obturator nerve block** (see Fig. 17.15). With the patient in the supine position, identify the pubic tubercle and insert a 3-inch needle 1.5 cm caudal and 1.5 cm lateral to the tubercle. After contacting the bone, withdraw the needle and redirect it slightly lateral and caudal while advancing 2 to 3 cm into the obturator foramen. After aspiration, inject 20 mL of local anesthetic while fanning lateral.

7. **Sciatic nerve block**

   a. **Indications**
      (1) **Surgery of the leg** when blocked proximally in combination with femoral nerve blockade.
      (2) **Surgery of the knee** when combined with blockade of the femoral, LFC, and obturator nerves.
      (3) **Foot and ankle surgery** when combined with saphenous nerve (femoral) blockade.

   b. **Classic posterior approach.** Place the patient in the Sims position (the lateral decubitus position with the leg to be blocked uppermost and flexed at the hip and knee; Fig. 17.17). Identify the posterior superior iliac spine and greater trochanter and draw a straight line connecting the two structures. At its midpoint, draw a perpendicular line inferiorly for 3 to 4 cm. Insert a 3.5-inch

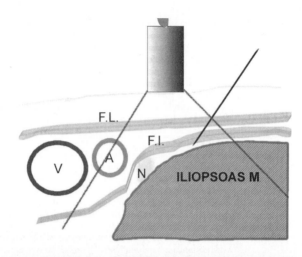

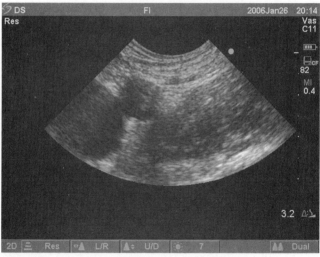

Figure 17.16. Fascia iliaca/femoral nerve block using ultrasound guidance. V = femoral vein; A = femoral artery; N = femoral nerve; F.L. = fascia lata; F.I. = fascia iliaca.

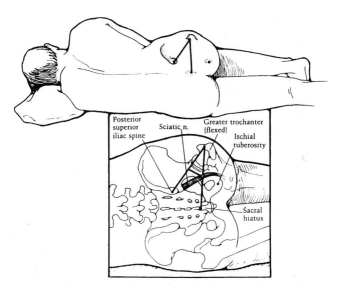

Figure 17.17. Sciatic nerve block, classic posterior approach. With the patient in the lateral position and the hip and knee flexed, the muscles overlying the sciatic nerve are stretched to allow easier identification. The nerve lies beneath a point 5 cm caudad along the perpendicular line that bisects the line joining the posterior superior iliac spine and the greater trochanter of the femur. This is also usually the intersection of that perpendicular with another line joining the greater trochanter and the sacral hiatus. (From Mulroy MF. *Regional anesthesia: an illustrated procedural guide*, 2nd ed. Boston: Little, Brown and Company, 1996:202, with permission.)

22-gauge needle perpendicularly to the skin, 3 cm below the midpoint, and connect the needle to a nerve stimulator set at an initial current of 2.5 mA. Advance the needle to a depth of approximately 3 cm to elicit a motor response in the sciatic distribution (contraction of hamstring or gastrocnemius, foot dorsi- or plantar flexion) or paresthesia in the leg or foot. If buttock contraction is observed, the inferior or superior gluteal nerves are being stimulated, and the needle is simply redirected. When an appropriate motor response is noted, decrease the stimulus current in a stepwise fashion to determine the threshold for stimulation. Reposition the needle until the goal of a stimulus threshold less than 1.0 mA is reached. After a test dose, inject 20 to 30 mL of local anesthetic, aspirating the syringe after each 5 mL injected. A double injection technique identifies and injects the tibial and peroneal components of the sciatic nerve separately, through the same skin wheal.

c. **Lithotomy approach.** With the patient supine, flex the lower extremity as far as possible at the hip and support it by stirrups or an assistant. Locate the midpoint of a line between the greater trochanter and the ischial tuberosity. Insert a 3.5-inch needle attached to a nerve stimulator perpendicular to the skin at this point and advance the needle until a motor response is seen, indicating sciatic nerve stimulation. Inject 20 to 30 mL of local anesthetic, aspirating intermittently.

   d. Sciatic block at the knee (Fig. 17.18). With the patient prone, flex the knee 30°. This outlines the borders of the popliteal fossa, which is bounded by the knee crease inferiorly, the long head of the biceps femoris laterally, and the superimposed tendons of the semimembranosus and semitendinosus muscles medially. Draw a vertical line on the skin, dividing the fossa into two equilateral triangles. Insert a needle 6 cm superior to the knee crease and 1 cm lateral to the line bisecting the fossa. Use a nerve stimulator to localize the nerve and inject 30 to 40 mL of local anesthetic, aspirating intermittently.

     (1) Sciatic nerve block at the knee using ultrasound guidance is performed with the patient preferably prone. The probe is placed at the level of the popliteal crease, and the popliteal artery should be seen in cross section. The artery is then followed cephalad 5 to 7 cm. The popliteal vein lies superficial and lateral to the artery, and the sciatic nerve lies even more superficial and lateral to the vein. The sciatic nerve appears as a bright, hyperechoic structure 10 to 18 mm in diameter (Fig. 17.19). The semimembranosus muscle is seen medial and the biceps femoris is seen lateral to the nerve. These muscles become more prominent with cephalad movement of the probe. The nerve should be followed caudad to ensure that it has not yet divided into the tibial and common peroneal nerves. With the sciatic nerve in the center of the image, a needle insertion site is chosen approximately 1 inch lateral to the probe and is infiltrated with local anesthetic. A 22-gauge 80-mm block needle is appropriate (although larger 17- to 20-gauge needles may be needed for more muscular or obese patients) and is inserted and advanced at a 45° angle to the skin until the tip is positioned at the 12 o'clock position of the sciatic nerve. After aspiration is performed and deemed negative for blood, 15 to 20 mL of local anesthetic is injected. Note that motor stimulation is *not* required provided the anatomy and spread of local anesthetic are easily appreciated. In fact, it has been observed that motor nerve response is generally not elicited until the needle tip is actually *impinging* upon the nerve.

8. Saphenous nerve block. The saphenous nerve (femoral) can be blocked at the ankle (see section VIII.C.9) or at the knee. At the knee, inject 10 mL of local anesthetic in the deep

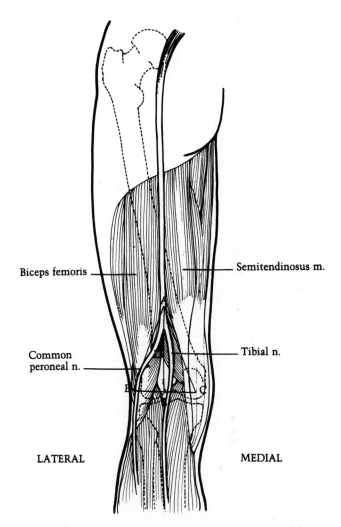

Figure 17.18. Popliteal fossa block. The two major trunks of the sciatic nerve bifurcate in the popliteal fossa 7 to 10 cm above the knee. A triangle is drawn using the heads of the biceps femoris and the semitendinosus muscles and the skin crease of the knee; a long needle is inserted 1 cm lateral to a point 6 cm cephalad on the line from the skin crease that bisects this triangle. (From Mulroy MF. *Regional anesthesia*. Boston: Little, Brown, 1989.)

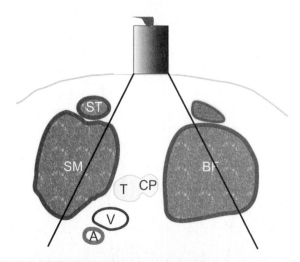

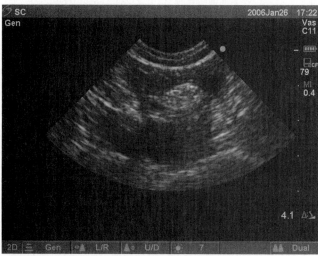

Figure 17.19.   Sciatic nerve block at the knee using ultrasound guidance. T = tibial nerve; CP = common peroneal nerve; SM = semimembranosus muscle; BF = biceps femoris muscle; ST = semitendinosus muscle; A = popliteal artery; V = popliteal vein.

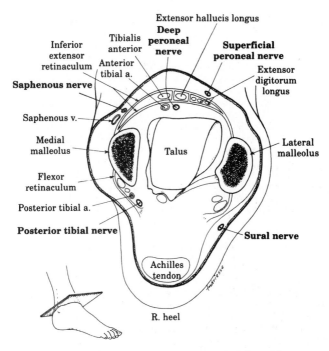

Figure 17.20. **Cross section at the level of the ankle.**

subcutaneous tissue, extending from the medial surface of the tibial condyle to the superimposed tendons of the semimembranosus and semitendinosus muscles.

9. **Ankle block** (Fig. 17.20)

   a. The five nerves supplying the foot can be blocked at the ankle. Elevate the foot on a pillow to provide easy access to both sides of the ankle.

   b. At the superior border of the malleoli, the **deep peroneal nerve** is situated between the anterior tibialis tendon and the extensor hallucis longus tendon, which are easily palpable with dorsiflexion of the foot and extension of the great toe. Insert a 1.5-inch needle just lateral to the anterior tibial artery between the two tendons until contacting the tibia and then withdraw the needle while depositing 5 to 10 mL of local anesthetic.

   c. Then, inject a 10-mL volume of local anesthetic subcutaneously across the anterior surface of the tibia, from malleolus to malleolus. This will block the **superficial peroneal nerve** laterally and the **saphenous nerve** medially.

   d. To block the **posterior tibial nerve,** insert a needle posterior to the medial malleolus, directed toward the inferior border of the posterior tibial artery. A paresthesia may be noted in the sole of the foot. Withdraw the needle 1 cm from the point of bony contact and inject 5 to 10 mL of local anesthetic in a fan-shaped area.

e. Block the **sural nerve** by inserting the needle midway between the Achilles tendon and the lateral malleolus, directing it toward the posterior surface of the lateral malleolus. After contacting bone, withdraw the needle and inject 5 mL of local anesthetic.

D. **Complications of lower extremity blocks** include epidural blockade with potential sympathectomy (psoas block), intravascular injection, inadvertent arterial puncture, and neural trauma (particularly if a paresthesia technique was performed).

SUGGESTED READINGS

Bailey SL, Parkinson SK, Little WL, et al. Sciatic nerve block. A comparison of single versus double injection technique. *Reg Anesth* 1994;19:9–13.

Cousins MJ, Bridenbaugh PO. *Neural blockade in clinical anesthesia and management of pain*, 3rd ed. Philadelphia: Lippincott-Raven, 1998.

Dalens B, Vanneuville G, Tanguy A. Comparison of the fascia iliaca compartment block with the 3-in-1 block in children. *Anesth Analg* 1989;69:705–713.

De Andres J, Sala-Blanch X. Peripheral nerve stimulation in the practice of brachial plexus anesthesia: a review. *Reg Anesth Pain Med* 2001;26:478–483.

Franco CD, Vieira ZEG. 1,001 subclavian perivascular brachial plexus blocks: success with a nerve stimulator. *Reg Anesth Pain Med* 2000;25:41–46.

Henderson CL, Warriner CB, McEwen JA, et al. A North American survey of intravenous regional anesthesia. *Anesth Analg* 1997;85:858–863.

Lanz E, Theiss D, Jankovic D. The extent of blockade following various techniques of brachial plexus block. *Anesth Analg* 1983;62:55–58.

Mulroy MF. *Regional anesthesia: an illustrated procedural guide*, 2nd ed. Philadelphia: Lippincott Williams & Wilkins, 1996.

Parkinson SK, Mueller JB, Little WL, et al. Extent of blockade with various approaches to the lumbar plexus. *Anesth Analg* 1989;68:243–248.

Pham-Dang C, Gunst J-P, Gouin F, et al. A novel supraclavicular approach to brachial plexus block. *Anesth Analg* 1997;85:111–116.

Raj PP. *Textbook of regional anesthesia*. New York: Churchill Livingstone, 2002.

Rorie DK, Byer DE, Nelson DO, et al. Assessment of block of the sciatic nerve in the popliteal fossa. *Anesth Analg* 1980;59:371–376.

Schroeder LE, Horlocker TT, Schroeder DR. The efficacy of axillary block for surgical procedures about the elbow. *Anesth Analg* 1996;83:747–751.

Scott DB, Hakansson L, Buckhoj P. *Techniques of regional anesthesia*. New York: McGraw-Hill, 1996.

Stan TC, Krantz MA, Solomon DL, et al. The incidence of neurovascular complications following axillary brachial plexus block using a transarterial approach. A prospective study of 1,000 consecutive patients. *Reg Anesth* 1995;20:486–492.

Urban MK, Urquhart B. Evaluation of brachial plexus anesthesia for upper extremity surgery. *Reg Anesth* 1994;19:175–182.

Vloka JD, Hadzic A, April E, et al. The division of the sciatic nerve in the popliteal fossa: anatomical implications for popliteal nerve blockade. *Anesth Analg* 2001;92:215–217.

Vongvises P, Panijayanond T. A parascalene technique of brachial plexus anesthesia. *Anesth Analg* 1979;58:267–273.

Wedel DJ. Nerve blocks. In: Miller RD, ed. *Anesthesia*, 5th ed. New York: Churchill Livingstone, 2000:1520–1548.

Wildsmith JAW, Armitage EN. *Principles and practice of regional anesthesia*, 2nd ed. Edinburgh: Churchill Livingstone, 1993.

18

Intra-anesthetic Problems

Deborah Stadfelt and Keith Baker

I. **Hypotension** is a significant decrease of arterial blood pressure below the patient's normal range. It may be due to a decrease in cardiac function (contractility), systemic vascular resistance (SVR), venous return, or dysrhythmias.

A. **Contractility**

   1. Most anesthetic agents, including inhalation agents, barbiturates, and benzodiazepines (see Chapter 11), cause dose-dependent direct myocardial depression. **Opiates** are not direct myocardial depressants in usual clinical doses.

   2. **Cardiac medications,** such as β-adrenergic antagonists, calcium channel blockers, and lidocaine, are myocardial depressants.

   3. **Acute cardiac dysfunction** may occur with myocardial ischemia or myocardial infarction (MI), hypocalcemia, severe acidosis or alkalosis, hypothermia less than $32°C$, cor pulmonale, vagal reflexes, and systemic toxicity from local anesthetics (particularly bupivacaine).

B. **Decreased SVR**

   1. **A decrease in SVR can be seen with many of the drugs used during anesthesia.**

      a. **Isoflurane** and, to a lesser extent, sevoflurane and desflurane produce a decrease in SVR.

      b. **Opiates** and propofol produce loss of vascular tone by reducing sympathetic nervous system outflow.

      c. **Benzodiazepines** may decrease SVR, particularly when administered at high doses with opiates.

      d. **Direct vasodilators** (e.g., nitroprusside, nitroglycerin, hydralazine).

      e. α-**Adrenergic blockers** (e.g., droperidol, chlorpromazine, phentolamine, labetalol).

      f. α-**Adrenergic agonists** (clonidine)

      g. **Histamine-releasing medications** (e.g., d-tubocurarine, mivacurium, morphine).

      h. **Ganglionic inhibitors** (e.g., trimethaphan).

      i. **Calcium channel blockers.**

      j. **Angiotensin-converting enzyme inhibitors and angiotensin receptor blockers.**

      k. **Milrinone**

   2. **Sympathetic blockade** frequently occurs during spinal and epidural anesthesia, leading to a decreased SVR.

   3. **Sepsis** causes release of vasoactive substances that mediate hypotension.

   4. **Vasoactive metabolites** (e.g., after bowel manipulation or tourniquet release) may cause hypotension.

   5. **Allergic reactions** (see section XVIII) may cause profound hypotension.

6. **Profound hypoxia**
7. **Adrenal insufficiency**

C. **Inadequate venous return**

1. **Hypovolemia** may be caused by blood loss, insensible evaporative losses, preoperative deficits (e.g., nothing-by-mouth status, vomiting, diarrhea, nasogastric tube suction, enteric drains, and bowel preparations), or polyuria (as a result of diuretics, diabetes mellitus, diabetes insipidus, or postobstructive diuresis).

2. **Caval compression** may result from surgical maneuvers, a gravid uterus, or increased intra-abdominal pressures during laparascopy.

3. **Increased venous capacitance** may occur with the following:
   a. Sympathetic blockade (e.g., ganglionic blockers or regional anesthesia)
   b. Direct vasodilators (e.g., nitroglycerin)
   c. Histamine-releasing medications (morphine, mivacurium, *d*-tubocurarine)
   d. Medications that reduce sympathetic outflow (e.g., barbiturates, propofol, and inhalational agents).

4. **Increased intrathoracic pressure** during mechanical ventilation with large tidal volumes, positive end-expiratory pressure (PEEP), or auto-PEEP (air trapping or dynamic hyperinflation) will impair venous return.

5. **Conditions with elevated central venous pressure**
   a. **Tension pneumothorax** causes a shift of the mediastinum, leading to compression of the heart and great vessels. This results in an elevated central venous pressure, decreased preload, and severe hypotension.
   b. **Cardiac tamponade** is a collection of fluid in the pericardial space causing compression of the heart, resulting in decreased filling secondary to elevated intracardiac pressures.

D. **Dysrhythmias (also see section III)**

1. **Tachydysrhythmias** often result in hypotension secondary to a decreased diastolic filling time.

2. **Atrial fibrillation, atrial flutter, and junctional rhythms** cause hypotension from loss of the atrial contribution to diastolic filling. This is particularly pronounced in patients with valvular heart disease or diastolic dysfunction, in whom atrial contraction may augment end-diastolic volume by more than 30%.

3. **Bradydysrhythmias** may cause hypotension if preload reserve is inadequate to maintain a compensatory increase in stroke volume.

E. **Treatment of hypotension** should be directed toward correcting the underlying cause and may include the following:

1. **Decreasing anesthetic depth**
2. **Volume expansion**
3. **Vasopressor support** to increase vascular resistance or decrease venous capacitance (e.g., phenylephrine, vasopressin if acidemic) and increase stroke volume (e.g., epinephrine).
4. **Correction of mechanical causes,** such as relief of pericardial tamponade, placement of a chest tube for

pneumothorax, reducing or eliminating PEEP, decreasing mean airway pressure, or relieving obstruction of the vena cava (e.g., left uterine displacement for a pregnant patient).

5. **Antidysrhythmic (see section III) or antiischemic medical therapy,** which may include beta blockers, calcium channel blockers, and amiodarone.

6. Inotropic support (e.g., dobutamine, dopamine, norepinephrine, epinephrine).

II. Hypertension

A. Etiologies

1. **Catecholamine excess,** which may be seen with inadequate anesthesia (especially during laryngoscopy, intubation, incision, and emergence), hypoxia, hypercarbia, patient anxiety, pain, and prolonged tourniquet use.

2. **Preexisting disease** (e.g., essential hypertension or pheochromocytoma).

3. **Increased intracranial pressure**

4. **Systemic absorption of vasoconstrictors** such as epinephrine and phenylephrine.

5. **Aortic cross-clamping**

6. **Rebound hypertension** from discontinuation of clonidine or β-adrenergic blockers.

7. **Drug–drug interactions.** Tricyclic antidepressants and monoamine oxidase inhibitors given with ephedrine may cause an exaggerated hypertensive response.

8. **Bladder distention**

9. **Administration of indigo carmine dye** (via an α-adrenergic effect).

B. Treatment of hypertension is directed toward correcting the underlying cause and may include the following:

1. Improving oxygenation and ventilatory abnormalities.

2. Increasing the depth of anesthesia.

3. Sedating an anxious patient or emptying a full bladder.

4. **Medications** (for further discussion, see Chapter 19).

   a. **β-Adrenergic blocking agents** (e.g., labetalol, 5- to 10-mg increments intravenously [IV]; propranolol, 0.5- to 1.0-mg increments IV; or esmolol, 5- to 10-mg increments IV).

   b. **Vasodilators** (e.g., hydralazine, 2.5- to 5-mg increments IV; nitroglycerin infusion starting at 30 to 50 μg/min IV and titrating to effect; nitroprusside infusion, 30 to 50 μg/min IV and titrating to effect.

   c. **Calcium channel blockers** (e.g., verapamil 2.5 to 5 mg IV, diltiazem 5 to 10 mg IV).

III. Dysrhythmias

A. Sinus bradycardia is a sinus node-driven heart rate of less than 60 beats/min. Unless there is severe underlying heart disease, hemodynamic changes are minimal. With slow rates, atrial and ventricular ectopic escape beats or rhythms may occur.

1. **Etiologies**

   a. **Hypoxia**

   b. **Intrinsic cardiac disease** such as sick sinus syndrome or acute MI (particularly inferior wall MI).

   c. **Medications** such as succinylcholine (especially in young children), anticholinesterases, β-adrenergic blockers, calcium channel blockers, digoxin, and narcotics.

d. **Increased vagal tone** occurs with traction on the peritoneum or spermatic cord, the oculocardiac reflex, direct pressure on the vagus nerve or carotid sinus during neck or intrathoracic surgery, centrally mediated vagal response from anxiety or pain, and Valsalva maneuvers.

e. **Increased intracranial pressure**

2. **Treatment of sinus bradycardia**

   a. Verify adequate oxygenation and ventilation.

   b. Bradycardia due to increased vagal tone requires discontinuation of the provocative stimulus. Atropine (0.5 mg IV) or epinephrine may be needed if the circulation is unstable. Glycopyrolate (0.2 to 0.6 mg IV) may be given for hemodynamically stable bradycardia.

   c. In patients with intrinsic cardiac disease, treatment should proceed with atropine (0.5 mg IV), chronotropes (e.g., ephedrine, dopamine), or cardiac pacing.

B. **Sinus tachycardia** is a sinus node-driven heart rate greater than 100 beats/min. The rate is regular and rarely exceeds 160 beats/min.

1. **Etiologies** include catecholamine excess, pain or light anesthesia, hypercarbia, hypoxia, hypotension, hypovolemia, medications (e.g., pancuronium, desflurane, atropine, ephedrine), fever, MI, pulmonary embolism, malignant hyperthermia, pheochromocytoma, and thyrotoxicosis.

2. **Treatment** should be directed toward correcting the underlying cause and may include the following:

   a. Correcting oxygenation and ventilatory abnormalities.

   b. Increasing the depth of anesthesia.

   c. Correcting hypovolemia.

   d. Medications such as narcotics and β-adrenergic blockers. Patients with active coronary artery disease and adequate blood pressure may benefit by treatment with β-adrenergic blockers to control heart rate while the cause is being determined.

C. **Heart block**

1. **First-degree atrioventricular (A-V) block** is prolongation of the PR interval for 0.2 second or longer. In first-degree block, every atrial pulse is transmitted to the ventricle.

2. **Second-degree A-V block** is divided into two types: Mobitz 1 (Wenckebach) and Mobitz 2.

   a. **Mobitz 1** usually occurs when a conduction defect is in the A-V node and is manifest by a progressive PR prolongation culminating in a nonconducted P wave. It is generally benign.

   b. **Mobitz 2** is a block in or distal to the A-V node with a constant PR interval and with randomly nonconducted P waves. It is more likely to progress to third-degree block.

3. **Third-degree heart block is** usually due to lesions distal to the His bundle and is characterized by the absence of

A-V conduction. Usually, a slow ventricular rate is seen (fewer than 45 beats/minute). P waves occur regularly but are independent of QRS complexes (A-V dissociation).

4. **Treatment** of heart block
   a. **First-degree heart block** does not usually require specific treatment. First-degree heart block in combination with a bifascicular block may warrant temporary pacing.
   b. **Second-degree heart block**
      (1) **Mobitz 1** requires treatment only if symptomatic bradycardia, congestive heart failure, or bundle branch block occurs. Transcutaneous or transvenous pacing may be necessary, particularly during inferior MIs.
      (2) **Mobitz 2** may progress to complete heart block, thus necessitating the use of a pacemaker.
   c. **Third-degree heart block** usually necessitates transcutaneous or transvenous pacing.

D. **Supraventricular tachycardias** originate at or above the bundle of His, and the resulting QRS complexes are narrow except during aberrant conduction.
   1. **Atrial premature contractions (APCs)** occur when ectopic foci in the atria fire before the next expected impulse from the sinus node. The P wave of an APC characteristically looks different from preceding P waves, and the PR interval may vary from normal. Early APCs may cause aberrant QRS complexes or be nonconducted to the ventricle if it is still in a refractory period. APCs are common, usually benign, and usually require no treatment.
   2. **Junctional or A-V nodal rhythms** are characterized by absent or abnormal P waves and normal QRS complexes. Although they may indicate ischemic cardiac disease, junctional rhythms are commonly seen in normal individuals receiving inhalation anesthesia. In the patient whose cardiac output depends heavily on the contribution from atrial contraction, stroke volume and blood pressure may decline precipitously. Treatment may include the following:
      a. Reduction of anesthetic depth.
      b. Increasing intravascular volume.
      c. Atropine in increments of 0.2 mg IV may convert a slow junctional rhythm to sinus rhythm, particularly if secondary to a vagal mechanism.
      d. Paradoxically, beta blockers may be used cautiously (propranolol, 0.5 mg IV; metoprolol, 1 to 3 mg).
      e. If the dysrhythmia is associated with hypotension, increasing the blood pressure with vasopressors (e.g., ephedrine or norepinephrine) may be required as a temporizing measure.
      f. If necessary, atrial pacing may be instituted to restore atrial contraction.
   3. **Atrial fibrillation** is an irregular rhythm with an atrial rate of 350 to 600 beats/min and a variable ventricular response. It may be seen with myocardial ischemia, mitral valvular disease, hyperthyroidism, excessive sympathetic stimulation, digitalis toxicity, after thoracic surgery, or when the heart

has been manipulated. Treatment is based on the hemodynamic status.

a. **Rapid ventricular rate with stable hemodynamics** can be treated initially with β-adrenergic blockade, such as propranolol (0.5-mg increments IV), metoprolol (2.5- to 5-mg increments), esmolol (5- to 10-mg increments), or a calcium channel blocker such as verapamil (2.5- to 5-mg increments) or diltiazem (10 to 20 mg IV). (see Chapter 37).

b. **Rapid ventricular rate with unstable hemodynamics** requires unsynchronized cardioversion. (360 J if monophasic or 150 to 200 J if biphasic) (see Chapter 37).

4. **Atrial flutter** is usually a regular rhythm with an atrial rate of 250 to 350 beats/min and a characteristic sawtooth electrocardiogram (ECG) configuration. It is often seen with underlying heart disease (i.e., rheumatic heart disease and mitral stenosis). A 2:1 block will result in a rapid ventricular rate (usually 150 beats/min). Treatment usually includes β-adrenergic or calcium channel blockade or synchronized cardioversion (see Chapter 37).

5. **Paroxysmal supraventricular tachycardia** is a tachydysrhythmia (atrial and ventricular rates of 150 to 250 beats/min) with reentry usually through the A-V node. This rhythm may be associated with **Wolff-Parkinson-White syndrome,** thyrotoxicosis, or mitral valve prolapse. Patients without heart disease may develop this dysrhythmia due to stress, caffeine, or excess catecholamines. Treatment includes **adenosine** (6 to 18 mg IV, 3 mg if given centrally), carotid sinus massage, or propranolol (1 to 2 mg IV). Synchronized cardioversion may be required for the hemodynamically unstable patient (also see Chapter 37).

E. **Ventricular dysrhythmias**

1. **Ventricular premature contractions (VPCs)** occur when ectopic foci in the ventricle fire before the next expected impulse arrives. They are characterized by widened QRS complexes. When coupled alternately with normal beats, ventricular bigeminy exists. VPCs are occasionally seen in normal individuals. Under anesthesia, they frequently occur during states of catecholamine excess, hypoxia, or hypercarbia. They may also signify myocardial ischemia or infarction, digitalis toxicity, or hypokalemia. **VPCs may require therapy when they are multifocal, occur in runs, increase in frequency, or occur on or near the preceding T wave (R-on-T phenomenon);** these situations may precede the development of ventricular tachycardia, ventricular fibrillation, and cardiac arrest. Treatment in an otherwise healthy individual may include deepening anesthesia and ensuring adequate oxygenation and ventilation. Patients with coronary artery disease who continue to have ventricular irritability should have the ischemia treated. If the ectopy continues, then **lidocaine** may be given, 1 mg/kg IV, followed by a lidocaine infusion at 1 to 2 mg/min.

Refractory ventricular ectopy may require further treatment (see Chapter 37).

2. **Ventricular tachycardia** is a wide-complex tachydysrhythmia at a rate of 150 to 250 beats/min. Unstable patients should be treated with cardiopulmonary resuscitation and cardioversion (360 J if monophasic or 150 or 200 J if biphasic). For stable patients the first-line treatment depends on whether the ventricular tachycardia is monomorphic or polymorphic. (If polymorphic, treat as if unstable.) In addition, the treatment may depend on the ejection fraction (see Chapter 37 for specific recommendations).

3. **Ventricular fibrillation** is chaotic ventricular activity resulting in ineffective ventricular contractions. Defibrillation and cardiopulmonary resuscitation are required (see Chapter 37 for specific recommendations).

4. **Ventricular preexcitation.** Wolff-Parkinson-White syndrome is due to an accessory pathway connecting the atria and ventricle. The most common mechanism is characterized by antegrade conduction through the normal A-V conduction system and retrograde conduction through the accessory pathway. Characteristic ECG findings include a short PR interval and a slurred delta wave at the onset of the QRS. Tachydysrhythmias are common. Treatment depends on whether the patient is hemodynamically stable (see Chapter 37). Unstable patients should receive synchronized cardioversion starting at 50 J (monophasic or biphasic). These patients are at high risk for ventricular fibrillation.

IV. **Hypoxemia** occurs when oxygen delivery to the tissues is insufficient to meet their metabolic demands.

A. **Intraoperative etiologies**

1. **Inadequate oxygen supply**

   a. Empty reserve oxygen tanks with loss of the main pipeline supply.

   b. An oxygen flowmeter that is not turned to a sufficient flow.

   c. Breathing system disconnection.

   d. Large leaks in the anesthesia machine, ventilator, carbon dioxide absorber, breathing circuit, or around the endotracheal tube. This may be managed acutely by using a self-inflating (Ambu) bag to deliver oxygen to the patient.

   e. Obstructed endotracheal tube.

   f. Malpositioned endotracheal tubes (e.g., esophageal or mainstem bronchial intubation).

2. **Hypoventilation** (see section V)

3. **Ventilation-perfusion inequalities or shunting**

   a. **Pulmonary**—as seen with atelectasis, pneumonia, pulmonary edema, aspiration, pneumothorax, bronchospasm, and other parenchymal pathologic states. In some cases, these inequalities may be corrected by increasing mean airway pressure or applying PEEP.

   b. **Cardiac**—Right-to-left cardiac shunt, as in tetralogy of fallot.

4. **Reduction in oxygen-carrying capacity.** Oxygen-carrying capacity is reduced with anemia, carbon monoxide poisoning, methemoglobinemia, and hemoglobinopathies despite a normal oxygen saturation as measured by pulse oximetry.

5. **Leftward shift of the hemoglobin-oxygen dissociation curve** results from hypothermia, decreased 2,3-diphosphoglycerate concentration, alkalosis, hypocarbia, and carbon monoxide poisoning.

B. **Treatment of hypoxemia**

1. If the patient is being mechanically ventilated, begin manual ventilation with 100% oxygen to assess pulmonary compliance. Evaluate breath sounds, check the surgical field for mechanical pressure on the airway, examine the endotracheal tube for obstruction or dislodgement, and confirm adequate movement of the chest wall or diaphragm. Elevated peak airway pressures may indicate bronchospasm, pneumothorax, or endobronchial intubation.

2. The breathing circuit, ventilator, and anesthesia machine should be checked for leaks. If present, ventilation should be started with 100% oxygen via an alternative source such as a self-inflating bag until the problem is rectified.

3. Adequate oxygen delivery to the patient should be confirmed with an in-line oxygen analyzer.

4. Further treatment is outlined in Chapter 36.

V. **Hypercarbia** is due either to inadequate ventilation or to increased carbon dioxide production and can lead to respiratory acidosis, increased pulmonary artery pressure, and increased intracranial pressure.

A. **Inadequate ventilation**

1. **Central depression of the medullary respiratory center** can be caused by medications (e.g., opioids, barbiturates, benzodiazepines, and volatile agents) or primary central nervous system pathology (e.g., tumor, ischemia, edema). Controlled ventilation or reversal agents (e.g., naloxone and flumazenil) may be required.

2. **Neuromuscular depression** may be seen with high spinal anesthesia, phrenic nerve paralysis, and muscle relaxants.

3. **Inappropriate ventilator settings** may result in a low minute ventilation.

4. **Increased airway resistance** may occur with bronchospasm, upper airway obstruction, mainstem intubation, kinked endotracheal tubes, severe chronic obstructive lung disease, congestive heart failure, and hemothorax or pneumothorax.

5. **Rebreathing of exhaled gases** may occur due to an exhausted carbon dioxide absorber, inspiratory or expiratory valve failure, or inadequate fresh gas flows in nonrebreathing systems.

B. **Increased carbon dioxide production** results from exogenous carbon dioxide (e.g., absorption of carbon dioxide from insufflation during laparoscopy), reperfusion, and hypermetabolic states (e.g., malignant hyperthermia).

C. **Treatment of hypercarbia** depends on the cause. Depending on the etiology, treatment may include increasing minute ventilation, respositioning the endotracheal tube, suctioning, treatment of bronchospasm, diuresis, or placing a chest tube.

VI. Abnormal urine output

   A. Oliguria is defined as urine output less than 0.5 mL/kg/hour. Prerenal, intrarenal, and postrenal causes are described in Chapter 4.

   1. Treatment includes ruling out mechanical causes (e.g., malpositioned or kinked Foley catheter).

   2. Hypotension should be corrected to improve renal perfusion pressure.

   3. Volume status should be assessed. A fluid bolus may be given if hypovolemia is suspected. If oliguria persists, central venous pressure measurement may help guide further fluid management. Patients with reduced ventricular function may require placement of a pulmonary artery catheter. Echocardiography may also help assess volume status.

   4. If oliguria persists despite an adequate volume status, urine output can be increased with the following:

   a. Furosemide, 2 to 20 mg IV.

   b. Dopamine infusion, 1 to 3 μg/kg/min IV.

   c. Mannitol, 12.5 to 25.0 g IV.

   d. Fenoldapam, 0.1 μg/kg/min to 0.4 μg/kg/min IV.

   5. Intraoperative diuretics may be required to preserve urine output in patients on chronic diuretic therapy.

   B. Anuria is a rare occurrence in the perioperative period. Mechanical causes, including Foley catheter malfunction or ureteral damage or transection, must be excluded and hemodynamic instability must be treated.

   C. High urine output may occur in response to vigorous fluid administration, but other causes must be considered, including hyperglycemia, diabetes insipidus, and exogenous diuretic administration. High urine output is not a problem unless associated with hypovolemia or electrolyte abnormalities. Treatment should be directed at the underlying cause, maintaining volume status, and correcting electrolyte abnormalities.

VII. Hypothermia is a common problem in the operative period.

   A. Heat loss may occur from any of the following mechanisms:

   1. Redistribution of heat from core areas (brain, heart, etc.) to peripheral tissues (limbs, skin, etc.). Redistribution results in a reduction in the core temperature with maintenance of the mean body temperature.

   2. Radiation. Radiant heat loss depends on cutaneous blood flow and exposed body surface area.

   3. Evaporation. Energy is lost as liquid vaporizes from mucosal and serosal surfaces, skin, and lungs. Evaporative losses depend on the exposed surface area and the relative humidity of ambient gas.

   4. Conduction, which is heat transfer from a warm to a cool object. This heat loss is proportional to the area exposed, difference in temperature, and thermal conductivity.

   5. Convection, which is the loss of heat by conduction to a moving gas. High air flow rates in the operating rooms (10 to 15 room volume changes per hour) may result in significant heat loss.

B. **Pediatric patients** are particularly susceptible to intraoperative hypothermia (see Chapter 29).

C. **Geriatric patients** are also more prone to hypothermia (see Chapter 27).

D. **Anesthetic effects.** Volatile anesthetics impair the thermoregulatory center located in the posterior hypothalamus and predispose to heat redistribution and heat loss due to their vasodilatory properties. Opioids will reduce the vasoconstriction mechanism for heat conservation because of their sympatholytic properties. Muscle relaxants reduce muscle tone and prevent shivering. Regional anesthesia produces sympathetic blockade, muscle relaxation, and sensory blockade of thermal receptors, which inhibit compensatory responses.

E. **Severe hypothermia** is associated with a number of physiologic changes:

1. **Cardiovascular.** Increased SVR, ventricular dysrhythmias, and myocardial depression may occur with severe hypothermia.

2. **Metabolic.** Decreased metabolic rate and decreased tissue perfusion (from catecholamine response) may occur.

3. **Hematologic.** Increased blood viscosity, leftward shift of the hemoglobin dissociation curve, impaired coagulation, and platelet dysfunction occur.

4. **Neurologic.** Decreased cerebral blood flow, increased cerebrovascular resistance, decreased minimum alveolar concentration, delayed emergence from anesthesia, drowsiness, and confusion may occur.

5. **Drug disposition.** Decreased hepatic blood flow and metabolism coupled with decreased renal blood flow and clearance result in decreased anesthetic requirement.

6. **Shivering** can increase heat production by 100% to 300% but with a concomitant increase in oxygen consumption of up to 500% and increased carbon dioxide production.

F. **Prevention and treatment of hypothermia**

1. **Maintain or increase ambient temperature.** Anesthetized patients frequently become hypothermic if the room temperature is below 21°C.

2. **Covering exposed surfaces** will minimize conductive and convective losses. Forced warmed air blankets (e.g., Bair Hugger and others) placed over the patient can provide both insulation and active warming.

3. **Warming transfused fluids and blood** is essential in cases with large fluid requirements (see Chapter 14).

4. **Use of closed or low-flow semiclosed circuit anesthesia** will decrease evaporative losses and modestly reduce heat loss.

5. **Heated humidifiers** added to the anesthetic circuit when high gas flow rates are used. These will warm and humidify inspired gas, minimizing evaporative loss from the lungs. The temperature of inspired gas must be monitored and kept below 41°C; otherwise, there is potential for airway burns. Alternatively, "artificial noses" (**passive heat and moisture exchangers**) can be placed between the endotracheal tube and the breathing circuit. These are hygroscopic

membrane filters with large surface areas that trap the humidity of expired air.

6. **Warming blankets** placed beneath the patient can increase body temperature by conduction from warm water pumped through the blanket. This method is most effective in children weighing less than 10 kg. The temperature should be kept below 40°C to avoid burns.

7. **Radiant warmers and heating lamps** warm patients by infrared radiation and are useful only for infants. The warming lamps should be kept at least 70 cm from the patient to avoid burns.

8. **Warming irrigation solutions** will reduce heat loss.

VIII. **Hyperthermia** is an increase in temperature of 2°C/hour or 0.5°C/15 min. It is uncommon for a patient to become hyperthermic because of maneuvers to conserve body heat in the operating room; therefore, any increase in temperature must be investigated. Hyperthermia and its accompanying hypermetabolic state produce an increase in oxygen consumption, cardiac work, glucose demand, and compensatory minute ventilation. Sweating and vasodilation will result in decreased intravascular volume and venous return.

A. **Etiologies**

1. **Malignant hyperthermia** must be considered during any perioperative temperature increase (see section XVII).

2. **Inflammation, infection, and sepsis** with release of inflammatory mediators may cause hyperthermia.

3. **Hypermetabolic states** such as thyrotoxicosis and pheochromocytoma may cause hyperthermia.

4. **Injury to the hypothalamic thermoregulatory center** from anoxia, edema, trauma, or tumor may affect temperature set points in the hypothalamus.

5. **Neuroleptic malignant syndrome** (NMS) from neuroleptics such as phenothiazines is a rare cause.

6. **Sympathomimetics** such as monoamine oxidase inhibitors, amphetamines, cocaine, and tricyclic antidepressants may produce a hypermetabolic state.

7. **Anticholinergics,** such as atropine, may suppress sweating.

B. **Treatment**

1. **If malignant hyperthermia is suspected,** dantrolene treatment must be initiated (see section XVII).

2. **Severe hyperthermia** can be treated by cooling exposed body surfaces (skin) with ice, cooling blankets, and reduced ambient temperature or by performing internal lavage (stomach, bladder, bowel, and peritoneum) with cold saline. Volatile liquids, such as alcohol, applied to the skin will promote evaporative heat loss. Conductive heat loss can be increased with vasodilators such as nitroprusside and nitroglycerin. Centrally active agents such as aspirin and acetaminophen can be given by nasogastric tube or rectally. Shivering can be prevented by maintaining neuromuscular blockade. When hyperthermia is profound, **extracorporeal cooling** can be used. Cooling should be stopped when body temperature reaches 38°C to avoid hypothermia.

IX. **Diaphoresis (sweating)** may occur in response to the sympathetic discharge caused by anxiety, pain, hypercarbia, or noxious stimuli in the presence of inadequate anesthesia. It may also be seen in conjunction with bradycardia, nausea, and hypotension as part of a generalized vagal reaction or as a thermoregulatory response to hyperthermia.

X. **Laryngospasm**

A. **Laryngospasm** is most commonly caused by an irritative stimulus to the airway during a light plane of anesthesia. Common noxious stimuli that may elicit this reflex include secretions, vomitus, blood, inhalation of pungent volatile anesthetics, oropharyngeal or nasopharyngeal airway placement, laryngoscopy, painful peripheral stimuli, and peritoneal traction during light anesthesia.

B. **Reflex closure of the vocal cords,** causing partial or total glottic obstruction, may be manifest in less severe cases by "crowing" respirations or stridor and, when complete, by a "rocking" obstructed pattern of breathing. In this situation, the abdominal wall rises with contraction of the diaphragm during inspiration, but because air entry is blocked the chest retracts or fails to expand. During attempted expiration, the abdomen falls as the diaphragm relaxes and the chest returns to its original position. With complete obstruction, the anesthetist will not be able to ventilate the patient.

C. The hypoxia, hypercarbia, and acidosis that result can cause hypertension and tachycardia. Hypotension, bradycardia, and ventricular dysrhythmias leading to cardiac arrest will ensue unless airway patency is restored within minutes. Children are particularly prone to these complications because of their small functional residual capacity and relatively high oxygen consumption.

D. **Treatment.** Deepening the anesthetic level and removing the stimulus (e.g., by suction, withdrawal of an artificial airway, or stopping peripheral stimulation) while administering 100% oxygen may be adequate to relieve laryngospasm. If laryngospasm is not relieved, **continuous positive pressure on the airway** with a jaw thrust may relieve the spasm; if not, a small dose of **succinylcholine** (e.g., 10 to 20 mg IV in an adult) will relax the striated muscles of the larynx. The lungs should be ventilated with 100% oxygen, and either the anesthetic level should be deepened before the noxious stimulation is resumed or the patient may be allowed to awaken if laryngospasm has occurred during emergence.

XI. **Bronchospasm**

A. **Reflex bronchiolar constriction** may be centrally mediated or may be a local response to airway irritation. Bronchospasm is common in anaphylactoid drug and blood transfusion reactions as well as in cigarette smokers and those with chronic bronchitis. Like laryngospasm, bronchospasm may be elicited by noxious stimuli such as secretions and endotracheal intubation.

B. **Wheezing** (usually more pronounced on expiration) characterizes bronchospasm and is associated with tachypnea and dyspnea in the awake patient. An anesthetized patient may be difficult to ventilate because of increased airway resistance. Decreased expiratory flow rates may produce air trapping and increase intrathoracic pressure, decreasing venous return, cardiac output, and blood pressure. The end tidal carbon dioxide curves often have an obstructive pattern (continual rise) during exhalation.

C. **Histamine-releasing drugs** (e.g., morphine, mivacurium, *d*-tubocurarine, atracurium) may exacerbate bronchoconstriction.

D. **Treatment**

1. The **endotracheal tube position** should be checked and, if carinal stimulation is the cause, withdrawn slightly.

2. **Deepening the anesthetic level** will frequently reverse bronchospasm that is secondary to "light anesthesia." This usually can be accomplished with an inhalation agent, but an IV agent may be necessary when ventilation is significantly impaired. Propofol produces fewer symptoms of bronchoconstriction than barbiturates and is usually preferable. Ketamine has the advantage of causing bronchodilatation by releasing endogenous catecholamines. The inspired oxygen concentration should be increased until adequate oxygenation is achieved.

3. **Medical treatment** includes administering inhaled or intravenous β_2-adrenergic agonists and anticholinergics (see Chapter 3). Inhaled bronchodilators have limited systemic absorption, which may minimize cardiovascular side effects. Nebulized forms may contain large particles, which deposit to a large extent in tubing and upper airways. The dosage of metered dose inhalers should be titrated to effect when administered into a breathing circuit. Large doses (10 to 20 puffs) may be necessary. If severe, ketamine or low-dose IV epinephrine should be started.

4. **Adequate hydration and humidification** of inspired gases will minimize inspissation of secretions.

XII. **Aspiration.** General anesthesia causes a depression of airway reflexes that predisposes patients to aspiration. Aspiration of gastric contents from vomiting or regurgitation may cause bronchospasm, hypoxemia, atelectasis, tachypnea, tachycardia, and hypotension. The severity of symptoms depends on the volume and pH of the gastric material aspirated. Conditions that predispose to aspiration include gastric outlet obstruction, gastroesophageal reflux, small-bowel obstruction, symptomatic hiatal hernia, pregnancy, severe obesity, and recent food ingestion.

A. **If vomiting or regurgitation occurs** in an anesthetized patient whose airway is not protected by an endotracheal tube, the patient should be placed in the Trendelenburg position to minimize passive flow of gastric contents into the trachea, the head should be turned to the side, the upper airway suctioned, and an endotracheal tube placed. Suctioning the endotracheal tube before instituting positive-pressure ventilation avoids forcing gastric contents into the distal airways. Evidence of significant aspiration includes wheezing, decreased lung compliance, and hypoxemia. A chest radiograph should be obtained, but radiographic evidence of infiltrates may be delayed. Bronchodilators may be useful.

B. **Bronchoscopy** should be performed if a clinically significant aspiration is suspected. The airways should be suctioned clear and foreign bodies such as teeth and food removed. Lavage with large volumes of saline is not helpful.

C. **Aspiration of blood,** unless of large volume, is usually benign.

D. **Administration of antibiotics** usually is not warranted unless the material aspirated contains a high bacterial load such as with bowel obstruction (see Chapter 7).

E. **A sputum specimen** should be obtained for Gram stain and culture.

F. **Steroids** are not useful for treating aspiration.

G. **If significant aspiration has occurred,** it is imperative that close postoperative observation be undertaken. This includes pulse oximetry and repeat chest radiography. Ventilatory support and supplemental oxygen may be necessary (see Chapter 36).

XIII. **Pneumothorax** is the accumulation of gas within the pleural space.

A. **Etiologies**

1. Spontaneous rupture of blebs and bullae.

2. Blunt or penetrating chest trauma.

3. Surgical entrance into the pleural space during thoracic, upper abdominal, or retroperitoneal surgery, tracheostomy, or surgery of the chest wall or neck.

4. As a complication of procedures such as subclavian or internal jugular vein catheter placement, thoracentesis, pericardiocentesis, or upper extremity nerve block.

5. During positive-pressure ventilation using high pressures and volumes, causing barotrauma and alveolar rupture. Patients with chronic obstructive pulmonary disease are at particularly high risk.

6. Malfunction of chest tubes.

B. **Physiologic effects** of pneumothoraces are largely a function of the gas volume and the rate of expansion. Small pneumothoraces may have no significant cardiopulmonary effect; larger ones may result in significant lung collapse and hypoxemia. A tension pneumothorax occurs when there is a one-way leak into the pleural space, causing a significant increase in intrapleural pressure. This can result in mediastinal shift and compression of the heart with subsequent hypotension and decreased cardiac output.

C. The **diagnosis** of pneumothorax can be difficult. Signs of pneumothorax include decreased breath sounds, a reduction in lung compliance, an increase in peak inspiratory pressure, and hypoxemia. Hypotension reflects the presence of a tension pneumothorax. A chest radiograph usually can confirm the diagnosis, but treatment of an unstable patient should not be delayed while waiting for a chest radiograph.

D. **Treatment.** Nitrous oxide should be discontinued, and the patient should be ventilated with 100% oxygen. Tension pneumothoraces require immediate evacuation. A large-bore catheter (14 to 16 gauge) on a 10-mL syringe can be inserted into the pleural space at the second intercostal space in the midclavicular line and aspirated to confirm the presence of air. A chest tube then can be placed at the fifth or sixth intercostal space in the midaxillary line.

XIV. **Myocardial ischemia**

A. **Etiology.** Myocardial ischemia is the result of an imbalance between myocardial oxygen supply and consumption and, if persistent, may lead to MI.

B. **Clinical features**

1. In the awake patient, myocardial ischemia may manifest as **chest pain, dyspnea, nausea and vomiting, diaphoresis, or shoulder and jaw pain. Asymptomatic ischemia is common** in the perioperative period, particularly in diabetic patients. In patients under general anesthesia, hemodynamic instability and ECG changes may occur with ischemia.

2. **ECG changes** such as **ST segment depression** greater than 1 mm or acute T-wave inversion may indicate subendocardial ischemia. **ST segment elevation** is usually seen with transmural myocardial ischemia. T-wave changes may also be seen with electrolyte abnormalities and thus are not particularly diagnostic of ischemia. Lead V_5 is the single most sensitive lead for detecting ischemia (see Chapter 10).

3. **Other indicators of ischemia** include the following:
   a. Hypotension.
   b. Changes in central filling pressures or cardiac output.
   c. Regional wall motion abnormalities as detected with transesophageal echocardiography.
   d. Dysrythmias, particularly ventricular ectopy.

C. **Treatment**

1. **Hypoxemia and anemia should be corrected** to maximize myocardial oxygen delivery.

2. **β-Adrenergic antagonists** (metoprolol in 1- to 3-mg increments IV or propranolol in 0.5- to 1.0-mg increments IV or esmolol in 5- to 10-mg increments IV) decrease myocardial oxygen consumption by decreasing heart rate and contractility.

3. **Nitroglycerin** (starting at 25 to 50 μg/kg/min IV or 0.15 mg sublingually) reduces ventricular diastolic pressure and volume through venodilation and thus decreases myocardial oxygen demand. Additionally, nitroglycerin may improve oxygen delivery by enhancing collateral coronary flow.

4. **Myocardial ischemia occurring in the setting of hypotension** may require a vasopressor such as phenylephrine (10 to 40 μg/min IV) or norepinephrine (2 to 20 μg/min IV) to improve myocardial perfusion pressure. Anesthetic depth may need to be decreased and intravascular volume optimized.

5. When myocardial ischemia results in a significant reduction in cardiac output and hypotension (cardiogenic shock), positive **inotropes** such as dopamine (5 to 20 μg/kg/min IV), dobutamine (5 to 20 μg/kg/min IV), milrinone (0.375 to 0.75 μg/kg/min after loading dose of 50 μg/kg) or norepinephrine (2 to 20 μg/min IV) are indicated. Intra-aortic balloon counterpulsation may be life-saving. A pulmonary artery catheter may be helpful in assessing ventricular function and response to therapy.

6. **Aspirin, heparin treatment, thrombolytic therapy, angioplasty, and coronary revascularization** may be considered in selected patients.

XV. **Pulmonary embolism** is the obstruction of pulmonary blood flow by thrombus, air, fat, or amniotic fluid.

A. **Thromboemboli** most commonly arise from the deep venous system of the pelvis and lower extremities. Predisposing factors for the development of thrombi are stasis, hypercoagulability, and vascular wall abnormalities. Associated conditions include pregnancy, trauma, carcinoma, prolonged bed rest, and vasculitis.

  1. **Physical findings** are nonspecific and may include tachypnea and tachycardia, dyspnea, bronchospasm, and fever.

  2. **Laboratory studies.** The ECG reveals a nonspecific tachycardia unless embolization is severe, in which case right-axis deviation, right bundle branch block, and anterior T-wave changes may be seen. The chest radiograph may be unremarkable unless pulmonary infarction has occurred. Typically, hypotension and hypoxemia are present. With a large embolism, the end-tidal carbon dioxide will be decreased. In spontaneously breathing patients, hypocapnia and respiratory alkalosis may result from the increased respiratory rate. Definitive diagnosis requires a pulmonary angiogram or high-resolution computed tomography of the chest (spiral computed tomography).

  3. **Intraoperative treatment** of a suspected pulmonary embolism is supportive. Oxygenation is increased. Intraoperative heparin treatment or thrombolytic therapy is usually not an option because of the risk of hemorrhage. In patients who are severely hypoxic or hypotensive, cardiopulmonary bypass and pulmonary embolectomy may be considered.

B. **Air embolism** occurs during entrainment of air into a vein or venous sinus. It occurs most commonly during intracranial surgery in the sitting position, where dural venous sinuses are stented open. Air embolism may also occur during liver transplantation, open cardiac procedures, and insufflation during laparoscopy.

  1. **Early indicators** include air seen by transesophageal echocardiography or heard with a precordial Doppler, a decrease in end-tidal carbon dioxide tension, and an increase in end-tidal nitrogen tension.

  2. **Additional indicators** include increased central venous pressure, hypoxemia, hypotension, ventricular ectopy, and a continuous "mill-wheel" precordial murmur.

  3. **Treatment** begins with limiting the entrainment of additional air by flooding the surgical field with saline or repositioning the patient so that venous pressure is increased. Nitrous oxide should be discontinued to avoid enlarging the size of bubbles within the circulation. Placing the patient in a left lateral decubitus position may help to reduce air lock. If a central venous catheter is in place, it should be aspirated in an attempt to remove air. Fluid and vasopressors are used to maintain blood pressure.

  4. **The use of PEEP** in the setting of air embolism is controversial. It will limit the entrainment of air by raising central venous pressure but at the expense of reducing venous return and possibly cardiac output. **Hyperbaric oxygen** may decrease the side effects of the bubbles.

C. **Fat embolism** occurs after trauma or surgery involving the long bones, pelvis, or ribs.

1. **Clinical features** are related to mechanical obstruction of the pulmonary circulation and are similar to those found with pulmonary thromboembolism. The release of free fatty acids may lead to diminished mental status, worsening hypoxemia, fat globules in the urine, thrombocytopenia, and petechial hemorrhages.

2. **Treatment is supportive,** with the administration of supplemental oxygen and ventilation as necessary.

D. **Amniotic fluid emboli** (see Chapter 30).

XVI. **Cardiac tamponade.** Accumulation of blood or other fluid within the pericardial sac may prevent adequate ventricular filling and reduce stroke volume and cardiac output. When the accumulation is rapid, cardiovascular collapse may occur within minutes.

A. **Cardiac tamponade** may be associated with the following:

1. Chest trauma.

2. Cardiac or thoracic surgery.

3. Pericardial tumor.

4. Pericarditis (acute viral, pyogenic, uremic, or postradiation).

5. Myocardial perforation by a central venous or pulmonary artery catheter.

6. Aortic dissection.

B. **Clinical features** include tachycardia, hypotension, jugular venous distention, muffled heart sounds, and a decrease in pulse pressure. An ECG may reveal **electrical alternans** and diffusely low voltage. **Pulsus paradoxis** (> a 10 mm Hg inspiratory decrease in systolic blood pressure) may be appreciated. There is **equalization of right and left heart pressures** as reflected in identical central venous pressure, right ventricular end diastolic pressure, pulmonary artery diastolic pressure, and pulmonary capillary wedge pressures. Radiographic findings may include an enlarged cardiac silhouette. An **echocardiogram** is diagnostic.

C. The **treatment** of a hemodynamically unstable patient with suspected cardiac tamponade is pericardiocentesis. Intravascular volume should be augmented and vasopressors that maintain chronotropy and inotropy (e.g., dopamine) are administered to maintain blood pressure. A long needle is inserted between the xiphoid process and the left costal margin and directed toward the left shoulder. If the precordial lead of the ECG is attached to the needle, an injury current (ST segment elevation) will be observed when the needle contacts the epicardium. The needle should be withdrawn slightly and aspirated. **Complications of pericardiocentesis** include pneumothorax, coronary artery laceration, and myocardial perforation. A surgical pericardial window is a more permanent approach to alleviating tamponade.

XVII. **Malignant hyperthermia**

A. **Etiology.** Malignant hyperthermia is a hypermetabolic syndrome occurring in genetically susceptible patients after exposure to an anesthetic triggering agent. **Triggering anesthetics** include all potent inhalational agents (e.g., halothane, enflurane, isoflurane, desflurane, sevoflurane) and succinylcholine. The syndrome is thought to be due to a reduction in the reuptake of Ca^{2+} by the sarcoplasmic reticulum necessary for termination of muscle contraction. Consequently, muscle contraction is sustained, resulting in signs of hypermetabolism, including tachycardia, acidosis, hypercarbia, muscle rigidity, tachypnea, hypoxemia, and hyperthermia. The first signs of malignant hyperthermia usually occur in the operating room but may be delayed until the patient reaches the postanesthesia care unit or even the postoperative floor.

B. Clinical features
1. Unexplained tachycardia.
2. Hypercarbia in the mechanically ventilated patient or tachypnea in the spontaneously breathing patient.
3. Metabolic acidosis.
4. Muscle rigidity even in the presence of neuromuscular blockade. Masseter spasm after giving succinylcholine is associated with malignant hyperthermia. However, not all patients who develop masseter spasm will develop malignant hyperthermia.
5. Hypoxemia.
6. Ventricular dysrhythmias.
7. Hyperkalemia.
8. Fever is a late sign.
9. Myoglobinuria.
10. The presence of a large difference between mixed venous and arterial carbon dioxide tensions confirms the diagnosis of malignant hyperthermia.

C. Treatment
1. **Summon help** as soon as malignant hyperthermia is suspected. Discontinue all triggering anesthetics, and hyperventilate with 100% oxygen. Surgery should be concluded as quickly as possible and the anesthesia machine should be changed when feasible.
2. **Administer dantrolene** (Dantrium), 2.5 mg/kg IV initially and repeated to a total of 10 mg/kg or more if signs of malignant hyperthermia persist. Dantrolene is the only known specific treatment for malignant hyperthermia. Its efficacy is due to its ability to inhibit Ca^{2+} release from the sarcoplasmic reticulum. Each ampule contains 20 mg of dantrolene and 3 g of mannitol and should be reconstituted with 50 mL of warm sterile water.
3. **Sodium bicarbonate administration** should be guided by pH and partial pressure of carbon dioxide (PCO_2) measurements.
4. **Hyperkalemia** may be corrected with insulin and glucose. However, hypokalemia may occur as the hypermetabolic state is brought under control. Calcium should be avoided.
5. **Dysrhythmias** generally subside with resolution of the hypermetabolic phase of malignant hyperthermia. Persistent dysrhythmias can be treated with procainamide.
6. **Hyperthermia** is treated by a variety of methods (see section VIII).
7. **Urine output** ideally should be maintained at 2 mL/kg/min to avoid renal tubular damage from myoglobin. This is done by maintaining adequate central filling pressures and administering furosemide or mannitol.

8. **Recrudescence, disseminated intravascular coagulation, and acute tubular necrosis** may occur after an acute episode of malignant hyperthermia. Therefore, dantrolene therapy (1 mg/kg IV or orally every 6 hours) and observation should be continued for 48 to 72 hours after an episode of malignant hyperthermia.

D. **Anesthesia for malignant hyperthermia-susceptible patients**

1. A **family history** of anesthetic problems suggesting susceptibility, such as unexplained fevers or death during anesthesia, should be sought in every patient.

2. **Malignant hyperthermia** may be triggered in susceptible patients who have had previous uneventful exposures to triggering agents.

3. **Pretreatment with dantrolene** generally is not recommended for malignant hyperthermia-susceptible patients. A malignant hyperthermia cart or other dantrolene supply, however, should be immediately available.

4. **The anesthesia machine** should be prepared by changing the carbon dioxide absorbent and fresh gas tubing, disconnecting the vaporizers, using a disposable breathing circuit, and flushing the machine with oxygen at a rate of 10 L/min for 5 minutes.

5. **Local or regional anesthesia** should be considered, but general anesthesia with nontriggering agents is acceptable. **Safe drugs** for induction and maintenance of general anesthesia include barbiturates, propofol, benzodiazepines, opioids, and nitrous oxide. Nondepolarizing neuromuscular blockers may be used and safely reversed.

6. **Close monitoring** for early signs of malignant hyperthermia such as unexplained hypercarbia or tachycardia is crucial.

E. **Associated syndromes.** An increased risk of malignant hyperthermia has been reported in association with a number of disorders. In many of these cases, the association is not well established. However, patients with the following disorders should be treated as though they are susceptible to malignant hyperthermia:

1. **Duchenne muscular dystrophy** and other **muscular dystrophies.**

2. **King-Denborough syndrome,** characterized by dwarfism, mental retardation, and musculoskeletal abnormalities.

3. **Central core disease,** a rare myopathy.

F. **NMS** is associated with the administration of neuroleptic drugs and shares many of the features of malignant hyperthermia.

1. **Clinical features.** NMS typically develops over 24 to 72 hours and is clinically similar to malignant hyperthermia, presenting as a hypermetabolic episode consisting of hyperthermia, autonomic nervous system instability, pronounced muscle rigidity, and rhabdomyolysis. Creatine kinase and hepatic transaminases often are increased, and mortality approaches 30%.

2. **Treatment** of NMS is with dantrolene, although benzodiazepines, dopamine antagonists like bromocriptine, and

nondepolarizing muscle relaxants will also decrease muscle rigidity.

3. **Anesthetic implications.** The exact relationship between NMS and malignant hyperthermia is unclear. Some patients with a history of NMS may be at risk for malignant hyperthermia, and a conservative approach may be warranted (e.g., avoidance of known triggering agents). Patients with NMS must be appropriately monitored for malignant hyperthermia during all anesthetics (e.g., temperature, end-tidal carbon dioxide). They should not be pretreated with dantrolene.

XVIII. **Anaphylactic and anaphylactoid reactions**
 A. **Anaphylaxis** is a life-threatening allergic reaction. It is initiated by antigen binding to preformed IgE antibodies on the surface of mast cells and basophils, which causes release of pharmacologically active substances. These include histamine, leukotrienes, prostaglandins, kinins, and platelet-activating factor.
 B. **Anaphylactoid reactions** are clinically similar to anaphylactic reactions, but they are not mediated by IgE and do not require prior sensitization to an antigen.
 C. **Clinical features** of anaphylactic or anaphylactoid reactions include the following:
  1. Urticaria and flushing.
  2. Bronchospasm or airway edema, which can produce respiratory failure.
  3. Hypotension and shock due to peripheral vasodilation and increased capillary permeability.
  4. Pulmonary edema.
 D. **Treatment**
  1. **Discontinue anesthetic agents** if circulatory collapse is present.
  2. **Administer 100% oxygen.** Assess the need to intubate and support ventilation.
  3. **Treat hypotension** with intravascular volume expansion.
  4. **Give epinephrine,** 50 to 100 μg IV. For overt cardiovascular collapse, epinephrine, 0.5 to 1.0 mg IV, is indicated, followed by an infusion if hypotension persists. Other catecholamines such as norepinephrine may be useful.
  5. **Steroids** (hydrocortisone, 250 mg to 1.0 g IV, or methylprednisolone, 1 to 2 g IV) may reduce the inflammatory response.
  6. **Histamine antagonists** (diphenhydramine, 50 mg IV, and ranitidine, 50 IV in the adult) may be useful as second-line therapy.
 E. **Prophylaxis for drug hypersensitivity reactions**
  1. **Histamine (H_1) antagonists.** Diphenhydramine (0.5 to 1.0 mg/kg or 50 mg IV in the adult) the night before and morning of exposure.
  2. **H_2 antagonists.** Cimetidine (150 to 300 mg IV or orally in the adult) or ranitidine (50 mg IV or 150 mg orally in the adult) the night before and the morning of exposure.
  3. **Corticosteroids.** Prednisone (1 mg/kg or 50 mg for adults) every 6 hours for four doses before exposure.

XIX. Fire and electrical hazards in the operating room

A. Fire in the operating room is a rare event that requires the presence of an ignition source, fuel, and an oxidizing agent.

1. **Lasers and electrocautery devices** are the most common ignition sources.

2. **Fuels** include alcohol, solvents, sheets, drapes, and plastic or rubber materials (including endotracheal tubes). Unlike diethyl ether and cyclopropane, modern potent inhalation anesthetics are not fuels. During an electrical fire, it is important to unplug the electrical source.

3. **Oxygen** is by far the most common oxidizing agent, although nitrous oxide will also support combustion. Materials that are only marginally combustible in air can produce a massive flame in the presence of a high oxygen concentration. Supplemental oxygen can accumulate under surgical drapes and should be administered only when medically indicated.

4. **Fire extinguishers** should be readily available in all anesthetizing locations. Carbon dioxide and Halon fire extinguishers offer the advantage of efficacy against a variety of fires without producing the particulate contamination associated with dry chemical extinguishers.

B. Electrical safety

1. **Macroshock** is an electrical injury caused when a large current passes through intact skin producing a thermal, neural, or muscular injury. It may disrupt normal physiologic function and cause cardiac or respiratory arrest. The level of injury varies with frequencies and individuals, but, in general, the following guidelines can be applied for an alternating current of 60 cycles/second:

    a. **1 mA for 1 second**—Threshold of perception

    b. **5 mA for 1 second**—Accepted as maximum harmless current intensity. Level at which line isolation monitors alarm.

    c. **10–20 mA for 1 second**—current that results in sustained muscular contraction, referred to as the "Let go current."

    d. **100 mA for 1 second**—Threshold for ventricular fibrillation.

2. **Microshock** occurs when small currents pass directly to the heart. This occurs intentionally when using cardiac pacemakers but can be harmful if it occurs inadvertently. Ventricular fibrillation can be produced by as little as **100 μA** of current applied to the myocardium. As this current is well below the 2 to 5 mA threshold of the line isolation monitor alarm, line isolation monitors do not protect a patient from microshcok. To minimize the likelihood of microshock, all equipment should be properly grounded with a three-prong plug, and connections to the patient should be electrically isolated. Battery operation does not ensure electrical isolation.

3. **Line isolation monitors** are designed to alarm the anesthesiologist when faulty ground connections place patients and operating room personnel at risk of potential exposure

to large currents (>2 to 5 mA). The line isolation monitor alarms when one of the two "hot" power lines becomes grounded, creating a first fault. This event signals that someone in the operating room may receive a macroshock if they touch any electrical equipment supplied by this circuit, as they now serve as the ground for the system, creating the second fault. If the line isolation monitor alarms, unplug the last appliance that was plugged in. Further investigation into the appliance or circuit will be necessary. Although line isolation monitors continue to be used in operating rooms, most electrical equipment used today has built-in electrical isolation.

4. **Burns from electrosurgical units** (Bovie) may result from poor contact between the dispersive electrode (grounding pad) and the patient, because electrical power dissipation is proportional to the resistance at the skin. Under such conditions, anything that is grounded may provide an alternative pathway for current to flow, resulting in burns at sites distant from the dispersive electrode. The risk of burns can be minimized by ensuring that the electrode gel is adequate, that the dispersive electrode is placed near the surgical site, and that the patient is insulated from possible alternative pathways for current flow.

SUGGESTED READING

Beebe JJ, Sessler DI. Preparation of anesthesia machines for patients susceptible to malignant hyperthermia. *Anesthesiology* 1988;69:395–400.

Gravenstein N, Kirby RR. *Complications in anesthesiology*. Philadelphia: Lippincott, 1995.

Levy JH. Allergic reactions during anesthesia. *J Clin Anesth* 1988;1:39–46.

Litt L, Ehrenwerth J. Electrical safety in the operating room: important old wine, disguised new bottles. *Anesth Analg* 1994;78:417–419.

Marik PE. Aspiration pneumonitis and aspiration pneumonia. *N Engl J Med* 2001;344:665–671.

Sessler DI. Complications and treatment of mild hypothermia. *Anesthesiology* 2001;95:531–543.

Stoelting RK, Dierdorf SF. *Anesthesia and co-existing disease*. New York: Churchill Livingstone, 2002.

Stoelting RK, Hillier S. *Pharmacology and Physiology in Anesthetic Practice*. Philadelphia: Lippincott–Raven, 2005.

19

Perioperative Hemodynamic Control

Vilma E. Ortiz and Phillip K. Lau

I. **Blood flow.** Systemic blood pressure is monitored as a reflection of
    local tissue perfusion. This is because pressure is much easier to mea-
    sure clinically than flow. Organs, however, require an adequate blood
    flow rather than a minimal blood pressure to meet their metabolic
    needs.
    A. **Ohm's law:** Pressure (i.e., blood pressure) = flow (i.e., cardiac
        output) × resistance
        Organ blood flow = (mean arterial pressure [MAP] – organ ve-
        nous pressure)/organ vascular resistance
    B. **Cardiac output** is influenced by heart rate, preload, afterload,
        and myocardial compliance and contractility. These variables are
        separate yet intimately interdependent and controlled by the au-
        tonomic nervous system and humoral mechanisms.
II. **Autoregulation.** The ability of an organ or vascular bed to maintain
    adequate blood flow despite varying blood pressure is termed autoregu-
    lation. Metabolic regulation controls about 75% of all local blood flow
    in the body. Organs have differing ability (autoregulatory reserve) to
    increase or decrease their vascular resistance to provide tight coupling
    between metabolic demand and organ blood flow. In general, anes-
    thetics inhibit autoregulation, making organ perfusion more pressure
    dependent. The most important of these organs are the brain, kidneys,
    heart, and lungs (see appropriate chapters for detailed discussions on
    each).
III. **Adrenergic receptor physiology.** Adrenergic receptors can be dis-
     tinguished by their response to a series of catecholamines. Recep-
     tors that demonstrate an order of potency so that norepinephrine >
     epinephrine > isoproterenol are termed α **receptors.** Those receptors
     that respond with the order of potency isoproterenol > epinephrine >
     norepinephrine are termed β **receptors.** Receptors that interact exclu-
     sively with dopamine are termed **dopaminergic.** Adrenergic receptors
     can be further subdivided based on their pharmacology and anatomic
     location.
     A. α_1 **receptors** are located postsynaptically in vascular smooth mus-
         cle and in the smooth muscle of the coronary arteries, uterus, skin,
         intestinal mucosa, iris, and splanchnic bed. Activation causes ar-
         teriolar and venous constriction, mydriasis, and relaxation of the
         intestinal tract. Cardiac α_1 receptors increase inotropy and de-
         crease heart rate.
     B. α_2 **receptors**
         1. **Presynaptic α_2 receptors** are located within the central ner-
             vous system, specifically the locus ceruleus and substantia
             gelatinosa. Activation causes inhibition of norepinephrine,
             acetylcholine, serotonin, dopamine, and substance P release.

Activation has been associated with hypnotic and sedative effects, antinociceptive action, hypotension, and bradycardia.

2. **Postsynaptic α_2 receptors** are located peripherally in vascular smooth muscle, the gastrointestinal tract, pancreatic beta cells, and within the central nervous system. Activation of peripheral postsynaptic a2 receptors causes vasoconstriction and a hypertensive (pressor) response, decreased salivation, and decreased insulin release. Activation of the central receptors is associated with analgesia and an anesthesia-sparing effect.

C. **β_1 receptors** are located in the myocardium, the sinoatrial node, the ventricular conduction system, adipose tissue, and renal tissue. Activation causes an increase in inotropy, chronotropy, myocardial conduction velocity, renin release, and lipolysis.

D. **β_2 receptors** are located in vascular, bronchial, dermal, and uterine smooth muscle as well as myocardium. Stimulation leads to vasodilation, bronchodilation, uterine relaxation, and possibly an increase in inotropy. β_2 receptor activation also promotes gluconeogenesis, insulin release, and potassium uptake by cells.

E. **β_3 receptors** are involved in lipolysis and regulation of metabolic rate.

F. **Dopaminergic receptors**
1. **Dopaminergic-1 receptors** are located postsynaptically on renal and mesenteric vascular smooth muscle and mediate vasodilation.
2. **Dopaminergic-2 receptors** are presynaptic and inhibit norepinephrine release.
3. **Dopaminergic-5** (similar to dopaminergic-1) and **dopaminergic-3 and 4** (similar to dopaminergic-2) **receptors** have been classified. Their clinical significance has not yet been identified.

G. **Receptor regulation.** There is an inverse relationship between receptor number and the concentration of circulating adrenergic agonist and the duration of exposure to that agonist. This is termed receptor up-regulation and down-regulation. Sudden cessation of beta-blockade therapy may be associated with rebound hypertension and tachycardia with resulting myocardial ischemia. This is a result of β-receptor proliferation (up-regulation) and consequent hypersensitivity to endogenous catecholamines.

IV. **Adrenergic pharmacology** (Table 19.1)
A. **α agonists**
1. **Phenylephrine** is a direct-acting α_1 agonist at normal clinical doses, with some β-receptor activity at extremely high concentrations. Phenylephrine causes both arterial and venous vasoconstriction. This dual action increases venous return (preload) and mean arterial blood pressure (afterload). Phenylephrine maintains cardiac output in patients with a normal heart but may decrease cardiac performance in an ischemic heart. Phenylephrine has a short duration of action that makes it easily titratable.
2. **Clonidine** is a centrally acting antihypertensive with relative selectivity for α_2 adrenoreceptors. Its actions include reducing sympathetic tone, increasing parasympathetic activity, reducing anesthetic and analgesic requirements, causing sedation, and decreasing salivation. It can be administered

Table 19.1. Drug dosages of commonly used vasopressors and inotropes

Drug Name (Trade Name)	IV Bolus	IV Infusion	Dose	Alpha	Beta	DA	V
					Adrenergic Effects		
Arginine vasopressin (Pitressin)	NR (septic shock) 40 U (cardiac arrest)	a. 50 units/250 mL b. 0.2 units/mL c. 0.01–0.1 unit/min d. 10–20 min					+++
Dobutamine (Dobutrex)	NR	a. 250 mg/250 mL b. 1000 μg/mL c. 2–20 μg/kg/min d. 5–10 min		+	+++		
Dopamine (Inotropin)	NR	a. 200 mg/250 mL b. 800 μg/mL c. 1–20 μg/kg/min d. 5–10 min	Low High	++	++	++ +++	
Ephedrine	5–10 mg	NR 5–10 min duration	++	++			
Epinephrine (Adrenaline)	20–100 μg (hypotension) 0.5–1 mg (cardiac arrest)	a. 1 mg/250 mL b. 4 μg/mL c. 0.5–5 μg/min d. 1–2 min	Low High	+ +++	+++ ++++		
Isoproterenol (Isuprel)	NR	a. 1 mg/250 mL b. 4 μg/mL c. 2–10 μg/min d. 5–10 min			+++		

continued

Table 19.1. (*continued*)

Drug Name (Trade Name)	IV Bolus	IV Infusion	Dose	Adrenergic Effects			
				Alpha	Beta	DA	V
Milrinone	NR	20 mg/250 mL of 0.9% NaCl; 50 μg/kg IV load over 10 min, then 0.375–0.75 μg/kg/min; dosage adjustment required for renally impaired patients			Nonsympathomimetic		
Norepinephrine (Levophed)	NR	a. 4 mg/250 mL b. 16 μg/mL c. 1–30 μg/min d. 1–2 min	Low High	++ ++++	+ ++		
Phenylephrine (Neosynephrine)	40–100 μg	a. 10 mg/250 mL b. 40 μg/mL c. 10–150 μg/min d. 5–10 min		++++			

a, mix in 5% dextrose in water; b, concentration; c, common IV dosage range; d, duration; DA, dopaminergic; V, vasopressin; NR, not recommended.

intravenously, intramuscularly, orally, transcutaneously, and into the intrathecal and epidural spaces.

3. **Dexmedetomidine** is a newer selective α_2 adrenoreceptor agonist currently approved for the intravenous sedation of mechanically ventilated patients in an intensive care setting. A potential advantage over other sedatives is its lack of respiratory depression. A decrease in blood pressure and heart rate can be attributed to a decrease in the level of circulating catecholamines.

B. **β agonists. Isoproterenol** is a direct-acting β-adrenergic agonist. It causes an increase in heart rate and contractility while reducing systemic vascular resistance (SVR). It is also a pulmonary vasodilator and a bronchodilator.

1. **Indications**

a. Hemodynamically significant, atropine-resistant bradycardia.

b. Atrioventricular block until temporary pacing can be instituted.

c. Low cardiac output states requiring fast heart rates (pediatric patients who have a fixed stroke volume, cardiac transplant recipients).

d. Status asthmaticus.

e. Beta-blockade overdose.

2. **Continuous electrocardiographic monitoring** is recommended with intravenous administration, which may be through a peripheral intravenous line.

3. Side effects include vasodilation, hypotension, and tachydysrhythmias.

C. **Mixed agonists**

1. **Epinephrine** is a direct-acting α- and β-receptor agonist produced by the adrenal medulla.

a. **Indications**

(1) Cardiac arrest.

(2) Anaphylaxis.

(3) Bronchospasm.

(4) Cardiogenic shock.

(5) Prolongation of regional anesthesia.

b. **The clinical effect of epinephrine is** the sum of its α- and β-receptor activation on various tissue beds, with β effects predominating at lower doses. At very low doses (e.g., $0.25 - 0.5 \ \mu g/min$), epinephrine causes primarily bronchodilation and is the most effective bronchodilator available. Increasing doses cause an increase in inotropy and chronotropy and vasoconstriction. As the dose of epinephrine increases, α effects predominate, and stroke volume may fall as SVR (afterload) increases. Significant tachycardia, dysrhythmias, and myocardial ischemia may limit the usefulness of epinephrine in the clinical setting. Volatile anesthetics (especially halothane) can sensitize the myocardium to circulating catecholamines to produce potentially life-threatening dysrhythmias. Epinephrine should be administered through a central intravenous line whenever possible because severe tissue necrosis can occur if it extravasates.

2. **Norepinephrine,** the neurotransmitter of the sympathetic nervous system, is the biosynthetic precursor of epinephrine. Norepinephrine is a potent α- and β_1-receptor agonist, with α effects predominating at lower doses. Compared with epinephrine, it has minimal effects on β_2 receptors. Norepinephrine increases blood pressure by increasing SVR (afterload), whereas cardiac output remains relatively unchanged. Myocardial performance may improve, if the increased blood pressure improves coronary blood flow and relieves myocardial ischemia. Norepinephrine increases the vascular resistance of most organs, thereby diminishing organ blood flow despite increases in MAP. It is useful in the setting of hypotension that is associated with mild myocardial depression. As with most vasoactive drugs, electrocardiogram and invasive monitoring are recommended to follow clinical effectiveness, and the drug should be administered centrally.

3. **Dopamine,** the immediate precursor of norepinephrine, produces a dose-related combination of α-, β-, and dopamine-receptor effects. It is a neurotransmitter in the basal ganglia and chemoreceptor trigger zone. At lower doses (approximately <4 $\mu g/kg/min$), renal and splanchnic vessel dopamine receptors are activated primarily, resulting in increased renal blood flow, glomerular filtration, and sodium (Na^+) excretion. As the concentration of dopamine is increased, β effects become apparent, leading to increases in myocardial contractility, heart rate, and arterial blood pressure. At high doses (>10 $\mu g/kg/min$), α_1 effects predominate, leading to marked increases in arterial and venous blood pressure and decreases in renal blood flow. Dopamine also causes release of norepinephrine from nerve terminals. Dopamine administration often increases urine output but does not prevent renal injury or alter its course. Dopamine may be indicated in states of shock associated with a failing myocardium, but tachycardia (often seen even at lower doses), increased myocardial oxygen consumption, and profound vasoconstriction may limit its clinical usefulness.

4. **Dobutamine** is a synthetic catecholamine that has β_1-, β_2-, and α_1-adrenergic receptor activity. Dobutamine is a mixture of stereoisomers; the L(–)-isomer stimulates α_1 receptors and the D(+)-isomer has β_1- and β_2-receptor activity. Dobutamine increases myocardial contractility through its effect on cardiac α_1 and β_1 receptors. In the peripheral vasculature, dobutamine is a vasodilator, because its β_2 effect overshadows its α_1 properties. Dobutamine increases heart rate secondary to the positive chronotropic effects of β_1 activation. It is a useful agent for treating low cardiac output states caused by myocardial dysfunction secondary to acute infarction, cardiomyopathy, or myocardial depression after cardiac surgery. Hemodynamic effects of dobutamine are similar to those of a combination of dopamine and nitroprusside. Dobutamine typically increases cardiac output and decreases SVR with minimal effects on arterial blood pressure and heart rate. Pulmonary vascular resistance (PVR) decreases, making dobutamine beneficial for patients with right heart failure. Systemic hypotension (dobutamine is an

inotrope, not a pressor), increased myocardial oxygen consumption, and tachydysrhythmias are the most common side effects.

5. **Ephedrine** is a plant-derived, noncatecholamine, direct, and indirect adrenergic agonist. Ephedrine causes the release of norepinephrine and other endogenous catecholamines stored within nerve terminals. Tachyphylaxis limits ephedrine use to bolus administration for the temporary treatment of hypotension associated with hypovolemia, sympathetic blockade, myocardial depression due to anesthetic overdose, and bradycardia.

D. **Nonadrenergic sympathomimetic agents**

1. **Inamrinone** (previously known as amrinone) and milrinone are synthetic, noncatecholamine, nonglycosidic, bipyridine derivatives. They act by inhibiting type III phosphodiesterase, thereby increasing cyclic adenosine monophosphate levels and causing increased contractility and peripheral vasodilation. Their action is independent of adrenergic receptors, and as such their effects are additive to that of adrenergic agents.

   a. **Inamrinone** produces a dose-dependent improvement in cardiac index, left ventricular work index, and ejection fraction. Heart rate and MAP remain constant. Time to peak effect is about 5 minutes, and hepatic elimination occurs with a half-life of 5 to 12 hours depending on the severity of cardiac disease. Side effects are uncommon and include dose-dependent but reversible hypotension, thrombocytopenia, hypokalemia, dysrhythmias, liver function test abnormalities, fever, and gastrointestinal distress.

   b. **Milrinone** is a derivative of inamrinone and has the same hemodynamic profile. Milrinone is 20 times more potent than inamrinone and lacks many of the side effects associated with its parent compound.

2. **Arginine vasopressin (AVP)** is a synthetic analog of antidiuretic hormone, which is produced by the posterior pituitary. AVP causes vasoconstriction by direct stimulation of smooth muscle V-1 receptors. It is a recommended alternative to epinephrine in the treatment of adult shock-refractory ventricular fibrillation as a one-time bolus [40 units intravenously (IV)]. It may also be beneficial as a low-dose (0.04 unit/min) IV infusion in the setting of catecholamine-resistant vasodilatory shock. AVP has a rapid onset with a duration of action of 10 to 20 min. Administration through a central line is recommended.

3. **Terlipressin** is a vasopressin analog currently under investigation in the United States for the treatment of hepatorenal syndrome as well as hypotension.

V. **β-Adrenergic antagonists** (Table 19.2)

A. **Propranolol** is a nonselective β_1- and β_2-adrenergic receptor antagonist available in both IV and oral forms. Propranolol is the prototype β-adrenergic antagonist against which other drugs in this class are judged. Propranolol is highly lipophilic, is almost entirely absorbed after oral administration, and undergoes up to 75% first-pass clearance by the liver. Hemodynamic

Table 19.2. β-Adrenergic antagonists

Drug Name (Trade Name)	Beta-1 Selectivity	Bioavailability (%)	Beta Half-life[a]	Elimination	Usual Oral Dose	IV Dose
Atenolol (Tenormin)	++	55	6–9 hr	R (85%)	50–100 mg qd	5-mg increments
Esmolol (Brevibloc)	++	–	9 min	Red blood cell esterase		10- to 20-mg bolus; 0.25–0.5 mg/kg load, then 50–200 μg/kg/min
Labetalol (Trandate, Normodyne)	0	25	3–8 hr	H	100 mg bid	5–10-mg bolus; 10–40 mg/hr titrated upward
Metoprolol (Lopressor)	++	50	3–6 hr	H	25–100 mg qd-qid	5–25-mg increments
Nadolol (Corgard)	0	20	14–24 hr	R (75%)	40–240 mg qd	NR
Propranolol (Inderal)	0	33	3–4 hr	H	10–40 mg bid-qid	0.25- to 1-mg increments
Timolol (Blocadren)	0	75	4–5 hr	H (80%) R (20%)	5–15 mg qd-bid	NR

H, hepatic elimination; R, renal elimination; NR, not recommended.
[a]Beta half-life may not be predictive of clinical duration of action.

effects of propranolol and other β-adrenergic antagonists are secondary to a reduction of cardiac output and suppression of the renin-angiotensin system. β-Adrenergic antagonists can be distinguished by their relative β_1 selectivity, their intrinsic sympathomimetic activity, and their pharmacologic half-lives.

B. **Metoprolol** is a selective β_1-adrenergic receptor antagonist available in both oral and IV forms. It may be used perioperatively to treat supraventricular tachycardias. It is also effective in the treatment of angina pectoris, in reducing mortality from myocardial infarction, and in treating mild to moderate hypertension. Metoprolol has an oral to IV beta-blockade ratio of 2.5:1.

C. **Esmolol** is a selective β_1-adrenergic receptor antagonist that is metabolized rapidly by an esterase located in the cytoplasm of red blood cells. The time to its peak effect is 5 minutes and its elimination half-life is 9 minutes. Esmolol is valuable perioperatively because it can be administered IV, has a fast onset, has a very short duration of action, and can be given to patients with asthma, chronic obstructive pulmonary disease, or myocardial dysfunction. The red blood cell esterase is different from plasma pseudocholinesterase and is not affected by anticholinesterases. Rapid administration of esmolol in large boluses has been associated with severe hypotension and cardiac depression, leading to cardiac arrest in some situations. Its diluent contains propylene glycol, which may cause an osmolar gap metabolic acidosis during prolonged infusions.

D. **Labetalol** is a mixed α- and β-adrenergic receptor antagonist with a β- to α-adrenergic receptor blockade ratio of 3:1 when given orally and of 7:1 when administered IV. Labetalol decreases PVR, blunts the reflex increase in heart rate, and minimally affects cardiac output. Labetalol is useful intraoperatively to blunt the sympathetic response to tracheal intubation and to control hypertensive episodes. Labetalol is also used in the management of patients with pheochromocytomas and the clonidine withdrawal syndrome.

VI. **Vasodilators** (Table 19.3)

A. **Sodium nitroprusside** is a direct-acting vasodilator that acts on arterial and venous vascular smooth muscle.

1. The mechanism of action of sodium nitroprusside is common to all nitrates. The nitroso moiety decomposes to release nitric oxide. Nitric oxide is an unstable short-lived free radical that activates guanylate cyclase. This results in an increase in the concentration of cyclic guanosine monophosphate, which causes smooth muscle relaxation.

2. The hemodynamic effects of sodium nitroprusside are principally afterload reduction by arterial vasodilation and some preload reduction by increasing venous capacitance. These effects typically cause a reflex increase in heart rate and myocardial contractility, an increase in cardiac output, and marked decreases in SVR and PVR. Sodium nitroprusside dilates cerebral blood vessels and should be used with caution in patients with decreased intracranial compliance.

3. Sodium nitroprusside dilates all vascular beds equally, increasing overall blood flow. A vascular steal phenomenon may be created where blood flow to an ischemic region that is maximally vasodilated may be shunted to nonischemic

Table 19.3. Vasodilator drugs

Drug Name (Trade Name)	IV Bolus	IV Infusion	Mechanism of Action
Fenoldopam (Corlopam)	NR	a. 10 mg/250 mL b. 40 μg/mL c. 0.05–1.5 μg/kg/min d. 1–4 hr	D1-receptor agonist; moderate α2-receptor affinity
Hydralazine (Apresoline)	2.5–5 mg q15 min, 20–40 mg IV q4–6 hr	NR	Direct-acting vascular smooth muscle dilation
Labetalol (Trandate, Normodyne)	5–10 mg q 5 min	a. 200 mg/250 mL b. 0.8 mg/mL c. 10–40 mg/hr d. 15 min	Alpha-receptor and beta-receptor blockade
Nitroglycerin	50–100 μg	a. 30 mg/250 mL[a] b. 120 μg/mL c. 0.5–15 μg/kg/min d. 4 min	Venous vasodilator
Nitroprusside (Nipride)	NR	a. 30 mg/250 mL[a] b. 120 μg/mL c. 0.2 μg/kg/min[b] d. 4 min	Arterial > venous vasodilator
Phentolamine (Regitine)	1–5 mg	NR	Alpha-receptor blockade
Prostaglandin E1 (Alprostadil)	NR	a. 1–2 mg/250 mL b. 4–8 μg/mL c. 0.05 μg/kg/min[b] d. 1 min	Direct vasodilator via prostaglandin receptors in vascular smooth muscle

a, mix in 5% dextrose in water; b, concentration; c, usual IV dosage range; d, duration; NR, not recommended.
[a]Massachusetts General Hospital infusion mix: 30 mg/250 mL of saline = 120 mg/1,000 mL = 120 μg/mL.
Infusion pump set at 20 mL/hour = 20/60 mL/min = 1/3 mL/min = 40 μg/min. Therefore, dose in μg/min is 2× the set infusion rate (2× mL/hour = μg/min).
[b]Dose may be titrated higher to desired effect.

regions that can vasodilate further. This is especially important in the coronary vasculature, where ischemia may be exacerbated with the use of sodium nitroprusside even though overall myocardial oxygen consumption has been reduced by afterload reduction.

4. Sodium nitroprusside is useful perioperatively because it has a fast onset time (1 to 2 min) and its effects dissipate within 2 minutes of discontinuation.

5. **Cyanide toxicity.** In vivo, sodium nitroprusside reacts nonenzymatically with the sulfhydryl groups in hemoglobin to release five cyanide radicals per molecule. Some of these can be converted to **thiocyanate** by tissue and liver rhodanese and excreted in urine. Thiocyanate has a half-life of 4 days and will accumulate in the presence of renal failure. Cyanide

radicals may also bind to intracellular cytochrome oxidase and disrupt the electron transport chain. This can lead to cell hypoxia and death even in the face of adequate oxygen tensions. In addition, cyanide can bind to methemoglobin, resulting in cyanmethemoglobin.

    a. Clinical features. Tachyphylaxis, metabolic acidosis, and elevated mixed venous oxygen tensions are early signs of cyanide toxicity, which typically occurs when more than 1 mg/kg has been administered within 2.5 hours or when the blood concentration of cyanide ion is greater than 100 μg/dL. Symptoms of cyanide toxicity include fatigue, nausea, muscle spasm, angina, and mental confusion.

    b. Treatment. Cyanide toxicity is treated by discontinuation of sodium nitroprusside and administration of 100% oxygen and **sodium thiosulfate** (a sulfur donor in the rhodanese reaction) 150 mg/kg dissolved in 50 mL of water, over 15 minutes. Severe cyanide toxicity (base deficit >10 mEq, hemodynamic instability) may require the additional administration of **amyl nitrate** (0.3 mL by inhalation) or **sodium nitrate**, 5 mg/kg IV over 5 minutes. These two compounds create methemoglobin, which will bind to the cyanide ion and form inactive cyanmethemoglobin.

B. Nitroglycerin is a potent venodilator that also relaxes arterial, pulmonary, ureteral, uterine, gastrointestinal, and bronchial smooth muscle. Nitroglycerin has a greater effect on venous capacitance than on arteriolar tone. This is nitroglycerin's major mechanism of decreasing MAP.

    1. Indications. Nitroglycerin is useful for treating congestive heart failure and myocardial ischemia by increasing coronary flow and improving left ventricular performance. Nitroglycerin increases venous capacitance, decreases venous return, and consequently decreases ventricular end-diastolic volume. By the law of Laplace (tension = pressure × radius), a decrease in end-diastolic volume is associated with a decrease in pressure and subsequently a decrease in ventricular wall tension, which reduces myocardial oxygen consumption.

    2. Reflex tachycardia frequently occurs and must be treated with beta-blockade to avoid increasing myocardial consumption and negating nitroglycerin's beneficial effects.

    3. Tachyphylaxis develops with continuous infusion.

    4. Complications. Nitroglycerin is metabolized by the liver and has no known toxicity in the clinical dose range. Extremely high doses and prolonged continuous use produce methemoglobinemia. Nitroglycerin produces cerebral vasodilation and should be used with caution in patients with low intracranial compliance.

C. Hydralazine is a direct-acting arterial vasodilator. It decreases MAP by a reduction of arteriolar tone and vascular resistance of the coronary, cerebral, renal, uterine, and splanchnic beds. This helps preserve blood flow to these organs. The vasodilation induced by hydralazine triggers a reflex increase in heart rate and causes activation of the renin-angiotensin system. These effects can be attenuated by the concomitant use of a beta-blocker. Hydralazine can be administered by an IV bolus to treat hypertensive emergencies or to augment other hypotensive agents. The time to peak effect of IV hydralazine is 15 to 20 minutes with an elimination half-life of 4 hours. Long-term use has been associated with a lupus-like syndrome, skin rash, drug fever, pancytopenia, and peripheral neuropathy.

D. **Calcium channel antagonists (verapamil, diltiazem, nifedipine)** alter calcium flux across cell membranes and cause various degrees of arterial vasodilation with minimal effect on venous capacitance. They decrease vascular resistance of peripheral organs and cause coronary artery vasodilation. They are also myocardial depressants and verapamil and diltiazem depress atrioventricular nodal conduction (see Chapter 37). Nifedipine is limited to oral administration for the treatment of hypertension. **Verapamil** and **diltiazem** additionally are indicated for the treatment of hemodynamically stable narrow-complex supraventricular tachydysrhythmias. The initial verapamil dose is 2.5 to 5.0 mg IV, with subsequent doses of 5 to 10 mg IV administered every 15 to 30 min. Diltiazem is given as an initial bolus of 20 mg. An additional dose of 25 mg and an infusion of 5 to 15 mg/hour can be administered if needed. Oral diltiazem is commonly used for chronic therapy of myocardial ischemia. Their vasodilator and negative inotrope properties can cause hypotension, exacerbation of congestive heart failure, bradycardia, and enhancement of accessory conduction in patients with Wolff-Parkinson-White (WPW) syndrome.

E. **Enalaprilat** is currently the only angiotensin-converting enzyme inhibitor available for IV use. It reduces systolic and diastolic blood pressure by inhibiting the conversion of angiotensin I to angiotensin II. Enalaprilat may be used to treat perioperative hypertension. It has an onset of action of approximately 15 minutes, peak effect of 1 to 4 hours, and overall duration of action of about 4 hours. Elimination is primarily renal and caution is recommended when used in the setting of renal dysfunction.

F. **Fenoldopam** is a synthetic dopamine (DA-1) receptor agonist. A continuous IV infusion may be used perioperatively for the management of severe hypertension in patients with impaired renal function. Fenoldopam acts by dilation of selective arterial beds while maintaining renal perfusion. Selective renal dose is 3 μg/kg per minutes. It also has diuretic and natriuretic properties. Initial hemodynamic response occurs within 5 to 15 minutes. The dose should be adjusted every 15 to 20 minutes until optimal blood pressure control is achieved. Side effects include dose-dependent tachycardia and occasional hypokalemia. Bolus administration is not recommended, and hypotension may occur with concomitant use of β-adrenergic receptor blockade.

G. **Adenosine** is an endogenous nucleotide that, in high doses, has inhibitory effects on cardiac impulse conduction through the atrioventricular node. Adenosine dilates cerebral blood vessels, impairs autoregulation, and is metabolized to uric acid. Its ability to slow conduction through the atrioventricular node has led to its use in diagnosing and treating supraventricular tachydysrhythmias. However, if atrial fibrillation/flutter and WPW are present, adenosine should be avoided as it may allow preferential conduction through the accessory pathway (WPW syndrome; see Chapter 37).

H. **Prostaglandin E_1 (PGE$_1$)** is a stable metabolite of arachidonic acid that causes peripheral and pulmonary vasodilation. It is used to dilate the ductus arteriosus in neonates and infants with ductal-dependent congenital heart disease (e.g., transposition of the great arteries). PGE$_1$ also has been used to treat pulmonary hypertension after mitral valve replacement and in patients with severe right heart failure.

I. **Phentolamine** is a short-acting selective α-adrenergic receptor antagonist that causes predominantly arterial and some venous vasodilation. Phentolamine is used mainly for states of norepinephrine excess (e.g., pheochromocytoma), as an adjuvant for induced hypotension, and for infiltration into skin where norepinephrine has been accidentally extravasated (5 to 10 mg diluted in 10 mL of saline).

VII. **Induced hypotension** is a technique used when control of bleeding improves operating conditions and facilitates surgical technique (e.g., middle ear microsurgery, cerebral aneurysm clipping, plastic surgery) or reduces or eliminates the need for transfusion (e.g., orthopedic surgery, patients with rare blood groups, religious constraints). It is also useful when reduction in MAP decreases the risk of vessel rupture (e.g., aortic dissection, resection of intracranial aneurysms, arteriovenous malformation surgery). This technique is not appropriate for patients with a history of vascular insufficiency to the heart, brain, or kidneys; cardiac instability (unless afterload reduction improves performance); uncontrolled hypertension; anemia; or hypovolemia. Hypotension can be achieved by neuraxial blockade, high concentrations of volatile anesthetics, use of a potent short-acting narcotic (e.g., remifentanil), and/or peripheral vasodilation (e.g., with nitroprusside or nitroglycerin).

VIII. **Drug dosage calculations.** Drug dosages frequently require conversion between units of measurement before bolus or continuous infusion administration to the patient.

A. A drug concentration expressed as Z % contains

Z mg/dL $= Z$ g/100 mL $= (10 \times Z)$ g/L $= (10 \times Z)$ mg/mL

Example: A 2.5% solution of sodium thiopental is equivalent to 25 g/L or 25 mg/mL.

B. A drug concentration that is expressed as a ratio is converted as follows:

1:1,000 $= 1$ g/1,000 mL $= 1$ mg/mL
1:10,000 $= 1$ g/10,000 mL $= 0.1$ mg/mL
1:100,000 $= 1$ g/100,000 mL $= 0.01$ mg/mL

C. Continuous drug infusions are calculated based on a simple formula:

Z mg/250 mL $= Z\ \mu$g/min at an infusion rate of 15 mL/hour or 15 drops/minutes

Standard drug mixes in use at Massachusetts General Hospital are shown in Table 19.1. The desired rate of infusion for any drug is easily calculated as either a fraction or multiple of 15 mL/hour or 15 drops/minutes.

Example: An 80-kg patient needs dopamine at 5 μg/kg/min:

$5 \times 80 = 400$

400/200 (number of milligrams in 250-mL solution) $\times$ 15 mL/h $= 30$ mL/hour

SUGGESTED READING

Barnes P. β-Adrenergic receptors and their regulation. *Am J Respir Crit Care Med* 1995;152:838–860.

Delmas A, Leone M, Rousseau S, Albanese J, Martin C. Clinical review: vasopressin and terlipressin in septic shock patients. *Crit Care* 2005 Apr; 9(2):212–222.

Frishman W, Hotchkiss H. Selective and nonselective dopamine receptor agonists: an innovative approach to cardiovascular disease treatment. *Am Heart J* 1996;132:861–870.

Gazmuri R, Ayoub I. Pressors for cardiopulmonary resuscitation: is there a new kid on the block? *Crit Care Med* 2000;28:1236–1238.

International Consensus on Science. Agents to optimize cardiac output and blood pressure. *Circulation* 2000;102[Suppl I]:I129–I135.

Kamibayashi T, Maze M. Clinical uses of α2-adrenergic agonists. *Anesthesiology* 2000;93:1345–1349.

Lawson N, Meyer D. Autonomic nervous system: physiology and pharmacology. In: Barash PG, Cullen BF, Stoelting RK, eds. *Clinical anesthesia*, 3rd ed. Philadelphia: Lippincott-Raven Publishers, 1997:243–309.

Rozenfeld V, Cheng J. The role of vasopressin in the treatment of vasodilation in shock states. *Ann Pharmacother* 2000;34:250–254.

Talke P, Richardson C, Scheinin M, Fisher DM. Postoperative pharmacokinetics and sympatholytic effects of dexmedetomidine. *Anesth Analg* 1997;85:1136–1142.

Varon J, Marik P. The diagnosis and management of hypertensive crises. *Chest* 2000;118:214–227.

Anesthesia for Abdominal Surgery

Marjorie A. Podraza and John J. A. Marota

I. **Preanesthetic considerations.** Patients undergoing abdominal surgery require a complete history and physical examination as outlined in Chapter 1. The following issues should be considered as well.

A. **Assessment of preoperative fluid status.** Surgical pathology may cause severe derangement in volume homeostasis, producing both hypovolemia and anemia. The main sources of fluid deficits are inadequate intake, sequestration of water and electrolytes into abdominal structures, and fluid loss.

1. **Mechanisms of fluid loss**

a. **Patients may have had decreased or no oral intake** for varying periods of time before surgery. NPO guidelines are reviewed in Chapter 1. Gastrointestinal tract obstruction may prevent adequate oral intake. Chronically ill patients may not have adequate oral intake for a prolonged period because of anorexia.

b. **Emesis or gastric drainage** may produce significant losses, especially in patients with bowel obstruction. Quantity, quality (presence of blood), duration, and frequency of emesis should be assessed.

c. **Sequestration of fluid** may occur either into bowel lumen from ileus or into interstitium from peritonitis.

d. **Bleeding** from gastrointestinal sources includes ulcers, neoplasms, esophageal varices, diverticula, angiodysplasia, and hemorrhoids. This may result in normovolemic or hypovolemic anemia; measured hematocrit may be falsely elevated due to hemoconcentration.

e. **Diarrhea** from intestinal disease, infection, or cathartic bowel preparation can cause significant extracellular fluid loss.

f. **Fever** increases insensible fluid loss.

2. **Physical signs of hypovolemia.** Postural changes in vital signs (increased heart rate and decreased blood pressure) may reveal mild-to-moderate hypovolemia; severe hypovolemia will produce tachycardia and hypotension. Dry mucous membranes, skin mottling, and decreased skin turgor and temperature indicate decreased peripheral perfusion secondary to hypovolemia.

3. **Laboratory analysis** including hematocrit, serum osmolality, blood urea nitrogen-creatinine ratio, serum and urine electrolyte concentrations, and urine output is sometimes helpful in estimating volume deficits. **No definitive laboratory test indicates intravascular volume status.**

4. If the intravascular volume status of a patient cannot be determined by clinical assessment alone, then **invasive monitoring** such as central venous pressure and pulmonary artery pressure measurements may be necessary.

B. **Metabolic and hematologic derangements** occur frequently in patients requiring emergency abdominal surgery. Hypokalemic metabolic alkalosis is common in patients with large gastric losses (emesis or nasogastric [NG] tube drainage); large losses from diarrhea or septicemia can cause metabolic acidosis. Sepsis can produce disseminated intravascular coagulopathy.

C. **Length of surgery** is influenced by history of previous abdominal surgery, intra-abdominal infection, radiation therapy, steroid use, surgical technique, and surgeon experience.

D. **All patients for emergency abdominal procedures are considered to have full stomachs.** A rapid sequence induction using cricoid pressure or an awake intubation technique is indicated with the goal of minimizing aspiration risk. Premedication with histamine (H_2) antagonist and oral nonparticulate antacid can decrease gastric acidity. Metoclopramide decreases gastric volume but should not be used in cases of bowel obstruction.

II. **Anesthetic techniques**

A. **General anesthesia** (GA) is the most commonly employed technique.

1. **Advantages** include protection of the airway, assurance of adequate ventilation, and rapid induction of anesthesia with controlled depth and duration.

2. **Disadvantages** include loss of airway reflexes, which increases the risk of aspiration during routine or emergency surgery, and potential adverse hemodynamic consequences of general anesthetics.

B. **Regional anesthetic techniques** for abdominal surgery include spinal, epidural, and caudal anesthesia and nerve blocks. Thorough discussion of the risks and benefits of regional anesthesia are discussed in Chapter 17. Patients commonly require supplementation with an anxiolytic to tolerate the operating room experience.

1. **Lower abdominal procedures** (e.g., inguinal hernia repair) can be performed with regional anesthesia techniques that produce a sensory level to T4-6.

a. **Epidural anesthesia** usually is performed with a continuous catheter technique. A "single-dose" technique is applicable for surgery of less than 3 hours.

b. **Spinal anesthesia** usually is performed with a single-dose technique, although spinal catheters can be placed. The duration of block is determined by the choice of local anesthetic and adjuvants (see Chapter 15).

c. **Nerve blocks** can also provide adequate anesthesia for abdominal surgery.

(1) Blockade of the ilioinguinal, iliohypogastric, and genitofemoral nerves produces a satisfactory field block for herniorrhaphy. These nerve blocks are easily performed by the anesthesiologist but may require direct supplementation of spermatic cord structures by the surgeon.

(2) Bilateral blockade of T8-12 intercostal nerves provides somatic sensory anesthesia, whereas celiac plexus block provides visceral anesthesia.

2. **Upper abdominal procedures** (above the umbilicus, T10) are not well tolerated under regional anesthesia alone.

a. **Spinal or epidural anesthesia** for upper abdominal procedures may require a sensory level to T2-4. Paralysis of intercostal muscles from a high thoracic level impairs deep breathing; although minute ventilation is maintained, patients often complain of dyspnea. Intraperitoneal air or upper abdominal exploration produces a dull pain referred to a C-5 distribution (usually over the shoulders) that is not prevented by regional anesthesia and may require supplementation with intravenous (IV) analgesics.

b. **Celiac plexus blockade** alone does not completely block upper abdominal sensation; visceral traction is poorly tolerated.

3. **Advantages**

   a. Patients maintain the ability to communicate symptoms (e.g., chest pain).

   b. Airway reflexes are maintained.

   c. Profound muscle relaxation and bowel contraction optimize surgical exposure.

   d. Sympathectomy increases blood flow to bowel.

   e. Continuous-catheter techniques provide a ready means for postoperative analgesia.

4. **Disadvantages**

   a. Local anesthetic toxicity from inadvertent IV injection or rapid absorption.

   b. Patient cooperation is necessary for institution of block and positioning during surgery.

   c. Failure necessitates intraoperative conversion to GA.

   d. Regional nerve blockade may be contraindicated in patients with abnormal bleeding profile or localized infection at the site of injection.

   e. Sympathectomy may lead to venodilation and bradycardia that can precipitate profound hypotension. Unopposed parasympathetic activity causes the bowel to contract and may make construction of bowel anastomoses more difficult; this can be reversed with glycopyrrolate, 0.2 to 0.4 mg IV.

   f. Blockade of upper thoracic nerves may compromise pulmonary function.

   g. It is not appropriate to delay emergent surgical intervention to perform regional anesthetic techniques.

   h. Awake patients often require frequent communication and reassurance; this may distract the anesthesiologist during complicated cases.

C. **A combined technique** makes use of an epidural anesthetic along with a light general anesthetic. This technique is commonly used for extensive upper abdominal surgeries.

1. **Advantages**

   a. Epidural anesthesia reduces the anesthetic requirement during GA, thereby minimizing myocardial depression and potentially decreasing emergence time and nausea.

   b. Combined techniques may reduce postoperative ventilatory depression and improve pulmonary function early after upper abdominal surgery, especially in patients at high risk for postoperative pulmonary complications (e.g., obese patients).

2. **Disadvantages**
   a. In addition to the disadvantages listed in section II.B.4., sympathectomy produced by regional anesthesia can complicate the differential diagnosis of intraoperative hypotension.
   b. Epidural catheter placement and testing add to preparation time, potentially offsetting time saved with faster recovery.

III. **Management of anesthesia**
   A. **Standard monitors** are used as described in Chapter 10.
   B. **Induction of anesthesia**
      1. Restoration of volume deficits before induction and careful titration of sedative premedications provide increased hemodynamic stability.
      2. **Rapid sequence induction** or awake intubation (see Chapter 13, section VII.A) is required for all patients considered "full stomachs." Indications include conditions in which gastric emptying is delayed, intra-abdominal pressure is increased, or lower esophageal tone is compromised. Examples include trauma, bowel obstruction or ileus, hiatal hernia, gastroesophageal reflux disease, pregnancy beyond the first trimester, significant obesity, ascites, and diabetes with gastroparesis and autonomic dysfunction.
   C. **Maintenance of anesthesia**
      1. **Fluid management** requires appropriate administration of maintenance fluids and replacement of both deficits and ongoing losses.
         a. **Bleeding** should be estimated both by direct observation of the surgical field and suction traps and by weighing sponges. Blood loss may be concealed (e.g., beneath drapes or within the patient).
         b. **Bowel and mesenteric edema** can result from surgical manipulation or intestinal pathology.
         c. **Evaporative losses** from peritoneal surfaces are proportional to the area exposed. Fluid replacement is guided by clinical judgment and/or invasive monitoring. Traditionally, very long cases with significant bowel exposure and preoperative hypovolemia required fluid replacement of up to 10 to 15 mL/kg/hour. New evidence, however, suggests that a more restrictive approach with as little as 4 mL/kg/hour plus bolus fluid supplementation for hypotension may be associated with faster recovery and fewer complications.
         d. **Abrupt drainage of ascitic fluid** with surgical entry into the peritoneum can produce acute hypotension from sudden decreases of intra-abdominal pressure and pooling of blood in mesenteric vessels, thus reducing venous return to the right heart. Postoperative reaccumulation of ascitic fluid can produce significant intravascular fluid losses.
         e. **NG and other enteric drainage** should be quantified and replaced appropriately.
      2. **Fluid losses** should be replaced with crystalloids, colloids, or blood products.
         a. Initially, fluid should be replaced by administration of an **isotonic salt solution.** There is no formula to calculate the volume required to correct extracellular fluid

depletion. Adequate repletion must be assessed clinically; blood pressure, pulse, urine output, and hematocrit are guides. Further management of electrolyte and acid-base abnormalities should be based on laboratory studies. When an isotonic crystalloid solution is used to replace blood loss, about two-thirds of administered volume will pass into the interstitial space and one-third will remain in the intravascular space; thus, a ratio of at least 3 mL of replacement per 1 mL lost is usually needed.

b. **Colloids** are fluids containing particles large enough to exert oncotic pressure. They remain in the intravascular space longer than crystalloids. Multiple studies comparing fluid resuscitation with crystalloids to colloids have reported no benefit (and perhaps even poorer outcome) with colloids. Colloid solutions are more expensive than crystalloids; thus, routine use is not justified. Albumin may be superior to crystalloid in patients with significant burns, hepatorenal disease, or acute lung injury.

c. Use of **blood products** should be guided by laboratory measurements of hematocrit, platelet count, and coagulation parameters (see Chapter 34).

3. **Muscle relaxation** is required for all but the most superficial intra-abdominal procedures; sufficient relaxation is critical during abdominal closure because bowel distention, edema, and organ transplantation can increase the volume of abdominal contents.

a. **Titrating relaxants** to obtain a single twitch by train-of-four monitoring should provide enough relaxation for surgical closure yet allow for reversal of muscle relaxants for extubation.

b. **Potent inhalational agents** block neuromuscular conduction and are synergistic with relaxants.

c. **Neuraxial blockade** with local anesthetics provides excellent abdominal muscle relaxation.

d. **Flexing the operating table** may decrease tension on transverse abdominal and subcostal incisions and facilitate surgical closure.

4. **Use of nitrous oxide** (N_2O) may cause bowel distention because N_2O diffuses into the bowel lumen faster than nitrogen can diffuse out; the amount of distention depends on the concentration of N_2O delivered, the blood flow to the bowel, and the duration of N_2O administration. Under normal conditions, the initial volume of bowel gas is small; doubling or tripling of this volume does not pose a significant problem. Use of N_2O is relatively contraindicated in bowel obstruction because the initial volume of bowel gas maybe large. Bowel distention can make closure difficult and increased intraluminal pressures may impair bowel perfusion.

5. **NG tubes** are frequently placed in the perioperative period.

a. **Preoperative placement** is indicated for decompression of the stomach, especially in trauma victims and patients with obstructed bowel; many patients arrive in the operating suite with an NG tube already in place. Although suction via a large-bore NG tube can reduce the volume of gastric contents, it does not completely evacuate the stomach and may facilitate aspiration by stenting open the lower esophageal sphincter. NG tubes may also compromise mask fit. Before induction, suction should be applied to NG tubes. During induction, tubes should be allowed to drain. Cricoid pressure may help to prevent passive reflux when an NG tube is present.

b. Intraoperative placement is required to drain gastric fluid and air during abdominal surgery. Naso- and orogastric tubes should never be placed with excessive force; lubrication and head flexion facilitate insertion. Tubes can be directed into the esophagus by using a finger within the oropharynx or with Magill forceps under direct visualization with a laryngoscope. If these methods fail, a large endotracheal tube (9.5 mm or larger), split lengthwise, can be used as an introducer. The split endotracheal tube is introduced orally into the esophagus and the NG tube is passed through the lubricated lumen of the tube into the stomach; the split tube is then removed while stabilizing the NG tube.

c. Complications of NG tube insertion include bleeding, submucosal dissection of the retropharynx, and placement in the trachea. Intracranial placement has been described in patients with basilar skull fracture. The NG tube should be secured carefully to avoid excessive pressure on the nasal septum or nares as this may cause ischemic necrosis.

6. Common intraoperative problems associated with abdominal surgery include the following:

a. Pulmonary compromise can be caused by surgical retraction of abdominal viscera to improve exposure (insertion of soft packs or rigid retractors), insufflation of gas during laparoscopy, or Trendelenburg positioning. These maneuvers may elevate the diaphragm, decrease functional residual capacity (FRC), and produce hypoxemia. Application of positive end-expiratory pressure (PEEP) may counter these effects.

b. Temperature control. Heat loss in open abdominal procedures is common. Potential sources and treatment are discussed in Chapter 18, section VII.

c. Hemodynamic changes as a result of bowel manipulation (i.e., hypotension, tachycardia, and facial flushing). Aprostanoid, prostaglandin $F_{1\alpha}$, found in vascular endothelial cells and luminal cells of the bowel has been implicated as a humoral element.

d. Opioids may aggravate biliary tract spasm. Although uncommon, opioids may produce painful biliary spasm in some patients when administered as a premedication or into the epidural space. Spasm rarely complicates surgical repair or interpretation of a cholangiogram and can be reversed with naloxone. Nitroglycerin and glucagon also relieve spasm by nonspecific smooth muscle relaxation.

e. Fecal contamination from perforation of the gastrointestinal tract can cause infection and sepsis.

f. Hiccups are episodic diaphragmatic spasms that may occur spontaneously or in response to stimulation of the diaphragm or abdominal viscera. Potential therapies include the following:

(1) Increasing depth of anesthesia to ameliorate reaction to endotracheal, visceral, or diaphragmatic stimulation.

(2) Removal of source of diaphragmatic irritation, such as gastric distention.

(3) Increasing depth of neuromuscular blockade; this may decrease the strength of spasms. Complete diaphragmatic paralysis is difficult to achieve and may be possible only with doses of relaxants in excess of those required for relaxation of abdominal musculature.

(4) Chlorpromazine titrated in 5-mg IV increments.

IV. Anesthetic considerations for specific abdominal procedures

A. Laparoscopic surgery. Due to advances in instrumentation and surgical techniques, laparoscopic approaches are applied to an increasing number of surgical procedures, including cholecystectomy, hernia repair, fundoplication, nephrectomy, and colon resection. Benefits of laparoscopic surgery include smaller incision, reduced postoperative pain, decreased postoperative ileus, early ambulation, shorter hospital stay, and earlier return to normal activities.

1. Operative technique involves intraperitoneal insufflation of CO_2 through a needle inserted into the abdomen via a small infraumbilical incision until intra-abdominal pressure reaches 12 to15 mm Hg. Patient positioning is used to facilitate operative exposure: steep reverse Trendelenburg improves visualization of upper abdominal structures; Trendelenburg helps to visualize lower abdominal structures.

2. Anesthetic considerations

a. Hemodynamic changes associated with laparoscopy are influenced by the intra-abdominal pressure needed for creation of pneumoperitoneum, volume of CO_2 absorbed, patient's intravascular volume status, positioning, and anesthetic agents used. Generally, intra-abdominal pressures of 12 to 15 mm Hg are well tolerated in healthy patients. Mean arterial pressure and systemic vascular resistance usually increase with creation of pneumoperitoneum in healthy patients; cardiac output is unaffected. Patients with coexisting cardiac disease may develop decreased cardiac output and hypotension associated with pneumoperitoneum. Absorption of CO_2 across the peritoneal surface can cause hypercarbia, resulting in sympathetic nervous system stimulation and increased blood pressure, heart rate, and cardiac output.

b. The **reduction in FRC** associated with GA is compounded by the creation of pneumoperitoneum. FRC may be further compromised by the Trendelenburg position because of increased pressure from abdominal viscera on the diaphragm. PEEP may be necessary to treat alveolar collapse. Pneumoperitoneum increases peak airway pressures. However, transalveolar pressure may not be increased because of decreased abdominal and chest wall compliance, leading to **decreased respiratory system compliance.** Because CO_2 is absorbed across the peritoneal surface, an increase in minute ventilation is necessary to maintain normocarbia.

c. Because patients may be positioned in steep Trendelenburg or reverse Trendelenburg, changes in venous return must be anticipated and monitored. Also, frequent attention must be given to patients' arms to prevent **brachial plexus injury.**

d. **Temperature control.** Heat loss may occur from intraperitoneal insufflation of cold gas.

e. Embryonic channels between the peritoneal and pleural/pericardial cavities may open with increased intraperitoneal pressure, resulting in **pneumomediastinum, pneumopericardium,** and **pneumothorax.** Diffusion of gas cephalad from the mediastinum can lead to **subcutaneous emphysema** of the face and neck.

f. **Vascular injuries** secondary to introduction of the needle or trocar can produce sudden blood loss and necessitate conversion to an open procedure to control bleeding.

g. **Venous gas embolism** is rare but may occur on induction of pneumoperitoneum if the needle or trocar is placed into a vessel or an abdominal organ or if gas is trapped in the portal circulation. The high capacity of blood to absorb CO_2 and its rapid elimination in the lungs increases the margin of safety in case of accidental IV injection of CO_2. Insufflation of gas under high pressure can lead to a "gas lock" in the vena cava and right atrium; this will decrease venous return and cardiac output and produce circulatory collapse. Embolization of gas into the pulmonary circulation leads to increased dead space, ventilation/perfusion mismatch, and hypoxemia. Systemic gas embolization (with occasionally devastating effects on cerebral and coronary circulation) can occur with massive gas entrainment or via a patent foramen ovale. Treatment consists of stopping gas insufflation, placing the patient on 100% O_2 to relieve hypoxemia, and positioning the patient in steep head-down left lateral decubitus to displace gas from the right ventricular outflow tract (see Chapter 18, section XV.B). Hyperventilation will increase CO_2 clearance.

3. **Anesthetic management.** GA is usually required for laparoscopy. Creation of pneumoperitoneum and steep Trendelenburg positioning can compromise ventilatory function; controlled ventilation is necessary to prevent hypercarbia. A urinary bladder catheter and an NG tube are inserted (usually after induction of general anesthesia) to improve visualization and reduce the risk of trauma to bladder and stomach with trocar insertion.

B. **Esophageal surgery** for gastroesophageal reflux disease can be performed via either an abdominal approach (see below) or a thoracic approach (discussed in Chapter 21).

1. **The Nissen fundoplication** is the more common procedure and involves wrapping the fundus of the stomach around the lower part of the esophagus. This creates a collar in which intragastric pressure serves to constrict the wrapped esophagus rather than pushing gastric contents into the esophagus. Hiatal

hernias, if present, are repaired at the time of surgery. This procedure is often performed by using laparoscopic techniques to decrease the duration of postsurgical hospitalization.

    a. **Anesthetic considerations:** This procedure is performed most commonly with GA or combined GA–epidural (for open procedures). Patients who come to surgery often have been treated medically with proton pump inhibitors, H_2-receptor antagonists, or prokinetic agents. These should be continued until the day of surgery. A rapid sequence induction or awake intubation is indicated because of the high risk of gastroesophageal reflux and the potential for aspiration.

    b. **An esophageal bougie** may be placed to calibrate fundoplication; this ensures an adequate esophageal lumen to minimize postoperative dysphagia. The stomach or esophagus may be perforated by passage of the bougie or NG tube. With the laparoscopic method, the bougie is directed into the stomach by observation alone. Correct angulation of the esophagus or stomach during this maneuver is extremely important in preventing injury. The dilator or NG tube should be passed slowly and should be directly visualized. Particular attention should be paid to patients with esophageal strictures.

C. **Gastric surgery** is usually performed with GA or combined GA–epidural. The high likelihood of aspiration in these patients necessitates rapid sequence or awake intubation. Large third-space losses and potential for hemorrhage should be anticipated.

    1. **Gastrectomy** or **hemigastrectomy with gastroduodenostomy** (Billroth I) or **gastrojejunostomy** (Billroth II) is usually performed for gastric adenocarcinoma or intractable bleeding from gastric or duodenal ulcers; rarely, it is necessary in Zollinger-Ellison syndrome.

    2. **Gastrostomy** can be performed through a small upper abdominal incision or percutaneously with an endoscope. Local anesthesia with sedation is often adequate in the debilitated elderly patient, although some require GA.

D. **Intestinal and peritoneal surgery**

    1. Indications for **small bowel resection** include penetrating trauma, Crohn disease, obstructing adhesions, Meckel diverticulum, carcinoma, and infarction (from volvulus, intussusception, or thromboemboli). Patients are usually hypovolemic (see section I.A.1) and are considered a full stomach.

    2. **Appendectomy** is performed through a small lower abdominal incision or via laparoscopy. Fever, poor oral intake, and vomiting may produce hypovolemia; IV hydration before induction is indicated. In rare cases where sepsis and dehydration are absent, a regional anesthetic may be appropriate; otherwise, GA with rapid sequence or awake intubation is necessary.

    3. **Colectomy or hemicolectomy** is used to treat colon cancer, diverticular disease, Crohn disease, ulcerative colitis, trauma, ischemic colitis, and abscess. Emergency colectomy on unprepared bowel carries a high risk of peritonitis from fecal contamination. Some emergencies involving the colon are treated with an initial diverting colostomy, followed later by bowel preparation and elective colectomy. Patients must be evaluated for hypovolemia, anemia, and sepsis. All emergency colectomies and colostomies should be treated as if at risk for aspiration. Combination general/regional anesthetics are preferable.

4. **Perirectal abscess** drainage, **hemorrhoidectomy,** and **pilonidal cystectomy** are relatively noninvasive and brief procedures. Pilonidal cysts are excised with patients positioned prone; abscess drainage and hemorrhoidectomy can be performed in either a prone or a lithotomy position. If GA is used, deep planes of anesthesia or use of muscle relaxants may be necessary to achieve adequate sphincter relaxation. Hyperbaric spinal anesthesia is used for procedures in the lithotomy position, whereas a hypobaric technique is useful for the flexed prone (jackknife) or knee–chest position. A caudal block may be performed for either position.

5. **Inguinal, femoral, or ventral herniorrhaphies** can be performed under local anesthesia, regional anesthesia (spinal, epidural, caudal, or nerve block), or GA. Maximum stimulation and profound vagal responses may occur during spermatic cord or peritoneal retraction. Communication with surgeons is important, as they may need to reduce traction if necessary. If GA is selected, either mask technique (e.g., laryngeal mask airway) or deep extubation should be considered to minimize coughing on emergence that can strain the repair.

E. **Hepatic surgery**
1. **Partial hepatectomy** is performed for hepatoma, unilobar metastasis of a carcinoma, arteriovenous malformation, or echinococcal cysts. Extensive hemorrhage should be anticipated; standard monitors are supplemented with placement of arterial and central venous catheters, and large-bore IV access. Blood loss during hepatic parenchymal division can be reduced by temporary occlusion of portal venous and arterial inflow at the level of the hepatic pedicle (Pringle maneuver). The normal liver has considerable reserve and extensive resection is required before clinical impairment of drug metabolism is evident. The effects of liver disease on anesthetic management are discussed in Chapter 5. Epidural catheters can be placed in patients with normal coagulation status.

2. Patients with **portal hypertension** may present with symptoms of liver failure and may be awaiting liver transplantation. Most patients are treated conservatively with pharmacotherapy (e.g., β-adrenergic blockers, vasodilators), endoscopic sclerotherapy or banding for acutely bleeding esophageal varices, and transjugular intrahepatic portosystemic shunts. Surgery may be required for palliation of bleeding varices and ascites. Surgery is associated with an increased risk of encephalopathy and does not significantly improve long-term outcome.

a. **Portacaval and splenorenal shunts** relieve portal hypertension by diverting portal blood flow into the inferior vena cava (IVC) either directly (portacaval) or indirectly through the renal veins (splenorenal) via a surgically created anastomosis. Because complete diversion of portal venous flow through the IVC results in rapid development of hepatic failure, incomplete "H"-type shunts are constructed to permit partial decompression of the portal venous system. Shunting can significantly increase ventricular preload and precipitate heart failure. Shunting procedures decompress esophageal varices and may be required if variceal bleeding remains refractory to sclerotherapy. Splenorenal shunts require complete dissection of the splenic vein as it crosses the pancreatic bed. Bleeding may be extensive and difficult to control with underlying coagulopathy. Shunting procedures have been replaced largely by the less invasive transjugular intrahepatic portosystemic shunt (see Chapter 32).

b. Peritoneovenous shunting is performed for intractable ascites. Valved conduits, such as **the LeVeen and Denver shunts,** divert ascitic fluid from the peritoneal cavity to the venous system. These procedures can be performed under local anesthesia or with a superficial cervical plexus block. Shunting is rarely performed because of the potential for superior vena cava thrombosis and fibrous peritonitis and a high rate of shunt obstruction requiring reoperation. Disseminated intravascular coagulopathy precipitated by shunting is a rare complication and requires prompt removal of the device. Postoperative care is directed toward preventing circulatory overload and requires aggressive diuretic management.

F. Biliary tract procedures

1. Cholecystectomy is a common procedure performed via either open laparotomy or laparoscopic techniques. GA is favored for either technique. During laparoscopic cholecystectomy, the patient is placed in a steep reverse Trendelenburg position and the gallbladder is dissected from the liver bed by using either cautery or laser. Muscle relaxants are required for adequate abdominal wall relaxation. The amount of hemorrhage is difficult to assess because of the limited field of view and high magnification of the laparoscope; heavy bleeding from the cystic or hepatic arteries may occur. Advantages of laparoscopic cholecystectomy include minimal postoperative pain and faster recovery. Most patients are discharged on the first postoperative day.

2. Biliary drainage procedures include **transduodenal sphincteroplasty** for extensive choledocholithiasis; **cholecystojejunostomy** for distal common bile duct obstruction from pancreatic cancer; and **choledochojejunostomy** for chronic pancreatitis, stone disease, and benign strictures of the distal bile duct. Endoscopic and transhepatic techniques are increasingly common, but open surgical drainage is occasionally required. Blood loss is usually minimal but fluid loss may be significant.

G. Pancreatic surgery

1. Although the initial treatment of acute pancreatitis is supportive, surgical intervention may be necessary for **complications of pancreatitis.** Surgical management is indicated for infected pancreatic necrosis and hemorrhagic pancreatitis unresponsive to resuscitation with blood products and correction of coagulopathy. Pancreatic pseudocysts may require drainage: the cyst may be anastomosed to a Roux-en-Y limb of jejunum, the posterior wall of the stomach, or duodenum. Surgical intervention can produce significant bleeding and third-space fluid losses. In severe acute pancreatitis, activation of inflammatory mediators can produce sepsis and multiple organ dysfunction that require fluid resuscitation, mechanical ventilation, and vasopressor support.

2. **Pancreatojejunostomy with gastrojejunostomy and chole-dochojejunostomy (Whipple procedure)** is performed for resection of adenocarcinoma of the pancreas, malignant cystadenoma, or refractory pancreatitis confined to the head of the pancreas. These procedures have a high potential for hemorrhage and fluid loss. Epidural catheters are generally helpful for postoperative pain control in the absence of contraindications.

H. **Splenectomy** may be performed emergently after blunt or penetrating trauma or electively for treatment of idiopathic thrombocytopenic purpura or staging Hodgkin lymphoma. GA and muscle relaxation are required. Large-bore IV access is necessary because major blood loss requiring transfusion can be encountered. A combined epidural and general anesthetic technique is appropriate with the caveat that significant hemorrhage in a patient with a sympathectomy may potentiate hypotension. Occasionally, a transthoracic approach to gain control of the hilar vessels of a very large spleen may be necessary. Splenectomy patients should receive polyvalent pneumococcal vaccine in the postoperative period.

I. **Intraoperative radiation therapy** for pancreatic or colonic adenocarcinoma may be performed during laparotomy for primary resection or tumor debulking. Specially designed operating rooms have been constructed to facilitate intraoperative radiotherapy. If transport to a separate radiation therapy suite is necessary, however, the anesthetized patient is transported before wound closure. The patient requires continuous monitoring and ventilation with 100% oxygen during transport; medications and resuscitation equipment must accompany the patient. Anesthesia can be maintained with IV agents (e.g., propofol). A previously prepared anesthesia machine must be available in the radiation therapy suite. The patients must be hemodynamically stable and have a stable ventilatory status as they are monitored by remote television outside the radiation area. Aortic or IVC compression may occur when the sterile cone of the radiation therapy device is positioned in the abdominal wound. Ventilation with 100% oxygen can maximize the sensitivity of the tumor to radiation therapy. Treatments usually require 5 to 20 minutes but can be interrupted in the event of problems with hemodynamics or ventilation. Wound closure may be performed either in the radiation suite or after transport back to the operating room.

J. **Surgery for the obese.** With more than 60% of the U.S. population considered overweight, obesity is a major health issue. The **body mass index** (BMI) is correlated to the relative amount of adipose tissue and is calculated as follows:

$$BMI = body\ weight\ (kilograms)/height^2\ (meters)$$

Patients are considered overweight if BMI is greater than 25, obese if BMI is greater than 30, and morbidly obese if BMI is greater than 35 to 40.

1. **Preanesthetic considerations**
   a. Obese patients have **increased circulating blood volume** and **increased cardiac output** to meet **increased oxygen consumption.** Depressed left ventricular function can be found even in young asymptomatic patients and is

correlated to the degree of obesity. **Hypertension** is also significantly correlated with obesity.

b. Obese individuals have a higher risk for **hypercholesterolemia,** a risk factor for development of atherosclerosis and coronary artery disease. Patients with several cardiac risk factors may require cardiology consultation to optimize medical therapy in the perioperative period and to determine the necessity for further cardiac evaluation.

c. Patients who have used the **appetite suppressant** dexfenfluramine or fenfluramine for more than 4 months have an increased risk of cardiac valve disorders, particularly aortic regurgitation. Pulmonary hypertension has also been associated with these drugs. A perioperative echocardiogram may be indicated to evaluate valve function.

d. **Respiratory system** compliance is decreased in obesity due to decreased chest wall compliance from extra weight. There is a slight decrease in lung compliance due to increased pulmonary blood volume. FRC is reduced. In the supine position, FRC may fall within the closing volume, leading to ventilation perfusion mismatch and hypoxemia. The higher metabolic demand of the obese person with concomitant increased oxygen consumption and CO_2 production requires increased minute ventilation to maintain normocapnia.

e. Increased submucosal fat in the pharynx predisposes to collapse of the hypopharynx during sleep, leading to **obstructive sleep apnea.** Long-standing hypoxemia, as suggested by polycythemia, can result in pulmonary hypertension and right heart failure. Patients with severe sleep apnea may benefit from intensive monitoring in the immediate postoperative period.

f. Increased gastric emptying time and elevated intraabdominal pressure and volume predispose to a higher incidence of symptomatic **gastroesophageal reflux.**

g. Type II **diabetes** with hyperglycemia, hyperinsulinemia, and insulin resistance is common in the obese. Because perfusion of adipose tissue is variable, IV insulin infusion may be necessary to control hyperglycemia. Guidelines for the management of glucose and insulin are covered in Chapter 6.

h. **Airway management** traditionally has been considered a challenge in the obese because of the large size of the neck and face. One study reported that obesity or BMI alone is not a predictor for difficult intubation, although increasing neck circumference and a Mallampati score ≥3 were associated with problematic intubation. However, in that study, the degree of neck size that justifies an awake fiberoptic technique was not determined. Careful assessment of neck and jaw mobility, inspection of the oropharynx, and examination of dental status is required. If tracheal intubation is expected to be difficult, an awake intubation should be considered and discussed with the patient. Positioning of the upper body so that the external auditory meatus is in line with the sternal notch has been shown to provide a superior view with direct laryngoscopy.

      i. Significant **psychological problems,** such as depression and low self-esteem, may occur in many of these patients.

2. **Bariatric surgery** is currently the most effective treatment of morbid obesity. Patients with a BMI of 35 or greater with obesity-related comorbidities or patients with a BMI of 40 or greater are candidates for surgery. Surgery is associated with a loss of at least 50% of excess body weight; increased physical activity; and a decreased rate of hypertension, diabetes, and sleep apnea. Currently, two basic types of bariatric surgery are performed.

    a. **Vertical banded gastroplasty** produces a small gastric pouch that restricts the volume of food that can be ingested. Long-term weight loss may be limited by maladaptive eating patterns (liquids with high caloric content) or by staple line disruption.

    b. **Roux-en-Y gastric bypass** surgery consists of formation of a small gastric pouch and anastomosis of the pouch to the proximal jejunum. Weight loss occurs because of both a restrictive anatomy as well as decreased absorption of calories because of the bypassed small intestine. Patients who undergo this surgery may experience a "dumping" syndrome in which ingestion of high-energy-density food leads to nausea, abdominal cramping, and diarrhea. This may serve as an impetus for behavioral modification. Patients who have undergone this surgery are at risk for iron and vitamin B_{12} deficiency. The Roux-en-Y gastric bypass can also be performed laparoscopically.

3. **Anesthetic management**

    a. **Standard operating tables** are often unable to accommodate the size and weight of the obese patient; tables specifically designed for obese patients should be used. Extra padding and skin protection are necessary even for short procedures.

    b. **Standard noninvasive monitoring,** with a urinary catheter, is acceptable in patients who are generally healthy. An appropriately sized blood pressure cuff is critical; a regular-sized cuff placed on the forearm may be more effective than an oversized cuff on the upper arm. Intra-arterial blood pressure monitoring is necessary only for strict blood pressure control or if frequent blood sampling is required. IV access may be challenging.

    c. **Clinical evaluation of hydration and blood volume** in the obese patient is difficult. While they have an increased total circulating blood volume, it is less than in normally sized patients as calculated per kilogram of body weight. Technical difficulties during surgery can lead to increased blood and fluid losses. Although fluid replacement guided by hemodynamics and urine output is generally safe in healthy individuals, invasive monitoring to guide fluid management may be necessary in some patients. Central venous pressure measurements can be falsely elevated due to transmission of increased intra-abdominal pressures to the thoracic cavity. Pulmonary artery catheterization may be indicated to monitor the volume status of patients with congestive heart failure or valvular disease. While transmitted intra-abdominal pressure can falsely elevate filling pressures, it does not alter the accuracy of cardiac output determinations.

d. **Regional anesthetic** techniques can be challenging because of difficulties in identifying anatomic landmarks. Nevertheless, use of epidural anesthesia in combination with a light general anesthetic may be advantageous. The postoperative analgesia is of superior quality and potentially avoids risks of oversedation with opioids that can produce hypoxemia and hypercarbia in patients with a marginal respiratory reserve. The midline of the spine may be more readily apparent in the sitting position than in lateral decubitus, thus facilitating catheter placement. Long epidural needles (5 inches) may be necessary. The volume of local anesthetic volume injected may need to be decreased in the patient with morbid obesity; the volume of the epidural space is decreased because of fatty infiltration and increased blood volume in the epidural venous system.

e. The morbidly obese may require either **rapid-sequence induction** or awake intubation.

  (1) Obese patients may be at increased risk for aspiration because of delayed gastric emptying, increased intra-abdominal pressures, and gastroesophageal reflux disease.

  (2) The combination of an increased metabolic demand and decreased FRC leads to **rapid, dramatic, and sometimes refractory desaturation** during apnea. Preoxygenation for 3 to 5 min is recommended; established oxygen reserve remains small.

  (3) **Mask ventilation** is often difficult with limited gas exchange. Use of an oropharyngeal airway or two-person bag-mask technique may be helpful.

f. **Tracheal intubation may be difficult** in the morbidly obese. Awake fiberoptic intubation is recommended when difficult intubation is anticipated. Proper "ramped" positioning with additional support under the upper thorax, neck, and head can significantly improve the view during laryngoscopy. Reverse Trendelenburg or sitting positions can also be helpful but may make it necessary for the anesthesiologist to use a stand. A variety of types and sizes of laryngoscope blades, laryngeal mask airways, and endotracheal tubes with stylets should be readily available. There are no specific recommendations for endotracheal tube size in the obese patient.

g. Morbidly obese patients have a greater reduction in lung volume than nonobese patients during GA; this promotes greater **atelectasis, airway closure,** and **hypoxemia.** Alveolar collapse may be treated with PEEP and larger tidal volumes. High airway pressures may result from decreased chest wall compliance.

h. **Drug dosages** are difficult to estimate in the obese patient due to alterations in baseline physiology (e.g., increased cardiac output) as well as pharmacokinetic parameters (e.g., volume of distribution, renal and hepatic clearances).

Doses in mg/kg based on actual body weight (TBW) may be excessive. Alternatively, requirements may exceed estimates based on ideal body weight (IBW).

(1) In general, dosages of drugs with distribution confined to lean tissues should be based on IBW. If distribution includes lean and fat tissues, dosage should be based on TBW. Dosage of maintenance infusions should be based on clearance of the drug in obese patients. Generally, short-acting drugs are recommended.

(2) Obese patients may have increased pseudocholinesterase activity; doses of succinycholine should be based on TBW.

(3) Loading and maintenance doses of propofol should be based on TWB.

(4) Doses of opioids, including remifentanyl, should be based on IBW.

(5) **Loading doses** for benzodiazepines should be based on TBW; infusions are calculated by IBW.

i. Titration of muscle relaxants may be difficult. Nerve stimulators may underestimate the need (due to thick subcutaneous tissues), leading to underdosing of relaxants. **Ketamine and clonidine** can be used as a narcotic-sparing technique. Clonidine, 0.1 mg by mouth upon arrival at the hospital on the day of surgery, can provide some preoperative sedation without respiratory depression. Ketamine, given 0.5 mg/kg IV at induction and then infused at a rate of 0.25 mg/kg/hour until about 1 hour before emergence, can reduce the total amount of narcotic required for postoperative pain control.

j. The patient should be **extubated** in the operating room when awake, with adequate cough reflexes, and after confirmation of adequate reversal of muscle relaxation. Because the supine position decreases FRC, obese patients should be placed in a sitting position as soon as possible. Patients requiring positive airway pressure by mask (noninvasive ventilation) for sleep apnea can resume this treatment as soon as necessary; gastric distention does not appear to be a problem.

k. **Postoperative intensive care** should be considered for patients with severe coronary artery disease, poorly controlled diabetes, and severe sleep apnea.

K. **Orthotopic liver transplantation** is a curative procedure for end-stage liver disease. Common etiologies include hepatoma, sclerosing cholangitis, Wilson disease, α_1-antitrypsin deficiency, primary biliary cirrhosis, and alcoholic cirrhosis. Unfortunately, the supply of donor organs, particularly for children, is limited. Currently, two strategies are used to expand the supply of liver grafts for children without affecting the supply for adults: removal of the left lateral liver segment from a **living-related donor** for transplantation into a child, or **split-liver transplantation** in which two grafts are made by dividing one liver from a cadaveric donor. Because ex vivo division of the liver allograft is lengthy, prolonged ischemic time can result in graft injury that predisposes to a high incidence of dysfunction. There is growing experience with grafts divided in situ in a living donor; patients who receive these grafts have similar survival rates to patients who received whole or reduced-sized grafts.

1. **Preanesthetic considerations** for the patient with liver disease are discussed in Chapter 5.

2. **Surgery for hepatic transplantation** proceeds in three distinct stages.

   a. **Recipient hepatectomy** includes resection of the gallbladder, hepatic veins, and sometimes a section of IVC.

   b. **Anhepatic phase** marked by decreased venous return from interruption of the IVC. Venovenous bypass (typically left femoral and portal to left axillary vein) can improve venous return.

   c. **Postanhepatic phase** marked by reperfusion of the donor liver that delivers hyperkalemic, hypothermic, and acidic solution to the central circulation. The patient's condition usually stabilizes after completion of vascular anastomoses. After biliary anastomoses are completed, donor cholecystectomy, choledochojejunostomy, and placement of a choledochal tube complete the surgery.

3. **Anesthetic considerations**

   a. **Hemorrhage** in the presence of baseline coagulopathy can produce dramatic blood loss (multiple blood volumes); recipient hepatectomy is usually the period of greatest hemorrhage. Fibrinolysis during the anhepatic phase may exacerbate preexisting coagulopathy. **Aminocaproic acid** (Amicar) and/or **aprotinin** may be helpful (see Chapter 34).

   b. **Hypothermia** should be avoided by aggressive warming starting before induction (see Chapter 18, section VII).

   c. Metabolic derangements are common.

      (1) **Oliguria** secondary to hypovolemia and hypoperfusion may produce renal failure and hyperkalemia.

      (2) **Large-volume transfusion of citrated blood products** may lead to hypocalcemia and hyperkalemia.

      (3) During the anhepatic phase, there is a theoretical risk of **hypoglycemia**, although **hyperglycemia** from administration of dextrose-containing solutions is more common. This phase of surgery is often marked by a progressive **metabolic acidosis.**

   d. **Hypoxia** can occur from intrapulmonary shunting, thoracic restriction from surgical retraction, and Trendelenburg position. Adequate oxygenation may require a high fraction of inspired oxygen (F_IO_2) and application of PEEP.

   e. **Hypotension** from hypovolemia or cardiac dysfunction should be anticipated. Vasopressors and inotropes are necessary until the underlying problem is corrected.

4. **Anesthetic management**

   a. **Standard monitors** plus an intra-arterial blood pressure monitor and a urinary catheter are essential. Most patients also require pulmonary artery catheter placement. Large-bore IV access is also necessary via central or peripheral means. **A rapid transfusion system** capable of delivering 1.0 to 1.5 L/min at 38°C should supply the largest catheter.

   b. **Rapid-sequence induction** of anesthesia is advised because these patients are at risk of reflux from a full stomach, ascites, or obtundation. Ketamine may be useful as an induction agent in hemodynamically unstable patients.

c. **Maintenance** of anesthesia is accomplished with a balanced technique including moderate- to high-dose opioids and a volatile agent. N_2O is avoided because of potential air embolism during venovenous bypass and to minimize bowel distention.

d. **Intraoperative laboratory studies** including arterial blood gas tensions, glucose, electrolytes, hematocrit, platelets, and coagulation profiles should guide therapy.

e. **Transfusion therapy** rests on both autologous transfusion of blood salvaged from the surgical field and banked products. Laboratory and clinical assessment of coagulation will determine the need for packed red blood cells, fresh frozen plasma, or other blood products. If possible, transfusion of platelets is delayed until after completion of venovenous bypass. Cryoprecipitate and aminocaproic acid are potential therapeutic adjuncts.

f. **Resuscitation from hemodynamic collapse** may be necessary during reperfusion. Malignant arrhythmias or cardiac arrest can result from the cold, hyperkalemic, acidemic washout of the donor organ, hypoperfused gut, and lower extremities. Normalization of serum potassium and acid-base status before reperfusion is helpful; administration of volume, sodium bicarbonate, diuretics, insulin, dextrose, and small doses of epinephrine (50 to 100 μg IV) may be necessary. Hyperventilation can be used to treat acidosis.

g. **After surgery,** the donor liver resumes function, coagulopathy generally improves, and ongoing fluid requirements diminish. Patients require additional opioids for analgesia and sedation.

L. **Renal transplantation** (see Chapter 26).

M. **Heterotopic pancreatic transplantation** is performed usually in conjunction with heterotopic renal transplantation. Although recipients may undergo a nephrectomy, their native pancreas is left intact. Anesthetic considerations are primarily related to renal transplantation and management of diabetes (see Chapters 6 and 26).

1. Surgery often entails anastomosis of the donor pancreas to the recipient's bladder via a portion of duodenum allowing exocrine pancreatic secretions to drain into the bladder. Blood glucose should be determined frequently because it rapidly falls to normal with perfusion of the pancreas. Because there is no pepsin present, trypsinogen and chymotrypsinogen are not activated. Gram-negative urinary tract infection can activate these enzymes and lead to bladder damage, requiring emergency removal of the transplanted pancreas. The pancreas secretes bicarbonate that is lost in the urine; severe metabolic acidosis can occur during renal failure.

2. **Pancreatic islet cell transplantation** remains an experimental procedure but holds promise for the treatment of diabetes. The procedure consists of purifying islets from cadaveric donors and injecting them into the liver via the portal vein. Transplantation can be performed percutaneously with local anesthesia.

N. Recovery of organs for transplantation after brain death

1. **A significant gap exists between the supply of suitable donated organs and the demand for these organs to treat end-stage disease.** To increase the donor pool, strict exclusion criteria (age, coexisting illnesses) are no longer used. In addition, some centers use aggressive care regimens for potential donors to prevent common perturbations in homeostasis that accompany brain death. An alternative is the non-heart-beating donor, who does not meet brain death criteria but has such a poor prognosis that a family might consider withdrawing life support. A transplant coordinator from an organ-procurement organization must screen all potential donors.

2. **Organs may be deemed unsuitable** based on donor age, organ injury, disease, or gross abnormalities.

3. Hormonal therapy using methylprednisolone, arginine vasopressin, and triiodothyronine can increase the number of successfully implanted organs and reduce graft dysfunction when administered to brain-dead donors who demonstrate resistance to conventional resuscitation as manifested by low cardiac output, inadequate organ perfusion, or worsening lactic acidosis.

4. **Anesthetic management** for harvesting organs should focus on optimizing organ perfusion and oxygenation. Multiple surgical teams are involved; effective communication among surgical teams, anesthesiologists, and operating room staff is essential and is facilitated by the organ and tissue donation coordinator. Specific protocols are usually required and depend on the circumstances of the donation.

   a. **Dissection** of organs usually occurs in the following order: heart (30 min), lungs (1 to 1.5 hours), liver (1 to 1.5 hours), pancreas (1 to 1.5 hours), and kidneys (30 min to 1 hour).

   b. Once all organs are mobilized, **heparin** (20,000 to 30,000 units IV in adult donors) is administered and the aorta is cross-clamped. The distal aorta and IVC are cannulated, and the harvested organs are perfused in situ, topically cooled, and exsanguinated via the IVC.

   c. **Ventilatory support** is discontinued after the aorta is cross-clamped, and the anesthesiologist's role is completed with the discontinuation of all monitoring and supportive care, except during heart and lung procurement, as discussed below.

   d. **Non-heart-beating organ donation,** also referred to as **donation after cardiac death,** is reserved for patients who are not declared brain dead but whose family has chosen to remove them from life support because their condition is considered "hopeless." Life-sustaining treatment (mechanical ventilation, pressors) is discontinued after the patient is prepared for surgery to remove the organs. Five minutes after asystole occurs, a physician who is not part of the transplant team declares death. The body is rapidly cooled with preservative solution via an aortic cannula, and the abdomen is entered and organs are removed expeditiously. This technique has the disadvantage of significant warm ischemia time before organ procurement begins. In addition, there are ethical debates about the appropriateness of interventions (heparin treatment) aimed at improving grafts before the donor's death. Currently, anesthesiologists in the intensive care unit at the Massachusetts General Hospital participate in the withdrawal of support and declaration of death; however, no anesthesiologist is present in the operating room during procurement.

5. **Organ-specific considerations**
   a. **Lung/heart-lung.** Arterial partial pressure of oxygen (Pao_2) is maintained above 100 mm Hg with $F_Io_2 \leq 0.4$ and PEEP of 5 cm H_2O, with the goal of minimizing the risk of oxygen toxicity. Early verification of the endotracheal tube position with the surgical team prevents possible mucosal injury at the site of anticipated suture lines. Heart or heart/lung procurement requires continued monitoring of F_Io_2 and low-rate mechanical ventilation according to surgical needs after the aorta is cross-clamped. Lungs are inflated with 100% oxygen just before removal. Suctioning and extubation are done at the end of this procedure.

6. **Specific management problems**
   a. **Hypoxemia** may be caused by atelectasis, pulmonary edema, aspiration, or pneumonia. The F_Io_2 and minute ventilation should be adjusted to maintain a $Pao_2 \leq 100$ mmHg and $Paco_2 = 35$ to 45 with pH 7.35 to 7.45. Arterial blood gases should be determined every 30 to 60 minutes. High levels of PEEP should be avoided to preserve cardiac output and avoid barotrauma. High F_Io_2 should be avoided in potential lung donors to minimize possible oxygen toxicity.
   b. **Poikilothermia** is common; hypothermia should be anticipated and early aggressive measures instituted to minimize heat loss.
   c. **Hypertension** often transiently accompanies brain death and can be dramatic; in addition, reflex hypertensive response to surgical stimulation may occur. Short-acting agents such as nitroprusside or esmolol should be used anticipating hypotension that is often more challenging to control during organ procurement.
   d. **Hypotension** is common and due to a combination of hypovolemia and neurogenic derangement of vasomotor control. Central venous or pulmonary artery catheterization may be necessary to optimize filling pressures. Hypovolemia can be treated with crystalloid, colloid solutions, and blood products as necessary. Hematocrit should be maintained >30%. After restoration of intravascular volume, a vasopressor such as dopamine, epinephrine, or norepinephrine may be necessary. Depressed myocardial function may be treated with dopamine or dobutamine.
   e. **Dysrhythmias** occur frequently, especially in the setting of electrolyte imbalance, hypothermia, increased intracranial pressure, hypoxemia and acidosis, and derangement of brainstem cardiovascular control centers. Standard therapy is indicated. Bradycardia is often resistant to atropine and may require pacing therapy.
   f. **Polyuria** may be secondary to volume overload, osmotic diuresis, or the diabetes insipidus resulting from

derangement of the hypothalamic-pituitary axis. An IV infusion of vasopressin or desmopressin may be titrated to treat severe diabetes insipidus (see Chapter 6, section VII.B.2) and should be done in consultation with the surgical team. If used, it is prudent to discontinue these infusions 1 hour before aortic cross-clamping to minimize the risk of uneven distribution or ischemic injury with the infusion of preservative solution.

    g. **Oliguria** should be treated by ensuring adequate intravascular volume. Dopamine is preferred for the initial treatment of hypotension. A brisk diuresis is preferred when the kidneys are to be harvested. If volume repletion and pressors are not effective in restoring adequate urine output, mannitol and/or furosemide may be used.

SUGGESTED READING

Ballantyne JC, Carr DB, deFerranti S, et al. The comparative effects of postoperative analgesic therapies on pulmonary outcome: cumulative meta-analyses of randomized, controlled trials. *Anesth Analg* 1998;86:598–612.

Brodsky JB, Lemmens HJ, Brock-Utne JG, Vierra M, Saidman LJ. Morbid obesity and tracheal intubation. *Anesth Analg* 2002;94(3):732–736.

Carton EG, Rettke SR, Plevak DJ, et al. Perioperative care of the liver transplant patient. Part 1. *Anesth Analg* 1994;78:120–133.

Carton EG, Plevak DJ, Kranner PW, et al. Perioperative care of the liver transplant patient. Part 2. *Anesth Analg* 1994;78:382–399.

Choi PT, Yip G, Quinonez LG, Cook DJ. Crystalloids vs. colloids in fluid resuscitation: a systematic review. *Crit Care Med* 1999;27:200–210.

Gridelli B, Remuzzi G. Strategies for making more organs available for transplantation. *N Engl J Med* 2000;343:404–410.

Jaffe RA, Samuels SI. *Anesthesiologist's manual of surgical procedures,* 2nd ed. Philadelphia: Lippincott Williams & Wilkins, 1999.

Lowham AS, Filipi CJ, Hinder RA, et al. Mechanisms and avoidance of esophageal perforation by anesthesia personnel during laparoscopic foregut surgery. *Surg Endosc* 1996;10:979–982.

Patel T. Surgery in the patient with liver disease. *Mayo Clin Proc* 1999;74:593–599.

Pelosi P, Ravagnan I, Giurati G, et al. Positive end-expiratory pressure improves respiratory function in obese but not in normal subjects during anesthesia and paralysis. *Anesthesiology* 1999;91:1221–1231.

Robertson KM, Cook DR. Perioperative management of the multiorgan donor. *Anesth Analg* 1990;70:546–556.

Shenkman Z, Shir Y, Brodsky JB. Perioperative management of the obese patient. *Br J Anaesth* 1993;70:349–359.

White PF. The changing role of non-opioid analgesic techniques in the management of postoperative pain. *Anesth Analg* 2005;101(5 Suppl):S5–S22.

21

Anesthesia for Thoracic Surgery

Jeanna D. Viola and Paul H. Alfille

I. **Preoperative evaluation**
   A. **Patients for thoracic surgery** should undergo the usual preoperative assessment as detailed in Chapter 1.
      1. Any patient undergoing elective thoracic surgery should be carefully screened for underlying bronchitis or pneumonia and treated appropriately before surgery.
         a. **Diagnostic procedures** such as bronchoscopy and lung biopsy may be indicated for persistent infection.
         b. **Infection beyond an obstructing lesion** may not resolve without surgery.
      2. In patients with **tracheal stenosis,** the history should focus on symptoms or signs of positional dyspnea, static versus dynamic airway collapse, and evidence of hypoxemia. The history may also suggest the probable location of the lesion.
   B. **An arterial blood gas (ABG)** may help to clarify the severity of underlying pulmonary disease but are not routinely necessary.
   C. **Pulmonary function tests** are useful in assessing the pulmonary risk of lung resection. Both exercise function (maximal oxygen uptake [$\dot{V}O_{2max}$]) and spirometry (forced expiratory volume in 1 second) have been used to stratify risks of resection. In marginal cases, split-function radionuclide scans and ventilation/perfusion ($\dot{V}/\dot{Q}$) scans can determine the relative contribution of each lung and individual lung regions.
   D. **Cardiac function** should be assessed if there is a question about the relative contribution of cardiac and pulmonary disease in the patient's functional impairment. **Echocardiography** can estimate pulmonary artery pressure and right ventricular function.
   E. **Imaging studies,** such as chest radiography, computed tomography (CT), and magnetic resonance imaging, are useful to determine the presence of tracheal deviation, the location of pulmonary infiltrates, effusion or pneumothorax, and the involvement of adjacent structures in the disease process.
   F. **Three-dimensional reconstruction** from CT is used to assess the caliber of stenotic airways and can be used to predict the size and length of the endotracheal tube that will be appropriate for the patient. Severe airway stenosis may change the anesthetist's plans for induction and intubation.

II. **Preoperative preparation**
   A. **Preoperative sedation** should be given carefully to patients with tracheal or pulmonary disease.
      1. **Heavy sedation** may impair postoperative deep breathing, coughing, and airway protection.
      2. Patients with poor pulmonary function will be more prone to hypoxemia when their respiratory drive is suppressed. When sedating these patients, it is prudent to monitor oxygenation and administer supplemental oxygen.

3. **In the presence of airway obstruction,** sedation must be carefully balanced. Oversedation may profoundly suppress ventilation, but an anxious patient may make exaggerated respiratory efforts. In this case, the increased turbulence may cause worsened airway obstruction, leading to increased anxiety. Benzodiazepines, reassuring words, careful monitoring, and an expeditious start to the procedure are the best approach. In patients with airway stenosis, heliox (a mixture of helium and oxygen) will lower the density of the respiratory gas and reduce airway resistance.

B. **Aspiration prophylaxis,** with an oral histamine-2 receptor antagonist, sodium citrate, and metoclopramide, should be considered in patients undergoing major thoracic surgery, as aspiration may significantly impair already poor lung function. Patients with esophageal disease should be considered at high risk for aspiration.

C. **Glycopyrrolate** (0.2 mg intravenously) may be given to decrease oral secretions.

III. **Monitoring**

A. **Standard monitoring** should be used as described in Chapter 10.

B. A **radial arterial catheter** should be placed in any patient undergoing major thoracic surgery.

1. Surgical exposure during thoracotomy and esophageal or pulmonary resection often compresses the heart and great vessels. Having continuous blood pressure readings allows for immediate feedback.

2. Peripheral thoracic surgery, such as thoracoscopic wedge resection, is less likely to rapidly impair cardiac function.

3. ABG measurements are helpful for tracheal surgery, especially in the postoperative period.

4. In the lateral position it is possible for blood flow to the dependent arm to be impaired. Pulsatile flow to the dependent arm should be monitored with an arterial catheter or a pulse oximeter.

5. During mediastinal surgery (e.g., tracheal reconstruction or mediastinoscopy), it is possible for the innominate artery to be compressed, stopping flow to the right carotid and brachial arteries. Perfusion to the right arm should be monitored by an arterial line or pulse oximeter. Immediate feedback to the surgeon will allow decompression of the innominate artery.

C. Further invasive monitoring is dictated by the patient's condition. If a pulmonary artery catheter is placed:

1. It is customarily inserted from the nondependent side of the neck. If the catheter interferes with the surgical resection, it can be retracted into the main pulmonary artery and readvanced when the artery on the operative side is clamped. Use of a long sterile sheath facilitates repositioning of the catheter during surgery.

2. Pressure measurements referenced to the atmosphere may be affected by lateral positioning and opening the chest. Trends in central venous pressure, pulmonary artery pressure, and pulmonary artery occlusion pressure can be followed, and cardiac output and stroke volume measurements remain accurate.

IV. **Endoscopic procedures** include direct or indirect visualization of the pharynx, larynx, esophagus, trachea, and bronchi. Endoscopy may be undertaken to obtain biopsy samples, delineate upper airway anatomy, remove obstructing foreign bodies, assess hemoptysis, place stents and guidewires, position radiation catheters, apply photodynamic therapy, and perform laser surgery.

A. **Flexible bronchoscopy** permits visualization from the larynx to the segmental bronchi.

   1. A "working lumen" is used for suction, administering drugs, and passing wire instruments.

   2. Ventilation must occur around the flexible bronchoscope. Bronchoscopes range in diameter from around 5 mm (a standard adult size) to 2 mm (neonatal bronchoscopes that lack a working lumen).

   3. **Topical anesthesia,** sometimes with the assistance of an anesthetist for monitoring and sedation, is a common anesthetic approach.

      a. The patient should meet fasting (nothing by mouth) guidelines.

      b. Lidocaine (4% spray) is applied to the oro- or nasopharynx, larynx, and vocal cords. The trachea can be sprayed with anesthetic through the bronchoscope or by transtracheal injection. If this is done patiently, no further anesthesia is required.

      c. Care should be taken with the total dose of local anesthetic due to high systemic absorption from the orotracheal mucosa.

      d. Premedication with atropine or glycopyrrolate will limit salivary dilution of the anesthetic and may improve the onset and efficacy of the anesthetic.

      e. Nerve blocks may be used to supplement airway anesthesia (see Chapter 13).

      f. The patient should have nothing by mouth until tracheal and laryngeal reflexes return (2 to 3 hours).

   4. **General anesthesia** may be indicated in anxious, compromised, or uncooperative patients or if bronchoscopy is part of a larger surgical procedure.

      a. Bronchoscopy is very stimulating but does not cause postoperative pain, so a potent short-acting anesthetic is preferable.

      b. Muscle relaxation or topical anesthesia to the trachea is generally needed to prevent coughing during the procedure.

      c. The endotracheal tube used should be sufficiently large (7 mm inner diameter or larger) to permit ventilation in the annular space around the scope.

      d. A laryngeal mask airway (LMA) has the additional advantage of allowing easy view of the cords and proximal trachea.

B. **Rigid bronchoscopy** permits visualization of the larynx to the mainstem bronchi.

   1. A rigid bronchoscope has better optics and a larger working channel than a flexible bronchoscope and can be used to dilate a stenotic airway, easing subsequent airway management.

   2. Ventilation is accomplished through the lumen of the scope, allowing better control of a marginal airway.

3. General anesthesia is required for rigid bronchoscopy. Either deep inhalation anesthesia or muscle relaxation is required to prevent movement and coughing.

4. Conventional ventilation can be used, with the anesthesia circuit attached to a side arm of the rigid bronchoscope. The proximal end of the rigid bronchoscope is closed by a clear lens or by a rubber gasket through which telescopes may be passed.

   a. A variable but potentially large leak requires an anesthesia machine capable of delivering high oxygen flows.

   b. An intravenous or a potent inhalational anesthetic technique can be used.

   c. Close coordination between the surgeon and anesthetist is needed because ventilation may need to be interrupted for surgery, and surgery in turn may be interrupted by the need to ventilate.

5. In cases of severely compromised airways (e.g., severe airway stenosis or airway disruption), maintenance of spontaneous ventilation is indicated. The patient may be given an inhalational induction with sevoflurane and the rigid bronchoscope may be introduced under a deep plane of anesthesia.

6. Ventilating gas usually leaks out around the bronchoscope so that measurements of end-tidal carbon dioxide may be inaccurate. Adequacy of ventilation should be assessed by observation of chest excursion, pulse oximetry, and, if necessary, blood gas analysis.

7. **Sanders rigid bronchoscopes** are designed for jet ventilation through a special small side lumen.

   a. The central lumen remains open. Severe barotrauma may occur if gas is not allowed to escape. Observation of chest movement during the expiratory phase is critical. Conversely, ventilation may be ineffective with noncompliant lungs.

   b. An intravenous anesthetic technique (see Chapter 14) must be used. Muscle relaxation is required for the jet to inflate the lungs adequately.

   c. Additional gas is added to the inspired gas by the Venturi effect. The inspired oxygen concentration is uncertain because the amount of room air entrained cannot be controlled.

   d. During laser surgery the inspired oxygen concentration should be reduced to below 0.4, either by jetting air or by using a gas blender for the jet intake.

   e. The advantage of the jet technique is that ventilation is not interrupted by suctioning or surgical manipulations because the proximal end of the bronchoscope is always open. This makes the Sanders bronchoscope suitable for use during laser surgery of the larynx, vocal cords, or proximal trachea.

   f. Automated jet ventilators carry the added safety feature of automatic hold when the airway pressure rises above a set threshold. This prevents breath stacking and subsequent barotrauma.

8. **Complications** of bronchoscopy include dental and laryngeal damage from intubation, injuries to the eyes or lips,

airway rupture, pneumothorax, and hemorrhage. Airway obstruction may be caused by hemorrhage, a foreign body, or a dislodged mass.

C. **Flexible esophagoscopy** may be performed under local anesthesia as described for flexible bronchoscopy (see section IV.A) or after the induction of general anesthesia and endotracheal intubation. Use of a smaller caliber endotracheal tube will allow the surgeon more room to work in the pharynx and proximal esophagus.

D. **Rigid esophagoscopy** is commonly performed under general anesthesia with muscle relaxation. As with flexible esophagoscopy, a smaller endotracheal tube is used.

E. **Laser surgery** is performed on upper and lower airway lesions, including laryngeal tumors, subglottic webs, and laryngeal papillomatosis. A laser's wavelength determines its penetration and tissue target. The surgery may be performed via rigid bronchoscopy, laryngoscopy with jet ventilation, or traditional endotracheal intubation.

V. **Mediastinal operations**

A. **Mediastinoscopy** is indicated to determine the extrapulmonary spread of pulmonary tumors and to diagnose mediastinal masses. Mediastinoscopy is performed through an incision just superior to the manubrium. A rigid endoscope is then introduced beneath the sternum, and the anterior surfaces of the trachea and the hilum are examined.

1. Any general anesthetic technique may be used, provided the patient remains immobile. Although the procedure is not very painful, intermittent stimulation of the trachea, carina, and mainstem bronchi occurs.

2. **Complications** include pneumothorax, rupture of the great vessels, and damage to the airways. Blood pressures measured in the right arm may demonstrate intermittent occlusion if the innominate artery is compressed between the mediastinoscope and the posterior surface of the sternum. The trachea may be intermittently compressed by the mediastinoscope, and the position of the patient and surgeon increases the chance of accidental disconnection of the breathing circuit.

B. **A Chamberlain procedure** uses an anterior parasternal incision to obtain lung or anterior mediastinal tissue for biopsy or to drain abscesses.

1. The procedure is performed with the patient in the supine position after induction of general anesthesia. If no ribs are resected, the procedure is usually not very painful. Infiltration of the incision with local anesthetic or administration of small doses of opioids usually is sufficient for analgesia.

2. One-lung ventilation is not required for lung biopsy, but manual ventilation in cooperation with the surgeon(s) can facilitate the procedure.

3. If the pleural space is evacuated as it is closed, a chest tube generally is not required postoperatively, although the patient should be monitored carefully for any signs of pneumothorax.

C. **Mediastinal surgery**

1. **Median sternotomy** is performed for resection of mediastinal tumors and for bilateral pulmonary resections. In descending order of frequency, mediastinal masses include

neurogenic tumors, cysts, teratodermoids, lymphomas, thymomas, parathyroid tumors, and retrosternal thyroids.

2. **Thymectomy** is performed by median sternotomy and may be performed to treat myasthenia gravis. Anesthetic considerations for the patient with myasthenia gravis are detailed in Chapter 12, section VI.C.

3. **General anesthesia** may be induced and maintained with any technique.

    a. **Muscle relaxants** are not required to maintain surgical exposure but may be a useful adjunct to general anesthesia. Relaxants are best avoided in the myasthenic patient.

    b. During the actual sternotomy, the patient's lungs should be deflated and motionless. Even so, complications of sternotomy include laceration of the right ventricle, atrium, or great vessels (particularly the innominate artery) and unrecognized pneumothorax in either side of the chest.

    c. **Postoperative pain** from a median sternotomy is significantly less than from a thoracotomy and may be managed with either an epidural or a parenteral opioids.

VI. Pulmonary resection

A. **Lateral or posterolateral thoracotomy** is the most common approach for the resection of pulmonary neoplasms or abscesses. Thoracotomy may be preceded by staging procedures such as bronchoscopy, mediastinoscopy, or thoracoscopy. If the staging procedures are performed at the same sitting, the anesthetic should be planned to accommodate the possibility of a shortened procedure if metastatic disease is discovered.

B. **Endobronchial tubes**. Placement of a double-lumen tube is indicated for lung protection (for significant hemoptysis or unilateral infection), bronchoalveolar lavage, or surgical exposure.

    1. **Choice**

        a. Double-lumen tubes range in size from 26 to 41 French. In general, a 39 or 41 French tube is chosen for adult males; a 35 or 37 French is chosen for adult females. Selection is also based on the patient's height.

        b. **Right- and left-sided double-lumen tubes** are available and are designed to conform to either the right or the left mainstem bronchus. Each tube has separate channels: one for ventilation of the bronchus and the other for the trachea and nonintubated bronchus. Right-sided tubes have a separate opening to permit ventilation of the right upper lobe.

        c. **The choice of a left- or right-sided tube** depends on the type and side of operation. If a mainstem bronchus is absent, stenotic, disrupted, or obstructed, the double-lumen tube must be placed on the opposite side, preferably under direct fiberoptic guidance. In most cases, the choice of a left- versus right-sided tube is not so absolute. Most surgical procedures can be performed with a left-sided double-lumen tube. It is our practice, however, to selectively intubate the dependent (nonoperative) bronchus. This ensures that the endobronchial tube will not interfere with resection of the mainstem bronchus if this is necessary. Also, if the nondependent lung is intubated, ventilation of the dependent lung through the tracheal lumen may be compromised by mediastinal pressure pushing the tube against the tracheal wall and creating a "ball-valve" obstruction.

2. **Insertion**

   a. The endobronchial tube, including both cuffs and all necessary connectors, should be carefully checked before placement. The tube may be lubricated, and a stylet should be placed in the bronchial lumen.

   b. After laryngoscopy, the endobronchial tube should be inserted initially with the distal curve facing anteriorly. Once in the trachea, the stylet should be removed and the tube rotated so that the bronchial lumen is toward the appropriate side. The tube is then advanced to an average depth of 29 cm at the incisors or gums (27 cm in females) or less if resistance is met.

   c. Alternatively, a fiberoptic bronchoscope can be passed down the bronchial lumen as soon as the tube is in the trachea and then used to guide the tube into the correct mainstem bronchus.

   d. Once the tube has been inserted and connected to the anesthesia circuit, the tracheal cuff is inflated, and manual ventilation is begun. Both lungs should expand evenly with bilateral breath sounds and no detectable air leak. The tracheal side of the adapter is then clamped and the distal tracheal lumen is opened to atmospheric pressure via the access port. The bronchial cuff is inflated to a point just sufficient to eliminate air leak from the tracheal lumen, and the chest is auscultated. Breath sounds should now be limited to the side that has been endobronchially intubated. Moving the clamp to the bronchial side of the adapter and closing the tracheal access port should cause only the nonintubated side to be ventilated.

   e. Once adequate lung isolation is achieved, the fiberoptic bronchoscope should be used to confirm position because physical examination may be difficult or misleading. When passed down the tracheal lumen, the bronchoscope should reveal the carina with the proximal edge of the bronchial cuff just visible in the mainstem bronchus. Passing the bronchoscope down the bronchial lumen should reveal either the left mainstem bronchus or the bronchus intermedius depending on whether a left- or right-sided tube has been placed. The orifice of the right upper lobe should be visible through the side lumen of a right-sided tube. A bronchoscope should be kept available throughout the case.

3. The most common error is positioning the tube too far into the bronchus so that the distal lumen is ventilating a single lobe.

4. The procedure for passing an endobronchial tube through an existing tracheostomy stoma is identical. Bronchoscopy will help to determine how far the tube should be advanced once it is in the trachea.

C. **Univent tubes** are large-caliber endotracheal tubes encompassing a small integrated channel for a built-in bronchial blocker. Indications for a univent tube include the need for post-op intubation, the desire to avoid changing from a DLT to an SLT, and situations in which placement of a double-lumen tube is difficult or contraindicated. A potential complication is inadvertent advancement and insufflation of the bronchial blocker into the trachea, causing complete obstruction to ventilation.

1. **Insertion.** The Univent tube is inserted into the trachea in the usual fashion and is rotated toward the operative lung. After inflation of the tracheal cuff, the bronchial blocker is advanced into the operative mainstem bronchus under fiberoptic guidance, and the cuff is inflated. Because the Univent tube is made of Silastic rather than polyvinyl chloride, thorough lubrication of the bronchoscope is required.

2. **Collapse of the operative lung** occurs through both exhalation via the small distal opening in the blocker and by progressive absorption of oxygen from the lung, which will produce alveolar collapse. This is a slow process but may be hastened by deflating the blocker and disconnecting the anesthesia circuit while observing the lung. Once collapse has occurred, the blocker can be reinflated and the circuit reconnected.

D. **Bronchial blockers** may be used in situations in which it is not possible to place an endobronchial tube, typically in pediatric patients, in those with difficult airway anatomy, or where satisfactory lung isolation cannot be achieved by other means.

1. **Insertion.** An appropriately sized Fogarty catheter (8 to 14 French venous occlusion catheter with a 10-mL balloon) is selected and placed into the trachea before endotracheal intubation. After intubation, the balloon tip is positioned with a fiberoptic bronchoscope in the appropriate mainstem bronchus and inflated. Lung collapse occurs slowly, via absorption of gases. The ability to suction or perform maneuvers such as continuous positive airway pressure (CPAP) to the nonventilated lung is lost.

2. The **Arndt blocker** is a bronchial blocker especially designed for lung isolation. Placement is facilitated by a distal loop that can be snared with a bronchoscope. The airway connector is well designed, with separate access ports for the blocker, bronchoscope, and ventilation circuit. Like the Univent tube, the blocker has a small central lumen that can be used for lung collapse or CPAP.

3. A blocker can be placed either intraluminal or extraluminal to the endotracheal tube. Generally, if an endotracheal tube is already in place, only the intraluminal approach is possible. Placing the blocker via the bronchoscope adapter through the tube is relatively easy, provided the lumen of the tube will accommodate both blocker and bronchoscope.

E. **Complications of lung isolation techniques** include collapse of obstructed segments of the lung, airway trauma, bleeding, and aspiration during prolonged efforts at intubation. Hypoxia and hypoventilation may occur both during placement efforts and as a result of malpositioning.

F. **Positioning.** Thoracotomies for lung resection are most commonly performed in the lateral decubitus position with the bed sharply flexed and the hemithorax of interest parallel to the floor.

1. The arms are usually extended in front of the patient and must be carefully padded to avoid compression on the radial and ulnar nerves or obstruction of arterial and venous cannulas. The dependent brachial plexus must be checked for excessive tension. Various devices exist for supporting the upper arm securely above the lower, leaving the anesthetist with good access to the lower arm. Neither arm should be abducted more than 90°.

2. The neck should remain in a neutral position, and the dependent eye and ear should be carefully checked to ensure that they are not under any direct pressure.

3. The lower extremities should be padded appropriately to avoid compression injuries. In male patients, the scrotum should be free of compressive forces.

4. During the positioning process, the vital signs should be closely observed because pooling of blood in dependent extremities may cause hypotension.

5. Changes in position can move the endobronchial tube or blocker and change $\dot{V}/\dot{Q}$ relationships. Lung compliance, lung isolation, and oxygenation should be reassessed after any change in position.

G. **One-lung ventilation.** General anesthesia, the lateral position, an open chest, surgical manipulations, and one-lung ventilation all alter ventilation and perfusion.

1. **Oxygenation**

a. The amount of pulmonary blood flow passing through the unventilated lung (pulmonary shunt) is the most important factor determining arterial oxygenation during one-lung ventilation.

b. Diseased lungs often have reduced perfusion secondary to vascular occlusion or vasoconstriction. This may limit shunting of blood through the nonventilated operative lung during one-lung ventilation.

c. Perfusion of the unventilated lung is also reduced by hypoxic pulmonary vasoconstriction.

d. The lateral position tends to reduce pulmonary shunting, because gravity decreases blood flowing to the nondependent lung.

e. Oxygenation should be continuously monitored by pulse oximetry.

2. **Ventilation**

a. **Arterial carbon dioxide tension** during one-lung ventilation is generally maintained at the same level as on two lungs. This should not be at the expense of hyperinflating or overdistending the ventilated lung.

b. **Controlled ventilation** is mandatory during open-chest operations.

c. **Plateau (or end-inspiratory) airway pressure** should generally be maintained below 25 cm H_2O to avoid overdistention of the lung. The occurrence of high airway pressure should be investigated immediately and is usually due to malpositioning of the tube or the presence of secretions.

d. A moderate increase of partial pressure of carbon dioxide in arterial blood is usually well tolerated. Respiratory rate can be increased to maintain minute ventilation if necessary (as long as intrinsic positive end-expiratory pressure [PEEP]) and air trapping are minimal).

e. When switching from two-lung to one-lung ventilation, manual ventilation allows instantaneous adaptation to the expected changes in compliance and facilitates assessment of lung isolation. Once tidal volume and compliance have been assessed by hand and lung collapse has been confirmed visually, mechanical ventilation can be reinstituted.

H. Management of one-lung ventilation

1. Anesthetic management. During one-lung ventilation, the use of nitrous oxide is limited or discontinued if there is any evidence of a significant decrease in partial pressure of oxygen in arterial blood (e.g., a decrease in oxygen saturation).

2. Difficulties with oxygenation during one-lung ventilation may be treated with a variety of maneuvers directed at decreasing blood flow to the nonventilated lung (decreasing shunt fraction), minimizing atelectasis in the ventilated lung, or providing additional oxygen to the operative lung.

a. Tube position should be reassessed by fiberoptic bronchoscopy and repositioned if necessary. Additionally, the tube should be suctioned to clear secretions and ensure patency.

b. CPAP can be applied to the nonventilated lung with a separate circuit. Under direct visualization, the collapsed lung is inflated and then allowed to deflate to a volume that will not interfere with surgical exposure (usually 2 to 5 cm H_2O CPAP).

c. PEEP may be added to the ventilated lung to treat atelectasis but this may lower arterial oxygen saturation if a greater proportion of blood flow is forced into the unventilated lung as a result.

d. Apneic oxygenation may be provided to the nonventilated lung by partially inflating it with 100% oxygen and then capping the exhalation port. In this way, a motionless partially collapsed lung is maintained. Reinstallation of oxygen will be necessary every 10 to 20 minutes.

e. In the event of persistent hypoxemia that is uncorrectable by combinations of the above therapies or a sudden precipitous desaturation, the surgeon must be notified and the operative lung reinflated with 100% oxygen. Two-lung ventilation should be maintained until the situation has stabilized, after which the operative lung can be allowed to collapse again. Periodic reinflations or manual two-lung ventilation may be required to maintain an adequate arterial oxygen saturation throughout some procedures.

    f. A total intravenous anesthetic (TIVA) technique may be preferred to the administration of a volatile anesthetic, because it is easier to maintain a constant depth of anesthesia while performing maneuvers to improve oxygenation and ventilation.

    g. If hypoxemia persists, the surgeon can minimize shunt by compressing or clamping the pulmonary artery of the surgical lung or any of its available lobes.

    h. Cardiopulmonary bypass can be instituted to provide oxygenation (see Chapter 23) in extreme situations.

3. When switching from one-lung back to two-lung ventilation, a few manual breaths with a prolonged inspiratory hold will help to reexpand collapsed alveoli.

I. Anesthetic technique. General anesthesia, in combination with epidural anesthesia, is the preferred technique. Thoracic epidural catheters are usually placed (see Chapter 16 for technique).

  1. General anesthesia is typically induced with propofol, a short-acting narcotic, and a muscle relaxant (such as cisatracurium) and maintained with a volatile agent in oxygen.

    a. Nitrous oxide may be used during the procedure to reduce the requirement for volatile agents.

      (1) During one-lung ventilation, shunting and hypoxemia may limit the use of nitrous oxide in some patients.

      (2) At the conclusion of the procedure with both lungs ventilated, nitrous oxide, in concentrations up to 70%, will provide a smoother emergence than a volatile agent alone. It is essential that the chest tubes are functioning.

    b. Muscle relaxants are useful adjuncts to general anesthesia. Although surgical exposure does not require muscle relaxation, movement and coughing carry some risk.

  2. Epidural analgesia is an effective method for postoperative pain relief after thoracotomy.

    a. Intraoperative use of the epidural can be with a local anesthetic, an opioid, or an anesthetic–opioid mixture. Phenylephrine should be used to counteract hypotension associated with epidural blockade.

    b. Stimulation caused by lung reexpansion, bronchoscopy, and bronchial dissection is not blunted by epidural analgesia and may provoke a sudden response in an otherwise well-anesthetized patient.

J. Emergence and extubation. The goal of the anesthetic technique selected is to have an awake, comfortable, and extubated patient at the end of the procedure.

  1. Before closing the chest, the lungs are inflated to 30 cm H_2O pressure to reinflate atelectatic areas and check for significant air leaks.

  2. Chest tubes are inserted to drain the pleural cavity and promote lung expansion. Chest tubes usually are placed under water seal and up to 20 cm H_2O suction, except after a pneumonectomy. After pneumonectomy, a chest tube, if used, should be placed under water seal only. Applying suction could shift the mediastinum to the draining side and reduce venous return.

3. **Prompt extubation** avoids the potential disruptive effects of endotracheal intubation and positive-pressure ventilation on fresh suture lines. If postoperative mechanical ventilation is required, the double-lumen tube should be exchanged for a conventional endotracheal tube with a high-volume low-pressure cuff. Inspiratory pressures should be kept as low as possible.

K. **Postoperative analgesia.** Lateral thoracotomy is a painful incision, involving multiple muscle layers, rib resection, and continuous motion as the patient breathes. Therapy for postoperative pain should begin before the patient emerges from general anesthesia.

1. **Epidural analgesia** has become the preferred approach for post-thoracotomy pain management (see Chapter 37). Shoulder pain that thoracotomy patients commonly note is referred pain from diaphragmatic irritation and is not covered by epidural analgesia but is well treated with nonsteroidal analgesics.

2. **Intercostal nerve blocks**
   a. Intercostal nerve blocks may be used when epidural analgesia is impractical or ineffective.
   b. Five interspaces are usually blocked: two above, two below, and one at the site of the incision.
   c. **Technique.** Under sterile conditions, a 22-gauge needle is inserted perpendicular to the skin in the posterior axillary line over the lower edge of the rib. The needle then is "walked" off the rib inferiorly until it just slips off the rib. After a negative aspiration for blood, 4 to 5 mL of 0.5% bupivacaine with 1:200,000 epinephrine is injected. The procedure is repeated at each interspace to be blocked. In addition, subcutaneous infiltration with bupivacaine is performed in a V-shaped pattern around each chest tube site to reduce the discomfort of chest tube movement.
   d. If a chest tube is not in place, the risk of pneumothorax from the block needs to be considered.

3. Parenteral narcotics, if required, should be administered judiciously.

4. **Nonsteroidal anti-inflammatory agents. Ketorolac** has proved effective as a supplemental analgesic but should be used with caution in the elderly, in patients with renal insufficiency, and in those with a history of gastric bleeding.

VII. **Tracheal resection and reconstruction**

A. **General considerations.** Surgery of the trachea and major airways involves significant anesthetic risks, including interruption of airway continuity and the potential for total obstruction of an already stenotic airway.

1. The surgical approach depends on the location and extent of the lesion. Lesions of the cervical trachea are approached through a transverse neck incision. Lower lesions necessitate an upper sternal split. Lesions of the distal trachea and carina may require a median sternotomy or a right thoracotomy.

    2. Extubation at the conclusion of the surgical procedure is the goal of the anesthetic because it will put less strain on the fresh tracheal anastomosis.

B. Induction

    1. The anesthetic technique must include a plan for preserving airway patency throughout induction and intubation and emergency plans and equipment for dealing with any sudden loss of airway control.

    2. If the airway is critically stenotic, spontaneous ventilation should be maintained throughout the induction because it may not be possible to ventilate the lungs by mask ventilation if apnea occurs. A volatile agent in oxygen is the preferred anesthetic and no muscle relaxants are used. Sevoflurane, with its lack of airway irritability, is suitable for inhalational induction. A deep plane of anesthesia must be achieved before instrumentation, and this may require 15 to 20 minutes in a patient with small tidal volumes and a large functional residual capacity. Hemodynamic support with phenylephrine may be required for an elderly or debilitated patient to tolerate the necessary high concentration of volatile agent.

    3. Patients with preexisting mature tracheostomies may be induced with intravenous agents followed cannulation of the tracheostomy with a cuffed, flexible, armored endotracheal tube. The surgical field around the tube is prepared, and the tube is removed and replaced with a sterile one by the surgeon.

C. Intraoperative management is complicated by periodic interruption of airway continuity by the surgical procedure.

    1. Rigid bronchoscopy is commonly performed before the surgical incision to delineate tracheal anatomy and caliber.

       a. If the surgeon determines that an endotracheal tube can be placed through the stenotic segment, this should be done as soon as the bronchoscope is withdrawn. Controlled ventilation can then be used safely.

       b. If the stenotic segment is too narrow or friable to allow intubation, spontaneous ventilation and anesthesia must continue through the bronchoscope until surgical access to the distal trachea is achieved. Alternatives include having the surgeon "core out" the tracheal lesion with the rigid bronchoscope, placing a tracheostomy distal to the stenotic segment, intubating the trachea above the lesion or placing a LMA and allowing spontaneous ventilation to continue, or using a jet ventilation system to ventilate the patient from above the lesion.

    2. When the airway is in jeopardy or ventilation is intermittent, 100% oxygen should be administered.

    3. For lower tracheal or carinal resections, a long endotracheal tube with a flexible armored wall can be used. This allows the surgeon to position the tip in the trachea or either mainstem bronchus and to operate around it without interrupting ventilation.

    4. When the trachea is surgically divided, the endotracheal tube must be retracted proximal to the division and a sterile armored tube placed into the distal trachea by the surgeon. A suture may be placed in the endotracheal tube before pulling it back into the pharynx to facilitate replacing it in the trachea at the end of the procedure.

    a. The tube is frequently removed and reinserted by the surgeons as they work around it. Manual ventilation during this portion of the procedure will help avoid leakage of gas from the circuit.

    b. Once the stenotic segment has been removed and the posterior tracheal reanastomosis completed, the transtracheal tube is removed and the endotracheal tube is readvanced from above. The distal trachea should be suctioned to remove accumulated blood and secretions. The patient's neck is then flexed forward, reducing tension on the trachea, and the anterior portion of the anastomosis is completed.

  5. **Jet ventilation** through a catheter held by one of the surgeons may be required during carinal resection if the distal airways are too small to accommodate an endotracheal tube.

    a. It is difficult to administer volatile agents by a jet ventilator so intravenous agents are needed during this portion of the surgery.

    b. Jet ventilation rate and pressure should be carefully titrated by direct observation of the surgical field. Obstruction of exhalation will lead to "stacking" of breaths, increased airway pressure, and barotrauma.

  6. **At the conclusion of the procedure,** a single large suture is placed from the chin to the anterior chest to preserve neck flexion and thereby minimize tension on the tracheal suture line. Several blankets under the head will help maintain flexion. Close attention during emergence, extubation, and transfer is essential.

D. Emergence and extubation

  1. **Spontaneous ventilation** should be resumed as soon as possible after the procedure to minimize trauma to the tracheal suture line. Most patients may be safely extubated, but in those for whom difficult anatomy or copious secretions make this undesirable, a small tracheostomy may be placed below the tracheal repair.

    a. The patient should be awake enough to maintain spontaneous ventilation and avoid aspiration but should be extubated before excessive head movement can damage the surgical repair.

    b. If tracheal collapse, airway edema, or secretions cause respiratory distress after extubation, the patient should be reintubated fiberoptically with a small uncuffed endotracheal tube, preferably with the head maintained in forward flexion.

  2. Frequent bronchoscopies at the bedside under local anesthesia may be required to remove secretions from the lungs in the postoperative period.

  3. Only relatively small amounts of intravenous opioids are usually needed to treat the mild pain from the neck incision. Analgesia usually is administered after the patient is wide awake and responsive and while monitoring for undesirable respiratory depression.

E. **Tracheal disruption** may be caused by airway instrumentation or thoracic trauma and may be signaled by hypoxia, dyspnea, subcutaneous emphysema, pneumomediastinum, or pneumothorax.

1. **The point of injury** is commonly at the cricoid, midtrachea, carina, or either mainstem bronchus. Several mechanisms of injury have been proposed, including high airway pressures, lateral stretch of the thoracic cavity, and deceleration injury.

2. **Positive-pressure ventilation** will exacerbate the air leak and rapidly worsen symptoms from pneumothorax or pneumomediastinum. If possible, the patient should be allowed to breathe spontaneously, following the protocol for the patient with critical tracheal stenosis.

3. **Tracheal damage** in the already anesthetized patient may be treated initially by advancement of a small endotracheal tube past the point of injury. In the case of a difficult airway in which the tube causes the injury, an immediate surgical tracheostomy must be performed and access to the distal trachea secured.

4. Once a tube has been placed across or distal to the site of tracheal disruption, controlled positive-pressure ventilation can begin. Further management is as for the patient undergoing elective airway surgery.

VIII. **Intrapulmonary hemorrhage.** Massive hemoptysis may be caused by thoracic trauma, pulmonary artery rupture secondary to catheterization, or erosion into a vessel by a tracheostomy, abscess, or airway tumor.

A. The trachea must be immediately intubated and the lungs ventilated with 100% oxygen.

B. An attempt should be made to suction the airway clear, ideally by rigid bronchoscopy.

C. **If a unilateral source is identified,** lung isolation may be undertaken to protect the uninvolved lung and facilitate corrective surgery. Techniques for lung isolation are described in section VI.B. Obstruction of the endotracheal tube is an ever present danger, and frequent suctioning may be necessary.

1. **Lung isolation** may be achieved by placing an endobronchial blocker or a double-lumen endobronchial tube. Choice of technique depends on experience, equipment at hand, and the extent of active bleeding. Active bleeding may obscure airway visualization during flexible bronchoscopy.

2. In an emergency, the existing endotracheal tube can be advanced into the mainstem bronchus of the uninvolved lung and the cuff inflated.

3. **Fiberoptic bronchoscopy** is essential for suctioning blood and confirming isolation.

D. Frequently, the source of bleeding is from the bronchial circulation. **Embolization** in the radiology suite is often attempted if the patient is stable.

E. Definitive treatment may require a thoracotomy and surgical repair.

IX. **Bronchopleural fistula** is a connection between a bronchial stump and the surrounding pleura. Symptoms include dyspnea, subcutaneous emphysema, persistent air leak, and purulent discharge from the chest tube.

A. **General considerations**
   1. Small fistulas may close spontaneously; a persistent leak indicates involvement of a larger bronchus.
   2. Treatment of subsequent sepsis involves antibiotics and chest tube drainage.
   3. Surgical approach varies, ranging from application of fibrin glue via bronchoscopy to thoracoplasty with a pedicled muscle flap.

B. **Anesthetic management**
   1. Positive pressure ventilation may be inadequate if most ventilation escapes through the fistula. A functional chest tube must be in place before induction and positive pressure ventilation.
   2. Patients often undergo inhalation induction with spontaneous ventilation and lung isolation via endobronchial intubation to minimize the amount of time spent ventilating the fistula.
   3. **High-frequency jet ventilation (HFJV)** has been used as an alternative to lung isolation to successfully decrease gas leak through the fistula by providing lower peak and mean airway pressures than with traditional positive pressure ventilation. HFJV is not effective in patients with noncompliant lungs such as acute respiratory distress syndrome patients. If mechanical ventilation via a standard endotracheal tube is to be used, flow redistribution may not be used to signal the end of a breath: the fistula will allow for gas flow at a constant velocity, causing the mechanical breath to continue indefinitely.

X. **Esophageal surgery** includes procedures for resecting esophageal neoplasms, antireflux procedures, and repairing traumatic or congenital lesions.

A. **General considerations**
   1. Patients may be chronically malnourished both from systemic illness (carcinoma) and anatomic interference with swallowing. Enteral or parenteral nutrition may have been begun preoperatively.
   2. Both esophageal carcinoma and traumatic disruption of the distal esophagus are associated with ethanol abuse; patients may have impaired liver function, elevated portal pressures, anemia, cardiomyopathy, and bleeding disorders.
   3. Patients who have difficulty swallowing may be significantly hypovolemic. Cardiovascular instability may be further exacerbated by preoperative chemotherapy with cardiotoxins.
   4. Most patients presenting for esophageal procedures will be at risk for aspiration. Appropriate preoperative prophylaxis should be given, and rapid sequence induction or awake intubation should be planned.
   5. Monitors should include a radial artery and urinary catheters. Central venous access may be desirable.
   6. Temperature conservation measures should be aggressively pursued. The use of a warmed air blanket over the lower body is routine.

B. **Operative approach and anesthesia**
   1. **An upper esophageal diverticulum** (Zenker's diverticulum) is approached through a lateral cervical incision, similar to

that for carotid surgery. This incision may also be used for upper esophageal myotomies for swallowing disorders.

a. **Positioning.** The patient is positioned supine with the neck extended and the head turned to the contralateral side.

b. **General anesthesia** may be induced and maintained with any technique after rapid sequence intubation. Postoperative pain and fluid shifts are usually minimal with a cervical incision, and patients may be safely extubated at the conclusion of the procedure. The surgeons may or may not elect to leave a nasogastric tube in place.

2. **Carcinoma**

a. Lesions of the upper esophagus are approached by a "three-hole" approach, which includes a transverse cervical incision, a laparotomy, and a right thoracotomy. The right-sided thoracic incision and abdominal incision are required to mobilize the stomach and lower esophagus. A cervical incision allows for anastomosis of the proximal esophagus and distal stomach.

b. **Lesions of the middle esophagus** are commonly approached with a right-sided thoracotomy, which allows for a proximal anastomosis above the level of the aortic arch. Mobilization of the stomach or jejunum is accomplished through a midline abdominal incision. This combination is known as an **Ivor-Lewis procedure.**

c. **Lower esophageal lesions** are approached through an extended left thoracoabdominal incision. After resection, the surgeon will perform a primary anastomosis of the esophagus and stomach. Occasionally, the stomach does not provide an adequate distal anastomosis and the surgeon instead brings up a roux-en-Y loop of jejunum.

d. Postoperative endotracheal extubation is performed when patients can protect their own airway from aspiration and they are fully awake. Immediate postoperative extubation can be considered in healthier patients after uncomplicated procedures.

e. Virtually any anesthetic technique may be used. Epidural analgesia is commonly used in the postoperative period.

f. If postoperative intubation is deemed necessary, it is usual to change from a double-lumen to a conventional endotracheal tube at the conclusion of the resection. Dependent tissue edema may significantly narrow the airway, rendering reintubation difficult.

3. **Traumatic damage to the entire esophagus** (as with lye ingestion) or extensive cancers may necessitate a total esophagectomy with subsequent interposition of a segment of colon or jejunum to serve as a conduit between the pharynx and stomach.

a. Surgical exposure may require two or three incisions. In some cases, the esophagus can be dissected bluntly from the posterior mediastinum through cervical and abdominal incisions, and no thoracotomy is necessary. This is known as a trans-hiatal esophagectomy.

b. These patients may have a prolonged postoperative course with significant fluid shifts and nutritional depletion and are at risk for aspiration pneumonia. The trachea may remain intubated at the conclusion of the surgery, if a complex procedure has done.

4. Fundoplication (e.g., Belsey Mark IV, Hill, or Nissen) is performed to relieve gastroesophageal reflux; the specific procedure depends on the surgeon's preference and the patient's anatomy.

   a. The surgical approach is transabdominal for the Hill and Nissen procedures and transthoracic for the Belsey. Collapse of the left lung is required for the latter procedure.

   b. Fluid shifts are usually less than after other esophageal surgeries and these patients may be safely extubated at the conclusion of the procedure. Postoperative analgesic requirements are determined by the specific incision made; most patients benefit from epidural medications.

XI. Lung transplantation is performed for end-stage nonmalignant lung disease. The most common indications are severe emphysema, α_1-antitrypsin deficiency, cystic fibrosis, pulmonary fibrosis, and pulmonary hypertension. Specific operations include living-related lobar lung transplant (LRLLTx), single-lung transplant (SLTx), double-lung transplant (DLTx), sequential single-lung transplant, and combined heart–lung transplantation. The etiology of the lung disease usually dictates the specific operation to be performed and the likelihood that cardiopulmonary bypass will be required; furthermore, the patient's position depends on the incision required for adequate surgical exposure (lateral decub/thoracotomy for SLTx, clamshell incision/supine for DLTx or LRLLTx). Hence, knowing the patient's preoperative diagnosis will suggest the required approach. Patients will have undergone preoperative counseling, exercise and cardiac testing, and a conditioning program along with other assessments outlined in section I. Because the optimal donor ischemic time is less than 4 hours, time is of the essence.

A. Monitors and equipment

   1. Transplant patients will be actively immunosuppressed; therefore, sterile technique for all procedures is paramount. In addition to the usual monitoring for pulmonary resection, a pulmonary artery catheter with atrioventricular pacing capabilities is placed, incorporating a long sterile protective sheath. A femoral arterial line is contemplated for patients who have a high likelihood of requiring cardiopulmonary bypass (CPB). A large-bore femoral nervous access line is also of use when CPB is contemplated. A bispectral index (BIS) monitor may also be useful given the technical troubles associated with a TIVA type anesthetic.

   2. Medications should be immediately available to treat bronchospasm, electrolyte disturbances, pulmonary hypertension, and right ventricular failure. Immunosuppressants, steroids, and antibiotics should also be administered. All blood products must be leukocyte depleted and transfused via a filter. Anticipation of a large transfusion requirement and maintenance of an ample supply of blood products are important.

3. An epidural catheter should be placed for postoperative pain management, unless there is a strong possibility that the patient will need cardiopulmonary bypass and full heparin treatment.

4. Rarely, an additional mechanical ventilator may be required to optimally ventilate each lung.

5. Equipment should be available for peripheral arteriovenous or venovenous bypass through an oxygenator if hypoxemia becomes a significant problem. (See Chapter 23 on cardiopulmonary bypass).

B. **Anesthetic technique.** Any technique that provides cardiovascular stability is appropriate. An intravenous technique may be preferable in the face of compromised ventilation. Organ availability is rarely planned, so most recipients will be considered "full stomachs."

1. **Lung isolation** is best achieved with a contralateral endobronchial tube. In the event of a DLT, a left-sided tube is used with the left-sided bronchial anastomosis performed distal to the tip. The endobronchial tube may be exchanged for a single-lumen endotracheal tube at the end of operation if the patient is expected to require postoperative ventilation.

2. **Capnography** may be misleading because of severe mismatching of ventilation to perfusion. Frequent measurements of ABG tensions are warranted to assess ventilation. Worsening acidemia may also signal inadequate tissue perfusion from a variety of causes (hypovolemia, airtrapping, decreased cardiac output).

3. **Full cardiopulmonary bypass** may be necessary for the patient with pulmonary hypertension who cannot tolerate unilateral pulmonary artery clamping. Indications for bypass include arterial oxygen saturation less than 90% after clamping of the pulmonary artery, cardiac index less than 3.0 L/min/m^2 despite therapy with dopamine and nitroglycerin, or a systolic blood pressure less than 90 mm Hg. Continuous cardiac output monitors may be used to assess cardiac function. Management of cardiopulmonary bypass is discussed in Chapter 23.

4. **The surgical approach** for a SLT is via a standard posterolateral incision. A bilateral subcostal thoracotomy is used for a DLT or LRLT.

5. The newly transplanted lung has impaired surfactant production and vascular endothelial permeability.

   a. PEEP and frequent recruitment maneuvers will be needed to prevent atelectasis.

   b. Pulmonary hypertension will cause increased hydrostatic pulmonary edema, worsening gas exchange and lung compliance.

C. **After surgery** the patient will require intensive care.

1. **Extubation** is possible in some patients after SLT and smooth intraoperative courses.

2. **Many** patients will remain intubated until the transplanted lung begins to function well and symptoms of reperfusion edema and acute rejection are controlled. The trachea is

extubated only when the patient is hemodynamically stable and breathing comfortably.

3. **Serial ABGs** are followed to document the function of the transplanted lung. Acute rejection may manifest as decreasing pulmonary compliance with worsening arterial oxygenation.

4. **The patient** must be observed for signs of toxicity from the immunosuppressive regimen, including acute renal failure.

5. **Cystic fibrosis patients** are observed for signs of sepsis, as that is a frequent complication.

D. **Repeated bronchoscopies and biopsies** of the transplanted lung are necessary after surgery and are managed under local anesthesia with intravenous sedation.

XII. **Lung volume reduction surgery** is performed on patients with severe bullous emphysema who experience incapacitating dyspnea despite maximal medical therapy. The goal is to relieve thoracic distention and improve the mechanics of ventilation. Patients are selected under strict criteria and undergo a period of cardiopulmonary conditioning before surgery. Patients have extremely limited respiratory reserve, complicating induction and extubation.

A. **The surgical approach** is via VATS, thoracotomy or median sternotomy. The least functional part of the lung, as determined by CT and intraoperative observation, is resected with staples that are buttressed with bovine pericardium to reduce air leaks.

B. **The anesthetic technique** is similar to lung resection (see section VI). Postoperatively, epidural analgesia is essential.

C. **Postoperative course.** The trachea should be extubated postoperatively and the patients admitted to an intensive care unit.

1. Patients will not usually meet classic extubation criteria.

2. Maneuvers such as sitting position, air admixture, nebulized bronchodilators, and deep extubation with assisted ventilation via mask or LMA as a bridge to full extubation may help.

D. It is not infrequent that the lungs have air leaks postoperatively. If intubation and mechanical ventilation are required, it is imperative to minimize stress on the lung and suture lines by using low airway pressures.

SUGGESTED READING

Alfille, PH. Anesthesia for tracheal surgery. In Grillo HC, ed. *Surgery of the trachea and bronchi.* Hamilton, Ontario: BD Decker, 2004:433–470.

Benumof JL. *Anesthesia for thoracic surgery,* 2nd ed. Philadephia: WB Saunders, 1995.

Bernard A, Deschamps C, Allen MS, et al. Pneumonectomy for malignant disease: factors affecting early morbidity and mortality. *J Thorac Cardiovasc Surg* 2001;121:1076–1082.

Bolliger CT, Perruchoud AP. Functional evaluation of the lung resection candidate. *Eur Respir J* 1998;11:198–212.

Bracken CA, Gurkowski MA, Naples JJ. Lung transplantation: historical perspective, current concepts, and anesthetic considerations. *J Cardiothorac Vasc Anesth* 1997;11:220–241.

Cicala RS, Kudsk KA, Butts A, et al. Initial evaluation and management of upper airway injuries in trauma patients. *J Clin Anesth* 1991;3:91–98.

Devitt JH, Boulanger BR. Lower airway injuries and anaesthesia. *Can J Anaesth* 1996;43:148–159.

Gruchnik KP, Clark JA. Pathophysiology of one-lung ventilation. *Thorac Surg Clin* 2005;15(1):85–103.

Hartigan PM, Pedoto A. Anesthetic Considerations for lung volume reduction surgery and lung transplant. *Thorac Surg Clin* 2005;15(1):143–157.

Kaplan JA. *Thoracic anesthesia,* 3rd ed. New York: Churchill Livingstone, 1991.

Sandberg W. Anesthesia and airway management for tracheal resection and reconstruction. *Int Anesthesiol Clin* 2000;38:55–75.

Anesthesia for Vascular Surgery

Michael D. Kaufman and Edward A. Bittner

I. **Preoperative assessment and management** Should be aimed at identifying coexisting disease, optimizing specific therapies, and anticipating intra- and postoperative problems.

   A. **Cardiovascular system.** Coronary artery disease is present in 40% to 80% of vascular surgery patients and is a major source of morbidity and mortality. Myocardial infarction (MI) accounts for about one-half of early postoperative deaths. Cardiac risk factors include congestive heart failure, MI, hypertension, valvular heart disease, angina, and dysrhythmias (see Chapter 2).

   1. **Coexisting medical conditions,** such as claudication, disability from a prior stroke, and emphysema limit the utility of exercise tolerance as a tool for assessing cardiac function.

   2. **Specialized cardiac testing,** such as exercise stress testing, pharmacologic stress testing with or without nuclear imaging, echocardiography, and cardiac catheterization help to stratify cardiac risk, as discussed in Chapter 2.

   3. Because of the widespread nature of **atherosclerosis,** the presence of major differences in blood pressure readings between arms is relatively common and should be determined preoperatively.

   4. **Risk stratification** may help with decisions about perioperative management. High-risk patients may benefit from additional preoperative medical therapy, coronary revascularization, and/or minimization of surgical procedures. Recent studies suggest that coronary revascularization does not improve survival after elective vascular procedures in patients with stable coronary artery disease and that aggressive medical treatment with beta-blocking agents lowers morbidity and mortality.

   B. **Respiratory system.** Many vascular patients have a significant smoking history, which compromises their pulmonary function (see Chapter 3).

   C. **Renal system.** Renal insufficiency is common. Important causes include atherosclerosis, hypertension, diabetes, inadequate perfusion, volume depletion, and angiographic, dye-related, acute tubular necrosis (see Chapter 4).

   D. **Central nervous system.** Patients should be examined for carotid bruits and questioned for a history of transient ischemic attacks (TIAs) and cerebrovascular accidents. Their presence warrants further evaluation before major vascular surgery.

   E. **Endocrine system.** Diabetics may manifest as diffuse, accelerated atherosclerosis, as well as distal small-vessel disease. Long-standing diabetics may have autonomic neuropathy, silent ischemia, diabetic nephropathy, and reduced resistance to infection. Preoperative insulin orders and related management are discussed in Chapter 6. Patients receiving **metformin** (Glucophage) should have the drug discontinued at least 48 hours before receiving intravenous (IV) contrast dye because of the potential for the development of severe lactic acidosis.

F. **Hematologic system.** Vascular surgical patients are often treated with anticoagulants (unfractionated or low-molecular-weight heparin, warfarin, dipyridamole, clopidogrel, ticlodipine, or aspirin). A history of easy bruising, petechiae, or ecchymosis should be sought and evaluated with a prothrombin time, partial thromboplastin time, and platelet count where appropriate. In patients with early thrombosis and rethrombosis, the presence of a hypercoagulable state can be evaluated. Patients with prior exposure to heparin can be tested for the presence of heparin antibodies. Underlying coagulopathies may affect the choice of anesthetic technique and intraoperative blood loss.

G. **Infection.** There is a high mortality rate associated with infection in patients with vascular grafts. Patients with any evidence of infection should receive appropriate antibiotics preoperatively, and consideration should be given to postponing cases in which heterologous graft materials will be used.

II. **Preoperative medication**
A. **Cardiac medications** should be continued up to the morning of surgery (see Chapter 2). It is particularly important to ensure the continuing administration of beta-blockers that the patient has taken preoperatively. If the patient has not been on beta-blockers, administration can begin in the induction room given that there are no known contraindications.

B. **Anticoagulation.** For patients on chronic anticoagulation therapy, warfarin should be discontinued at least 3 days before surgery and, if indicated, heparin therapy started. If regional anesthesia is planned, unfractionated heparin generally is withheld 4 hours before surgery, in consultation with surgical staff. Low-molecular-weight heparin should be withheld for 24 hours before a regional anesthetic. **Clopidogrel** should be withheld for 1 week before surgery and **ticlodipine** should be withheld for 10 to 14 days before elective surgery (see Chapter 16).

C. **Sedatives.** The goals and regimens for sedative premedication generally are the same as for elderly patients undergoing other major procedures (see Chapter 1).

III. **Carotid endarterectomy**
A. **General considerations.** Carotid endarterectomy is performed in patients with stenotic or ulcerative lesions of the common carotid artery and its internal and external branches. These lesions often present as carotid bruits and may produce TIAs or strokes.
    1. Widespread atherosclerotic disease (especially coronary vessels) is often present.
    2. The baseline blood pressure and heart rate should be determined by reviewing the medical record.
    3. **Preexisting neurologic deficits** should be documented so that new deficits can be determined postoperatively. Patients may exhibit neurologic symptoms with extreme neck motion, necessitating careful positioning for surgery.

B. **Monitoring**
    1. **An arterial catheter,** in addition to standard monitors, is used. In rare cases, a pulmonary artery (PA) catheter may be placed when needed (see Chapter 10). Sites for placement include

the subclavian, antecubital, and contralateral internal jugular veins.

2. **An electroencephalogram** (EEG) is used during general anesthesia to ensure adequate perfusion during carotid cross-clamping and to identify patients who may require shunting to preserve cerebral blood flow (see Chapter 24).

C. **Anesthetic technique**
   1. **Regional anesthesia**
      a. Regional anesthesia may be performed with superficial and deep cervical plexus blocks (see Chapter17); both have potential complications.
      b. This technique requires an alert, cooperative patient who is able to tolerate lateral head positioning under the surgical drapes. It is important to properly position and drape the patient to provide access to the head and control of the airway, which may be necessary at any time. An appropriately sized laryngeal mask airway should be readily available.
      c. Continuous neurologic assessment is facilitated with an awake patient.
      d. Our preference is to use a superficial block with supplementation by the surgeons as needed. This minimizes the potential complications associated with the deep block, especially phrenic nerve paralysis.
   2. **General anesthesia**
      a. **General anesthesia** provides control of ventilation, oxygenation, and reduced cerebral metabolic demand.
      b. **A baseline EEG** is obtained in the preinduction period.
      c. **Blood pressure** should be maintained at the patient's high-normal range and may require a vasopressor such as phenylephrine.
      d. **Induction** requires the slow titration of anesthetic drugs to preserve cerebral perfusion while minimizing hemodynamic alterations. Ventilation should be adjusted to avoid hypocapnic cerebral vasoconstriction. Hypercarbia, however, has no clinical benefit.
      e. A steady state of "light" anesthesia generally does not interfere with EEG monitoring and facilitates early postoperative neurologic examination. Muscle relaxants should be carefully titrated to minimize movement that can interfere with EEG interpretation.

D. **Carotid cross-clamping**
   1. **Surgical traction on the carotid sinus** may cause an intense vagal stimulus, leading to hypotension and bradycardia. Infiltration with local anesthetic may abolish the response. Release of traction and administration of anticholinergics may be required. Prophylactic local infiltration should be considered for patients with significant preoperative cardiac conduction problems, critical aortic stenosis, and unstable angina in which treatment with an anticholinergic would potentiate myocardial ischemia.
   2. **Heparin** (5,000 units IV) is administered before cross-clamping.

3. **A shunt** is placed if the patient's neurologic exam changes while under regional anesthesia, if EEG changes occur, or routinely in cases without neurologic monitoring.

4. **Blood pressure** may be temporarily increased by use of a vasopressor, which may increase cerebral perfusion via the circle of Willis.

5. **Unclamping** may produce reflex vasodilation and bradycardia. Vasopressors may be required as the baroreceptors adapt. Their use may also be required in the postoperative period.

6. Protamine is administered if needed, in coordination with the surgeon, although is rarely needed to reverse heparin as the superficial small incision makes exposure to the field very easy to control any bleeding sites.

E. **Postoperative neurologic deficits** may occur from hypoperfusion or emboli (from shunts or ulcerated plaques). Minor neurologic changes usually resolve, but sudden major changes require immediate evaluation and possible reexploration.

F. **Postoperative management.** Patients are monitored during transport to the postanesthesia care unit, where they remain for observation. Major concerns include neurologic status, control of blood pressure and heart rate, and evidence of postoperative hemorrhage, which may lead to rapid airway obstruction. Occasionally, plaque removal alters the baroreceptor response with resultant hypotension requiring vasopressor (phenylephrine), which may extend into the recovery room period. This hypotension does not reflect hypovolemia, and excessive fluid replacement to manage this low pressure is inappropriate.

G. **The International Carotid Stenting Study** is under way to compare the risks and benefits of primary carotid stenting with those of conventional carotid endarterectomy in patients at high risk for stroke.

IV. **Peripheral vascular (arterial) surgery**

A. **General considerations.** Peripheral vascular surgery is performed to bypass occlusive disease or aneurysms, remove emboli, and repair pseudoaneurysms and catheter injuries. Although peripheral vascular surgery is less of a physiologic insult than aortic surgery, their perioperative cardiac risks are comparable.

B. **Femoral-popliteal and distal lower extremity bypass grafting.** Lower-extremity, occlusive arterial disease is most often bypassed with an autologous saphenous vein graft. If this is not available or is of unacceptable quality, an arm vein or cryopreserved cadaveric vein may be used. Preparation of the vein and subsequent anastomoses to the arterial circulation may be time-consuming but rarely place significant hemodynamic stress on the patient. The use of synthetic grafts (e.g., Gore-Tex) in selected patients may shorten these procedures. Although blood loss is usually minimal, revision of previous peripheral vascular procedures and surgically difficult cases may result in significant blood loss.

1. **Monitoring.** Most types of peripheral vascular procedures require similar monitoring, unless noted otherwise. In relatively healthy patients undergoing limited surgery, routine monitoring, as outlined in Chapter 10, is sufficient. As a case proceeds, hemodynamic lability, excessive blood loss, low urine output, or cardiac ischemia may dictate placement of invasive

monitors (arterial, central venous, or PA catheters). A Foley catheter is placed routinely.

2. **Regional anesthesia.** A continuous lumbar epidural catheter is commonly used. It provides excellent anesthesia and a route to administer postoperative analgesia. Spinal anesthesia is appropriate if the length of the procedure can be predicted with some assurance. A continuous spinal technique is useful during prolonged procedures for patients in whom epidural anesthesia proves technically difficult or unsatisfactory. For procedures limited to a single limb, combined lumbar plexus and sciatic nerve block may be used.

   a. **An α-adrenergic agent** (e.g., phenylephrine) should be available to treat the hypotension associated with sympathetic blockade.

   b. **Anticoagulation**

      (1) The anticoagulated patient must have his or her clotting abnormality corrected (with fresh-frozen plasma, vitamin K, or protamine) before catheter insertion or must receive a general anesthetic.

      (2) There is no evidence that heparin treatment after epidural catheter placement increases the risk of epidural hematoma formation. If postoperative warfarin therapy is needed, the epidural should be removed before the onset of the anticoagulant effect (within 24 hours of administration of the first dose).

   c. **Regional anesthesia** may help detect myocardial ischemia, because the patient can complain of chest pain or other symptoms.

   d. **Attention to patient comfort** is particularly important when regional techniques are used during long procedures. Appropriate back and shoulder padding and freedom of the neck and arms should be provided. Sedation should reduce patient anxiety without producing confusion, respiratory depression, or unresponsiveness. Blankets and other warming measures are important, because heat loss from vasodilated extremities is significant. Shivering not only is unpleasant but may also be detrimental as it increases oxygen consumption in an already stressed patient.

3. **General anesthesia.** Any technique is appropriate provided hemodynamic stability is maintained.

C. **Iliofemoral and iliodistal bypass grafting** may be performed with spinal or epidural anesthesia. A higher anesthetic level is needed (i.e., T-8) because of proximal extension of the incision and peritoneal retraction for exposure of the iliac artery.

D. **Peripheral embolectomy and femoral pseudoaneurysm** repair frequently involve patients with unstable cardiovascular disease (e.g., recent MI). Some of these patients are anticoagulated or recently have received thrombolytic agents, thus precluding regional anesthesia. If not, lumbar plexus blockade provides adequate coverage. Field blocks with local anesthesia are sometimes appropriate. Surgical embolectomy and flushing of the thrombi from an obstructed artery may be associated with significant blood loss and hypotension.

E. **Femoral-femoral bypass grafting** is used to treat symptomatic unilateral iliac occlusive disease.

F. **Peripheral aneurysms,** such as popliteal aneurysms, rarely rupture but are associated with a high rate of thrombosis and embolism.

G. **Axillofemoral bypass grafting** provides arterial blood flow to the lower extremities. This approach is chosen when there is an active abdominal infection or an infected aortic bypass graft, or when a patient is medically unfit for abdominal aortic surgery. Routine monitoring is supplemented by an arterial catheter, which should be placed in the arm opposite the surgery. Central venous and PA lines are used as necessary.

H. **Vascular surgery of the upper extremity** usually includes distal embolectomy and repair of traumatic injuries. The surgery is localized, but there may be a need to harvest a vein graft at a site distant from the vascular repair. Possible anesthetic techniques include field block, regional, or general anesthesia. Proximal vascular surgical procedures (e.g., thoracic outlet syndrome and vertebral stenosis) may require an intrathoracic approach and/or temporary interruption of carotid blood flow.

I. **Postoperative care.** These patients require careful hemodynamic control and adequate analgesia. Graft occlusion in the immediate postoperative period may occur, requiring reexploration. Epidural catheters are left in place for the postoperative period.

J. **Percutaneous balloon angioplasty and stenting** have gained wide acceptance in the treatment of atherosclerotic and other vascular stenotic disease. Procedures on upper and lower extremities are typically performed in the operating room angiography suites and are done under sedation or general anesthesia. The procedures are typically associated with administration of large amounts of IV dye, and require maneuvers to prevent contrast-induced nephropathy (CIN). In our institution, patients routinely receive *N*-acetylcysteine and sodium bicarbonate infusions (see Chapter 4).

V. **Abdominal aortic surgery**

A. **Infrarenal aortic surgery**

1. **Abdominal aortic surgery** may be required for atherosclerotic occlusive disease or aneurysmal dilation. These processes can involve any portion of the aorta and its major branches and lead to ischemia, rupture, and exsanguination. Ninety-five percent of all abdominal aortic aneurysms (AAAs) occur below the level of the renal arteries. Patients with AAAs more than 5 cm in diameter, especially those shown to be expanding, have a better prognosis if they undergo elective resection. The annual risk of rupture of an expanding 5-cm aneurysm is about 4%. The operative mortality for elective AAA resection is less than 2%, while the overall mortality of aneurysm rupture is 70% to 80%.

2. **Surgical technique.** Compared with a transabdominal approach, the retroperitoneal approach may result in a lower incidence of postoperative ileus, pulmonary complications, cardiovascular complications, and fluid shifts. The approach is technically advantageous in morbidly obese patients and in those who have had previous abdominal procedures.

3. **Monitoring.** A large peripheral IV (14 gauge), electrocardiogram (ECG) (leads II and V5), a central venous catheter,

arterial line, and Foley catheter, in addition to the usual monitoring, are required. PA catheters are used when indicated, as outlined in Chapter 10. Most monitoring catheters (except the Foley) are inserted before induction, and initial baseline values are obtained to guide anesthetic management. A central venous catheter can be placed after induction and is usually dictated by patient's comorbidities. Vasoactive agents (e.g., nitroglycerin and phenylephrine) must be available for every case. Other vasoactive agents should be available based on a patient's comorbid conditions.

4. **Anesthetic technique**

   a. **General considerations.** Most patients receive combined general and epidural anesthesia using a midthoracic epidural catheter. Although general anesthesia alone is acceptable, a combined technique reduces anesthetic requirements, facilitates immediate extubation, and provides for postoperative analgesia.

   b. **Induction.** The epidural catheter is injected with 2% lidocaine and a sensory level is confirmed before administration of general anesthesia. Reduced blood pressure associated with the onset of epidural anesthesia is treated with phenylephrine. General anesthesia is induced in a slow and controlled fashion, titrating drugs to the desired hemodynamic and anesthetic effect. Because immediate postoperative extubation is usually planned, high-dose opioid techniques are generally avoided.

   c. **Maintenance**

      (1) **Anesthesia** is provided primarily by epidural blockade with 2% lidocaine. This is supplemented by nitrous oxide, muscle relaxants, and a low inspired concentration of a volatile anesthetic. A continuous epidural infusion of dilute 0.1% bupivacaine with an opioid (dilaudid or fentanyl) is begun during the procedure.

      (2) **Heat conservation.** Heat loss during aortic procedures may be considerable. Strategies for heat conservation are discussed in Chapter 18.

      (3) **Bowel manipulation** is necessary to gain access to the aorta during a transabdominal approach and may be accompanied by skin flushing, decreased systemic vascular resistance, and profound hypotension. These changes may be caused by release of prostaglandins and vasoactive peptides from the bowel and last for 20 to 30 min. Treatment consists of IV phenylephrine, volume expansion, and reducing anesthetic depth.

      (4) **Fluid management.** Intravascular volume is depleted by hemorrhage, insensible losses into the bowel and peritoneal cavity, and evaporative losses associated with large abdominal incisions.

         (a) **Crystalloid solutions** are used for volume replacement at an approximate rate of 10 to 15 mL/kg per hour.

    (b) **Colloid solutions** are rarely necessary and are reserved for patients who are unresponsive or intolerant of large amounts of crystalloid.

    (c) Serum **hemoglobin** should be maintained above the 10-g/dL range. With blood losses >2,000 mL, coagulation profiles should be monitored and platelets, clotting factors, and calcium replaced, guided by laboratory evaluation.

    (d) **Autotransfusion devices** should be used intraoperatively to scavenge shed blood. Autotransfused blood is deficient in plasma, clotting factors, and platelets.

(5) **Aortic cross-clamping**

    (a) **Heparin** (5,000 units IV) is given several minutes before applying an aortic cross-clamp.

    (b) **Increased afterload following aortic cross-clamping** is well tolerated by patients with normal hearts. Those with compromised left ventricular function may exhibit a decreased cardiac output and/or myocardial ischemia. The use of nitroglycerin or, rarely, nitroprusside may improve myocardial oxygen supply–demand balance.

(6) **Renal preservation.** The incidence of renal failure is 1% to 2% for infrarenal aortic surgery. Preoperative angiographic dye studies and preexisting renal disease increase this risk. Patients with chronically elevated creatinine levels (>2 mg/dL) have substantially greater morbidity and mortality after vascular surgery. Renal cortical blood flow and urine output may decrease with infrarenal aortic cross-clamping, possibly because of circulatory derangements, effects on the renin-angiotensin system, and microembolization. Maintenance of adequate hydration and urine flow is extremely important. If the urine output falls in spite of adequate hydration, IV mannitol, furosemide, or fenoldopam (3 μg/kg per min) may be given.

(7) **Aortic unclamping.** Intravascular volume must be maintained in the normal to hypervolemic range, anticipating a fall in systemic vascular resistance and venous return after release of the aortic cross-clamp. Volume loading, decreasing anesthetic depth, discontinuing vasodilators, infusing a vasopressor, and a slow, controlled release of the aortic cross-clamp will minimize hypotension. Reperfusion of the lower extremities, resulting in washout of anaerobic products and systemic acidosis, may produce a negative inotropic effect, which is related to the duration of cross-clamp time and degree of collateral flow. Sodium bicarbonate administration is rarely necessary. Minute ventilation can be adjusted to allow for more CO_2 elimination if deemed necessary.

- **(8)** **Emergence.** Most patients are extubated at the end of the procedure. Patients with unstable cardiac or pulmonary function, ongoing bleeding, or severe hypothermia ($<33°C$) are left intubated. Hypertension, tachycardia, pain, and shivering should be anticipated and treated.
- **(9)** **Transport.** All patients should receive supplemental oxygen and continuous monitoring of blood pressure and ECG.

B. Suprarenal abdominal aortic surgery. The surgical procedure may involve cross-clamping of the aorta at various levels above the renal arteries. Anesthetic considerations are similar to those for infrarenal aortic surgery (see section V.A), with the following caveats:

1. PA catheters are used more frequently.
2. Blood loss is potentially greater.
3. Renal perfusion is at greater risk because of longer cross-clamp times and potential for cholesterol embolization.
4. Cross-clamping above the celiac and superior mesenteric arteries can produce visceral ischemia and profound acidosis. Sodium bicarbonate is given routinely during the cross-clamping before opening.
5. IV mannitol and fenoldopam are administered before cross-clamping with the aim of minimizing ischemic renal injury.

C. Renal artery surgery. Renal artery stenoses or aneurysms are repaired with a variety of techniques. Aortorenal bypass and transaortic endarterectomy require aortic cross-clamping; hepatorenal (right) and splenorenal (left) bypass procedures avoid cross-clamping. The anesthetic considerations are the same as for abdominal aortic surgery (see section V.A). Postoperative concerns include ongoing hypertension and deterioration in renal function.

D. Endovascular abdominal aneurysm repair (EVR) (Fig. 22.1)

1. EVR of an AAA involves deployment of an expandable, prosthetic graft within the lumen of the aneurysm, thus excluding the aneurysm from the circulation and reducing the risk of its rupture. The graft usually is deployed, under fluoroscopic guidance, from sheaths placed in the femoral arteries via cutdown arteriotomies. Compared with conventional AAA repair, EVR involves less blood loss and a lower incidence of perioperative morbidity, including pulmonary, cardiovascular, and renal complications. The use of EVR has resulted in fewer postoperative intensive care unit admissions, earlier ambulation, and shorter hospital stays.
2. **Patient selection** and stent graft sizing depend on detailed preoperative imaging. Up to 60% of patients with known infrarenal AAAs may be amenable to EVR.
3. **Monitoring.** In addition to standard monitors (Chapter 10), a large peripheral IV (14- to 16-gauge), arterial catheter, and Foley catheter are used. Conversion to an open procedure is relatively rare, but each case should be set up for the possibility of an emergent AAA repair (see below).
4. **Anesthetic technique.** Most patients receive an epidural or combined spinal and epidural anesthetic. IV sedation with

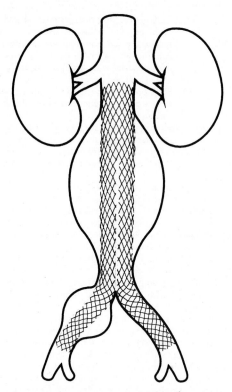

Figure 22.1. Endovascular graft repair of an infrarenal abdominal aortic aneurysm. (From Kaufman JA, Geller SC, Brewster DC, et al. Endovascular repair of abdominal aortic aneurysm: current status and future directions. *Am J Roentgenol* **2000;175:289–302, reprinted with permission from the American Journal of Roentgenology.)**

propofol and/or benzodiazepines and short-acting narcotics is titrated to patient comfort.

5. **Complications of EVR** include failure to exclude the AAA from the arterial system (endoleak), embolism, arterial injury, graft kinking, limb ischemia, and infection. Patients with impaired renal function are at risk for CIN, and both *N*-acetylcysteine and sodium bicarbonate infusion are given routinely as described above.

E. **Emergency abdominal aortic surgery.** Patients present with a wide spectrum of signs and symptoms and can be divided into two groups:

1. **The hemodynamically stable patient** with an expanding contained rupture has the same anesthetic considerations as described above (see section V.A), but the preoperative preparation must proceed expeditiously.

     a. **Foley catheter and nasogastric tube insertion** should be delayed until after induction, to avoid Valsalva maneuvers (or hypertension) that may aggravate bleeding or cause frank rupture. Placement of a central venous pressure or PA line is undertaken while the patient is awake.

     b. **Induction** proceeds after preoxygenation, using placement of cricoid pressure and careful titration of hypnotic agents, opioids, and muscle relaxants. Hypertension must be avoided and anesthesia may be supplemented with vasoactive drugs.

2. **The hemodynamically unstable patient** (ruptured aneurysm) requires resuscitative measures. Mortality can be limited by restoration of intravascular volume, judicious use of vasoconstrictors, and rapid surgical control. Under the best of situations, there is a 40% to 50% mortality, usually resulting from the physiologic consequences of hypotension and massive blood transfusion. The incidence of MI, acute renal failure, respiratory failure, and coagulopathy is high.

     a. **General considerations**

         (1) **Large-bore IV access** is paramount.

         (2) **Blood samples** should be sent immediately for cross-matching and any other pertinent laboratory studies. Blood components should be ordered immediately, but universal donor-type blood (type O-negative in women of child-bearing age, type O-positive in all others) should be obtained if type-specific blood is unavailable. Colloid solutions should be available. The autotransfusion team should be notified and equipment set up.

     b. **Surgical technique.** The immediate surgical priority will be to control bleeding by cross-clamping the aorta in the chest or abdomen.

     c. **Monitoring.** Minimum monitoring standards (see Chapter 10) should be applied during the initial volume resuscitation, followed by placement of invasive monitors as time and hemodynamics permit. Placement of monitors and fluid resuscitation should not delay definitive surgical control of a rupture in an unstable patient.

     d. **Anesthetic technique**

         (1) **Induction**

            (a) In **moribund patients,** endotracheal intubation should be performed immediately.

            (b) In **hypotensive patients,** a rapid careful induction is indicated, but the patient may be able to tolerate only small doses of scopolamine, ketamine, etomidate, and/or a benzodiazepine and a relaxant.

         (2) **Maintenance**

            (a) Once the aorta has been clamped to control bleeding, resuscitative efforts should continue until hemodynamic stability is achieved. Incremental doses of opioid and supplemental anesthetics are given as tolerated.

(b) **Blood products** (including fresh-frozen plasma and platelets) are administered when available. Serial laboratory studies should guide further management. Fluid warmers capable of infusing large volumes should be available.

(c) **Hypothermia** is common and contributes to the acidosis, coagulopathy, and myocardial dysfunction that complicate aortic aneurysm repair. Methods of heat conservation and warming are discussed in Chapter 18.

(d) **To prevent renal failure,** aggressive efforts should be made to preserve urine output with volume replacement, mannitol, and fenoldopam. Mortality in patients developing renal failure following a ruptured AAA is high.

(3) **Emergence.** Large fluid shifts; hypothermia; and acid-base, electrolyte, and coagulation abnormalities make the immediate postoperative period complex. Most patients remain intubated and mechanically ventilated at the end of the procedure.

VI. **Thoracic aortic surgery.** Causes of thoracic aorta disease include atherosclerosis, degenerative disorders of connective tissue (e.g., Marfan and Ehlers-Danlos syndromes, and cystic necrosis), infection (e.g., syphilis), congenital defects (e.g., coarctation and congenital aneurysms of the sinus of Valsalva), trauma (e.g., penetrating and deceleration injuries), and inflammatory processes (e.g., Takayasu aortitis). The most common problem affecting the thoracic aorta is **atherosclerotic aneurysm** of the descending portion, accounting for about 20% of all aortic aneurysms. When such aneurysms dissect proximally, they may involve the aortic valve or coronary ostia. Distal dissection may involve the abdominal aorta or renal or mesenteric branches. The next most frequent problem is **traumatic disruption** of the thoracic aorta. Adventitial false aneurysms may form distal to the left subclavian artery at the insertion of the ligamentum arteriosum, because of penetrating or deceleration injuries. These false aneurysms may dissect anterograde and involve the arch and its major branches.

A. **Ascending aortic aneurysms** are approached by median sternotomy and require cardiopulmonary bypass with arterial cannulation through the femoral artery, the distal ascending aorta, or the aortic arch.

B. **Transverse aortic arch repair** requires median sternotomy, cardiopulmonary bypass, and hypothermic total circulatory arrest.

C. **Descending thoracic aortic aneurysms** often are approached by a left lateral thoracotomy with the cross-clamp placed distal to the left subclavian artery.

D. **Thoracoabdominal aneurysms** are approached by a thoracoabdominal incision.

1. **Crawford classification** of thoracoabdominal aneurysms (Fig. 22.2).

a. **Type I.** Aneurysm of the descending thoracic aorta distal to the subclavian artery, ending at or above the origin of the visceral vessels.

b. **Type II.** Aneurysm from the origin of the subclavian artery to the distal abdominal aorta.

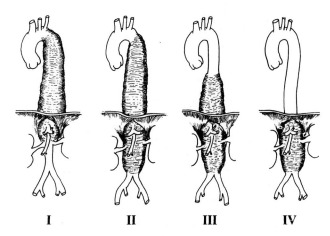

I   II   III   IV

Figure 22.2. Crawford classification of descending thoracic aortic aneurysms.

  c. **Type III.** Aneurysm from the mid-descending thoracic aorta to the distal abdominal aorta.

  d. **Type IV.** Aneurysm from the diaphragm down to the distal aorta.

2. **Associated findings**

  a. **Airway deviation or compression,** particularly of the left mainstem bronchus, producing atelectasis.

  b. **Tracheal displacement or disruption,** producing difficulties with endotracheal intubation and ventilation. Long-standing aneurysms may damage the recurrent laryngeal nerves, resulting in vocal cord paralysis and hoarseness.

  c. **Hemoptysis,** because of erosion of the aneurysm into an adjacent bronchus.

  d. **Esophageal compression** with dysphagia and an increased risk of aspiration.

  e. **Distortion and compression of central venous and arterial anatomy,** producing markedly asymmetric pulses and difficult internal jugular vein cannulation.

  f. **Hemothorax and mediastinal shift** from rupture or leakage, producing respiratory and circulatory compromise.

  g. **Reduced distal perfusion** secondary to aortic branch vessel occlusion, producing renal, mesenteric, spinal cord, or extremity ischemia.

3. **Surgical technique.** During repair of the aneurysm, the affected aortic segment is isolated, and an interposition graft is inserted. Proximal blood flow to collateral vessels provides the only distal perfusion. Additional distal perfusion may be provided via a heparin-bonded Gott shunt or pump-assisted bypass. The **inclusion technique** involves using the portion of native aorta containing the celiac, superior mesenteric, and renal ostia as a component of the bypass graft.

4. **Spinal cord protection**
   a. **Anatomic concerns**
      (1) **The anterior spinal artery** arises from the vertebral arteries at the base of the skull and anastomoses with aortic radicular arteries. The latter arise segmentally (a few in the lumbar and lower thoracic regions, but none or one in the upper thoracic region).
      (2) The dominant vessel is the **artery of Adamkiewicz** (usually found between T-8 and T-12); cross-clamping of the aorta may compromise flow through this vessel, and in turn through the anterior spinal artery, and produce spinal cord ischemia.
   b. **Anterior spinal artery syndrome.** Manifestations of the anterior spinal artery syndrome are paraplegia, rectal and urinary incontinence, and loss of pain and temperature sensation with maintenance of vibratory and proprioceptive sensation. The incidence of paraplegia resulting from anterior spinal artery syndrome ranges from 1% to 41%, depending on the type of aneurysm, among other factors. Risk factors include the duration of the cross-clamp, the location of proximal and distal cross-clamps, increased body temperature, the degree of collateralization of the spinal cord circulation, reperfusion with cross-clamp removal, and previous thoracoabdominal aneurysm surgery. It may be possible to detect spinal cord ischemia by monitoring somatosensory evoked potentials (see Chapter 24), but that is not routinely done at Massachusetts General Hospital.
   c. **Preservation**
      (1) Steroids, barbiturates, free radical scavengers, cerebrospinal fluid (CSF) drainage, intrathecal papaverine, magnesium, naloxone, thiopental, and reanastomosis of intercostal vessels have all been tried without convincing evidence that any technique reduces the incidence of paraplegia.
      (2) **Hypothermia** has been shown to be protective. Using a protocol developed at Massachusetts General Hospital (see Davison et al. 1994 in Suggested Readings), regional spinal cord cooling is begun before cross-clamping and continued until the graft is reperfused.
      (3) **Lowering CSF pressure** may promote spinal cord perfusion. Therefore, a lumbar CSF catheter is inserted to monitor and control CSF pressure.
      (4) **Glucose-containing solutions are avoided,** because experimental evidence suggests that hyperglycemia is detrimental during ischemia and may worsen neurologic outcome. Although no data on intraoperative glycemic control are available, hyperglycemia can be treated with insulin infusion.
      (5) **Monitoring.** Routine monitoring is supplemented with the following:
         (a) Right radial arterial catheter (a high cross-clamp may compromise left subclavian artery flow).

     (b) PA catheter.

     (c) Number 8.5 French (Fr) introducer used for volume infusions.

     (d) Number 4 Fr epidural cooling catheter at spinal level T-12 to L-1.

     (e) Number 4 Fr subarachnoid catheter, with thermistor, at spinal levels L-2, L-3.

     (f) Foley catheter.

(6) Anesthetic technique

     (a) Vasopressors (phenylephrine and nore-pinephrine), **vasodilators** (nitroglycerin and nitroprusside), and **renal preservation agents** (mannitol and fenoldopam) should be available before induction.

     (b) A thoracic epidural and a lumbar subarachnoid catheter are inserted preoperatively, and a sensory level is achieved with 2% lidocaine via the epidural catheter.

     (c) General anesthesia is induced as detailed in section V.A.4.b.

     (d) A right-sided, double-lumen endo-bronchial tube is placed to facilitate surgical access and protect the left lung from trauma during left thoracotomy (see Chapter 21). Alternatively, the patient is intubated with a single-lumen tube and an endobronchial blocker (Arndt), or an occlusive catheter (Fogarty) is used to achieve lung isolation.

     (e) Muscle relaxation is usually provided by a cisatracurium infusion.

(7) Positioning. The patient is turned to the right lateral decubitus position and prepared for incision.

(8) Maintenance

     (a) Anesthesia is continued as in section V.A.4.c, and one-lung ventilation is begun as described in Chapter 21.

     (b) Fluid management is limited to fresh-frozen plasma, red blood cells, platelets, and colloids after induction in an attempt to limit the development of a coagulopathy and excessive edema. An autotransfusion device and a blood warmer capable of high flow rates are used.

(9) Aortic cross-clamping

     (a) Before cross-clamping, CSF pressure is adjusted and the spinal cord is cooled according to protocol.

     (b) Marked hypertension is universal with a proximal aortic cross-clamp and is treated with epidural anesthesia, nitroglycerin, and nitroprusside.

     (c) Renal function is preserved by infusion of iced saline solution through a catheter placed by the surgical team into the orifices of the renal arteries.

(10) **Aortic unclamping** produces hypotension by the mechanism discussed in section V.A.4.c.(7). Volume administration before and during unclamping, slow release of the cross-clamp, and use of vasopressors are continued until myocardial function and vascular tone have returned to normal.

(11) **Use of shunts**

(a) Mesenteric shunt-proximal side-arm graft sewn on to graft before aortic cross-clamp. After proximal anastomosis is complete, flow through a coronary artery catheter in to this sidearm is established to the mesentery through the celiac or superior mesenteric artery. This provides temporary perfusion while the intercostal vessels and the visceral and renal vessel are anastomosed.

(b) Atrial (or pulmonary vein) to left femoral artery bypass with the use of an inline roller pump. Distal aortic perfusion is monitored by placement of a right femoral artery catheter. This permits retrograde perfusion up to the level of an aortic clamp placed distal to the initial aortic clamp. This clamp can be sequentially placed more distally, as the operation proceeds.

(12) **Systemic acidosis** is universal after release of the aortic cross-clamp. An infusion of bicarbonate during the cross-clamping period will help prevent severe acidosis during reperfusion.

(13) **Emergence.** The patient is asked to move all four extremities, and once a satisfactory neurologic examination has been completed, the patient is again sedated and the double-lumen tube is replaced with a standard endotracheal tube. In cases in which a bronchial blocker was used it is simply removed and the existing endotracheal tube is left in place. Dependent tissue edema may significantly narrow the airway, making reintubation difficult.

(14) **Transport.** The patient remains sedated for transport to the intensive care unit. Both ECG and blood pressure are monitored.

5. **Endovascular repair.** Certain traumatic disruptions, dissections, and aneurysms of the thoracic aorta are now amenable to endovascular stenting. Precise imaging is obtained to ensure that vital arteries (carotid, subclavian, mesenteric, and renal arteries) are not excluded after stent deployment. Endovascular stenting of the thoracic aorta is often combined with less invasive open surgical procedures to ensure that vital organ vascular supply is maintained through extra-anatomic grafts when the aortic stent graft excludes the normal anatomic supply. Such bypass procedures that may be done before, or combined with, the endovascular stent graft include ascending aorta to inominate and/or carotid bypass, carotid to subclavian bypass, and distal aortic/iliac to mesenteric or renal artery bypass.

VII. **Postoperative considerations.** Intensive care is required after most vascular surgical procedures. Attention to urine output, cardiac output, distal extremity perfusion, respiratory adequacy, hematocrit, and hemostasis is required. Postoperative complications include MI, renal failure, bowel ischemia or infarction, pancreatitis, sepsis, disseminated intravascular coagulation, peripheral embolization, respiratory insufficiency, and paraplegia. Hypotension in the postoperative period increases the risk of delayed onset paraplegia and should be avoided.

SUGGESTED READING

Allain R, Marone LK, Meltzer J, et al. Carotid endarterectomy. *Int Anesth Clin* 2005;43(1):15–38.

Barnett HJM, Taylor DW, Eliasziw M, et al. Benefit of carotid endarterectomy in patients with symptomatic moderate or severe stenosis. *N Engl J Med* 1998;339:1415–1425.

Baron JF, Bertrand M, Barre E, et al. Combined epidural and general anesthesia versus general anesthesia for abdominal aortic surgery. *Anesthesiology* 1991;75: 611–618.

Brewster DC, Kaufman JA, Geller SC, et al. Initial experience with endovascular repair: comparison of early results with conventional open repair. *J Vasc Surg* 1998;27:992–1005.

Cambria RP, Davison JK. Regional hypothermia with epidural cooling for spinal cord protection during thoracoabdominal aneurysm repair. *Sem Vasc Surg* 2000;13:315–324.

Chitilian HV, Isselbacher EM, Fitzsimons MG. Preoperative cardiac evaluation for vascular surgery. *Int Anesth Clin* 2005;43(1):1–14.

Christopherson R, Beattie C, Frank SM, et al. Perioperative morbidity in patients randomized to epidural or general anesthesia for lower extremity vascular surgery. *Anesthesiology* 1993;79:422–434.

Crawford ES, Crawford JL, Safi HJ, et al. Thoracoabdominal aortic aneurysms: preoperative and intraoperative factors determining immediate and long-term results of operations in 605 patients. *J Vasc Surg* 1985;3:389–404.

Davison JK, Cambria RP, Vierra DJ, et al. Epidural cooling for regional spinal cord hypothermia during thoracoabdominal aneurysm repair. *J Vasc Surg* 1994;20:304–310.

Gelman S. The pathophysiology of aortic cross-clamping and unclamping. *Anesthesiology* 1995;82:1026–1060.

Isaacson IJ, Lowdon JD, Berry AS, et al. The value of pulmonary artery and central venous monitoring in patients undergoing abdominal aortic reconstructive surgery. *J Vasc Surg* 1990;12:754–760.

Kashyap VP, Cambria RP, Davison JK, et al. Renal failure after thoracoabdominal aortic surgery. *J Vasc Surg* 1997;26:949–955.

Kaufman JA, Geller SC, Brewster DC, et al. Endovascular repair of abdominal aortic aneurysm: current status and future directions. *Am J Roentgenol* 2000;175: 289–302.

Levine WC, Lee JJ, Black JH, Cambria RP, Davison JK Thoracoabdominal aneurysm repair, anesthetic management. *Int Anesth Clin* 2005;43(1):39–60.

Mangano ET, Layug EL, Wallace A, et al. Effect of atenolol on mortality and cardiovascular morbidity after noncardiac surgery. *N Engl J Med* 1996;335: 1713–1720.

Pierce ET, Pomposelli FB, Stanley GD, et al. Anesthesia type does not influence early graft patency or limb salvage rates of lower extremity arterial bypass. *J Vasc Surg* 1997;25:226–233.

Raby KE, Goldman L, Creager M, et al. Correlation between preoperative ischemia and major cardiac events after peripheral vascular surgery. *N Engl J Med*
1989;321:1296–1300.

Rao TLK, El-Etr AA. Anticoagulation following placement of epidural and
subarachnoid catheters: an evaluation of neurologic sequelae. *Anesthesiology*
1981;55:618–620.

Riddell JM, Black JH, Brewster DC, Dunn PF. Endovascular abdominal aortic
aneurysm repair. *Int Anesth Clin* 2005;43(1):79–92.

Tuman KJ, McCarthy RJ, March RJ, et al. Effects of epidural anesthesia and analgesia on coagulation and outcome after major vascular surgery. *Anesth Analg*
1991;73:696–704.

Wallace A, Layug B, Tateo I, et al. Prophylactic atenolol reduces postoperative
myocardial ischemia. *Anesthesiology* 1998;88:7–17.

Wesner L, Marone LK, Dennehy KC. Anesthesia for lower extremity bypass. *Int
Anesth Clin* 2005;43(1):93–110.

Wozniak MF, LaMuraglia GM, Musch G. Anesthesia for open aortic aneurysm
surgery. *Int Anesth Clin* 2005;43(1):61–78.

Anesthesia for Cardiac Surgery

George A. Mashour and Edwin G. Avery, IV

I. **Preanesthetic assessment**

A. **Issues pertinent to cardiac surgical procedures** as well as the physiologic impact of cardiopulmonary bypass (CPB) and elective arrest include the following:

   1. **Prior surgery** in the chest technically complicates cardiac surgery.

   2. **Prior admissions for peripheral vascular disease,** including transient ischemic attacks or cerebral vascular accidents, and the results of noninvasive and invasive vascular studies should be noted. Symptomatic or documented carotid arterial disease may warrant endarterectomy before or concomitantly with the cardiac operation.

   3. **A history of bleeding or prothrombotic** tendencies may reveal a condition responsive to perioperative therapy.

   4. Patients with a history of **heparin-induced thrombocytopenia** (HIT) may develop life-threatening thrombotic complications when exposed to heparin; a plan for anticoagulation during CPB should be determined preoperatively.

   5. **Renal insufficiency** may indicate the need for intraoperative renal protective measures.

   6. **Post-CPB pulmonary dysfunction** can be life threatening; patients with pulmonary disease may benefit from preoperative antibiotics, bronchodilators, steroids, or chest physical therapy.

B. **Cardiac evaluation** should determine the major anatomic and physiologic characteristics of the cardiovascular system; this allows one to predict the likelihood of intraoperative ischemia and to determine the functional reserve of the heart.

   1. **Radionuclide imaging** may demonstrate the regions and extent of myocardium at risk for ischemia.

   2. **Radionuclide ventriculography** characterizes cardiac chamber volume, ejection fraction, and right-to-left stroke volume ratios.

   3. **Echocardiography** provides an assessment of ventricular function and valve function. Regional wall motion abnormalities may reflect ischemia or prior myocardial infarction.

   4. **Cardiac catheterization** provides anatomic and functional data often not available from noninvasive studies.

      a. **Anatomic data.** Coronary angiography reveals the location and extent of coronary stenoses, distal runoff, collateral flow, and coronary dominance. **Significant stenosis** implies a greater than 70% reduction in luminal diameter. The **dominant coronary artery** supplies the atrioventricular node and the posterior descending coronary artery.

      b. **Functional data.** Ventriculography may demonstrate wall motion abnormalities, mitral regurgitation, and

Table 23.1. Normal intracardiac pressure and oxygen saturation

	Pressure (mm Hg)	O_2 Saturation (%)
Superior vena cava	—	71
Inferior vena cava	—	77
Right atrium (mean)	1–8	75
Right ventricle (systolic/diastolic)	15–30/0–8	75
Pulmonary artery (systolic/diastolic)	15–30/4–12	75
Pulmonary artery occlusion pressure (mean)	2–12	—
Left atrium (mean)	2–12	98
Left ventricle (systolic/diastolic/ end-diastolic)	100–140/0–8/2–12	98
Aorta (systolic/diastolic)	100–140/60–90	98

intracardiac shunts. Left ventricular (LV) ejection fraction is normally greater than 0.6. Impaired ventricular performance is a useful predictor of increased surgical risk.

   c. **Hemodynamic data** are compiled from both right and left heart catheterization. Intracardiac and pulmonary vascular pressures reflect volume status, cardiac valve function, and the presence of pulmonary vascular disease (normal values are presented in Table 23.1). An elevated LV end-diastolic pressure (LVEDP) (measured at the base of the "a" wave) may be due to ventricular failure and dilation, volume overload (mitral or aortic insufficiency [AI]), poor compliance from ischemia or hypertrophy, or a constrictive process. The LVEDP may rise substantially in patients with coronary artery disease (CAD) after dye injection for ventriculography or coronary angiography, despite otherwise normal hemodynamic values.

   d. **Left-to-right intracardiac shunts** are demonstrated by an arterial oxygen saturation (Sao_2) "step up" in the right heart. Systemic and pulmonary flow and flow ratios can be calculated by Fick principles (see section IV.C.1.d for equations).

   e. **Cardiac output** is determined by thermodilution, and hemodynamic indices can be derived (Table 23.2).

5. **High-resolution (64-slice) computed tomographic scanning** serves as a useful noninvasive imaging modality to assess patients for coronary vascular disease. This modality is a useful screening tool in patients who are not ideal candidates for cardiac catheterization.

C. **Laboratory studies.** Routine studies for patients undergoing a cardiac operation include a complete blood count, prothrombin time, activated partial thromboplastin time, platelet count, electrolytes, blood urea nitrogen, creatinine, glucose, aspartate aminotransferase, lactate dehydrogenase, creatine kinase, urinalysis, chest

Table 23.2. Ventricular function indices

Formula	Units	Normal Value
$SV = \dfrac{CO}{HR} \times 1{,}000$	mL/beat	60–90
$SI = \dfrac{SV}{BSA}$	mL/beat/m^2	40–60
$LVSWI = \dfrac{1.36(MAP - PCWP)}{100} \times SI$	$\dfrac{\text{gram-meters/m}^2}{\text{beat}}$	45–60
$RVSWI = \dfrac{1.36(PAP - CVP)}{100} \times SI$	$\dfrac{\text{gram-meters/m}^2}{\text{beat}}$	5–10
$SVR = \dfrac{MAP - CVP}{CO} \times 80$	dynes-sec/cm^5	900–1,500
$PVR = \dfrac{PAP - PCWP}{CO} \times 80$	dynes-sec/cm^5	50–150

BSA, body surface area; CO, cardiac output; CVP, mean central venous pressure; HR, heart rate; LVSWI, left ventricular stroke work index; MAP, mean systemic arterial pressure; PAP, mean pulmonary artery pressure; PCWP, pulmonary capillary wedge pressure; PVR, pulmonary vascular resistance; RVSWI, right ventricular stroke work index; SI, stroke index; SV, stroke volume; SVR, systemic vascular resistance.

radiograph, and a 12-lead electrocardiogram (ECG) with a rhythm strip. A heparin platelet factor 4 antibody detection assay should be considered for patients with a low or rapidly falling platelet count who are receiving heparin, as these patients are at risk for developing HIT.

II. **Anesthetic management**
  A. **Patient education.** Anxieties are often allayed by an explanation of what is to be expected, both immediately before and after surgery. It is important to emphasize that the patient will be comfortable.
  B. **Premedication**
   1. **Cardiac medications**
     a. **Beta-Adrenergic antagonists, calcium channel blockers, and nitrates,** including intravenous (IV) nitroglycerin, routinely are continued on schedule until the patient's arrival in the operating room (OR).
     b. **Digitalis** preparations are commonly held for 24 hours preoperatively because of inherent toxicity (especially in the presence of hypokalemia) and a long elimination half-life. When rate control is critical, however, as in mitral stenosis (MS), digitalis should be continued.
     c. **Antihypertensives,** including angiotensin-converting enzyme (ACE) inhibitors and diuretics, are usually held the morning of surgery. Patients with significant LV dysfunction are more likely to develop vasodilatory shock when they receive an ACE inhibitor preoperatively. If the patient's blood pressure is extremely labile, however, the antihypertensives may need to be continued.
     d. **Antiarrhythmics** are generally continued until the time of surgery. Type I agents (e.g., quinidine, procainamide,

and disopyramide) may suppress automaticity and conduction, especially when patients are hyperkalemic. **Amiodarone** has a half-life of 30 days; discontinuation within a few days of surgery will have little effect on serum levels. Amiodarone use may be associated with pulmonary toxicity, decreased atrioventricular nodal conduction, atropine-resistant bradycardia, and myocardial depression in the perioperative period.

e. **Aspirin** has been discontinued 7 to 10 days before heart surgery in the past. Recent evidence suggests that aspirin does not increase perioperative bleeding. Moreover, aspirin has a positive effect on graft patency. It may be prudent to continue aspirin therapy in patients who have significant CAD. Bleeding related solely to aspirin therapy can be overcome with platelet transfusion provided the drug has been cleared from the circulation. Aspirin has a 15 to 20 minute half-life in patients with normal hepatic function. Patients with cardiovascular pathology may be receiving multiple antiplatelet agents that may or may not be reversible (Table 23.3). An accurate medication history is required for cardiac surgical patients to determine the risk of perioperative coagulopathy and hemorrhage.

f. **Warfarin** should be held 2 to 3 days preoperatively. A normal prothrombin time should be documented before surgery. Vitamin K (10 mg subcutaneously) or 2 to 4 units of fresh-frozen plasma (FFP) may be used emergently to correct coagulopathy; however, FFP will only transiently correct a warfarin-induced coagulopathy due to the relatively longer half-life of warfarin compared with the vitamin K-dependent cofactors (factors II, VII, IX, and X), thus putting the patient at risk for rebound coagulopathy.

g. **Heparin** infusions initiated for unstable angina or for patients with left main coronary disease are routinely continued preoperatively. The anticoagulant effects of unfractionated heparin are acutely reversible with IV protamine administration. In contrast, the anticoagulant effects of low molecular weight heparin preparations are not fully reversible with protamine administration and have been associated with increased perioperative hemorrhage in cardiac surgical patients.

2. **Sedation and analgesia** are warranted in almost all cardiac surgical patients. Combinations of benzodiazepines and morphine provide excellent amnesia and analgesia for preinduction catheter insertion, with an acceptable degree of cardiorespiratory depression in all but the most debilitated patients.

a. For full-sized adults with good LV function, **lorazepam,** 1 to 2 mg orally, is given the night before and again 1 hour before arrival in the OR, and **morphine,** 0.1 to 0.15 mg/kg intramuscularly (or subcutaneously if the patient is anticoagulated), is given at least 1 hour before induction.

b. Even a small amount of premedication-induced hypotension can be hazardous to patients with severe aortic stenosis (AS) or left main CAD. Drug dosages should be reduced in these patients.

Table 23.3. Antiplatelet agents

Drug	Inhibits	Half-life	Duration of Effects	Reversible Effects?	Methods to Restore Function
Aspirin	Cyclooxygenase	15–20 minutes	7 days	No	Platelet transfusion
Abciximab (Reopro)	Glycoprotein IIb/IIIa receptor	30 minutes	48 hours	Yes, but only partial	Platelet transfusion
Eptifibatide (Integrilin)	Glycoprotein IIb/IIIa receptor	2.5 hours	4–8 hours	Yes	Delay surgery 2 hours after stopping drug
Tirofiban (Aggrastat)	Glycoprotein IIb/IIIa receptor	1.5–3 hours	4–8 hours	Yes	Discontinue drug as soon as possible before surgery
Clopidogrel (Plavix)	Adenosine diphosphate receptor	8 hours	7 days	No	Blood and product transfusion as needed[c]
Ticlopidine (Ticlid)	Adenosine diphosphate receptor	12 hours to 5 days with repeated dosing	7 days	No	Blood and product transfusion as needed
Dipyridamole[a] (Persantine)	Adenosine uptake; Phosphodiesterase	9–13 hours	4–10 hours	Yes	Platelet transfusion
Cilostazol (Pletal)	Phosphodiesterase III	11–13 hours	48 hours	Yes	Blood and product transfusion as needed
Herbal Therapies[b]	Platelet aggregation	Variable	Variable	Variable	Limited data available

[a] Dipyridamole is available in a formulation with aspirin (Aggrenox).
[b] Includes garlic, ginkgo, ginseng, ginger, feverfew, fish oil, dong quai.
[c] Administration of aprotinin has been associated with a reduction of bleeding in Plavix-treated cardiac surgical patients.

    c. Patients with MS may develop life-threatening pulmonary hypertension with sedation-induced hypoventilation and hypoxemia. Because these patients may also be extremely sensitive to the central effects of sedation, no or minimal premedication is administered until the patient arrives in the OR.

    d. Patients requiring anesthesia transport to the OR may be given IV premedication by the transport team.

  3. Supplemental oxygen therapy is given primarily to patients with severe LV dysfunction, valvular disease, and compromised pulmonary function.

C. Monitoring

  1. Standard monitors (see Chapter 10).

    a. ECG. Continuous display of both leads II and V_5 with ST segment trend analysis will facilitate the diagnosis of ischemia and rhythm disturbance.

    b. Temperature monitoring includes measurement of the "core" temperature, measured in the nasopharynx and reflective of brain and other highly perfused tissues; the blood temperature, measured by the pulmonary artery catheter; and the "shell" temperature, measured in the rectum or on the epidermis, reflective of less perfused regions.

  2. Central venous and pulmonary artery pressures

    a. Patients with normal ventricular function undergoing cardiac surgery can be effectively managed with central venous pressure (CVP) monitoring. Cardiac output and filling pressure data obtained from a pulmonary artery (PA) catheter, however, facilitate rational drug and volume therapy throughout the perioperative period.

    b. Pacing PA catheter and Paceport catheters provide pacing capability for the management of a variety of valvular lesions (AI and mitral regurgitation) and conduction disorders and for "redo" operations during which rapid access for epicardial pacing may not be possible. **Mixed venous oxygen saturation** ($Smvo_2$) monitoring is available continuously with PA catheters specially equipped with a fiberoptic-linked oximeter. A decrease in $Smvo_2$ is the result of either decreased cardiac output, decreased hemoglobin, increased oxygen consumption, or decreased Sao_2.

  3. Intraoperative transesophageal echocardiography (TEE) can be very helpful for the following:

    a. Preoperative evaluation of valve pathology to help the surgeon determine whether a repair, rather than a replacement, is possible.

    b. Preoperative evaluation for intracardiac thrombi, intracardiac shunts, and intra-aortic plaques. The combination of TEE and epiaortic echocardiography helps the surgeon determine the best location to cannulate the aorta in the presence of aortic plaque. In patients with severe atheromatous disease in the proximal aorta, the femoral artery or axillary artery may be cannulated or off-pump coronary artery bypass grafting (CABG) can be performed.

    c. Perioperative evaluation of aortic dissection.

    d. Perioperative evaluation of ventricular anatomy and function.

    e. Evaluation of intracardiac air before terminating CPB.

    f. Postoperative evaluation of valve repair or replacement and intracardiac shunt repair.

    g. There are many ways to perform a comprehensive TEE exam. The Society of Cardiovascular Anesthesiologists/American Society of Echocardiography TEE guidelines are helpful in ensuring that all necessary views are obtained.

4. Neurologic monitors such as transcranial Doppler, multichannel electroencephalography, and cerebral oximetry may improve neurologic outcome by alerting the clinician to perfusion imbalances during CPB. Use of the BIS monitor allows appropriate titration of sedative-hypnotic anesthetic agents for cardiac surgical patients that are being considered for intraoperative extubation or "fast track" anesthesia pathways.

D. Preinduction. Upon the patient's arrival in the OR, vital signs are checked, an adequate SpO_2 is ensured, and additional premedication (1 to 2 mg of midazolam), if indicated, is titrated.

1. Peripheral venous access is established. In adults, one large-bore (14-gauge) peripheral IV catheter is sufficient. If excessive bleeding is expected (e.g., a redo operation or a patient with a preexisting coagulopathy), a second peripheral line will facilitate blood product administration.

2. Arterial cannulation is performed with either an 18- or 20-gauge catheter.

    a. When possible, in patients undergoing left internal mammary dissection, the right radial artery is cannulated so that the left arm may be safely tucked.

    b. Bilateral radial artery cannulation is often performed for complex aortic arch surgery, particularly in the setting of an aortic dissection.

    c. Cannulation distal to a previous brachial artery cutdown site should be avoided. Pressure gradients may occur across arteriotomies, especially during and after CPB.

    d. If blood pressure measurements are asymmetric, the arterial catheter should be placed on the side with the higher value.

    e. Be certain to note whether the surgeon will use the radial artery as a conduit for CABG surgery.

    f. Femoral artery cannulation is a safe and reliable alternative to radial artery cannulation. Preoperative femoral artery cannulation in patients with severe CAD and poor LV function provides a site for postoperative intra-aortic balloon (IABP) insertion, if it becomes necessary. Brachial and axillary artery cannulations are third and fourth choices.

    g. Intra-aortic balloon central lumen pressure can be transduced as a monitor of central arterial pressure.

3. Central venous access may be established before or after induction, depending on the clinical situation.

4. A defibrillator and external pacemaker generator must be available, as should a magnet to regulate pacemakers or implantable cardioverter defibrillators (ICDs), if applicable.

5. Typed and cross-matched packed red blood cells (2 to 4 units) must be present and checked.

6. **Baseline hemodynamics,** including cardiac output and a 7-lead ECG are recorded.
7. Readily available medications should include heparin, calcium chloride, lidocaine, amiodarone, inotropes, vasopressors, vasodilators, and nitroglycerin. Protamine should never be drawn up until the patient is safely separated from CPB.

E. **Induction** is one of the critical times in the anesthetic management of the patient. A surgeon should be available, and the CPB pump should be ready in the event that a hemodynamic emergency occurs. The choice of agents and sequence of events depend on the specific cardiac lesions, the patient's underlying condition, and the surgical plan. A systematic, gradual induction with frequent assessment of the degree of cardiovascular depression and depth of anesthesia (as determined by hemodynamic response to graded stimuli including oral airway insertion and Foley catheterization) will minimize hemodynamic instability.

1. **Agents** useful in the induction and maintenance of anesthesia in the cardiac surgical patient include the following:

   a. **IV opioids** produce various degrees of vasodilation and bradycardia without significant myocardial depression. A high-dose technique utilizes fentanyl (50 to 100 μg/kg) or sufentanil (10 to 20 μg/kg) as both the induction and primary maintenance agents. Alternatively, a smaller induction bolus (fentanyl 25 to 50 μg/kg) may be supplemented with a continuous narcotic infusion, or even lower doses (fentanyl 10 to 25 μg/kg, or sufentanil 1 to 5 μg/kg) may be used in conjunction with other central nervous system depressants as part of a "balanced technique."

   b. **Sedative hypnotics and amnestics,** including thiopental, propofol, and etomidate may be useful as coinduction agents in particular situations. Of these drugs, etomidate causes the least myocardial depression.

   c. **Volatile inhalation anesthetics** are useful supplementary agents, especially in the treatment of hypertension.

   d. **Muscle relaxants** with minimal cardiovascular effects are commonly chosen (e.g., vecuronium, cisatracurium). Pretreatment with a "priming dose" and early relaxant administration help to counteract chest wall rigidity often encountered during narcotic-based inductions. **Succinylcholine** is used in modified rapid sequence inductions for patients with reflux or a full stomach. **Pancuronium** is used to counteract the bradycardic effects of opioids.

2. **Specific considerations for valvular heart disease** (see also Chapter 2).

   a. **Aortic stenosis.** Hemodynamic goals include adequate intravascular volume, slow heart rate with sinus rhythm, and maintenance of contractility and systemic vascular tone. The thick, noncompliant left ventricle associated with AS often requires high filling pressures (LVEDP of 20 to 30 mm Hg). Anesthetic agents that reduce vascular tone or myocardial contractility (e.g., thiopental) should be avoided. An infusion of a vasopressor (e.g., norepinephrine) can be started 1 to 2 minute before induction to decrease the risk of developing significant hypotension associated with induction. Dysrhythmias must be treated aggressively.

b. Aortic insufficiency. Hemodynamic goals include adequate intravascular volume, maintenance of an increased heart rate and contractile state, and decreased systemic vascular tone to facilitate forward flow. Patients with AI often are highly dependent on endogenous sympathetic tone. Patients with coexisting CAD may decompensate with significant bradycardia (very low diastolic perfusion pressure); a rapid method for pacing should be available.

c. Mitral stenosis. Hemodynamic goals mandate maintenance of a slow rhythm, preferably sinus, and adequate intravascular volume, contractility, and systemic resistance. Elevated pulmonary vascular resistance (PVR), often secondary to hypoventilation or positive end-expiratory pressure (PEEP), must be avoided. Patients with severe MS and elevated PVR are challenging to induce. Insertion of a PA line before induction is recommended.

d. Mitral regurgitation. Hemodynamic goals include maintenance of adequate volume, contractility, a normal to elevated heart rate, and a reduction of systemic vascular tone. Increased PVR should be avoided. Anesthesia-induced decreases in systemic vascular resistance are usually well tolerated.

e. In patients with mixed valvular lesions, the most hemodynamically significant lesion will predominate the management goals. The addition of CAD to mixed valve lesions makes planning even more complex (e.g., AS with AI and CAD). In all situations, determine the three most likely problems that could occur during induction and plan the management for each.

3. **Specific considerations for emergent inductions**

   a. Pulmonary embolus. Induction and positive pressure ventilation can precipitate cardiovascular collapse. It is prudent to prepare and drape the unstable patient before induction. Cannulation of the femoral vessels under local anesthesia for initiation of cardiopulmonary bypass is indicated for patients with poor right ventricular function.

   b. Pericardial tamponade. Similar concerns are present for patients with pericardial tamponade. Adequate volume administration is essential. Starting an inotropic agent and a vasopressor before induction may be helpful. Acute sternotomy may be required if hemodynamic collapse occurs with anesthesia induction. Insertion of a pericardial drain may be needed before anesthesia induction to prevent hemodynamic collapse.

   c. Aortic dissection. Hypertension can precipitate aortic rupture. Blood must be available before induction. Proximal extension of the dissection can occur and cause coronary ischemia or tamponade.

   d. Ventricular septal defect (VSD) and papillary muscle rupture after myocardial infarction. Patients may present with extreme hypotension. Rapidity in establishing CPB is essential. Preinduction initiation of intra-aortic balloon counterpulsation therapy is indicated in many of these patients.

e. Blood pressure may fall precipitously during the induction of critically ill patients. Cardiopulmonary resuscitation should not be delayed while waiting for pharmacologic therapy to work. If the patient does not recover quickly with chest compressions and defibrillation, consider initiating CPB immediately.

F. The prebypass period is characterized by variable levels of stimulation during preparation for the initiation of CPB. Particularly stimulating periods include sternal splitting and retraction, pericardial incision, and aortic root dissection and cannulation. Spontaneous cooling will occur.

1. A blood sample should be obtained to check the baseline arterial blood gas (ABG) tensions and pH, hematocrit, and a baseline activated clotting time (ACT). Phlebotomy and acute normovolemic hemodilution may be considered in otherwise healthy patients with a starting hematocrit of 40% or greater, thus providing fresh autologous whole blood for transfusion following CPB and heparin reversal.

2. The lungs are deflated during sternal splitting. Anatomic changes in chest wall configuration produce ECG changes, especially T-wave changes, which should be noted to avoid confusion with ischemia-induced changes.

3. Left internal mammary artery dissection may produce blood loss into the left chest that can negatively affect pulmonary function in patients with reduced pulmonary reserve.

4. Anticoagulation for cannulation

a. Before induction of anesthesia, heparin, 350 international units (IU)/kg (500 IU/kg if the patient is on IV heparin or being treated with IABP counterpulsation therapy), should be prepared in case emergency initiation of CPB is necessary. Administer the heparin through a centrally placed catheter, aspirating blood both before and after injection to confirm patency.

b. Vasodilation often follows the heparin bolus and should be anticipated.

c. The **ACT,** determined approximately 5 min after heparin administration, is used to monitor the degree of anticoagulation. Baseline values are 80 to 150 seconds. Heparin treatment sufficient to prevent microthrombus formation during CPB correlates with an ACT of more than 400 seconds (at higher than 35°C). An ACT value of greater than 450 seconds is preferred, given the inherent variance that exists in this point-of-care test. Patients on continuous IV heparin preoperatively, or being treated with IABP counterpulsation may become relatively "heparin resistant." If an ACT longer than 400 seconds is not achieved with standard heparin dose regimens, an additional 200 to 300 IU/kg is administered. If this fails, antithrombin concentrate (500 to 1,000 IU) or 2 to 4 units of FFP may be necessary to correct a probable antithrombin deficiency.

d. Patients with a diagnosis of HIT type 2 or HIT with thrombotic syndrome (HITTS) require special anticoagulation management during CPB. The classification of HIT is determined by immune involvement. HIT type 1 is a non-immune-mediated reaction of heparin with platelets that causes a mild thrombocytopenia. HIT type 2 is an immune-mediated phenomenon that activates platelets, resulting in platelet aggregation. Biochemical mediators from activated platelets can induce the generation of thrombin, leading to HIT-mediated thrombotic syndrome. For patients with HIT type 2 or HITTS, two alternatives to standard heparin treatment exist (Table 23.4); each has significant limitations that should be discussed with the surgeon and a hematologist before use.

(1) All forms of heparin are removed preoperatively. (Saline is used to flush pressure transducers, and citrate is used to wash salvaged blood during the centrifugation process.)

(2) A heparin-free PA catheter is used.

(3) Alternative anticoagulant regimens may be used. These include bivalirudin, or unfractionated heparin in combination with an antiplatelet agent (see Table 23.4). The safe management of anticoagulation for CPB with bivalirudin should not be attempted without consulting a clinician experienced with this technique.

(4) If unfractionated heparin is used, then a bypass dose of porcine heparin is administered before aortic cannulation (to minimize the likelihood of a repeat dose of heparin).

(5) Aspirin is administered early in the postoperative period, and initiation of systemic anticoagulation with a direct thrombin inhibitor and coumadin may be indicated to prevent both early and late postoperative thromboembolic complications.

5. **Preparation for CPB** begins with aortic cannulation. **Epiaortic scanning** is used to sonographically direct the cannulation site in patients with known atherosclerotic disease (by history or intraoperative TEE). Maintaining a systolic blood pressure near 100 mm Hg during aortic cannulation decreases the risk of dissection.

6. Some surgeons will perform the proximal saphenous vein graft anastomoses before going on CPB. An improperly placed side-biting clamp may occlude more than 50% of the aortic lumen and markedly increase afterload, causing myocardial decompensation. The early signs are hypotension, elevation of PA pressures, and ST-segment changes.

7. One or two venous return cannulas are inserted via the right atrium. A catheter is frequently inserted into the proximal ascending aorta for antegrade cardioplegia delivery.

8. A retrograde cardioplegia cannula is often inserted into the coronary sinus. Placement of this cannula may precipitate a supraventricular dysrhythmia that can result in acute hemodynamic decompensation requiring immediate synchronized cardioversion or initiation of CPB. Placement of this cannula can be guided by TEE.

Table 23.4. Alternative cardiopulmonary bypass anticoagulation in patients with HIT

Drug	Mechanism	Half-life	Lab Monitor	Reversible?
Bivalirudin (Angiomax)[a]	Direct thrombin inhibitor	25 minutes (normal renal function)	ACT	No
Tirofiban (Aggrastat) + Unfractionated heparin[a]	Glycoprotein IIb/IIIa receptor inhibitor prevents platelet aggregation in HIT	1.5–3 hours	ACT (platelets and D-dimer if HIT thrombosis is suspected)	No

[a] Additional training is required to safely use this anticoagulation technique for patients requiring CPB.

G. Cardiopulmonary bypass

1. **CPB circuit.** In the typical primary CPB circuit, blood is transferred by gravity through plastic tubing from the right atrium to a venous reservoir. A pump (roller or centrifugal) propels the venous blood into a heat exchanger and an oxygenator that adds oxygen and removes carbon dioxide. The arterialized blood passes through a filter before entering the patient's ascending aorta via the aortic cannula. The CPB machine also includes a circuit for the delivery of cardioplegia and one or more for aspirating blood from the surgical field. Approximately 1,600 mL of crystalloid is added to "prime" the primary circuit. This will decrease the patient's hematocrit (Hct) proportionately: Hct = [patient weight (kg) × 70 mL/kg × Hct]/[patient weight × 70 mL/kg + pump prime (mL)]. As a general rule, a cardiac anesthetist should be able to prepare the CPB machine in an emergency and to anticipate and manage potential CPB-related problems (e.g., clotted membrane oxygenator, inadequate pump occlusion, and air embolus).

2. **Initiation of CPB.** After adequate heparin treatment is established (an ACT of 400 to 480 seconds), the bypass is initiated when the surgeon releases the clamp on the venous line. After the perfusionist is convinced that the venous return is adequate, he or she will turn on the pump and progressively increase the speed to a flow of 2.0 to 2.4 L/minute/m^2 or roughly 50 mL/kg/minute for adults. A mean arterial pressure (MAP) of 40 to 120 mm Hg may be achieved by such flow, depending on vascular resistance, intravascular volume, and blood viscosity. Observe the bright red blood entering the aorta during this initiation to confirm that the membrane oxygenator is working properly. Once adequate flows and venous drainage are established, volatile anesthetics from the anesthesia machine, IV fluids, and pulmonary ventilation are discontinued. Muscle relaxants are supplemented to prevent shivering. Anesthesia is maintained by IV agents or by inhalation agents administered through a vaporizer in the fresh gas line of the circuit. It is advisable to pull the PA catheter back 1 to 5 cm to prevent the catheter tip from migrating into a wedge position during CPB. If two venous return lines are used and tourniquets are applied to achieve complete CPB, the CVP should be measured in the most proximal position possible (i.e., side arm of the PA-line introducer). Because cerebral perfusion pressure is equal to MAP minus the superior vena cava (SVC) pressure, obstruction of the SVC cannula and consequent increasing SVC pressures must be detected to avoid neurologic injury. After fibrillation or arrest, mean PA pressures are displayed. A vent cannula may be inserted into the left ventricle to prevent distention.

3. **Maintenance of CPB**

   a. **Myocardial protection** during the cross-clamp period is achieved primarily by reducing myocardial oxygen consumption through hypothermia, hyperkalemic arrest, or both.

      (1) **Cardioplegia solutions** may be delivered antegrade through the aortic root, coronary ostia, or vein graft or retrograde through the coronary sinus.

(2) **Intermittent cold cardioplegia** currently is a commonly used technique. Cold (4°C to 6°C) hyperkalemic solution with or without blood is delivered to the coronary circulation approximately every 20 min (or sooner if cardiac electrical activity returns). Systemic cooling of the patient and topical cooling of the heart augment the protection.

(3) The **warm cardioplegia technique** delivers a warm (32°C to 37°C) hyperkalemic solution mixed with blood at approximately a 1:5 ratio. The solution is delivered continuously during the cross-clamp period with a few interruptions to allow visualization of the anastomotic sites. Mild systemic cooling to 32°C to 34°C is frequently used. Lidocaine or esmolol may be used to augment the protection. Serum glucose levels will increase dramatically and are treated with IV insulin.

(4) The **cold fibrillating technique** (no aortic cross-clamp) may be used for CABG procedures. This technique requires elevated systemic pressure (MAP greater than 80 mm Hg), continuous measurement of LV vent pressure, and a continuous nitroglycerin infusion to ensure adequate myocardial perfusion.

b. **Hypothermia** (20°C to 34°C) is commonly used during CPB. Oxygen consumption, and thereby flow requirements, are reduced while blood viscosity increases, thus counteracting prime-induced hypoviscosity. Adverse effects of hypothermia include impaired autoregulatory, enzymatic, and cellular membrane function; decreased oxygen delivery (leftward shift of the hemoglobin oxygen dissociation curve); and potentiation of coagulopathy.

c. **Hemodynamic monitoring** during CPB is the shared responsibility of the perfusionist, anesthetist, and surgeon.

(1) **Hypotension** during initiation of CPB usually is due to hemodilution and hypoviscosity. Other important causes include inadequate pump flow, vasodilation, acute aortic dissection, and incorrect placement of the aortic cannula (e.g., directing flow toward the innominate artery not supplying the cannulated radial artery). The PA pressure and LV vent flow rate should be inspected to ensure that aortic incompetence has not compromised forward pump flow. (The venous cannula can potentially increase AI by compressing the noncoronary cusp of the aortic valve.) A phenylephrine infusion may be required to treat transient hypotension. During the course of CPB, a pressure gradient (as high as 40 mm Hg) may develop between the radial artery and the aorta. The lower radial artery pressure could lead to unnecessary administration of vasopressors if this is not recognized. In the presence of carotid stenosis, MAP should be maintained at a higher level than usual (e.g., 80 to 90 mm Hg), and hypocarbia should be avoided.

(2) **Hypertension** (MAP higher than 90 mm Hg) may be due to excessive flow rates or increased vascular resistance, which may be treated with vasodilators or anesthetics.

(3) **Elevated PA pressures** indicate left heart distention, which may be due to inadequate venting, AI, or inadequate isolation of venous return. Severe distention may result in myocardial damage.

d. **Metabolic acidosis and oliguria** suggest inadequate systemic perfusion. Additional volume (blood or crystalloid depending on hematocrit) may be required to achieve increased flow. Brisk urine output should be established during the first 10 min of CPB.

(1) **Oliguria** (less than 1 mL/kg/hour) should be treated with a trial of increased perfusion pressure and/or flow, mannitol (0.25 to 0.5 g/kg), or dopamine (1 to 5 μg/kg/minute). Patients on chronic furosemide therapy may require their usual dose during CPB to sustain diuresis. Fenoldopam, a selective dopamine agonist, will promote natriuresis and may provide renoprotective effects during CPB.

(2) **Hemolysis** during CPB usually is due to physical trauma to red blood cells by the pump suction. Released pigments may cause acute renal failure postoperatively. For hemoglobinuria, diuresis is maintained with mannitol or furosemide. In severe cases, the urine is alkalinized by administering sodium bicarbonate at 0.5 to 1.0 mEq/kg.

e. **Additional heparin** may be needed for prolonged CPB. A 100-IU/kg hourly reinforcement dose is given beginning 2 hours after the initial dose. An artificially elevated ACT is seen during aprotinin therapy when using celite ACT tubes. Hypothermia prolongs both the celite and the kaolin ACT. The duration of heparin anticoagulation may be shorter in patients on chronic heparin therapy or during cases in which systemic hypothermia is not used. The ACT does not correlate well with plasma heparin levels when the patient is on CPB, but many centers routinely monitor the ACT during hypothermic (25°C to 34°C) CPB.

H. **Discontinuing CPB** implies transferring cardiopulmonary function from the bypass system back to the patient. In preparation for this transition, the anesthetist must examine and optimize the patient's metabolic, anesthetic, and cardiorespiratory status.

1. **Preparation for discontinuing CPB begins during rewarming.** The arterial blood is warmed. The core temperature should reach but not exceed 37°C, and the shell (rectal or epidermal) temperature, reflective of less highly perfused tissues, should reach 35°C to 36°C before discontinuation from CPB.

a. **Laboratory data** to acquire during rewarming include ABG tensions and pH, potassium, calcium, glucose, hematocrit, and ACT. ABG tensions and pH can be reported both at 37°C (the temperature of the sample in the blood gas machine) and corrected to the patient's temperature. Clinical decisions concerning pH usually are made according to the values measured at 37°C (**alpha-stat** management). The topic remains controversial, and some anesthetists act on the values reported at the patient's temperature (**pH-stat** management).

   b. **Adequate anticoagulation** during rewarming and separation from CPB is ensured with additional heparin if necessary.

   c. **Metabolic acidosis** should be treated with sodium bicarbonate, and appropriate ventilatory changes should be instituted by the perfusionist.

   d. **Hyperkalemia,** commonly seen following the use of cardioplegia, frequently corrects spontaneously by redistribution and diuresis. If not, the administration of IV insulin, sodium bicarbonate, and glucose will lower serum potassium.

   e. **Severe hyperglycemia** (blood glucose higher than 400 to 500 mg/dL), most commonly seen in diabetic patients following a warm cardioplegia technique, requires an insulin infusion.

   f. A **hematocrit** over 20% should be achieved before separation, either by transfusion or hemoconcentration, as indicated by the CPB reservoir volume. A higher or lower hematocrit may be appropriate, depending on the patient's age and condition.

   g. **FFP** should be thawed before separation from bypass (requiring 30 to 45 minutes) if the patient is at risk for postoperative bleeding. **Platelets** should also be readily available for these patients.

2. **Anesthetic considerations** during rewarming include maintenance of adequate neuromuscular blockade, analgesia, and amnesia. Supplementary relaxants, narcotics, and benzodiazepines may be given. Pressure transducers are rezeroed. If MAP is elevated, sodium nitroprusside may be used for blood pressure control as well as to facilitate rewarming.

3. **Separation from CPB**

   a. After procedures in which the heart has been opened (e.g., valve replacements), **"de-airing maneuvers"** under TEE guidance are used to prevent air embolism to the cerebral or coronary circulations. Positive-pressure ventilation accompanied by clamping of the venous return lines will move air forward from the pulmonary veins. Air in the ventricular trabeculae can be liberated by shifting the OR table from side to side and lifting the apex of the heart; it can then be evacuated by needle aspiration of the apex. Direct aspiration of air bubbles visible within coronary artery vein grafts may help prevent ischemia.

   b. **Aortic cross-clamp removal** reestablishes coronary perfusion. A lidocaine bolus may be given followed by an infusion (1 mg/minute). Nitroglycerin is started in CABG or CABG/valve patients.

   c. **Defibrillation** may be spontaneous; ventricular fibrillation is treated with directly applied 10- to 30-joule DC countershock. (If using a device capable of delivering a biphasic waveform, 7 to 10 joules is commonly adequate.) Failure may indicate inadequate warming, graft problems, a metabolic disturbance, or inadequate myocardial protection. Additional lidocaine, magnesium (1 g IV slowly), or amiodarone (150-mg IV bolus followed by infusion at 1 mg/min for 6 hours, then 0.5 mg/minute) may be required.

d. **Rhythm is assessed.** With slow rhythms, atrial pacing is established through epicardial wires, but if the **PR** interval is prolonged or if there is complete heart block, ventricular pacing is added. Hypothermia as well as hypocalcemia, hyperkalemia, and hypermagnesemia caused by cardioplegia solutions may contribute to a high incidence of reversible heart block immediately after CPB. Atrial tachycardia may indicate inadequate anesthesia and may be treated with fentanyl. Other atrial dysrhythmias may be treated with overdrive pacing, cardioversion, and then, if necessary, antidysrhythmics (e.g., esmolol, propranolol, amiodarone, verapamil, or rarely digoxin).

e. **The ECG should be inspected** for evidence of ischemia possibly related to intracoronary air or inadequate revascularization.

f. **LV filling** may be guided during separation from CPB by mean PA, PA occlusion pressure, or a surgically placed LA line. Right ventricular (RV) filling is indicated by the CVP or direct RV visualization. The determination of target postbypass filling pressures should consider the patient's preoperative pressures, the degree of left ventricular hypertrophy (LVH), the adequacy of the myocardial revascularization, and the anticipated physiologic effects of corrective valvular surgery. A normotensive patient without LVH probably needs a LA pressure of 10 mm Hg or a mean PA pressure of 20 mm Hg. A patient with severe LVH and inadequate revascularization may need an LA pressure of 20 mm Hg or a mean PA pressure of 30 mm Hg. TEE is particularly helpful in assessing LV filling.

g. **Comparison** is made between central (aortic) and peripheral (radial) arterial pressures to ensure that no significant pressure gradient exists.

h. **Compliance and resistance of the lungs** is tested with a few trial breaths (ventilation should be reestablished when LV ejection, even on bypass, occurs). To facilitate expansion of the lungs, the stomach is suctioned, and, if previously opened, the pleural cavities are drained. If the lungs are difficult to ventilate, suctioning or bronchodilators may be indicated (see Chapter 18, section XI).

i. **Visual inspection of the heart** confirms atrioventricular synchrony; contractility is assessed both by gross appearance and by systolic performance, as estimated by peak systolic and pulse pressure, taking into account pump flow and LA and PA pressure. If poor myocardial performance is demonstrated or anticipated (e.g., impaired preoperative function or intraoperative ischemia), initiation of inotropic support before separation from CPB may be indicated. Pump flow rate is checked and compared with the patient's preoperative cardiac output. Significantly higher flows indicate the need to increase vascular tone (using agents such as norepinephrine and phenylephrine).

    j. **Ionized Ca^{2+}** may be corrected slowly 15 minutes after cross-clamp removal. Rapid Ca^{2+} administration, especially in the presence of myocardial ischemia, is associated with Ca^{2+}-induced myocardial injury. Calcium will increase both contractility and systemic vascular resistance (SVR).

I. **At the time of actual separation from CPB,** venous lines are slowly clamped, allowing the heart to gradually fill and eject with each contraction. Prolonged partial venous line occlusion allows for "**partial bypass,**" during which time cardiopulmonary function is shared and hemodynamics are assessed. After complete venous line occlusion, once adequate filling pressures are achieved, perfusion through the aortic cannula is stopped, and the heart alone provides systemic perfusion. Manual ventilation with full tidal volumes and short inspiratory times facilitates RV performance.

    1. **Pressure maintenance.** Transfusion from the CPB reservoir maintains the LA pressure or mean PA pressure at an optimal level. Care is taken not to overdistend the heart. Should overdistention occur, the surgeon may "empty" the heart by transiently unclamping a venous line. Alternatively, the patient may be temporarily placed in reverse Trendelenberg position to decrease venous return to the overdistended heart.

    2. **After bypass has been terminated, assess the following:** ECG, systemic blood pressure (SBP), left-sided filling pressure (LFP), right-sided filling pressure (RFP), and the cardiac output. Compare these values with the target values for the patient. If the patient is not doing well, correct any pacing problems, ask the surgeon to assess the adequacy of the grafts, and use TEE to assess the valve replacement or repair. Assuming there is no surgically related cause, the unstable patient will usually fall into one of the following situations:

        a. **SBP low, cardiac output low, LFP low, RFP low: hypovolemia.** Give volume from the bypass reservoir. If the patient cannot tolerate the low blood pressure (e.g., a patient with severe LVH and distal coronary disease), use a pressor transiently until the volume resuscitation is adequate.

        b. **SBP low, cardiac output low, LFP high, RFP low: left heart failure.** Give a positive inotrope. A common first-line agent is dopamine, started at 200 to 300 μg/minute IV and titrated as necessary. Milrinone, a phosphodiesterase III inhibitor, is added when additional support is necessary (load 25 to 50 μg/kg followed by an infusion at 0.375 to 0.750 μg/kg/minute). The patient may need to go back on CPB temporarily. If inotropes are ineffective, an IABP (see section V.A) is inserted. The final intervention is insertion of an LV assist device (LVAD) (see section V.B).

        c. **SBP low, cardiac output low, LFP low, RFP high: right heart failure.** This situation can be caused by primary RV failure (inadequate myocardial protection or intracoronary air) or secondary RV failure (severe protamine reaction, inadequate ventilation, fixed elevation in PVR). Management includes the following:

            (1) If achievable, a rapid increase in systemic perfusion pressure using norepinephrine or epinephrine may reverse primary RV failure.

(2) Treat known causes of elevated PVR: light anesthesia, hypercarbia, hypoxemia, and acidemia. Vasopressors and calcium chloride may be administered through an LA line if available.

(3) Vasodilator therapy, including nitroglycerin, sodium nitroprusside, or prostaglandin E_1 (begin 0.05 μg/kg/minute IV, titrate as necessary) through a right-sided line. Systemic vasodilatation often necessitates compensatory vasopressor support through an LA line. Alternatively, inhaled nitric oxide can be used to avoid the systemic hypotension.

(4) Inotropic support is maintained with milrinone or dobutamine for maximal pulmonary vasodilatation. Mechanical support (IABP if right ventricular ischemia is the etiology of right heart failure or RV assist devices [RVADs; see sections V.A and B]) may be necessary.

d. SBP low, cardiac output low, LFP high, RFP high: biventricular failure. Management includes maneuvers to treat left and right heart failure, as outlined above. Frequently, the patient will need to go back on bypass.

e. SBP low, cardiac output high, LFP low, RFP low: low SVR. Initial management consists of administration of a pressor such as norepinephrine or phenylephrine. Epinephrine may be necessary. In certain patients with vasodilatory shock (e.g., after heart transplant or LVAD insertion), arginine vasopressin is used starting with an infusion at 0.03 unit/minute.

f. SBP high, cardiac output low, LFP normal, RFP normal: high SVR. Hypertension with adequate cardiac output should be treated to prevent bleeding at suture lines and cannulation sites. Vasodilators (e.g., nitroprusside), narcotics, or volatile anesthetics may be appropriate.

g. If a return to CPB is necessary in any of the above situations, adequate anticoagulation must be ensured, and a full heparinizing dose is indicated if any protamine has been given.

J. Postbypass period

1. Hemodynamic stability is the primary goal, since myocardial function has been impaired by CPB. Maintain adequate volume status, perfusion pressure, and appropriate rate and rhythm. Continuously monitor and reassess the surgical field.

2. Hemostasis. Once cardiovascular stability has been achieved and the surgeon is confident that the bleeding is under control, protamine administration begins. Initially, 25 to 50 mg is given over 2 to 3 minutes, and the hemodynamic response is observed. Protamine often causes systemic vasodilation that depends on the rate of administration; hence, slow infusions are prudent. Rarely, an anaphylactic or anaphylactoid reaction or catastrophic pulmonary hypertension is encountered. Upon severe reaction, protamine is immediately discontinued, appropriate resuscitative measures are used, and, if necessary, the patient is retreated with heparin (with a full loading dose), and CPB is reinitiated. If forward flow is compromised, ask the surgeon to inject the heparin into the right atrium.

    a. It is advisable to monitor PA pressures while administering protamine (even if LA pressure is available).

    b. In general, 1 mg of protamine is administered for each mg (100 IU) of heparin administered throughout the procedure. Alternatively, the administered protamine dose can be determined by assessing the patient's whole blood heparin level and calculating the required protamine dose for complete heparin neutralization.

    c. After protamine, the ACT is measured and compared with baseline. Further protamine is given to return the ACT toward control. The activated partial thromboplastin time also serves as a sensitive indicator of residual circulating heparin.

    d. During transfusion of blood obtained from the hemoconcentrator, additional protamine (25 to 50 mg) is given to reverse the heparin. Blood obtained from autotransfusion devices (cell saver) is devoid of heparin.

    e. Desmopressin, aminocaproic acid, tranexamic acid, aprotinin, and various blood products may be of value in the treatment of post-CPB coagulopathy.

    f. Maintenance of normothermia through the use of a patient temperature management system can reduce the severity of post-CPB coagulopathy.

3. Pulmonary dysfunction may follow CPB. Aggressive treatment of bronchospasm before sternal closure is imperative.

4. Pulmonary hypertension may arise during the post-CPB period. See section II.I.2.c for approaches to management.

5. Sternal closure may precipitate acute cardiovascular decompensation. **Cardiac tamponade** may develop from compression of the heart and great vessels in the mediastinum.

    a. Volatile anesthetics and other negative inotropes are reduced in anticipation of sternal closure. Intravascular volume should be optimized.

    b. Immediately after sternal closure, the filling pressures and cardiac output are compared with preclosure values, and appropriate adjustments in volume or drug infusions are made.

    c. Mediastinal and pleural tubes are placed on suction to prevent tamponade and quantify blood loss. Blood drainage of greater than 300 mL in 30 minutes warrants consideration of surgical reexploration.

    d. The LA waveform and the ability of pacemakers to capture are rechecked to verify that displacement has not occurred.

    e. If the patient is hemodynamically unstable or ventilation is inadequate, management should begin with early reopening of the sternum. The patient may require transfer to the intensive care unit (ICU) with the sternum open.

K. Transfer to the ICU

1. Patients should always be hemodynamically stable before transport. Immediately after transferring the patient from the OR table to the bed, reassess vital signs and confirm that drug infusions are still infusing. The patient's bed should be equipped with a full cylinder of oxygen, an Ambu bag, mask, intubation equipment, defibrillator, and essential monitors. Drugs for resuscitation should accompany the patient during transport and include calcium chloride, lidocaine, a vasopressor, and a vasodilator.

2. During transfer, the ECG, arterial and PA pressures, and oxygen saturation are monitored.

3. Upon arrival at the ICU, mediastinal and pleural drainage tubes are attached to suction. An anteroposterior chest radiograph and a 12-lead ECG are obtained, and blood samples are sent for ABG, electrolytes, hematocrit, platelet count, prothrombin time, and activated partial thromboplastin time. Before leaving the ICU, the anesthetist should review the ECG and ABG and should check the chest radiograph for the presence of abnormal findings (e.g., atelectasis, pneumothorax, malpositioned tubes and catheters, widened mediastinum, or pleural effusion).

III. Postoperative care

A. **Warming.** Most cardiac surgical patients will be hypothermic upon arrival in the ICU, and their initial course is notable for warming and vasodilation. A temperature overshoot phenomenon is common, and patients will, on average, reach a maximal temperature (39°C) at 6 to 12 hours into their ICU stay. Pressor and volume requirements should be anticipated. Adequate sedation, by either periodic bolus or continuous infusion, will prevent early waking and shivering during this period.

B. **Extubation.** Ventilatory support is withdrawn coincident with emergence from anesthesia. Intracardiac cannulas and chest tubes are removed, and hemodynamic support is then gradually withdrawn.

C. **Complications**

1. **Dysrhythmias and myocardial ischemia** are common in the immediate postoperative period. Diagnosis and management are discussed in Chapter 18.

2. **Unexplained profound hypotension,** unresponsive to volume and pharmacologic resuscitation, is an indication for immediate reopening of the chest in the ICU. The OR should be notified and blood products requisitioned.

3. **Cardiac tamponade** may occur insidiously. Most often, an accumulation of blood in the mediastinum and inadequate chest tube drainage secondary to clot are responsible. Placing mediastinal tubes on suction as soon as the sternum is closed and frequent "stripping" of the tubes will help to prevent the development of tamponade. Reopening the sternum may be lifesaving. The diagnosis is considered with hypotension or low-output syndrome. Equilibration of mean CVP, PA, and PA occlusion pressures is rarely present because the pericardium is open.

IV. Pediatric cardiac anesthesia

A. **Transition from fetal to adult circulation.** The transition from fetal to adult circulation is a transformation from a parallel to a series circulation (see Chapter 27). In utero, there is right-to-left shunting of blood across the ductus arteriosus. After birth, as the lungs are expanded and alveolar oxygen tension rises, the PVR decreases. Simultaneously, the SVR increases in association with the loss of the low-resistance placental circulation. The net effect of the PVR falling beneath the SVR is a reversal of ductus flow. The ductus arteriosus will contract and functionally close in the first 10 to 15 hours of life. This is caused by a loss of placental-produced prostaglandins and an increase in neonatal blood oxygen tension. Accompanying the decrease in PVR is an increase in pulmonary blood flow, an improvement in RV compliance, and a decrease in right-sided pressures relative to the left. This drop in right atrial pressure results in the closure of the foramen ovale. With the closure of the ductus arteriosus and the foramen ovale, the circulation assumes an adult configuration. These changes in the neonatal period are transitional, however, and reversion to a fetal circulation can occur during periods of abnormal physiologic stress. Persistence of elements of fetal circulation is common in many cases of congenital heart disease (CHD) and can occasionally be lifesaving.

B. Differences between neonatal and adult cardiac physiology

1. In infants, there is **parasympathetic nervous system dominance** that reflects the relative immaturity of the sympathetic nervous system. Infant hearts are more responsive to circulating catecholamines than to sympathetic nervous stimulation.

2. Neonatal hearts have more inelastic membrane mass than elastic contractile mass. Consequently, infant hearts have less myocardial reserve, a greater sensitivity to drugs causing myocardial depression, and a greater sensitivity to volume overload. The relatively noncompliant ventricles make stroke volume less responsive to increases in preload or demand. As such, **increases in cardiac output largely depend on increases in heart rate.**

3. The right and left ventricles are equal in muscle mass at birth. A left to right muscle mass ratio of 2:1 is not achieved until the age of 4 to 5 months.

C. CHD. In CHD, the clinical presentation depends on both the anatomy and the physiologic changes secondary to intracardiac shunts and obstructive lesions.

1. **Shunt classification.** A shunt is an abnormal communication between the systemic and pulmonary circulations.

   a. **Simple shunts** are not associated with anatomic obstruction to ventricular outflow. Pulmonary and systemic blood flow is determined by both the size of the shunt and the relative PVR/SVR ratio.

   b. **Complex shunts** are accompanied by an anatomic obstruction to blood flow. The direction and magnitude of blood flow are determined by the presence of the obstructive lesion. Blood flow depends less on the PVR/SVR ratio and more on the resistance of the obstructive lesion.

   c. **Balanced shunts** are characterized by right and/or LV output that can be directed to either the pulmonary or the systemic circulation. The amount of pulmonary and systemic blood flow depends solely on the PVR/SVR ratio.

   d. **Shunt flow calculation.** The amount of systemic arterial desaturation due to CHD is determined by the relative amount of pulmonary-to-systemic blood shunting ($\dot{Q}p/\dot{Q}s$) and the saturation of the venous blood.

$$\dot{Q}p/\dot{Q}s = (Sao_2 - Smvo_2)/(Spvo_2 - Spao_2)$$
$$\dot{Q}p/\dot{Q}s > 1 \text{ left-to-right shunt}$$
$$\dot{Q}p/\dot{Q}s < 1 \text{ right-to-left shunt}$$

where $\dot{Q}p$ is pulmonary blood flow, $Smvo_2$ is mixed venous oxygen saturation, $\dot{Q}s$ is systemic blood flow, $Spvo_2$ is pulmonary venous oxygen saturation, Sao_2 is systemic arterial oxygen saturation, and $Spao_2$ is pulmonary artery oxygen saturation. Because we are calculating the ratio of flows, oxygen saturation can be used instead of oxygen content. To simplify the calculation, if systemic blood is fully saturated, one can approximate that there is no significant right-to-left shunting and that pulmonary venous oxygen saturation is equal to systemic oxygen saturation ($Spvo_2 = Sao_2$).

2. **The effect of left-to-right shunts** on the cardiovascular system includes ventricular volume overload and dysfunction, increased pulmonary blood flow and PA pressures, and the potential for permanent increases in PVR. The net effect on the pulmonary system is pulmonary edema, with associated decreases in compliance and ventilatory reserve. **Right-to-left shunting** can produce hypoxemia.

3. **Clinical presentation**

   a. **Cyanosis** due to CHD is caused by inadequate pulmonary blood flow. This may be caused by a simple shunt with right-to-left flow (e.g., VSD with Eisenmenger syndrome), a complex shunt with right-to-left flow (e.g., tetralogy of Fallot or tricuspid atresia), or balanced shunts complicated by inadequate pulmonary blood flow (e.g., single ventricle lesions or truncus arteriosus).

   b. **Congestive heart failure** (CHF) and/or hypotension may be caused by either left-to-right shunting with excessive pulmonary blood flow (e.g., atrial septal defect [ASD], VSD, or patent ductus arteriosus [PDA]) or LV outflow obstruction and pressure overload (e.g., congenital subvalvular, valvular, or great-vessel obstruction).

   c. **Balanced shunts** (e.g., truncus arteriosus or hypoplastic left heart syndrome) can cause a combination of cyanosis due to mixing and/or systemic hypotension from pulmonary overcirculation.

D. **Anesthetic management**

1. **Preoperative evaluation**

   a. The **history** should provide an assessment of the extent of cardiopulmonary impairment (e.g., presence of cyanosis or CHF, exercise tolerance, cyanotic spells, activity level, feeding and growth patterns, associated syndromes, and anatomic abnormalities).

   b. **Physical examination** should make note of skin color, activity level, respiratory pattern and frequency, and appropriateness of development for given age. The heart and lungs should be auscultated and close attention given to the patient's airway and IV access. Peripheral pulses should be palpated and blood pressure obtained in both arms and the lower extremities if coarctation is suspected.

   c. The **chest radiograph** is examined for evidence of increased heart size, presence of CHF, decreased pulmonary blood flow, abnormalities in heart position, and the presence of any thoracic cage abnormalities.

   d. The **ECG** may be normal even in the presence of CHD. However, abnormalities can be important clues to underlying cardiac lesions.

   e. **Echocardiography** will show anatomic abnormalities and, with Doppler, provide information about flow patterns and pressure gradients.

   f. **Cardiac catheterization** can define anatomy, pulmonary and systemic shunt flows, vascular resistances, and intracardiac chamber pressures.

2. **Premedication.** Infants younger than 6 months of age, cyanotic or dyspneic children, and patients who are critically ill generally receive no premedication. Older or more vigorous children may be given oral midazolam (0.5 to 1.0 mg/kg); oral ketamine (5 to 7 mg/kg) may be added for a deeper level of sedation. An alternative intramuscular regimen is ketamine (3 to 5 mg/kg) in combination with midazolam (0.5 to 1.0 mg) and glycopyrrolate (0.1 to 0.2 mg) given in the preanesthetic holding area. Dosages are reduced in cases in which decreasing SVR would increase right-to-left shunting. Fasting guidelines must be adjusted based on the patient's age and cardiac condition (see Chapters 1 and 29). Cyanotic infants are usually polycythemic and may be prone to vital organ thrombi if not hydrated with IV fluids preoperatively.

3. **Monitoring and equipment** (Table 23.5). In addition to the standard monitoring required for all patients, a precordial or esophageal stethoscope and three temperature probes (tympanic membrane, esophageal, and rectal) should be available. Intra-arterial pressure monitoring usually is necessary. (Note that previous surgical procedures [e.g., classic Blalock-Taussig shunt or coarctation repair] may influence the choice of site for radial artery cannulation.) Central venous catheters are inserted regularly for infusion of vasoactive drugs, CVP measurement, and volume administration; a 4-French double-lumen catheter can be used for infants weighing 10 kg or less and a 5-French, triple-lumen catheter can used for larger children. A warming/cooling blanket, radiant heating lamps, and a heated humidifier are useful perioperatively. TEE is an important diagnostic and perioperative management tool.

4. **Resuscitation drugs** and infusions of inotropic medications appropriate for pediatric use must be available. **Air bubbles** must be meticulously removed from IV lines and syringes. **Air filters** should be used whenever possible. Even in the absence of shunts, paradoxical air emboli may traverse a probe-patent foramen ovale.

5. **Induction.** The choice between an inhalation and IV induction is based primarily on ventricular function and the degree of patient cooperation. A slow, carefully titrated induction by either technique usually provides for a safe and stable anesthetic. Theoretically, patients with right-to-left shunts may have a slower rate of induction with volatile anesthetics, because blood is shunted past the lungs. Similarly, arterial concentrations of IV anesthetic may increase faster in patients with a significant right-to-left shunt. For the uncooperative child or a child surviving primarily on sympathetic stimulation, intramuscular ketamine (3 to 5 mg/kg) along with an antisialagogue such as

Table 23.5. Equipment and drug checklist for pediatric cardiac surgery

Equipment

Pediatric anesthesia machine with air tank (full) and extra oxygen tanks

Pediatric circle circuit (appropriate for children of all sizes) 500-mL, 1-L, 2-L, and 3-L breathing bags

Heated humidifier or in-line passive humidifier

Sevoflurane, and isoflurane vaporizers (full)

Full ECG and invasive hemodynamic monitoring display

Pediatric ECG leads

Appropriate pressure transducer and flush systems

Two noninvasive automatic blood pressure machines

Neonatal, infant, and pediatric blood pressure cuffs

Two pulse oximeters and probes (infant and pediatric sizes)

Appropriate size masks, airways, laryngoscope blade, ETT cuffed and uncuffed, adult and pediatric stylets, Magill forceps

Lidocaine/phenylephrine solution (for nasal ETT and nasogastric tube insertion)

Nasogastric tubes

Tympanic/esophageal temperature probe and monitor

Rectal/bladder temperature probe and monitor

Esophageal stethoscope with integral temperature probe

Hat

Padded head rest

Capnograph with agent analyzer

End-tidal capnograph connector

Precordial stethoscope and stickers (when appropriate)

Suction catheters

TEE machine

Pediatric and adult biplane or omniplane (if available) TEE probes

Drugs

Calcium gluconate (100 mg/mL)

Cisatracurium

Dopamine, dobutamine, epinephrine, milrinone, isoproterenol, nitroglycerin, and prostaglandin E_1 drips as needed

Epinephrine (1, 10, and 100 μg/mL concentration syringes)

Fentanyl (up to 100 μg/kg)

Ketamine (50 or 100 mg/mL concentration for PO, IM, or IV use)

Midazolam (1 or 5 mg/mL concentration for PO, IM, or IV use)

Morphine sulfate

Pancuronium

Phenylephrine (1, 10, and 100 μg/mL concentration syringes)

Sodium bicarbonate

Succinylcholine (4 mg/kg for emergent IM use)

Thiopental

ECG, electrocardiographic; ETT, endotracheal tubes; TEE, transesophageal echocardiography; IM, intramuscular; PO, oral.

atropine (0.02 mg/kg) or glycopyrrolate (0.01 mg/kg) may be used.

E. **Cardiopulmonary bypass**
1. **Pump prime volume** ranges between 150 and 1,200 mL. Packed red blood cells frequently are added to the prime to yield an initial hematocrit of circa 25% when on bypass. For smaller children, the red cells may be washed to remove potassium, lactic acid, and citrate-phosphate-dextrose-adenine preservative. Cells may be leukocyte-depleted to decrease patient exposure to cytomegalovirus. Typical constituents of pump prime include sodium bicarbonate (to counteract acidosis), mannitol (to promote diuresis), heparin, and calcium (to offset the effects of the citrate in blood). Albumin solutions and FFP may be added to the prime for neonates.
2. **Infants and children** generally lack vasoocclusive disease. Consequently, blood flow during CPB is more important than arterial pressure. Flows as high as 150 mL/kg/minute may be used in infants weighing less than 5 kg, while MAP as low as 30 mm Hg is well tolerated provided that SVC pressure is low (indicating that venous drainage is adequate).
3. **Deep hypothermic circulatory arrest** is used extensively for infants weighing less than 10 kg. Up to 1 hour of circulatory arrest is tolerated without neurologic injury at a core and brain temperature of 15°C to 20°C. Where appropriate, low-flow CPB may offer advantages over circulatory arrest. Management points include the following:
   a. Adequate brain hypothermia (e.g., packing the head with ice packs).
   b. Hemodilution.
   c. Acid-base balance.
   d. Muscle relaxation.
   e. Avoidance of increased blood glucose.

F. **Procedures not requiring CPB**
1. **Closed-heart cases** without the use of CPB include PDA ligation, coarctation repair, PA banding, and most shunts designed to increase pulmonary blood flow (e.g., modified Blalock-Taussig shunt).
2. **Open-heart cases** without CPB include those that can be accomplished through normothermic caval inflow obstruction, such as pulmonary valvotomy, aortic valvotomy, and creation of ASDs. Increasingly, these procedures can be accomplished with transvenous techniques in the catheterization laboratory.

G. **Management of specific CHD lesions** (Table 23.6).
1. **Lesions with decreased pulmonary blood flow (cyanotic lesions)** can occur via an anatomic obstruction to pulmonary blood flow and/or right-to-left shunting and include tetralogy of Fallot, tricuspid atresia, pulmonary atresia, and pulmonary hypertension.
   a. **Management goals** are to decrease PVR, increase pulmonary blood flow, maintain SVR, and maintain central volume.
   b. **Anesthetic maneuvers** include modest hypocarbia, increased inspired oxygen concentration, maintaining normal functional residual capacity, and avoiding acidosis.

Table 23.6. Specific congenital cardiac lesions

Lesion	Anatomy	Pathophysiology	Surgical Correction	Anesthetic Considerations
Atrial septal defect	Three varieties: 1. Ostium secundum: defect in septum (most common). 2. Ostium primum: endocardial cushion defect. 3. Sinus venosus: caval-atrial defect often with partial anomalous pulmonary venous return.	Left to right shunt. RV volume overload. Potential for right to left shunting (e.g., during valsalva maneuver) with paradoxical embolus risk. Minimal symptoms until later age, when CHF may develop.	Suture or patch closure. Percutaneous catheterization device closure.	Inhalation or intravenous induction. Potential extubation at end of procedure. Avoid air bubbles.

(continued)

Table 23.6. (*Continued*)

Lesion	Anatomy	Pathophysiology	Surgical Correction	Anesthetic Considerations
Ventricular septal defect	Supracristal, membranous canal, and muscular subtypes.	Left to right shunt. Increased pulmonary blood flow. Pulmonary hypertension and reversal of shunt as a late effect (Eisenmenger syndrome).	Dacron patch closure of singular or multiple defects. Muscular defects may be difficult to locate. Selected defects may be amenable to percutaneous catheterization device closure.	Hypocarbia and low F_{IO_2} to decrease pulmonary blood flow. Avoid myocardial depressants. Avoid air bubbles. Potential for postoperative AV block and pacing requirement. Potential need for post-repair inotropic support.
Coarctation of the aorta	Narrowing usually distal to origin of left subclavian artery. May be pre- or post-ductal in location. Often associated with a VSD.	Increased blood flow to upper extremities and head. Systemic hypoperfusion. Pressure overload of LV.	Left thoracotomy approach. Subclavian artery flap angioplasty or resection and end-to-end anastomosis.	Non-CPB case. Arterial line on right Suitable for regional anesthesia-supplementation. Potential for post-repair hypertension.

Patent ductus arteriosus	Patent ductus arteriosus.	Right to left shunt when PVR is high. Left to right shunt as PVR decreases. Necessary for survival with certain lesions (e.g., hypoplastic left heart syndrome).	Left thoracotomy vs thoracoscopic approach. Ligation and occasional division of PDA. Potential for percutaneous catheterization coil embolization.	Usually premature infants with concomitant pulmonary disease. Avoid high Fio_2 (risk of retrolental fibroplasia). Risk of recurrent laryngeal nerve damage.
Tetralogy of Fallot	1. VSD. 2. Pulmonary outflow tract obstruction. 3. RV hypertrophy. 4. Overriding aorta.	Right to left shunting through VSD into overriding aorta. Fixed (pulmonic stenosis) and dynamic (infundibular hypertrophy) RV outflow obstruction components. Systemic desaturation ("Tet" spell).	Patch closure of VSD. RV outflow tract reconstruction/augmentation. Excision of infundibular muscle band (when appropriate).	Management of "Tet spell": augment intravascular volume, minimize PVR (increase Fio_2, decrease $Paco_2$), increase SVR (knee-chest position, phenylephrine), consider negative inotropes (halothane, beta-blockade). Potential need for postoperative pacing.

(continued)

Table 23.6. *Continued*

Lesion	Anatomy	Pathophysiology	Surgical Correction	Anesthetic Considerations
Transposition of the great arteries	Transposition of both the aorta to the RV and the PA to the LV resulting in isolation of pulmonary and systemic circulations.	ASD, VSD, and/or PDA required for pulmonary and systemic blood mixing and, hence, survival.	Atrial switch procedure (Mustard, Senning): rarely performed. Arterial switch procedure (Jatene). When associated with a VSD and pulmonic stenosis, a Rastelli procedure (LV to aorta baffle closure via the VSD, and RV to PA allograft conduit).	Ductus/mixing lesion dependent CHD lesion. Prostaglandin E_1 to maintain ductus patency (when appropriate).
Truncus arteriosus	Single great artery that gives rise to the aorta, PA, and coronary arteries. Associated VSD.	Mixing of pulmonary and systemic blood. Most commonly presents with pulmonary overcirculation.	VSD closure. RV to PA valved conduit. Valvuloplasty of truncal valve.	Increase PVR/decrease pulmonary blood flow precorrection (based on degree of pulmonary overcirculation). Normalize PVR postcorrection. Potential need for inotropic support post-repair.

Lesion	Anatomy	Physiology	Surgical repair	Anesthetic considerations
Atrioventricular canal defect	Common AV valve. Deficiency of atrial and ventricular septae.	Mixing of blood at the atrial and ventricular level. Usually presents with pulmonary overcirculation.	Closure of ASD and VSD. Mitral/tricuspid valvuloplasty.	Manipulate PVR to balance/optimize pulmonary systemic blood flow. Anticipate need for inotropic support postrepair. Associated with Down syndrome (potential airway issues).
Hypoplastic left heart syndrome	Atretic/hypoplastic mitral valve, aortic valve, LV, and ascending aorta.	Left to right shunt (obligatory) at atrial or ventricular level for mixing. Ductus arteriosus dependent for right to left (i.e., systemic) perfusion.	Palliative, staged repair: 1. Norwood I: atrial septectomy, reconstruction of aortic arch, PA plasty, creation of systemic to pulmonary shunt.	Critically ill neonates. Preoperative (ICU) management will impact outcome. Prostaglandin E_1 to maintain ductal patency. Inotropes often necessary pre- and postrepair.

(continued)

Table 23.6. *Continued*

Lesion	Anatomy	Pathophysiology	Surgical Correction	Anesthetic Considerations
			2. Bidirectional Glenn: takedown of systemic to pulmonary shunt, creation of SVC to PA (cavopulmonary) shunt. **3.** Modified Fontan procedure: creation of an IVC to PA anastomosis via an intra-atrial baffle; creates total cavopulmonary continuity. Alternatively, cardiac transplantation is an option.	Avoid myocardial depressants. Fentanyl >50 μg/kg prior to sternotomy. Manipulate PVR via adjustments in Fio_2 and Pco_2 to balance/optimize pulmonary vs systemic perfusion. Target goal: MAP = 40, pH = 7.40, Pao_2 = 40, $Paco_2$ = 40.

ASD, atrial septal defect; AV, atrioventricular; CHD, congenital heart disease; CHF, congestive heart failure; CPB, cardiopulmonary bypass; Fio_2, fraction of inspired oxygen; ICU, intensive care unit; IVC, inferior vena cava; LV, left ventricle; MAP, mean arterial pressure; PA, pulmonary artery; Pao_2, partial pressure of oxygen; $Paco_2$, partial pressure of carbon dioxide; PDA, patent ductus arteriosus; PVR, pulmonary vascular resistance; RV, right ventricle; SVC, superior vena cava; SVR, systemic vascular resistance; VSD, ventricular septal defect.

    c. **For tetralogy of Fallot,** a negative inotrope (e.g., propranolol) may be used to relax dynamic infundibular stenosis and improve pulmonary blood flow. Adequate volume loading is critical in the management of a "tet spell." Prostaglandin E_1 (0.1 μg/kg/minute IV) may be helpful in supporting ductus arteriosus patency (when possible), decreasing PVR, and increasing pulmonary blood flow. A peripheral vasoconstrictor (e.g., phenylephrine) should be available.

2. **Lesions with increased pulmonary blood flow** and left-to-right shunting include ASD, VSD, and PDA.

    a. **Management goals** are to avoid myocardial depressants and excessive pulmonary blood flow.

    b. **Anesthetic maneuvers** include IV induction (e.g., opiates or ketamine), avoiding negative inotropes (e.g., inhalation agents or propofol), maintaining normocarbia to slight hypercarbia, limiting inspired oxygen concentration, and PEEP.

3. **Balanced shunts** have the potential for a ventricle's output to be directed to the pulmonary or systemic circulation and include hypoplastic left heart syndrome, truncus arteriosus, double-outlet RV, and complete AV canal defect. The direction of blood flow is governed by relative resistances (PVR/SVR ratio).

    a. Management goals are to manipulate pulmonary blood flow to maintain adequate systemic perfusion. Often both a low-normal blood pressure (i.e., MAP = 40 mm Hg) and a low Pao_2 (i.e., 40 mm Hg) must be tolerated.

    b. **Anesthetic maneuvers** depend on the balance of systemic versus pulmonary blood flow. These include the following:

      (1) (1) Normal to slightly elevated $Paco_2$, consideration of PEEP and limiting inspired oxygen concentration to increase PVR, decrease pulmonary blood flow, and favor systemic blood flow.

      (2) (2) Normal to slightly decreased $Paco_2$ and increased inspired oxygen concentration to decrease PVR and increase pulmonary relative to systemic blood flow.

H. Anesthesia for cardiac catheterization. The goal is to provide sufficient sedation to allow the procedure to be completed without excessive movement while avoiding sedative-induced hemodynamic changes and hypoventilation.

1. **An anesthesia machine** (fitted with compressed air as well as oxygen) and standard monitoring equipment, resuscitation drugs, airway management equipment, and a defibrillator (with appropriately sized paddles) must be present.

2. **Premedication** is similar to that mentioned in section IV.D.2. Patients generally are well sedated and maintain a good airway with a continuous infusion of ketamine (2 mg/kg/hour) and midazolam (0.1 mg/kg/hour) supplemented with additional boluses as needed. Alternatively, a low-dose propofol infusion (25 to 100 μg/kg/minute) may be used.

3. **General endotracheal anesthesia** may be used in children prone to airway obstruction (trisomy 21 or nasopharyngeal

defects) and in children with suprasystemic RV pressures where cyanosis from pulmonary hypertension may improve after anesthesia reduces sympathetic tone. IV techniques utilizing a combination of remifentanil (0.1 to 0.5 μg/kg/minute) and propofol (50 to 100 μg/kg/minute) for amnesia can provide a rapidly titratable anesthetic.

V. Mechanical support devices

A. The **IABP** provides circulatory assistance for the failing or ischemic heart. Inflation augments aortic diastolic pressure and drives blood toward the coronary ostia, thus augmenting coronary perfusion, particularly to the LV (which receives most of its blood supply in diastole). Deflation of the balloon reduces the impedance to LV ejection and so reduces myocardial oxygen consumption. **Preoperative indications** include unstable angina that is refractory to medical therapy; LV failure due to myocardial infarction, ruptured papillary muscle, or VSD; and prophylaxis for a high-risk patient with severe left main disease. **Postbypass indications** include refractory LV failure preventing successful termination of CPB and refractory ST-segment elevation.

1. The IABP is inserted through a femoral artery and advanced until the tip is 1 to 2 cm distal to the left subclavian artery in the descending thoracic aorta (positioning can be guided by TEE). It can be placed transthoracically if iliofemoral disease precludes use of a femoral artery.

2. **Inflation of the IABP** is synchronized with the patient's ECG, a pacemaker potential, or else the arterial blood pressure trace. Balloon inflation occurs early in diastole (at the dicrotic notch of the arterial pressure waveform). **Balloon deflation** occurs during isovolumic contraction. Intraoperative triggering directly from a pacemaker generator will eliminate interference otherwise caused by electrocautery or blood sampling.

3. **Relative contraindications** include severe AI, aortic aneurysm, and severe peripheral vascular disease.

4. **Complications** of IABPs include distal embolization, aortic dissection or rupture, and lower extremity ischemia.

B. Ventricular assist devices (VAD) may be classified as either extracorporeal or implantable. Although both types of devices require cannulation of the heart, extracorporeal devices employ a pump that is positioned outside of the patient.

1. **Extracorporeal devices** (e.g., ABIOMED BVS 5000 and Thoratec VAD).

   a. Indications include postcardiotomy support, cardiogenic shock, and bridge to transplant.

   b. These devices can provide biventricular support. Inflow cannulation sites include the LV or LA for left-sided support and the RV or right atrium for right-sided support. Corresponding outflow cannulas are inserted into the ascending aorta and main pulmonary artery. The cannulas (inflow and outflow) are connected to an external pump. Surgical time and dissection are significantly less with these than with implanted devices.

   c. Both the ABIOMED BVS 5000 and the Thoratec VAD utilize pneumatically driven pumping sacs. Whereas the ABIOMED BVS 5000 depends on gravity for venous drainage, the Thoratec VAD is equipped with vacuum-assisted drainage. The primary difference between the two devices is patient mobility. Patients with the ABIOMED BVS 5000 must lie supine; patients with the Thoratec may ambulate.

2. **Implantable devices** (e.g., Novacor V-E, HeartMate V-E, HeartMate Pneumatic, and Heartmate II).

   a. These devices are typically used for patients who have cardiogenic shock and are candidates for transplantation.

   b. These devices are designed for LV support only. They consist of an inflow cannula (inserted into the LV apex), a pump, and an outflow cannula (inserted into the ascending aorta). A drive line that is tunneled through the skin connects the implanted pump to the external console. CPB is always necessary.

   c. The Novacor V-E, HeartMate V-E, and Heartmate II devices are electrically driven; the rechargeable power source fits into a backpack or holsters and allows the patient to leave the hospital. The Heartmate II is 60% smaller than the Heartmate V-E, making it appropriate for use in a wider range of patients. Because of its axial flow characteristics, it provides a significantly reduced degree of pulsatile arterial perfusion.

3. **Anesthetic considerations**

   a. Patients will have **marginal cardiac function;** extreme care is required during induction to minimize decreases in contractility and preload.

   b. **Bleeding** can be problematic, especially with the implanted devices. Establish adequate IV access for volume administration and consider using an antifibrinolytic drug.

   c. If the patient is receiving the device as a bridge to transplant, transfuse with leukocyte-depleted cellular blood products to minimize HLA-antigen exposure.

   d. **TEE is required.** Determine the degree of AI (if significant, a tissue valve may need to be inserted), the degree of tricuspid regurgitation, the presence of a patent foramen ovale, the presence of an ASD or VSD, the degree of right heart dysfunction (the patient may require mechanical RV support), and the presence of thrombus. Postoperative TEE examination is used to assess whether the inflow cannula is properly inserted (look for the absence of turbulent flow) and ensure that any air is removed from the heart.

   e. Patients receiving an LVAD frequently require RV support. Inotropes, nitric oxide, and occasionally an RVAD are required.

   f. Most devices function best in the automatic mode after chest closure. The flow will then depend largely on venous return. Decreased venous return will be signaled by a decreased pumping rate because the devices will pump only when adequately filled. Volume administration or a pressor agent should be given.

VI. **Other cardiac procedures**

A. **Off-bypass CABG** is performed to avoid the complications associated with CPB and to minimize aortic manipulation. Proximal grafts are performed using either a partial aortic cross-clamp technique or a specifically designed proximal anastamosis device that precludes aortic clamping. Distal grafts are performed using one of several heart stabilizing devices. Considerations for this procedure include the following:

1. **Temperature management.** Warm the room and consider using a patient warming system (e.g., hydrogel energy conduction pads or a convective forced-air warming blanket).

2. Patients can be **extubated early** after the surgery, so the anesthetic should be tailored to allow early extubation (e.g., fentanyl 5 to 10 μg/kg, volatile anesthetic, then propofol infusion).

3. **Heparin** 350 IU/kg IV is given, and the ACT is maintained above 400 seconds. This allows the patient to emergently go on CPB if necessary. Antifibrinolytic therapy is avoided. A small dose of protamine (50 to 100 mg) is given after the procedure.

4. Drugs that might provide beneficial ischemic preconditioning to the myocardium include nitroglycerin, morphine (0.25 to 0.50 mg/kg), and isoflurane (0.5% to 1.0%). Hyperglycemia (>300 mg/dL) is avoided because it inhibits ischemic preconditioning.

5. **Monitoring the ECG** is difficult because the heart is placed in nonanatomical positions. Nonetheless, it is important to establish a baseline ECG (for each position) and to monitor the ST-segments.

6. **Hemodynamic instability** is common, particularly when the surgeon is performing the distal anastomoses. Grafts to vessels that have lesser disease tend to be associated with more instability than those to vessels that are occluded. Medical support for the ischemic heart during the distal anastamosis includes increasing the perfusion pressure to provide adequate coronary flow to the remainder of the coronary arterial system. Occasionally, repositioning of the heart is required to permit augmented right-sided filling when hemodynamic instability is due to obstruction of right heart inflow. Coronary shunting is indicated when hemodynamically intolerable ischemia results during creation of the distal anastamosis.

7. **IV volume requirements** tend to be high. A full heart tends to tolerate the positioning better. A diuretic may be required at the end of the operation.

8. **Patented immobilizers** are used to stabilize the heart; they virtually eliminate the need for drug-induced heart rate slowing.

9. **Dysrhythmias** may be a problem. Lidocaine, amiodarone, and magnesium (0.5 g/hour) infusions are frequently used. Potassium is maintained above 4.0 mEq/L.

B. **"Redo" cardiac surgery**

1. **Mediastinal structures,** including the heart, major vessels, vascular grafts, or lungs may be adherent to the underside of the sternum and can be lacerated during sternotomy. Blood must be in the OR and checked before sternotomy. An extra 14-gauge IV catheter or a rapid infusion catheter should be placed to facilitate volume resuscitation. Because the patient may need to go on CPB emergently, heparin must be in a syringe ready to administer immediately. In emergency situations, venous return may be supplied from the pump suction line on the field ("sucker bypass").

2. Line insertion may be difficult at sites previously used for catheters.

3. Insertion of a PA line equipped with pacing capability is prudent because emergent epicardial pacing may not be possible during chest opening. Transcutaneous defibrillation pads should be applied to the lateral aspects of the patient's chest because the surgeon will not be able to use internal paddles before the heart is exposed.

4. **Diffuse bleeding** from extensive dissection of scar tissue may occur after CPB. Use of an antifibrinolytic drug is encouraged. Ascertain whether the patient has received aprotinin in the past, because reexposure is associated with an increased risk of anaphylaxis. Aprotinin should not be administered at any dose until the aorta, or femoral artery, has been prepared for bypass cannulation in order to avoid the potentially fatal complications of an anaphylactic reaction.

5. **Careful ECG monitoring** is imperative because manipulation of atheromatous grafts may send emboli to the coronary circulation. Because myocardial protection is more challenging in patients with previous coronary grafts, postbypass myocardial dysfunction is more likely.

C. **Cardiac tamponade and constrictive pericarditis**

1. The **major goals** are to avoid decreases in myocardial contractility, peripheral vascular resistance, and heart rate. **Pericardiocentesis** may be advisable before induction in patients with tamponade (unless associated with an aortic dissection).

2. **"Lines"** should include an arterial line, a large-bore IV catheter, and preferably a PA line (if the patient can tolerate its insertion).

3. Useful **induction agents** include etomidate and ketamine. A dopamine infusion during induction and the skin-prepping phase is helpful.

4. A method for **backup atrial pacing** (transesophageal or transvenous) should be available.

5. **In severe cases,** consider an awake intubation and/or having the patient surgically "prepped and draped" before induction.

D. **Cardiac transplantation**

1. **Management of the donor** (see Chapter 20).

2. **Anesthetic management of the recipient**

   a. **The key to patient survival** is minimizing the time that the donor heart is ischemic. Consequently, expeditious preparation of the recipient and good communication with the surgeons is essential.

   b. **Preoperative evaluation** of the recipient should determine whether the patient had previous chest surgery (more time required), whether the patient has elevated PVR, and whether the patient is coagulopathic.

   c. **Invasive monitoring** should include an arterial line and a triple-lumen central venous catheter; a PA catheter is used when the patient has severe increases in PVR. **Aseptic technique** is critical because the patient will be immunocompromised after the surgery.

   d. **Precautions for a full stomach** may be necessary during induction. Etomidate and fentanyl are good choices to provide hypnosis and analgesia, respectively. If the patient is receiving inotropic infusions, consider increasing their doses before induction. If a VAD is present, venous return must be maintained for the pump to maintain its flow rate.

e. **Right heart failure and coagulopathy** are common problems during the rewarming phase of bypass. Transfusion requirements should be anticipated; cellular blood products should be leukocyte-depleted to minimize foreign HLA-antigen exposure.

f. When weaning from CPB, the donor heart will be unresponsive to interventions mediated by the recipient's nonhumoral autonomic nervous system. The optimal heart rate is between 80 and 110 beats per minute. This is accomplished with epicardial pacing, or a dopamine infusion is used to achieve this pharmacologically.

g. **Immunosuppressants** will be necessary and are administered in consultation with the surgeon and transplant cardiologist.

E. **Circulatory arrest** may be necessary for surgery on the distal ascending aorta or aortic arch (for an aneurysm or aortic dissection). Management issues include the following:

1. Systemic cooling to 18°C and application of ice around the head.

2. Supplemental administration of drugs such as pentothal, magnesium, ketamine, methylprednisolone, mannitol, and additional heparin before circulatory arrest.

3. Trendelenburg (head down) position.

4. Retrograde cerebral perfusion (with arterialized blood) through the SVC cannula with pressure monitoring through the sidearm of the PA-line introducer (pressure maintained at 25 mm Hg, and blood flow at 300 to 600 mL/minute).

F. **Antidysrhythmia surgery** may involve aneurysmectomy (with or without electrophysiologic mapping), cryoablation, endocardial resection, or implantation of an ICD system.

1. **Aneurysmectomy.** It is crucial to prevent hyperdynamic responses; stress on the ventricular suture line is life threatening. Large resections may compromise ventricular stroke volume. Thus, patients may be rendered highly rate dependent to achieve adequate cardiac output.

2. **ICD surgery.** Modern ICDs consist of an endocardial lead system and a pectoral pulse generator. Older systems used epicardial lead systems and abdominal generators. Recently, the proven benefits of cardiac resynchronization therapy have resulted in increased intraoperative placement of epicardial leads for combination biventricular pacemaker-ICD devices.

a. Most devices are now placed under local anesthesia in the electrophysiology laboratory. A brief period of general anesthesia is necessary for testing of the device once it is implanted; **IV propofol** and spontaneous ventilation with airway support are suitable. Patients with severe reflux, a difficult airway, or agitation may need endotracheal intubation. Standard monitoring is used. Intubation equipment, a bag and mask, emergency drugs, oxygen, suction, and a defibrillator must be present.

b. Patients sometimes go to the OR for epicardial electrode placement. These patients are often hemodynamically compromised; it is helpful to have a large-bore IV catheter, an arterial line, and a line for vasoactive medications (either a separate IV or a central line). Emergency drugs, including epinephrine, must be immediately available.

VII. **Anesthesia for cardioversion and electrophysiology procedures**

A. **Cardioversion.** The patient will usually fall into one of three categories:

1. **Hemodynamically stable and fasting.** After careful airway assessment, propofol (or etomidate) can be given in small doses until the patient loses consciousness. A prolonged drug delivery time should be anticipated. Phenylephrine or ephedrine, succinylcholine, airway equipment, and suction should be immediately available.

2. **Hemodynamically stable and a full stomach.** The patient and cardiologist are given two choices: rapid sequence induction with general endotracheal anesthesia or waiting until the patient has been fasting for 6 to 8 hours. Usually, the decision is made to wait the necessary time for gastric emptying to occur.

3. **Hemodynamically unstable.** The patient should be cardioverted as soon as possible, and administration of general anesthesia may be risky. Provision of sedation and an amnestic should be considered for conscious patients.

B. **Noninvasive programmed stimulation** is used to test the function of an ICD after it has been implanted. An ICD programmer is used to induce the irregular rhythm (ventricular fibrillation or tachycardia). The device then is checked for proper sensing and dysrhythmia termination. Because this is an elective situation, the patient should be fasting, and propofol anesthesia is used as described in section VI.F.2.a.

SUGGESTED READING

Diaz LK, Andropoulos DB. New developments in pediatric cardiac anesthesia. *Anesthesiol Clin North Am* 2005;23(4):655–676.

El-Marghabel I. Ventricular assist devices and anesthesia. *Semin Cardiothorac Vasc Anesth* 2005;9(3):241–249.

Gravlee GP, Davis RF, Kurusz M, Utley JR. *Cardiopulmonary bypass,* 2nd ed. Philadelphia: Lippincott Williams & Wilkins, 2000.

Hensley FA, Martin DE, Gravlee GP. *A practical approach to cardiac anesthesia,* 3rd ed. Philadelphia: Lippincott Williams & Wilkins, 2002.

Karl TR. Neonatal cardiac surgery. Anatomic, physiologic, and technical considerations. *Clin Perinatol* 2001;28(1):159–185.

Konstadt S, Shernan S, Oka Y. *Clinical transesophageal echocardiography: a problem-oriented approach.* 2nd ed. Philadelphia: Lippincott Williams & Wilkins, 2003.

Murkin JM. Perioperative multimodality neuromonitoring: an overview. *Semin Cardiothorac Vasc Anesth* 2004;8(2):167–171.

Myles PS, McIlroy D. Fast-track cardiac anesthesia: choice of anesthetic agents and techniques. *Semin Cardiothorac Vasc Anesth* 2005;9(1):5–16.

Reul H, Akdis M. Temporary or permanent support and replacement of cardiac function. *Expert Rev Med Devices* 2004;1(2):215–227.

Riess FC. Anticoagulation management and cardiac surgery in patients with heparin-induced thrombocytopenia. *Semin Thorac Cardiovasc Surg* 2005;17(1):85–96.

Serna DL, Thourani VH, Puskas JD. Antifibrinolytic agents in cardiac surgery: current controversies. *Semin Thorac Cardiovasc Surg* 2005;17(1):52–58.

Speiss BD. *Perioperative transfusion medicine,* 2nd ed. Philadelphia: Lippincott Williams & Wilkins, 2005.

Thys D. *Textbook of cardiothoracic anesthesiology.* New York: McGraw-Hill, 2001.

Warkentin TE, Koster A. Bivalirudin: a review. *Expert Opin Pharmacother* 2005; 6(8):1349–1371.

Woo YJ. Cardiac surgery in patients on antiplatelet and antithrombotic agents. *Semin Thorac Cardiovasc Surg* 2005;17(1):66–72.

Anesthesia for Neurosurgery

George A. Mashour and Michele Szabo

I. **Physiology**
   A. **Cerebral blood flow** (CBF) is equal to cerebral perfusion pressure divided by the cerebral vascular resistance. **Cerebral perfusion pressure is defined as the difference between mean arterial pressure (MAP) and intracranial pressure (ICP) or central venous pressure, whichever is higher.** CBF averages 50 mL/100 g of brain tissue per min in the normal brain and is affected by blood pressure, metabolic demands, $Paco_2$, Pao_2, blood viscosity, and neurogenic regulation.

   1. **CBF** is maintained at a constant level by constriction and dilation of arterioles (autoregulation) (Fig. 24.1) when the MAP is between 50 and 150 mm Hg. When MAP is outside these limits, CBF varies directly with MAP. Chronic hypertension shifts the autoregulatory curve to the right, rendering hypertensive patients susceptible to cerebral ischemia at blood pressures considered normal in healthy individuals. Chronic antihypertensive therapy may normalize the autoregulatory range. Cerebral ischemia, trauma, hypoxia, hypercarbia, edema, mass effect, and volatile anesthetics attenuate or abolish autoregulation and may make blood flow to the affected area dependent on MAP.

   2. **$Paco_2$** has profound effects on CBF by its effect on the pH of brain extracellular fluid (ECF). CBF increases linearly with increasing $Paco_2$ in the range from 20 to 80 mm Hg, with an absolute change of 1 to 2 mL/100 g per minute for each mm Hg change in $Paco_2$. The effect of $Paco_2$ on CBF decreases over 6 to 24 hours because of slow adaptive changes in brain ECF bicarbonate concentration. Sustained hyperventilation causes cerebrospinal fluid (CSF) bicarbonate production to decrease, allowing CSF pH to gradually normalize. Rapid normalization of $Paco_2$ after a period of hyperventilation results in a significant CSF acidosis with vasodilation and increased ICP.

   3. **Pao_2.** Hypoxia is a potent cerebral vasodilator; CBF increases markedly below a Pao_2 of 60 mm Hg. Pao_2 in the range of 60 to >300 mm Hg has little influence on CBF.

   4. **Neurogenic regulation.** The role of the extensive sympathetic/parasympathetic innervation of the cerebral vasculature is not well established. It is likely that increased sympathetic tone in hemorrhagic shock shifts the autoregulatory curve to the right and results in lower CBF at a given MAP.

   5. **Viscosity.** Normal hematocrit (33% to 45%) in a normal brain has little influence on CBF. In the setting of focal cerebral ischemia, reduction in viscosity by hemodilution (hematocrit 30% to 34%) may increase CBF to ischemic territories.

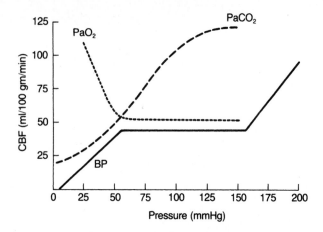

Figure 24.1. Autoregulation maintains a constant level of cerebral blood flow (CBF) over a wide range of carotid artery mean blood pressures. Independent of this effect, CBF is elevated by hypercarbia (PaCO₂) and hypoxemia (PaO₂); hypocarbia diminishes CBF.

B. **Cerebral metabolic rate** ($CMRO_2$) and CBF are coupled, because the brain requires a constant supply of substrate to meet its relatively high metabolic demands. Regional or global increases in $CMRO_2$ elicit a corresponding increase in CBF, probably mediated by signaling molecules such as nitric oxide. Other factors that modulate $CMRO_2$ (and CBF through this mechanism) include the following:

   1. **Anesthetics** (see sections II.A and B).
   2. **Temperature.** Hypothermia decreases $CMRO_2$ 7% per 1°C, and hyperthermia increases it.
   3. **Seizures**
   4. **Pain or arousal**

C. **ICP** reflects the relationship between the volume of the intracranial contents (brain, blood, and CSF) and the volume of the cranial vault. **Normal ICP is 5 to 15 mm Hg.** A sustained elevation of ICP >15 to 20 mmHg in the setting of intracranial pathology is considered abnormal.

   1. **The cranial vault is rigid,** and its capacity to accommodate increases in intracranial volume is limited. A developing intracranial mass (e.g., tumor, edema, hematoma, or hydrocephalus) initially displaces one or more of the intracranial components and ICP remains relatively normal (Fig. 24.2). As intracranial volume increases further, intracranial compliance decreases and ICP rises rapidly (see Figure 24.2). Thus, patients with decreased compliance may develop marked increases in ICP even with small increases in intracranial volume (i.e., cerebral vasodilation due to anesthesia, hypertension, or carbon dioxide retention) (see Fig. 24.2).
   2. **Clinical features of elevated ICP.** ICP elevation usually decreases cerebral perfusion pressure and may cause ischemia in regions of the brain where autoregulation is defective and

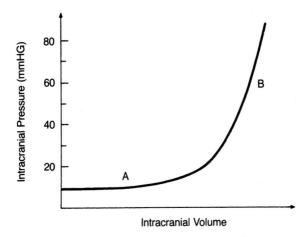

Figure 24.2. The intracranial compliance curve. In the normal intracranial pressure (ICP) range (*A*), increases in intracranial volume produce minimal changes in ICP. Further small increases in ICP after the "elbow" of the curve can produce abrupt increases in ICP (*B*).

CBF depends on cerebral perfusion pressure. Early signs and symptoms of increased ICP include headache, nausea, vomiting, blurred vision, papilledema, and decreased levels of consciousness. As ICP continues to increase, distortion and ischemia of the brainstem and/or brain herniation may occur. This may result in hypertension with bradydysrhythmia or tachydysrhythmia, irregular respiration, oculomotor (third cranial) nerve palsy leading to ipsilateral pupillary dilation with no light reflex, abducens (sixth cranial) nerve palsy, contralateral hemiparesis or hemiplegia, and ultimately coma and respiratory arrest.

3. **Treatment of elevated ICP** involves strategies aimed at decreasing the volume of the intracranial components:

   a. **Hypoxia and hypercarbia cause cerebral vasodilation** and should be avoided. Hyperventilation to a $Paco_2$ of 25 to 30 mm Hg produces cerebral vasoconstriction and is useful as a temporizing measure in the management of acutely increased ICP. However, hyperventilation is potentially deleterious and can cause ischemia in injured brain where CBF is low and should be withdrawn when effective definite therapy is established.

   b. **Decrease jugular venous pressure.** Elevating the head at least 30° promotes venous drainage and decreases intracranial venous blood volume. Avoid excessive flexion or rotation of the neck and prevent increases in intrathoracic pressure (e.g., coughing, straining, and elevated intrathoracic pressure). Positive end-expiratory pressure should be minimized to the lowest level that provides adequate lung recruitment.

    c. **Control CMOR$_2$.** Barbiturates are potent vasoconstrictors that decrease cerebral blood volume while decreasing CMRO$_2$. Prevent increases in CMOR$_2$ due to arousal/seizures with adequate sedation and seizure prophylaxis where indicated.

    d. **Maintaining high serum osmolality** (305 to 320 mOsm/kg) may reduce cerebral edema and decrease brain volume. Fluid management is designed to achieve this goal (see section V.D). In addition, **mannitol** (0.5 to 2.0 g/kg intravenous [IV]) and **furosemide** produce a hyperosmolar state and are effective in the acute reduction of ICP. Hypertonic saline is becoming an alternative to mannitol for managing raised ICP.

    e. **CSF volume can be reduced by** draining CSF through ventriculostomy catheter or needle aspiration intraoperatively.

    f. Surgical removal of tumor, hematoma, or decompressive craniectomy reduces intracranial volume and ICP.

II. Pharmacology. Agents used in anesthesia may affect CMRO$_2$ and CBF.

    A. **Inhalation anesthetics** produce a dose-related reduction in CMRO$_2$ while causing an increase in CBF.

        1. The effect of **nitrous oxide** can cause increases in CMRO$_2$, CBF, and ICP. This effect can be greatly attenuated or abolished when it is administered in conjunction with IV anesthetic agents. Nitrous oxide should be avoided when intracranial airspaces (e.g., pneumocephalus) exist, because it diffuses more rapidly into such spaces than nitrogen diffuses out and may produce an acute increase in ICP.

        2. Volatile agents cause increases in CBF due to their direct vasodilatory actions. Autoregulation can be attenuated or abolished by increasing the concentrations of these drugs, but responsiveness to carbon dioxide seems to be preserved (Table 24.1). The vasodilatory effect of inhalational agents

Table 24.1. Cerebral physiologic effects of inhalational anesthetics

	Nitrous Oxide	Desflurane	Sevoflurane	Isoflurane
Cerebral Blood Flow	⇑	⇑⇑	⇑	⇑⇑
Cerebral Perfusion Pressure	⇓	⇓⇓	⇓	⇓⇓
Intracranial Pressure	⇔/⇑	⇔/⇑	⇔/⇑	⇔/⇑
Metabolic Demands	⇑	⇓	⇓	⇓
CO$_2$ Reactivity	⇔	⇔	⇔	⇔
Seizure Threshold	⇓	⇓	⇓	⇓

is clinically insignificant in patients with normal intracranial compliance. These agents should be used with caution in patients with compromised intracranial compliance (e.g. large intracranial mass lesion, acute intracranial hematoma).

3. Volatile anesthetics produce dose-dependent reductions in metabolism ($CMRO_2$), probably by depressing neuronal electrical activity. Isoflurane is the most potent in this respect and is the only volatile agent that induces an isoelectric electroencephalogram (EEG) at clinically relevant concentrations (2 × MAC).

B. Most **IV anesthetics** (e.g., barbiturates, benzodiazepines, opioids, etomidate, propofol, and dexmetetomidine) cause coupled reduction in CBF and $CMRO_2$ in a dose-dependent manner. This is due to depression of cerebral metabolism. **Barbiturates, etomidate,** and **propofol** markedly decrease CBF and $CMRO_2$ and can produce isoelectric EEGs. Etomidate has been associated with seizures and is best avoided in seizure-prone patients. **Ketamine** increases CBF and $CMRO_2$ and is used infrequently in neuroanesthesia. **Opioids** produce minimal changes in CBF and $CMRO_2$. **Lidocaine** in therapeutic doses decreases both CBF and $CMRO_2$. Autoregulation and carbon dioxide responsiveness appear to be preserved with IV agents.

C. **Muscle relaxants** have no direct effect on CBF and $CMRO_2$. They may alter cerebral hemodynamics indirectly through their effects on blood pressure. **Succinylcholine** produces a transient increase in ICP, likely caused by arousal phenomena, which can be attenuated by prior administration of a barbiturate or a defasciculating dose of a nondepolarizing muscle relaxant.

D. **Vasoactive drugs**

1. **Adrenergic agonists.** α-Adrenergic agonists and low-dose β-adrenergic agonists have little influence on CBF. Larger doses of β-adrenergic agonists can produce an increase in $CMRO_2$ and CBF that can be exaggerated in the setting of a defect in the blood–brain barrier. Dopamine causes an increase in CBF with little change in $CMRO_2$.

2. **Vasodilators.** Sodium nitroprusside, nitroglycerin, hydralazine, nimodipine, and nicardipine can increase CBF and ICP by direct cerebral vasodilation if arterial blood pressure is maintained. β-Adrenergic blocking agents probably have minimal effects. Despite these profiles, all these agents have been used safely during neuroanesthesia, particularly if cerebral perfusion pressure is maintained.

E. **Cerebral protection**

1. **Focal versus global cerebral ischemia:**

   a. **Focal,** characterized by densely ischemic tissue in the center of an arterial occlusion, the presence of surrounding nonischemic brain, and possible collateral flow to the penumbral margins, which may allow neurons to survive for varied periods of time (e.g., thrombolysis within 3 hours after stroke onset may prevent a full infarct due to reperfusion).

   b. **Complete global,** characterized by absent CBF (e.g., cardiac arrest). Tolerance for surviving global ischemia is on the order of minutes.

2. **Agents**
   a. **IV anesthetic agents:** High-dose **barbiturates** may slightly improve neurologic recovery from focal ischemia, possibly by decreasing metabolic rate or more likely by a direct pharmacologic effect. The protective benefit may likely be achieved with an induction dose of barbiturate (thiopental 3 to 7 mg/kg IV). **Propofol** may also reduce focal ischemic cerebral injury, although it is not as extensively studied as the barbiturates. Etomidate aggravates ischemic brain injury. Early clinical reports suggest that prophylactic low-dose **lidocaine** may have neruoprotective effects in nondiabetic patients.
   b. The neuroprotective effects of **volatile anesthetic agents** are equivocal, although they appear to provide protection relative to the unanesthetized state. It is unclear whether this neuroprotection is sustained.
   c. **Nimodipine's** beneficial effects on vasospasm after subarachnoid hemorrhage (SAH) are well established and are likely mediated through neuronal, rather than vascular, effects. Clinical trials failed to detect a beneficial effect for acute stroke patients.
   d. **Steroids** have not been found to be beneficial after stroke or severe head injury.
   e. **Magnesium** confers significant neuroprotection in animal studies. However, a large clinical trial did not show protection in acute stroke victims.
   f. **Hypothermia,** which can reduce metabolism for both neuronal and cellular functions, is the established protective technique for circulatory arrest procedures. In the laboratory, mild hypothermia (a 2°C to 4°C reduction) can confer significant cerebral protection during focal ischemia while minimizing associated risks. Induced mild hypothermia (12 to 24 hours) has been shown to be effective in reducing morbidity in patients who sustain cardiac arrest. In contrast, two clinical studies did not demonstrate improved outcome when induced mild hypothermia was used in patients after significant head injury or intraoperatively for aneurysm surgery.
   g. **Hyperthermia** profoundly worsens outcome from focal cerebral ischemia and should be avoided.
   h. Moderate **hyperglycemia** (>170 mg/dL) exacerbates neurologic injury after an ischemic insult. Experimentally, correction with insulin reduces ischemic brain damage. Confirmatory clinical trials are lacking.
   i. **Other physiologic variables:** In addition to the abovementioned variables of temperature and glucose, meticulous management of perfusion pressure, pCO_2, pO_2, pH normalization, and seizure prophylaxis contribute significantly to improved neurologic outcome in the setting of cerebral ischemia. Maintenance of a high normal cerebral perfusion pressure (CPP) can augment collateral CBF. In contrast, hypotension reduces CBF and exacerbates the injury. Normocapnia should be maintained. Seizures, which can increase CBF and ICP and decrease CPP, should be prevented and rapidly treated.

III. Electrophysiologic monitoring

A. **Electroencephalography** measures electrical activity of the neurons of the cerebral cortex and is thus used as a threshold marker for detecting ischemia due to inadequate CBF. It is used frequently during procedures that jeopardize cerebral perfusion, such as carotid endarterectomy, or to ensure electrical silence before circulatory arrest.

1. Normal CBF in gray and white matter averages 50 mL/100 g/minute. With most anesthetic techniques, the EEG starts to become abnormal when the CBF decreases to 20 mL/100 g/minute. Isoflurane is distinct as the EEG becomes abnormal when CBF is much lower at 8 to 10 mL/100 g/minute. Cellular survival is endangered when CBF decreases to 12 mL/100 g/minute (lower with isoflurane). Thus, EEG changes can warn of ischemia before CBF becomes insufficient to maintain tissue viability. Prompt detection of EEG changes may be treated with increases in perfusion pressure or shunting to restore CBF to prevent infarction.

2. The EEG may exhibit changes intraoperatively with no demonstrable neurologic deficit during postoperative examination. Cerebral ischemia can produce electrical dysfunction without causing neuronal cell damage because the blood flow threshold for electrical failure is higher than that needed to maintain cellular integrity.

3. Factors other than anesthetics that may affect the EEG include hypothermia (which may limit the usefulness of EEG during cardiopulmonary bypass), hypotension, hypoglycemia, hypoxia, tumors, vascular abnormalities, and epilepsy. An abnormal EEG in patients with preexisting neurologic deficits, strokes in evolution, and recent reversible ischemic neurologic deficits can also make it difficult to interpret new changes.

4. **Anesthetic effects on the EEG** are generally global, which often helps distinguish them from the focal changes of ischemia. A predominance of slow activity is seen as the anesthetic depth increases. "Deep" anesthesia may cause marked EEG slowing, making detection of superimposed ischemic changes during critical periods difficult to interpret. Maintaining a constant level of anesthesia during critical periods (e.g., carotid clamping) facilitates EEG interpretation.

B. **Evoked potential monitoring**

1. **Sensory-evoked potentials** (EPs) are electrical potentials generated within the neuraxis in response to stimulation of a peripheral or cranial nerve. As they travel from the periphery to the brain, these potentials can be recorded by electrodes placed over the scalp and along the transmission pathway. EPs have lower voltage than background EEG activity, but summation of hundreds of signals using computerized devices makes it possible to extract them by averaging out the random background EEG. A normal response implies that the conduction pathway is intact. **Damage to the pathway generally decreases the amplitude or prolongs latency** (i.e., the time from peripheral stimulus to arrival of potentials at the recording site) of the waveform peaks. EPs are classified according to the nerve tract being evaluated.

a. **Somatosensory-evoked potentials (SSEPs)** are obtained by stimulating a peripheral nerve (e.g., median nerve at the wrist or posterior tibial nerve at the ankle or in the popliteal fossa) and recording the elicited signals over the spinal cord (spinal SSEPs) or cerebral cortex (cortical SSEPs). SSEPs are used most commonly to monitor spinal cord function during spinal cord or vertebral column surgery (e.g., major spine surgery with instrumentation) and may be used during peripheral nerve, brachial plexus, or thoracic aortic surgery (to detect spinal ischemia during aortic cross-clamping). Because SSEPs are conducted primarily by the dorsal column in the spinal cord, there are concerns about the reliability of SSEP monitoring for detecting threatened motor function (i.e., anterior spinal cord ischemia). For this reason, the "wake-up test" is used in some centers (see section VII.A.2), as well as motor-evoked potential (MEP) monitoring.

b. **Brainstem–auditory-evoked potentials (BAEPs)** are recorded by delivering an auditory stimulus to one ear through an ear-insert headphone. BAEPs reflect the transmission of electrical impulses along the auditory pathway and are monitored during posterior fossa surgery in an attempt to avoid brainstem or auditory (eighth cranial) nerve damage.

2. **Motor-evoked potentials.** Monitoring the integrity of the motor tracts within the spinal cord may be more reliable than SSEP monitoring during spinal surgery. The ventral motor columns of the spinal cord may be more susceptible to ischemia than the posterior proprioceptive fibers. Motor impulses can be generated by transcranial electrical stimulation. The evoked responses are measured as a potential over the spinal cord below the surgical field and in the muscle of interest. Anesthetics substantially modify transcranially induced potentials, but less so if the stimulus is measured in the spinal cord below the surgical field.

3. **Electromyography** (EMG) records muscle responses to stimulation of motor nerves. EMG is used frequently when there is risk of facial nerve injury during cerebellopontine angle surgery (e.g., posterior fossa surgery for meningioma). Because the EMG records motor responses to stimulation, neuromuscular blocking agents are avoided during the periods of electrical stimulation.

4. **Confounding factors.** Interpretation of EP changes is confounded by factors similar to those that affect the EEG (e.g., anesthetics, temperature, hypotension, hypoxia, anemia, preexisting neurologic lesions). Volatile anesthetics can depress SSEPs by reducing the amplitude or prolonging the latency of the SSEPs and can abolish the far more sensitive MEPs. BAEPs appear to be more resistant to the depressive effects of anesthetics than cortical SSEPs. IV anesthetics have less of an effect; barbiturates, propofol, and fentanyl/or remifentanil are compatible with effective monitoring of cortical SSEPs, BAEPs, and MEPs.

5. **False positives.** Changes in EPs occur frequently and often are not associated with postoperative neurologic complications. Further work is required to establish the nature, magnitude, and duration of EP changes associated with irreversible damage.

IV. Preoperative considerations for neurosurgical procedures

A. **Intracranial compliance** may be decreased by intracranial mass lesions (e.g., tumor, hematoma, or abscess). Surrounding normal brain tissue may be compressed, leading to blood–brain barrier compromise, cerebral edema, and loss of cerebral autoregulation. Signs and symptoms of increased ICP are discussed in section I.C.3.

B. **A computed tomography (CT) or magnetic resonance imaging scan** should be reviewed. Midline shift and compressed ventricles or cisterns suggest the presence of diminished intracranial compliance. The degree of brain edema surrounding the mass and the site of the lesion in relation to major intracranial vessels and structures should be noted. Lesions near the dural venous sinuses may require exposure of the sinuses to the atmosphere and may be associated with a higher risk of venous air embolism (see section VI.D.3).

C. **The pathology of the mass** is important in anticipating possible perioperative problems. Vascular lesions (e.g., meningiomas and some metastatic brain tumors) may bleed profusely. Infiltrating malignant tumors may render the patient particularly prone to postoperative cerebral edema.

D. **Preoperative fluid and electrolyte imbalances** and glucose intolerance may be present due to poor oral intake, use of diuretics and steroids, and centrally mediated endocrine abnormalities.

E. **Anticonvulsants** may be required to control seizures. **Corticosteroids** may be necessary to treat edema. These drugs should be continued preoperatively.

F. **Premedication** should be prescribed cautiously, because patients with intracranial disease may be extremely sensitive to the effects of central nervous system (CNS) depressants. Frequently, no premedication is given. If sedation is needed, diazepam (0.1 to 0.2 mg/kg orally) can be used. Additional sedation can be given once the patient arrives in the operating room. If the patient has impaired intracranial compliance and/or a high ICP, opioids should be avoided because of their respiratory depressant effects and the increases in CBF that occur with hypercarbia.

G. In addition to standard monitoring (see Chapter 10), arterial catheters are used in most patients undergoing craniotomy. Capnography is particularly useful when reducing ICP by hyperventilation. A urinary catheter is placed to aid fluid management and diuretic therapy. Invasive monitoring (e.g., pulmonary artery catheter) may be indicated for patients with severe cardiac, renal, or pulmonary disease in the context of marked diuretic-induced fluid shifts. Because access to the neck is limited during neurosurgery, placing central lines by brachial or subclavian approaches should be considered. A second IV catheter for drug administration is often useful.

V. Intraoperative management. Anesthetic goals for intracranial procedures include hypnosis, amnesia, immobility, control of ICP and cerebral perfusion pressure, and a "relaxed brain" (i.e., optimal surgical conditions). Whenever possible, the anesthetic plan should provide an awake, extubated patient who can be evaluated neurologically at the end of the procedure.

A. **Induction of anesthesia** must be accomplished without increasing ICP or compromising CBF. Hypertension, hypotension, hypoxia, hypercarbia, and coughing should be avoided.

1. While thiopental (3 to 7 mg/kg), propofol (2.0 to 2.5 mg/kg), midazolam (0.2 to 0.4 mg/kg), and etomidate (0.3 to 0.4 mg/kg) are all reasonable IV induction agents, the hemodynamic effects caused by these agents should be anticipated.

2. **An adequate mask airway** is essential. After induction, hyperventilation by mask is started with either a nitrous oxide–oxygen mixture or 100% oxygen.

3. An intubating dose of muscle relaxant is given. Nondepolarizing agents are commonly chosen. Adequate relaxation should be obtained before laryngoscopy and intubation to avoid coughing and straining during these procedures.

4. **Opioids** cause minimal changes in cerebral hemodynamics and are useful in blunting responses to intubation and craniotomy. Because intubation, placement of head pins, and craniotomy (skin incision and manipulation of the periosteum) represent the most stimulating periods during intracranial procedures, generous doses of narcotics are given before these manipulations. Fentanyl (5 to 10 μg/kg) and remifentanil are most commonly used, because both have rapid onset and high potency. Lidocaine (1.5 mg/kg IV) can also be used to attenuate the cardiovascular and ICP responses to intubation.

5. **Low concentrations of a potent volatile agent** occasionally are added to prevent hypertension during the initial surgical stimulation.

6. **After intubation,** the eyes are covered with watertight patches to prevent irritation from surgical preparation solutions, the head is carefully checked after final positioning to ensure good venous return, and **close attention is paid to thoroughly securing the airway, because access to the airway is limited during neurosurgical procedures.** Breath sounds and ventilation should be checked after final positioning to ensure proper placement of the endotracheal tube, and all connections in the breathing circuit should be securely tightened.

B. **Maintenance**

1. **Adequate brain relaxation** is necessary before opening the dura. This is achieved by ensuring adequate oxygenation, venous return, muscle relaxation, anesthetic depth, a $Paco_2$ of 33 to 35 mm Hg (hyperventilation if dictated by surgical field), and often the administration of furosemide (10 to 20 mg IV) and mannitol (0.5 to 1.5 g/kg IV) before the craniotomy is completed. The surgeon can assess the need for further brain relaxation by checking the tension of the dura. If necessary, additional IV thiopental can be administered or CSF can be drained through a previously placed lumbar subarachnoid catheter.

2. **Anesthetic requirements** are substantially lower after craniotomy and dural opening, because the brain parenchyma is devoid of sensation. If supplemental narcotics are needed, small doses of morphine or fentanyl can be given. A continuous infusion of propofol (50 to 150 μg/kg per minute) and/or remifentanil (0.1 to 0.5 μg/kg per minute) produces a stable level of anesthesia and allows a rapid emergence. Large doses of **long-acting narcotics and sedatives are usually avoided during the last 1 to 2 hours of the procedure** to facilitate neurologic examination at the end of surgery and avoid potential drowsiness and hypoventilation.

3. **Muscle relaxants** are frequently continued throughout the procedure to prevent movement. Patients receiving anticonvulsants (e.g., phenytoin) may require more frequent administration of muscle relaxants.

C. **Emergence** should occur promptly without straining or coughing. IV lidocaine may be administered to suppress the cough reflex but may delay emergence. Toward the end of the procedure, $Paco_2$ is normalized gradually. Hypertension should be controlled to minimize bleeding; rapidly acting IV agents such as labetalol, esmolol, sodium nitroprusside, and nitroglycerin are often used. Muscle relaxation is usually maintained until the head dressing is completed and then reversal agents are administered. Before leaving the operating room, the patient should be awake so that a brief neurologic examination can be performed. The differential diagnosis of persisting unconsciousness after discontinuation of all anesthetics should include residual anesthesia, narcosis, hypothermia, hypoxia, hypercapnia, partial neuromuscular blockade, and surgically induced increases in ICP (bleeding, edema, and hydrocephalus). Physostigmine (0.01 to 0.03 mg/kg IV) or naloxone (0.04 to 0.4 mg IV) may help antagonize pharmacologically induced CNS depression. The presence of new localized or generalized neurologic deficits should be immediately addressed and may be evaluated by CT and/or surgical reexploration.

D. **Perioperative fluid management** is designed to decrease brain water content, thereby reducing ICP and providing adequate brain relaxation, while maintaining hemodynamic stability and cerebral perfusion pressure.

1. **The blood–brain barrier** is selectively permeable. Gradients for osmotically active substances ultimately determine the distribution of fluids between the brain and intravascular spaces.

a. **Water freely passes through the blood–brain barrier.** Intravascular infusion of free water may increase brain water content and may elevate ICP. Iso-osmotic glucose solutions (e.g., 5% dextrose in water) have the same effect, because the glucose is metabolized and free water remains. These are usually avoided during neurosurgery.

b. **The blood–brain barrier is impermeable to most ions** including Na^+. Unlike the peripheral vasculature, total osmolality, rather than colloid oncotic pressure, determines the osmotic pressure gradient across the blood–brain barrier. Consequently, maintenance of high normal serum osmolality can decrease brain water content, while administration of a large amount of hyposmolar crystalloid solution may increase it.

    c. Large, polar substances cross the blood–brain barrier poorly. Albumin has little effect on brain ECF, because the colloid oncotic pressure contributes to only a small portion of total plasma osmolality (approximately 1 mOsm/L).

    d. If the blood–brain barrier is disrupted (e.g., by ischemia, head trauma, or tumor), permeability to mannitol, albumin, and saline increases so that these molecules have equal access to brain ECF. Under such circumstances, iso-osmolar colloid and crystalloid solutions seem to have similar effects on edema formation and ICP.

2. Severe fluid restriction can produce marked hypovolemia, leading to hypotension, reduced CBF, and ischemia of the brain and other organs, while only modestly decreasing brain water content. **Excessive hypervolemia** may cause hypertension and cerebral edema.

3. Specific treatment recommendations. The overall goal is to maintain normal intravascular volume and to produce a hyperosmolar state.

    a. Fluid losses. The fluid deficit incurred by an overnight fast is usually not replaced. Physiologic maintenance fluids are given. Third-spacing of fluids during intracranial surgery is minimal and usually does not warrant replacement. Two-thirds to total intraoperative urine output is replaced with crystalloid. If signs of hypovolemia develop, additional fluid is administered.

    b. Assessment of blood loss may be difficult during intracranial procedures because significant amounts can be hidden under the drapes. Also, irrigating solutions are used generously by the neurosurgeon.

    c. The serum osmolality is increased to 305 to 320 mOsm/kg. If large fluid requirements are anticipated, iso-osmolar crystalloid solutions such as 0.9% normal saline (309 mOsm/kg) may be preferable to hyposmolar solutions such as lactated Ringer's (272 mOsm/kg). However, large volumes of 0.9% normal saline may cause a metabolic acidosis. Therefore, it is prudent to follow the arterial blood gases and change to lactated Ringer's if indicated. Mannitol (0.5 to 2.0 g/kg IV) and/or furosemide (5 to 20 mg IV) is also administered. The marked diuresis produced by these agents demands close monitoring of intravascular volume and electrolytes.

    d. Hypokalemia may develop from the use of steroids or potassium-wasting diuretics and is exacerbated by hyperventilation. Nevertheless, intraoperative administration of potassium is rarely necessary.

    e. Hyponatremia may be produced by diuretics or syndrome of inappropriate antidiuretic hormone secretion (SIADH).

    f. Hyperglycemia may worsen neurologic outcome after ischemia (see section II.E.2.d). Glucose-containing solutions are avoided in patients at risk for CNS ischemia.

E. **Immediate postoperative care.** Patients are observed closely in an intensive care setting after most intracranial neurosurgical procedures.

1. **The head of the bed** should be elevated 30° to promote venous drainage.

2. **Neurologic function,** including the level of consciousness, orientation, pupillary size, and motor strength should be assessed frequently. Deterioration of any of these may indicate development of cerebral edema, hematoma, hydrocephalus, or herniation.

3. **Adequate ventilation and oxygenation** are essential in patients with reduced consciousness.

4. **Continuous monitoring of ICP** may be indicated if intracranial hypertension exists at the time of dural closure or is anticipated in the postoperative period.

5. **Serum electrolytes and osmolarity** should be checked.

6. **SIADH** can be diagnosed by hyponatremia and serum hyposmolality with high urine osmolality and is treated by restricting free water intake.

7. **Diabetes insipidus** may occur after any intracranial procedure but is most common after pituitary surgery. **Polyuria** is associated with hypernatremia, serum hyperosmolality, and urine hyposmolality. Conscious patients can compensate by increasing their fluid intake; otherwise, adequate IV replacement is mandatory. **Aqueous vasopressin** (5 to 10 USP units subcutaneously or 3 units per hour by IV infusion) may be given. Larger doses may cause hypertension. Alternatively, **desmopressin** (1 to 2 μg IV or subcutaneously every 6 to 12 hours) can be used and is associated with a lower incidence of hypertension.

8. **Seizures** may indicate the presence of an expanding intracranial hematoma or cerebral edema. If a seizure occurs, airway patency, oxygenation, and ventilation must be ensured. The patient should be protected from injury and the IV secured. For acute therapy, thiopental (50 to 100 mg IV), midazolam (2 to 4 mg IV), or lorazepam (2 mg) may be used. Fosphenytoin (15 to 20 mg/kg IV, 100 to 150 mg per min) can be administered to prevent recurrence.

9. **Tension pneumocephalus** may occur and should be suspected after failure to awaken from anesthesia. Skull radiographs or head CT scans confirm the diagnosis; treatment consists of opening the dura to release the air.

F. **Awake craniotomy**

1. Recommended for removal of tumors involving or adjacent to speech and/or motor cortex in cooperative patients. Functional mapping is planned.

2. The goals are to minimize patient discomfort with adequate analgesia, sedation, and careful patient positioning as well as to ensure patient responsiveness and cooperation with neurologic testing during cortical stimulation. Many diverse techniques are successful for this procedure.

3. Be prepared to treat a **cortical stimulation-induced seizure.** If one occurs, ask the neurosurgeons to irrigate the cortex with iced saline. Next, the seizure may be aborted with either midazolam or a small amount of barbiturate (thiopental 50

Table 24.2. Classification of patients with intracranial aneurysms according to surgical risk (Hunt and Hess classification)

Grade	Characteristics
I	Asymptomatic or minimal headache and slight nuchal rigidity
II	Moderate to severe headache, nuchal rigidity, no neurologic deficit other than cranial nerve palsy
III	Drowsiness, confusion, mild focal deficit
IV	Stupor, moderate to severe hemiparesis, possibly early decerebrate rigidity, vegetative disturbances
V	Deep coma, decerebrate rigidity, moribund

    mg IV). These small doses may stop the seizure and not overly sedate the patient so that testing may continue. It is important that the IV catheter is not placed across a joint, which may be flexed and ineffective during a grand mal seizure. Before the procedure, the patient's anticonvulsant level should be checked to ensure that it is therapeutic.

    4. Allow adequate access to the patient's airway. This should include sufficient room to provide mask ventilation and laryngeal mask airway insertion should the circumstances require these interventions.

VI. Specific neurosurgical procedures
  A. Patients with **intracranial aneurysms** present for surgery electively or emergently following **SAH.**

    1. Preoperative evaluation of patients with SAH should include all components of a routine preoperative evaluation (see Chapter 1), with attention to known associated physiologic perturbations. These include the **neurologic grade** (Table 24.2); presence of **vasospasm** (and the hemodynamic parameters that have been effective in relieving clinical symptoms), degree of hydrocephalus, ICP elevation, and concurrent drug therapy such as calcium channel blockade with nimodipine, which may cause moderately lower systemic pressures intraoperatively. **Electrocardiographic changes** are common after SAH and include arrhythmias and fluctuating ST-segment, QT-interval, and T-wave changes. These are probably caused by subendocardial injury following the autonomic discharge that occurs in association with the initial SAH. Provided these are not associated with cardiac dysfunction, no modification of patient management is necessary.

    2. Current practice is to intervene early during the first 72 hours after SAH for patients with neurologic grades I to III, which decreases the risk of rebleeding and facilitates the hypertensive management of vasospasm.

    3. Specific anesthetic considerations include the following:
      a. Avoidance of hypertension, which may increase the risk of aneurysm rupture, before aneurysm clipping. Prophylactic use of agents such as IV nicardipine, fentanyl, β-adrenergic blockers, lidocaine, or additional doses of

barbiturates or propofol will often attenuate the blood pressure response to noxious stimulus such as intrahospital transport, laryngoscopy, and intubation.

b. **Avoidance of hypotension** to maintain adequate cerebral perfusion pressure in the recently insulted brain with resultant altered autoregulation and often marginally perfused areas of brain.

c. **Providing adequate brain relaxation** to optimize surgical exposure. Rapid reductions in ICP may affect transmural pressure and increase the risk of aneurysm rupture. This should be done cautiously before dural opening.

d. **Induced hypertension** may be requested during temporary clipping to improve collateral blood flow to regions that were perfused by the clipped arteries. Often IV phenylephrine is used for this purpose. It is critical that hypertension be induced only **after** the temporary clip has been placed.

e. **Intraoperative aneurysm rupture** can produce rapid and **massive blood loss** requiring large-bore IV access for volume resuscitation. Accurate estimation of blood loss is essential to guide volume repletion. Induced hypotension, adenosine planned arrest, or, occasionally, manual pressure on the ipsilateral carotid artery in the neck may be helpful during the desperate situation of a large and uncontrolled premature rupture.

f. **Mild hypothermia** (34°C) traditionally has been used as a protective strategy for the brain during periods of cerebral ischemia. **Recent data suggest, however, that hypothermia does not improve neurologic outcome in low-grade neurologic injured patients after SAH who undergo aneurysm surgery.** Given the cardiac and infectious morbidity associated with hypothermia, it is now a matter of controversy whether hypothermia is the desired physiologic goal for aneurysm surgery.

g. Once the permanent clips have been placed on the aneurysm, prevention of postoperative vasospasm becomes important. Blood pressure is increased moderately, and fluids are administered to achieve a mildly positive fluid balance.

h. When appropriate, the anesthetic should be designed for a prompt emergence from anesthesia to enable an immediate neurologic exam to ensure good clip placement that does not compromise the parent vessel.

B. **An arteriovenous malformation** (AVM) is a direct communication between cerebral arteries and veins without an intervening capillary bed. Because an AVM is a high-flow, low-resistance system, surrounding brain regions may be hypoperfused by the diversion of blood through the AVM ("steal" phenomenon). The most common presentations of an AVM are SAH, seizures, headaches, and, rarely, progressive neurologic deficits due to steal phenomenon.

1. Patients with AVMs may require anesthetic care for embolization procedures or surgical resection.

a. **Embolizations** are usually done to decrease blood flow to the AVM before surgical resection. Embolization may decrease the risk of intraoperative bleeding and postoperative reperfusion hyperemia.

b. Embolizations can be done under general anesthesia or sedation with monitored anesthesia care, which has the advantage of permitting continuous neurologic evaluation.

c. The anesthetist should be prepared for adverse reactions to the contrast dye (anaphylaxis; osmotic load that may cause congestive heart failure), vessel perforation (sudden and rapid blood loss requiring immediate craniotomy), and neurologic changes.

2. **Anesthetic management for surgical resection** of an AVM is similar to that for cerebral aneurysms.

a. The primary focus is on tight blood pressure control, because hypotension can lead to ischemia of hypoperfused regions. Hypertension can exacerbate perfusion pressure breakthrough, a poorly understood phenomenon that is thought to be caused by abrupt diversion of the AVM's blood flow to adjacent, previously marginally perfused brain, which produces sudden cerebral engorgement and hemorrhage. Should perfusion pressure breakthrough and brain swelling occur, they are commonly treated with barbiturates, hypothermia, and modest lowering of blood pressure.

b. Potential for large blood loss occurs in cases in which the AVM is large, has arterial feeders from more than one part of the cerebral arterial vasculature, or when the preoperative embolization has been unsuccessful.

c. **Postoperative angiography** to confirm complete AVM resection is usually done immediately after surgery, sometimes within the operating room. Should any residual AVM be detected, further resection is indicated.

C. **Posterior fossa surgery**

1. **Posterior fossa tumors** may cause cranial nerve palsies, cerebellar dysfunction, and hydrocephalus due to obstruction of the fourth ventricle. Tumors or surgery around the glossopharyngeal and vagus nerves may impair the gag reflex and increase the risk of aspiration. Tumor resection that results in edema in the floor of the fourth ventricle may damage respiratory centers and necessitate postoperative mechanical ventilation.

2. **Cardiovascular instability** resulting from surgical manipulation is common. Sudden severe bradycardia and hypertension occur if the trigeminal nerve is stimulated. Bradycardia, asystole, or hypotension may follow stimulation of the glossopharyngeal or vagus nerve. In such cases, the surgeon should be notified immediately, because the instability usually resolves with cessation of the stimulus. Pharmacologic treatment (e.g., atropine, glycopyrrolate, or ephedrine) is rarely necessary.

3. A **sitting position** is occasionally used for posterior fossa surgery. The advantages include better surgical exposure; improved venous and CSF drainage; diminished bleeding

due to lower venous pressures; and improved access to the airway, chest, and extremities for the anesthetist. The sitting position is also associated with a higher incidence of venous air embolism and cardiovascular instability. Modified supine, prone, and three-quarter prone positioning may be substituted for the sitting position because of these concerns.

   a. **Venous air embolism** is a risk whenever the operative site is above the level of the heart and there is an open noncollapsible vein. Under these circumstances, an open venous sinus can entrain air and produce hypoxia, hypercarbia, bronchoconstriction, hypotension, and ultimately cardiovascular collapse. Systemic arterial air embolism is a risk whenever right-to-left shunts occur and can cause myocardial and cerebral ischemia. Monitoring devices for the detection of air embolism and central venous catheters for aspiration of air are often placed when there is risk for venous air embolism.

   b. **Methods used to monitor for venous air embolism** include Doppler ultrasound (which reveals a characteristic "mill wheel" murmur when air is entrained), capnography (which may reveal a sudden decrease in end tidol CO_2), mass spectroscopy, and transesophageal echocardiography.

   c. **If air is detected,** the focus is to prevent further air aspiration and treatment of the adverse consequences. First, the surgeons are notified so they can eliminate the source of air (close the dural opening, place bone wax, or flood the surgical field), nitrous oxide is discontinued, and air is aspirated from the central venous pressure catheter. If the patient remains stable, the prevention of further air entry may be all that is needed. If hypotension develops, Trendelenburg positioning, fluid administration, and inotropic support may be required.

  4. At the end of surgery, the adequacy of the airway and respiration should be verified before extubation. Surgical manipulation may have caused damage to the cranial nerves or respiratory centers in the brainstem with resulting pharyngeal or respiratory dysfunction. Postoperative infarction, edema, or hematoma formation in the posterior fossa can cause rapid clinical deterioration. Close observation and prompt support including intubation, mechanical ventilation, and circulatory management may be required.

D. **Transsphenoidal resection of the pituitary gland** is performed through either a nasal or a labial incision.

  1. Although nonfunctioning **pituitary adenomas** are the most common tumor type, some patients have endocrine deficiencies due to hypothalamopituitary compression. Various hyperpituitarism syndromes may accompany functioning adenomas, including Cushing syndrome, acromegaly (with associated airway difficulties), and amenorrhea-galactorrhea (see Chapter 6).

  2. ICP is not a concern as these tumors are usually small and unlikely to compromise intracranial compliance.

3. **Uncontrollable bleeding** is rare but can be massive and catastrophic due to lack of exposure. Frontal craniotomy ultimately may be required to achieve hemostasis.

4. **Monitoring.** The operating microscope obstructs access to the patient's head, so the endotracheal tube must be firmly secured. Continuous monitoring of ventilation is essential. Arterial monitors are usually not indicated.

5. **Throat packs** will prevent blood from accumulating in the stomach and may reduce postoperative vomiting. The throat pack must be removed before extubation.

6. At the conclusion of surgery, nasal breathing will be obstructed by packs. Patients should be prepared for this preoperatively.

7. **Diabetes insipidus** may occur after transsphenoidal hypophysectomy (usually 4 to 12 hours postoperatively). Treatment with IV fluids or vasopressin may be necessary (see section V.E.7). Some patients may develop postoperative adrenal insufficiency and require corticosteroids postoperatively.

E. **Stereotactic surgery** is performed through a burr hole, using a three-dimensional reference grid attached to the head with pins placed in the outer table of the skull. This approach allows localization of a discrete area of brain for biopsy or ablation. In most cases, the procedure can be performed under local anesthesia with IV sedation. Because the stereotactic apparatus precludes full access to the airway, sedation must be given with caution. If general anesthesia is needed after the frame is placed, the technique for securing the airway is selected based on the urgency of airway management and whether the stereotactic frame interferes with the mask or laryngeal mask airway. Because the frame may also prevent optimal head positioning for mask ventilation and direct laryngoscopy, laryngeal mask airways and equipment for awake intubation, preferably with a fiberoptic laryngoscope, should be available. The stereotactic frame can be removed in an emergency; newer models can be quickly removed to provide access to the airway.

F. **Epilepsy surgery** is performed in patients with epilepsy of focal origin who are refractory to medical therapy or intolerant of the side effects of anticonvulsants. The procedures include excision of a seizure focus or interruption of epileptiform pathways. Electrophysiologic mapping of the epileptic focus and other cortical areas (e.g., language, memory, or sensorimotor) is often performed to maximize the resection of the epileptogenic lesion while minimizing the neurologic deficits. Awake craniotomy with IV sedation and local anesthesia of the scalp permits performance of the mapping procedure, which requires patient cooperation. General anesthesia offers the advantages of patient comfort, immobility, a secure airway, and ability to control $Paco_2$ and other variables. The anesthetic technique is chosen for its ability to augment (e.g., enflurane, methohexital, etomidate, or ketamine) or attenuate (e.g., benzodiazepines, barbiturates, or isoflurane) the seizure focus and its compatibility with intraoperative monitoring (see section III). Because there is often an initial increase in seizure activity postoperatively, anticonvulsants should be resumed promptly.

G. Head trauma. Anesthetic management of the patient with head trauma is complicated by the challenging combination of a "tight" head, full stomach, and potentially unstable cervical spine. While following the "ABCs" of resuscitation, the anesthesiologist should ascertain the mechanism and extent of injury. **Cervical spinal cord injury** must be suspected and the neck stabilized until cervical vertebral fracture is excluded.

1. Patients who are responsive and ventilating adequately should receive supplemental oxygen and be observed closely for evidence of neurologic deterioration.

2. Comatose patients require immediate endotracheal intubation for airway protection and to avoid hypercarbia and hypoxia, which can exacerbate increases in ICP and contribute to secondary brain injury.

3. **Endotracheal intubation** should be accomplished rapidly, with blood pressure stability and without coughing or straining.

   a. **A rapid sequence induction** is usually performed. If a cervical spine fracture has not been excluded, the neck should be immobilized with manual in-line stabilization. The anterior part of the cervical collar may be removed to apply gentle cricoid pressure (excessive pressure may displace a fracture) and obtain sufficient mouth opening. A short-acting induction agent such as propofol, thiopental, or etomidate is used to induce anesthesia, which is immediately followed by an intubating dose of muscle relaxant. Succinylcholine can be used safely unless contraindicated for other reasons (see section II.C and Chapter 12). Nondepolarizing relaxants also may be used.

   b. **Awake intubation** (e.g., blind nasal or fiberoptic) may be advocated because of full-stomach considerations, the potential for worsening neck injuries during manipulation of the airway, and anticipation of a difficult airway due to associated facial injuries. Awake approaches are often impractical or unwise in head-injured patients because of lack of cooperation, airway bleeding, and increases in ICP that can be induced by hypertension, coughing, and straining.

   c. **Nasal intubation and nasogastric tube placement** are relatively contraindicated in the presence of a basilar skull fracture (e.g., CSF rhinorrhea, otorrhea, or Le Fort III facial fracture).

4. **Hypertension** in head-injured patients may be the body's compensatory effort to maintain cerebral perfusion pressure in the face of increased ICP. Perfusion pressure (MAP-ICP) should be maintained at 60 mm Hg. **Hypotension can be detrimental** in patients with elevated ICP and when combined with tachycardia should lead one to suspect bleeding from other injuries. Interventions to stop bleeding and restore intravascular volume should precede or proceed in concert with surgical treatment of the head injury.

5. Hypoxia should be aggressively treated as it presence dramatically worsens neurologic outcome in head injured patients.

6. Hyperglycemia should be treated to improve neurologic outcome.

7. **ICP monitoring** can be performed if severe or progressive intracranial hypertension is suspected (see section I.C.2).

8. **Seizures** may accompany direct cerebral injury or signal the expansion of an intracranial hematoma.

9. **Brain contusion** is the most common type of head injury. Surgery is usually reserved for acute epidural hematomas and acute subdural hematomas. Subdural hematomas are much more common than epidural hematomas and carry a worse prognosis. Intracranial hypertension is frequently seen even after evacuation of hematomas because of severe brain swelling.

10. **Penetrating brain injuries** require early debridement of injured tissue and removal of bone fragments and hematoma. Skull fractures may require debridement, cranioplasty, and repair of dural lacerations.

11. **Anesthetic management** follows the general rules of maintaining cerebral perfusion pressure and reducing ICP and cerebral edema. Postoperative intubation and ventilatory support frequently are required for ICP control and airway protection in patients with prolonged loss of consciousness or an inadequate gag reflex. Preoperative alteration in the level of consciousness is helpful in predicting the need for postoperative intubation.

12. **Disseminated intravascular coagulation** is a frequent complication of an acute head injury, particularly those associated with a subdural hematoma. Frequent monitoring of patient's coagulation status is recommended throughout the procedure.

13. **Corticosteroids are not indicated for head trauma** and according to recent data may increase morbidity and mortality.

H. **Deep brain stimulators** are inserted in patients with movement disorders (mostly Parkinson disease) who have failed medical therapy. Microelectrodes are inserted through burr holes to a precise location in either the subthalamic nuclei, globus pallidum or thalamus. A stereotactic headframe is required to identify and locate the electrode target.

1. Patients do not receive their morning dose of either dopaminergic or anticholinergic medications to improve electrode recordings that guide electrode placement to a specific cell layer.

2. Patients are awake and not sedated during the electrode placement. Sedatives alter the electrode recordings. Once the electrodes are secure, appropriate sedation is desirable.

I. **CSF shunts** are inserted in patients with hydrocephalus. A VP shunt is the most common treatment for hydrocephalus. A ventricular catheter is placed through a frontal burr hole and is attached to a subcutaneous reservoir and valve. These are then attached to the draining catheter which is tunneled subcutaneously to the upper abdomen where a minilaparotomy is performed to insert the catheter under direct supervision.

1. The anesthetic management of these patients is determined primarily by the acuity of their disease. Acute hydrocephalus is a neurosurgical emergency where rapidly rising ICP could

cause ischemic neurologic damage. Management should focus on measures which will reduce the patient's ICP, maintain a perfusion pressure of at least 60 mmHg and will enable rapid neurosurgical decompression. Anesthetic management of elective VP shunt insertion or revision employs a standard, well managed, and safe anesthetic where factors which cause extreme ICP elevation are avoided.

2. Some patients with a trapped ventricle can be treated with a ventriculostomy that is inserted through a frontal burr hole. A perforation is made in the ventricular septum under direct vision. These patients are anesthetized with general anesthesia as the ICP sometimes increases with the infused irrigating solution. This could potentially cause patient discomfort or altered consciousness

VII. **Surgery on the spine and spinal cord** is undertaken for a variety of conditions, including intervertebral disk diseases, spondylosis, stenosis, neoplasm, scoliosis, and trauma. The physiology of the spinal cord and brain is similar, even though absolute rates of blood flow and metabolism are lower in the spinal cord. Maintaining spinal cord perfusion pressure (which equals MAP minus extrinsic pressure on the cord) and reducing cord compression are clinical management objectives.

A. **The prone position** is frequently used. Most patients can be anesthetized on a stretcher and "log rolled" onto the operating room table after endotracheal intubation. Awake intubation should be considered for patients with tenuous neurologic conditions that may be worsened by laryngoscopy/intubation or positioning (e.g., patients with unstable cervical or thoracic spine injuries). Under these circumstances, an abbreviated neurologic examination should be performed after intubation and transfer to ensure that injury has not occurred. The anesthetist should ensure that all pressure points are padded; neck and extremities are in neutral positions; eyes, ears, nose, and genitalia are free from pressure; and all monitors and lines are secured in place and functioning. Special attention should be paid to the endotracheal tube, since it can move or kink in the process of positioning. **Ischemic optic neuropathy is a potential complication** of prone cases associated with length of procedure (usually >5 hours), blood loss (usually >2 L), hypotension, and fluid resuscitation. Increased facial swelling may alter venous hemodynamics in the globe, leading to optic nerve ischemia and postoperative visual deficits. There are no standard preventive guidelines, but frequent eye checks to assess for direct pressure on the globe and maintenance of adequate perfusion are likely beneficial.

B. **Surgery to correct scoliosis** can be accompanied by significant blood loss. Various techniques can be used to reduce homologous blood transfusion, including preoperative autologous donation, intraoperative hemodilution, use of intraoperative blood-scavenging techniques, and meticulous patient positioning to prevent increased abdominal and intrathoracic pressures that can increase venous bleeding. Because of concern of neurologic sequelae, induced hypotension may not be advantageous in this procedure. Scoliosis surgery is accompanied by a 1% to 4% incidence of serious postoperative neurologic complications. Spinal instrumentation and distraction can cause spinal cord ischemia and result in paraplegia. Intraoperative monitoring of spinal cord function is used routinely.

1. **SSEP and MEP monitoring** provide continuous evaluation of spinal cord function (see section III.B).

2. **The selective wake-up test.** Intraoperatively, if there is uncertainty about the neurophysiolic monitoring a, the presence of neuromuscular function is assured when patients are awakened briefly and asked to move their legs. If there is no leg movement, the spine distraction is released until movement is observed. Patients should be prepared for this event preoperatively. Wake-up tests can be performed in older children.

3. **Total IV anesthesia** with remifentanil and propofol is often selected because it is less likely to interfere with neurophysiologic monitoring than volatile anesthetics; however, it does not provide for a reliably fast intraoperative wakeup test. Alternatively, children, who often have robust nerve conduction, may be anesthetized with desflurane, with or without nitrous oxide and short-acting narcotics to achieve a much faster intraoperative wake up. Communication of anesthetic interventions with the clinical neurophysiologist or technician is important.

C. **After acute spinal cord injury,** surgery may be required to decompress and stabilize the spinal cord. The primary goal in the initial management of acute spinal cord injury is to prevent secondary damage to the injured cord. This is accomplished by stabilizing the spine and correcting circulatory and ventilatory abnormalities that can exacerbate the primary injury. The presence of cervical cord injury should lead one to suspect associated head, face, or tracheal trauma; thoracic and lumbar spine injuries often are associated with chest and intra-abdominal trauma.

1. **Spinal shock** is characterized by vasodilation and hypotension. If the lesion involves the sympathetic cardiac accelerator nerves (T-1 to T-4), bradycardia, bradyarrhythmias, atrioventricular block, and cardiac arrest can occur due to unopposed vagal activity. Spinal shock occurs because of functional transection of sympathetic innervation below the level of the injury and may persist for days to weeks. Bradycardia can be treated by atropine. Hypotension can be treated by fluid, vasopressors, or both. A pulmonary artery catheter may be helpful when other injuries are present and volume status is uncertain. Patients with high spinal cord injury may be unusually sensitive to the cardiovascular depressant effects of anesthetics because of an inability to increase sympathetic tone.

2. **Lesions above C-3 to C-4 necessitate intubation and mechanical ventilatory support** because of loss of innervation to the diaphragm (C-3 to C-5). Lesions below C-5 to C-6 may still cause as much as a 70% reduction in vital capacity and FEV_1 with impaired ventilation and oxygenation.

3. **Atony of the gastrointestinal tract and urinary bladder** necessitates a nasogastric tube and indwelling urinary catheter, respectively. These patients are also **prone to heat loss** because of inability to vasoconstrict.

4. **Methylprednisolone** (30 mg/kg IV loading dose, followed by an infusion of 5.4 mg/kg per hour for 23 hours) may

improve the functional recovery of patients with acute spinal cord injuries if treatment is begun within the first 3 hours after injury. There is some controversy surrounding this therapy for spinal cord injury and some centers do not follow this protocol.

5. **Chronic spinal cord injuries** are discussed in Chapter 26.
6. **Airway management** of patients with cervical spine injury is discussed in section VI.H.

VIII. Neuroradiological procedures are performed in suites often remote from the main operating room. For a detailed discussion of anesthetic issues pertaining to the patient having a magnetic resonance imaging or interventional radiologic procedures, see sections IV and V in Chapter 32.

SUGGESTED READING

Cottrell JE, Smith DS, eds. *Anesthesia and neurosurgery,* 4th ed. St. Louis: Mosby, 2001.

Drummond JC, Patel PM. *Neurosurgical anesthesia.* In Miller RD, ed. *Miller's Anesthesia.* Philadelphia: Churchill Livingstone, 2005;813–858 and 2127–2174.

25

Anesthesia for Head and Neck Surgery

Tzuhao Harry Wu and Martin Andrew Acquadro

I. **Anesthesia for ophthalmic surgery**
   A. **General considerations**
      1. **Intraocular pressure** (IOP; normal ranges from 10 to 22 mm Hg; abnormal is greater than 25 mm Hg) is determined mainly by the rate of production of aqueous humor in relation to its rate of drainage.
         a. **Factors that may increase IOP** include hypertension, hypercarbia, hypoxia, laryngoscopy and endotracheal intubation, venous congestion, vomiting, coughing, straining, bucking, external pressure on the eye, succinylcholine, and ketamine.
         b. **Factors that may decrease IOP** include hypocarbia, hypothermia, central nervous system depressants, ganglionic blockers, most volatile and intravenous (IV) anesthetics, nondepolarizing muscle relaxants, mannitol, diuretics, acetazolamide, and head elevation.
      2. **Glaucoma**
         a. **Open-angle glaucoma** usually arises from chronic obstruction of aqueous humor drainage and is characterized by a progressive insidious course that may not be associated with pain.
         b. **Closed-angle glaucoma** results from acute aqueous outflow obstruction caused by a narrowing of the anterior chamber as a result of pupillary dilation or lens edema and is painful.
      3. **Oculocardiac reflex**
         a. The oculocardiac reflex can be triggered by increased pressure on the globe or by traction on the extrinsic eye muscles, causing cardiac arrhythmias (e.g., bradycardia or asystole). Administration of ocular regional anesthesia may also elicit this response.
         b. The **afferent arc** of this reflex is mediated by the trigeminal (fifth cranial) nerve and the **efferent arc** is mediated by the vagus (tenth cranial) nerve. The oculocardiac reflex should be promptly treated by cessation of the stimulus. Atropine (0.01 to 0.02 mg/kg IV) administration minimizes these arrhythmias. Atropine prophylaxis does not always prevent the reflex. If the reflex persists, infiltration of local anesthetic near the extrinsic eye muscles or placing a peribulbar or retrobulbar block is effective. The reflex fatigues quickly with repeated stimulation.
      4. **Commonly used drugs**
         a. **Topical.** Most ophthalmic medications are highly

concentrated solutions that are administered topically and may produce systemic effects.

(1) **Mydriatics**

    (a) **Phenylephrine** eye drops may cause hypertension and reflex bradycardia, especially when administered as a 10% solution. For this reason, a 2.5% solution is commonly used. It dilates the pupil and constricts periocular blood vessels.

    (b) **Cyclopentolate** may produce central nervous system toxicity (e.g., confusion, seizures). It dilates the pupil and prevents lens accommodation.

(2) **Miotics.** Cholinergic drugs (e.g., pilocarpine 0.25% to 4% solution) may produce bradycardia, salivation, bronchorrhea, and diaphoresis.

(3) **Drugs that decrease IOP**

    (a) **Topical β-adrenergic antagonists** (e.g., timolol or betaxolol) may cause bradycardia, hypotension, congestive heart failure, and bronchospasm.

    (b) **Anticholinesterases,** such as echothiophate, depress plasma cholinesterase activity for 2 to 4 weeks, and may prolong recovery from succinylcholine and mivacurium.

  b. **Systemic. Acetazolamide,** a carbonic anhydrase inhibitor, is administered systemically to control aqueous humor secretion. Chronic use can lead to the development of hyponatremia, hypokalemia, and metabolic acidosis.

B. Anesthetic management

  1. **Preoperative evaluation.** Patients undergoing eye surgery often present with significant concomitant diseases that require careful evaluation (i.e., the formerly premature infant with bronchopulmonary dysplasia for retinal surgery or the elderly patient with cardiovascular disease for cataract excision).

  2. **Premedication**

    a. Visually impaired patients may be apprehensive about surgery and require constant verbal communication.

    b. Ophthalmic procedures performed with ocular regional anesthesia require a calm and cooperative patient.

    c. Common premedications do not increase IOP. There is no evidence that premedication with customary doses of parenteral atropine causes increased IOP, even in glaucoma patients.

    d. **Benzodiazepines** are effective anxiolytics with amnestic properties. Diazepam (5 to 10 mg orally) or lorazepam (0.5 to 2 mg orally), 1 hour preoperatively, can be used. Alternatively, midazolam (0.5 to 2 mg) IV before administration of anesthesia is very effective for adults. For children, oral midazolam (0.5 mg/kg) can be given 20 min preoperatively.

    e. Opioids, if used, can be given in combination with an antiemetic such as metoclopramide, droperidol, or ondansetron. Use of antidopaminergic agents in elderly patients may be associated with confusion.

3. **Avoidance of coughing, sudden movement, or straining is essential.** Unexpected patient or eye movements during delicate microscopic intraocular surgery can lead to increased IOP, choroidal hemorrhage, expulsion of vitreous material, or loss of vision.

4. **Regional anesthesia (retrobulbar or peribulbar block)**

   a. Ophthalmic procedures such as cataract extraction, corneal transplant, and anterior chamber irrigation can be performed under regional anesthesia and light conscious sedation.

   b. Patient cooperation and lack of head motion are important for the success of this technique. Patients who are unable to understand because of extreme age, impaired hearing, psychosis, or a language barrier or who are unable to maintain a relatively motionless position because of chronic cough, tremor, or arthritis may not be candidates for regional anesthesia for delicate eye surgery.

   c. The advantages of regional anesthesia include a lower incidence of coughing, straining, and emesis. The technique is useful for ambulatory patients and provides postoperative analgesia.

   d. **IV sedation** may be used perioperatively. Midazolam (0.25 to 1 mg IV), fentanyl (10 to 50 μg IV), remifentanil (0.25 to 0.5 μg/kg IV), or propofol (5 to 20 mg IV) can be administered just before the regional injection. Patients should be monitored during regional block placement and receive supplemental oxygen if indicated.

   e. **Technique.** Intraocular surgery requires adequate sensory and motor block of the eye and often the eyelids as well. Anesthesia of the eye is accomplished by injecting local anesthetic into either retrobulbar or peribulbar space, facilitating neural blockade of cranial nerves II through VI. The **retrobulbar block** is achieved by injecting 4 to 6 mL of a 50:50 mixture of 2% lidocaine and 0.75% bupivacaine (with 1:200,000 to 1:400,000 epinephrine) within the muscle cone formed by the four recti muscles and the two oblique muscles. With the eye in a neutral position, a 23- or 25-gauge needle is inserted through the lower lid or conjunctiva at the level of the inferior orbital rim in the inferotemporal quadrant. The needle is first advanced slightly inferiorly and temporally approximately 1.5 cm; once past the equator of the eye, the needle is then directed superiorly and nasally toward the apex of the orbit to a depth of approximately 3.5 cm, while feeling for a "pop" as the needle penetrates through the muscle cone. With the **peribulbar block,** there is no attempt made to enter the muscle cone. The needle is advanced along the inferior orbital floor to a depth of approximately 2.5 cm. Between 8 and 10 mL of local anesthetic is required, and hyaluronidase (3.75 to 15 units/mL) frequently is added to help facilitate spread through the muscle cone. Careful aspiration before injection is required for both blocks, followed by gentle massage or orbital compression to promote spread of the anesthetic. If desired, the facial nerve can also be blocked by infiltration of 2 to 4 mL of additional local anesthetic along the inferior and superior orbital rim to help prevent squinting. The retrobulbar block provides faster, more reliable anesthesia and akinesia but has a higher complication rate than the peribulbar block.

   f. **Complications** are infrequent but include direct optic nerve trauma, retrobulbar hemorrhage, transient globe compression with increased IOP, globe perforation, and stimulation of the oculocardiac reflex. Hyaluronidase is toxic to the eye if injected into the globe. Intravascular injection of local anesthetic may cause seizures or myocardial depression. Rarely, the local anesthetic may dissect proximally along the neural sheath of the optic nerve and cause temporary (15 minutes) loss of consciousness without seizures. The patient may become apneic briefly; treatment is supportive.

   g. During the procedure, **fresh air** at a flow rate of 10 to 15 L per minute is provided to the patient under the drapes using a large face mask. This helps to remove exhaled carbon dioxide and helps offset the sense of suffocation or claustrophobia some patients may experience. **Oxygen** may be used if indicated but the surgeon should be notified not to use electrocautery while oxygen is flowing. During supplementation of IV sedation, the patient should not become unresponsive; undue restlessness may be a sign of oversedation in the elderly. End-tidal carbon dioxide monitoring through the face mask can be used or a precordial stethoscope can be applied because observation of ventilation can be obscured by drapes.

5. General anesthesia

   a. The eye is highly innervated and very sensitive. Eye surgery requires sufficient depth of general anesthesia to prevent eye motion, coughing, straining, or hypertension. General anesthesia with an inhalation agent, supplemented by a nondepolarizing muscle relaxant, is usually satisfactory. Coughing or straining with an open eye can lead to catastrophic choroidal hemorrhage or vitreous extrusion.

   b. The lack of access to the airway during the procedure necessitates endotracheal intubation or a laryngeal mask airway. If intubation is planned, IV lidocaine (1.0 to 1.5 mg/kg) or 4% lidocaine spray to the larynx and trachea may help to attenuate the response to laryngoscopy (i.e., straining, bucking, or increase in IOP). The endotracheal tube should be firmly supported and taped in place to prevent disconnection, extubation, and stimulation of a cough reflex by motion.

   c. **Ketamine** can cause blepharospasm, nystagmus, and vomiting. It may increase arterial pressure and IOP. For these reasons, ketamine usually is a poor choice for most ophthalmic surgery. Low doses of ketamine, however, do not increase IOP and may be useful as a supplement to IV sedation for retrobulbar or peribulbar block.

    d. **Smooth emergence and extubation** are particularly desirable after ophthalmic surgery. This may be facilitated by thorough posterior pharyngeal suctioning while the patient is still deeply anesthetized, administration of an opioid to reduce the cough reflex, and IV lidocaine (1 to 1.5 mg/kg) 5 minutes before planned extubation. The patient may then be extubated awake with intact airway reflexes. Deep extubation is also an option but does not guarantee a smooth emergence.

C. Specific procedures

    1. Open-eye injury. Penetrating eye trauma is a surgical emergency, frequently occurring in patients who have recently eaten. It requires a carefully conducted anesthetic designed to prevent aspiration and favorably affect IOP (see section I.A.1). A sudden increase in IOP can result in extrusion of ocular contents and cause permanent vision loss. Trauma to the eye and orbit, long duration and complex surgery, and a crying patient with a full stomach usually mandate general endotracheal anesthesia. Orbital pressure from face masks should be avoided.

        a. **Succinylcholine** administered during a rapid sequence induction causes an increase in IOP of approximately 10 mm Hg for 5 minutes. Pretreatment with nondepolarizing muscle relaxants may attenuate but does not ablate this response. Nevertheless, succinylcholine often is the drug of choice to quickly establish adequate intubating conditions in the eye surgery patient with a full stomach. Alternatively, nondepolarizing muscle relaxants can be used, but adequate intubating conditions may not be achieved for 60 to 90 seconds.

        b. An adequate depth of anesthesia and degree of neuromuscular blockade must be ensured before laryngoscopy and intubation to minimize increases in IOP (which may rise to 40 to 50 mm Hg) secondary to straining, coughing, and bucking.

        c. In children, if an IV cannot be placed, an inhalation induction using cricoid pressure and nonirritating volatile anesthetics (e.g., nitrous oxide, sevoflurane, or halothane) may be necessary.

    2. Strabismus repair is a common pediatric operation whereby the lengths of the extraocular muscles are altered by recession or resection.

        a. **Succinylcholine administration** can interfere with the forced duction test for up to 20 minutes; therefore, laryngoscopy and intubation are facilitated by a nondepolarizing muscle relaxant or adequate inhalation anesthesia

        b. Surgical manipulation frequently elicits **the oculocardiac reflex** (see section I.A.3).

        c. **Postoperative nausea and vomiting** are very common (80% incidence in untreated patients). The following measures should be considered to decrease the incidence of postoperative nausea and vomiting prophylactically:

           (1) Minimal use of opioids for pain management.

           (2) Antiemetics given 30 minutes before surgery

(metoclopramide [0.1 to 0.15 mg/kg IV)] dexamethasone [0.5 mg/kg IV, maximum of 10 mg], droperidol [25 to 30 μg/kg IV], ondansetron [0.15 mg/kg IV]).

(3) Stomach is decompressed with an orogastric tube.

(4) Adequate hydration of the patient with IV crystalloids.

(5) If possible, avoidance of nitrous oxide.

(6) Consider a propoful infusion.

d. Patients with musculoskeletal abnormalities may be at increased risk for **malignant hyperthermia.** Children with strabismus may be at risk for development of masseter muscle spasm and malignant hyperthermia. A thorough family history should be obtained. Heart rate, endtidal carbon dioxide, ventilatory parameters, and temperature should be carefully monitored for early detection of malignant hyperthermia. Masseter muscle spasm arising from the use of succinylcholine may be a harbinger of malignant hyperthermia; therefore, a cautious approach to anesthetic management is needed (see Chapter 18).

3. **Retinal surgery for detachment and vitreous hemorrhage** often is performed on premature infants with retinopathy of prematurity. Concomitant medical problems are often present; meticulous attention to airway management, fluid status, normothermia, and postoperative transport is crucial (see Chapter 29). Premature infants, especially less than 60 weeks postconceptional age, are at risk for postoperative central apnea. They should demonstrate a 12-hour apneafree interval before discharge. Patients with diabetes or sickle cell anemia also may require retinal surgery (see Chapters 6 and 34).

a. **Regional anesthesia** is suitable for short procedures (<2 hours) in cooperative patients, although unexpected movement during the delicate retinal repair may result in vision loss. If **general anesthesia** is administered, deep inhalational anesthesia, IV anesthesia with an opioid and/or propofol, use of a remifentanil infusion, or a balanced technique with an adequate degree of neuromuscular blockade is recommended. Postoperative coughing, straining, and vomiting should be avoided (see section I.C.2c).

b. An intravitreal gas bubble containing an inert, high-molecular-weight, low-diffusivity gas such as SF_6, C_3F_8, C_4F_8, or air, may be injected at the conclusion of surgery to reduce intravitreal bleeding. Nitrous oxide should be discontinued at least 20 minutes before bubble injection. The presence of nitrous oxide will rapidly expand the bubble and increase IOP; cessation of nitrous oxide at the end of the procedure shrinks the bubble, with resulting loss of its mechanical advantage. Because these gas bubbles remain for various periods of time, readministration of nitrous oxide should be avoided for 5 days after an air injection, 10 days after SF_6 injection, and 60 days after C_3F_8 injection.

II. **Anesthesia for otorhinolaryngologic procedures**
 A. **General considerations**
  1. **Airway.** For many otorhinolaryngologic (ORL) surgical procedures, the airway must be shared with the surgeon. Pathology, scarring from previous surgery or irradiation, congenital deformities, trauma, or manipulation can produce chronic or acute airway obstruction, bleeding, and a potentially difficult airway. Preoperative discussion with the surgeon and analysis of previous anesthetic records regarding perioperative airway management, endotracheal tube size and position, patient positioning, and use of nitrous oxide and muscle relaxants are essential. The patient may require an awake examination of the airway under sedation and topical anesthesia or an awake fiberoptic intubation before induction of general anesthesia.
  2. Patients presenting for ORL surgery may have a history of heavy smoking, alcohol abuse, obstructive sleep apnea, and chronic upper respiratory tract infections. Preoperative laboratory testing, imaging, and evaluation of cardiac, hepatic, and pulmonary function may be necessary.
  3. In addition to standard monitors, major procedures may require intra-arterial blood pressure monitoring and urine output.
  4. **Extubation** after any upper airway surgery requires careful planning. Throat packs are removed, the pharynx is suctioned, and the patient is oxygenated. Extubation is performed when full protective laryngeal reflexes return. Excessive upper airway bleeding, edema, or pathology may preclude extubation in the operating room.
 B. **Ear surgery**
  1. **Preoperative considerations**
   a. **Ear surgery** often involves dissecting and preserving the **facial (cranial nerve VII) nerve.**
   b. The **middle ear** communicates with the oropharynx via the Eustachian tube. If Eustachian tube patency is compromised by trauma, edema, inflammation, or congenital deformity, normal venting of middle ear pressure cannot occur. In this situation, a high concentration of nitrous oxide can increase middle ear pressure to 300 to 400 mm Hg in 30 minutes. Conversely, acute cessation of nitrous oxide can result in rapid resorption and a net negative pressure in the middle ear. These changes may result in alteration of middle ear anatomy, rupture of tympanic membrane, disarticulation of artificial stapes, disruption of surgical grafts, and postoperative nausea and vomiting.
   c. **Positioning.** During surgery, the patient's head often is elevated and turned to the side. Extremes of head position should be assessed preoperatively to determine limits of range of motion, especially in patients with arthritis or cerebrovascular disease. Eyes should be taped closed and padded.
  2. **Anesthesia** is induced with a hypnotic and short-acting muscle relaxant or by inhalation and usually is maintained with a volatile anesthetic. The use of nitrous oxide should

be discussed with the surgeon; nitrous oxide should be discontinued at least 30 minutes before placement of a tympanic membrane graft.

a. Delicate microsurgery of the ear requires adequate hemostasis. Volatile anesthetics and α- or β-adrenergic antagonists work well to induce mean arterial pressures of 60 to 70 mm Hg. Elevation of the head of the bed to approximately 15° to decrease venous congestion and local application of epinephrine for vasoconstriction usually improve operating conditions.

b. Myringotomy with tube placement is one of the most frequently performed outpatient pediatric surgeries. These procedures are short and can usually be performed under mask anesthesia with or without an IV placement. No muscle relaxant is needed. If the procedure is performed without an IV line, intranasal fentanyl (1 to 2 μg/kg) and preoperative oral acetaminophen (20 mg/kg) can be used for postoperative pain management.

c. Antiemetics should be given because postoperative vomiting is very common with ear surgery (see section I.C.2c).

C. Nasal surgery

1. **Anesthetic technique.** Nasal surgery can be performed with local or general anesthesia. With either technique, the surgeon may initially apply 4% cocaine to the nasal mucosa, followed by injection of 1% to 2% lidocaine with 1:100,000 to 1:200,000 epinephrine for hemostasis. These agents may cause tachycardia, hypertension, and arrhythmias, especially in the presence of halothane. In a healthy adult, the cocaine dose should not exceed 1.5 mg/kg (each drop of a 4% solution contains about 3 mg of cocaine). Smaller doses should be used when administered with epinephrine, in the presence of halothane, or in patients with cardiovascular disease. General anesthesia may be needed to provide immobility, airway protection, or amnesia.

2. After **nasal cosmetic surgery,** the nose is unstable and application of a face mask is undesirable. Smooth emergence and extubation are important to decrease postoperative bleeding and to avoid laryngospasm and the need for positive pressure ventilation by mask.

3. **Blood loss** during nasal surgery may be substantial and difficult to estimate. A throat pack may help decrease postoperative nausea and vomiting by preventing passage of blood into the stomach. The throat pack must be removed before extubation. An orogastric tube may be placed to evacuate the stomach of any swallowed blood.

4. Patients with **severe epistaxis** presenting for internal maxillary artery ligation or embolization often are anxious, tired, hypertensive, tachycardic, and hypovolemic. These patients need reassurance, hydration, and prompt care. They are assumed to have a full stomach and induction of anesthesia and endotracheal intubation should be planned accordingly. Hypertension should be controlled to reduce blood loss. Posterior nasal packing, while helpful, can cause edema and hypoventilation. Because the extent of blood loss is difficult to

assess, adequate IV access (14- or 16-gauge IV) and blood for transfusion should be available. Removal of the posterior packing can be associated with substantial blood loss.

D. Upper airway surgery

1. Tonsillectomy and adenoidectomy

a. **Preoperative evaluation** should seek a history of bleeding disorders, obstructive sleep apnea, and loose teeth. Coagulation studies are performed. Patients with obstructive sleep apnea may be obese, and ventilation and intubation may be difficult. Many patients have chronic or recurrent upper respiratory tract infections. If the patient has an acute infection that is accompanied by fever, productive cough, lower respiratory symptoms, additional comorbidities, or age <1 year, consider postponing the procedure or requesting a postoperative intensive care unit for observation.

b. **Most children** receive an inhalation induction, followed by placement of an appropriately sized IV. A technique consisting of a volatile agent, supplemented with an opioid (e.g., morphine 0.1 mg/kg IV) usually is performed. Glycopyrrolate (5 to 10 μg/kg IV) sometimes is administered to decrease secretion, and antiemetics should be considered. Muscle relaxation facilitates intubation but is not mandatory. Inadvertent endotracheal tube obstruction, disconnection, or dislodgment can occur during head and mouth gag manipulation. Oral rae tube provides better oral access for the surgeons and causes less kinking with the placement of retractors. Oral rae tube, as with other endotracheal tubes, should be firmly secured at the midline of the mandible for surgical access.

c. **At the end of surgery,** the throat pack should be removed, an orogastric tube should be placed to empty the stomach of any swallowed blood, and the pharynx should be suctioned thoroughly. Extubation may be performed under deep anesthesia or when the patient is awake with intact airway reflexes. Coughing on the endotracheal tube may be attenuated by the administration of lidocaine (1 to 1.5 mg/kg IV) 5 minutes before planned extubation. The use of an oropharyngeal airway after surgery can cause surgical wound disruption and bleeding if not carefully placed in the midline. Nasal airways are useful alternatives.

d. **After extubation,** patients are placed on their side, in a slight Trendelenburg position, and administered 100% oxygen. Auscultate for unobstructed breathing before transport to the postanesthesia care unit (PACU). Transport patients with supplemental oxygen. In the PACU, patients are given humidified oxygen by mask, monitored according to recovery room protocol, and checked for a dry pharynx before discharge.

2. Bleeding tonsil

a. **Rebleeding** after a pediatric tonsillectomy usually occurs within 24 hours after surgery but may be delayed for 5 to 10 days. Hematemesis, tachycardia, frequent swallowing, pallor, and airway obstruction may be seen.

The extent of blood loss is often underestimated because the blood is swallowed.

b. The induction of anesthesia in a bleeding, hypovolemic child can result in severe hypotension or cardiac arrest. Adequate IV access is necessary and the patient should be adequately resuscitated (with blood products if necessary) before reoperation. Hematocrit, coagulation studies, and availability of blood products should be ascertained. Doses of anesthetic agents may need to be reduced in the setting of hypovolemia.

c. Because the stomach is full of blood, ideally a **rapid-sequence induction** with cricoid pressure and in a slight head-down positioning of the patient should be performed to protect the trachea and glottis from aspiration of blood or stomach fluid. Two working suctions and an additional styletted endotracheal tube one size smaller than anticipated should be available. The surgeon should be present. Extubation is safest with the patient awake.

3. **A tonsillar or parapharyngeal abscess** may present with trismus, dysphagia, and a distorted, compromised airway. The surgeon may be able to decompress the abscess with needle aspiration before induction of anesthesia. If needed, an awake fiberoptic intubation may be performed. Anesthetic management and extubation procedures are similar to those for tonsillectomy (see section II.D.1). In Ludwig angina, a cellulitis of the submandibular and sublingual spaces may extend to the anterior compartments of the neck. Trismus, airway edema, and distorted anatomy often make visualization by direct laryngoscopy of the glottic opening difficult. General anesthesia is contraindicated if stridor occurs at rest. Consider tracheostomy under local anesthesia through the area of cellulitis, although not ideal, to secure the airway.

4. **Direct laryngoscopy** is indicated for diagnostic (biopsy) or therapeutic (vocal cord polyp removal) purposes and may involve potentially compromised airways. Evaluation of imaging studies (magnetic resonance imaging or computed tomography) and laboratory studies (pulmonary flow-volume loops) may help identify airway abnormalities and potential perioperative problems. Many patients have a history of smoking and cardiopulmonary disease.

a. **Anesthetic management** is described in Chapter 21, section IV.

b. **Postoperative airway edema** may develop. If anticipated, dexamethasone, 4 to 10 mg IV, may be given. Additional treatment includes head elevation, humidified oxygen by mask, and nebulized racemic epinephrine. Occasionally, cessation of nebulized racemic epinephrine is associated with the return of airway edema.

5. **Laser** (**l**ight **a**mplification by **s**timulated **e**mission of **r**adiation) produces a high-energy, high-density beam of coherent light that generates focused heat on contact with tissue. The emission media used to produce the monochromatic light determines the wavelength.

a. **Short wavelength (1 μm) laser** (argon gas, ruby, yttrium aluminum garnet [YAG]) emissions in the red–green visible part of the electromagnetic spectrum are poorly absorbed by water but well absorbed by pigmented tissues such as the retina and blood vessels.

b. **Infrared (10 μm) carbon dioxide laser** emissions are well absorbed by water and superficial surface cells and commonly are used to treat laryngeal lesions. They cannot be transmitted through fiberoptics.

c. **Eyes must be protected** from the laser beam. Operating room personnel must wear appropriate safety goggles (green-tinted for argon, amber for YAG, and clear for carbon dioxide) and the patient's eyes should be taped closed and covered with wet gauze.

d. **The most serious complication of laser airway surgery is airway fire.** The likelihood of fire depends on the gas environment of the airway, the energy level of the laser, the manner in which the laser is used, the presence of moisture, and the type of endotracheal tube used. Oxygen and nitrous oxide both support combustion. A safe gas mixture during laser upper airway surgery is oxygen/air or oxygen/helium to achieve a fraction of inspired oxygen of 25% to 30%.

e. **Safe laser use.** Lasers should be used intermittently, in the noncontinuous mode, and at moderate power (10 to 15 watts). Surgeons should not use the laser as a cautery and should share responsibility for fire prevention by limiting the energy input, allowing time for heat dispersal, packing aside nontarget tissue and endotracheal tube cuffs with moist gauze, and maintaining moisture (as a heat sink) in the field.

f. **Airway options during laser surgery.** Specially designed, fire-resistant, impregnated or shielded endotracheal tubes (e.g., Xomed-Treace Laser-Shield II endotracheal tube) are used and the cuff is filled with blue saline. For some procedures, intubation is not possible because the surgeon requires free access to the surgical field. Options include the following:

   (1) Jet-Venturi technique. This technique eliminates the need for endotracheal tube but airway fire may still occur due to the dry tissue igniting. All patients are at risk for barotrauma; pediatric patients, patients with emphysema, and patients with chronic obstructive pulmonary disease are at highest risk.

   (2) Ventilation and apneic oxygenation. The surgeon operates during periods of apnea and stops intermittently to allow the anesthesiologist to ventilate and oxygenate the patient.

g. **If an airway fire occurs,** stop ventilation and immediately disconnect the endotracheal tube from the breathing circuit, remove the tube, pour saline in the pharynx to absorb the heat, suction, and reintubate with a new endotracheal tube. While ventilating with 100% oxygen, examine the airway by bronchoscopy. **Complications** include airway edema, inhalation injury, tracheal and laryngeal granulation tissue formation, and airway stenosis.

    h. The **anesthetic technique** for laser surgery is similar to that described for endoscopy (see Chapter 21 and section in airway options during laser surgery). Goals include adequate surgical exposure, fire prevention, and return of protective airway reflexes before extubation. Surgeons may or may not request muscle relaxants for vocal cord examination or manipulation; therefore, communication with the surgical team is essential before proceeding with induction. Endotracheal intubation, jet ventilation, intermittent mask, or total intravenous anesthesia may be used; regardless of the technique, a mixture of oxygen/air is used (<30% oxygen). Because airway edema may occur, the patient is given humidified oxygen postoperatively and is observed closely in the PACU. Corticosteroids or aerosolized racemic epinephrine may be necessary.

III. Anesthesia for head and neck procedures

  A. **The primary anesthetic concern** during head and neck surgery is establishing and maintaining a secure airway.

    1. An **armored endotracheal tube** (e.g., Tovell) may be necessary to prevent kinking.

    2. An **elective tracheostomy** under local anesthesia may be performed before induction of general anesthesia for some extensive procedures or for those with the potential for acute airway obstruction.

    3. **Vocal cord paralysis.** Injury to one recurrent laryngeal nerve may cause unilateral vocal cord paralysis, a benign condition limited to hoarseness and a weak voice. Bilateral vocal cord paralysis, however, usually leads to increasing upper airway obstruction and stridor, and the patient will be unable to phonate. Obstruction may be relieved by positive-pressure ventilation while preparations are being made for reintubation. The patient may require tracheostomy for long-term airway management.

    4. **Bleeding** at the operative site after thyroid or parathyroid surgery may compress the trachea and cause airway obstruction. Opening the wound by placing a sterile hemostat through the incision allows egress of trapped blood. If this maneuver fails, the obstruction may be secondary to acute lymphedema and may necessitate immediate reintubation.

    5. **Teflon injection of the vocal cords** must be performed during awake laryngoscopy to continuously assess voice quality. The procedure should be performed with adequate local anesthesia and light sedation.

  B. **Radical neck dissection**

    1. **Patient condition.** These patients are often elderly, chronically debilitated, and malnourished and often have a history of tobacco and alcohol use. The severity of cardiac, pulmonary, renal, and hepatic disease will determine the extent of preoperative evaluation and choice of perioperative monitoring. Radical neck dissection in previously irradiated patients may be associated with large blood loss and difficult airway.

2. **Anesthetic technique.** A volatile anesthetic without a muscle relaxant is preferred to allow the surgeon to identify nerves with a nerve stimulator. A 15° to 30° head up-tilt and mild hypotension (mean arterial pressure 60 to 70 mm Hg), facilitated by a volatile anesthetic, vasodilators, or β-adrenergic antagonists, may help reduce blood loss. However, prolonged, profound hypotension and anemia may increase the risk of blindness.

3. During dissection, traction or pressure on the carotid sinus can cause **arrhythmias** such as bradycardia or asystole. Treatment is immediate cessation of the stimulus. If necessary, the surgeon can infiltrate local anesthetic near the sinus. Atropine (0.01 to 0.02 mg/kg IV) or glycopyrrolate (0.01 mg/kg) can be given if arrhythmias persist.

4. The patient is at risk for pneumothorax and venous air embolism during surgical dissection.

5. If airway compromise is anticipated postoperatively, the endotracheal tube is left in place or elective tracheostomy is performed.

6. Avoidance of hypothermia, adequate hydration with crystalloids, and minimizing the use of vasoconstrictors are desirable during reconstructive flap transfer surgery.

C. **Dentistry and oral and maxillofacial surgery**

1. Patients requiring general anesthesia for dentistry may be young children, adults with severe phobias, or the mentally or physically impaired; thus, they often require premedication. Oral midazolam (0.5 to 1.0 mg/kg) or rectal methohexital (25 mg/kg as a 10% solution) is suitable for children less than 5 years old. Intramuscular ketamine (3 to 5 mg/kg) with midazolam (0.05 to 0.1 mg/kg) and glycopyrrolate (0.01 mg/kg) may be necessary for the agitated or uncooperative patient.

2. **Nasal intubation** is usually preferred; care must be taken not to damage the turbinates or adenoids. Prior intubation, topicalization of the nasal mucosa with oxymetazoline (Afrin), use of a lubricant, and warming/softening the endotracheal tube before insertion may help to reduce epistaxis. The use of undiluted phenylephrine (1% solution) may cause profound hypertension and lead to pulmonary edema. The endotracheal tube should be securely taped, pressure on the nasal ala avoided, and eyes protected and padded.

3. Patients with maxillomandibular skeletal anomalies, temporomandibular pathology, facial fractures, intermaxillary fixation, or trismus may require fiberoptic intubation.

4. **Hypotensive anesthesia** (mean arterial pressure 60 to 70 mm Hg) for orthognathic surgery may reduce blood loss and can be facilitated by volatile anesthetics, α- and β-adrenergic blockers, nitroprusside, and head elevation. The overall medical condition of the patient may preclude the use of controlled hypotension.

5. If intermaxillary fixation with wires is present, the endotracheal tube is removed only when the patient is awake, edema has subsided, and bleeding is controlled. Administration of an antiemetic and decompression of the stomach with a nasogastric tube before extubation are recommended. Wire cutters

are kept at the bedside should emergent access to the mouth be necessary. Oral pharynx should be suctioned before extubation and before the jaw is wired.

SUGGESTED READING

Brimacombe J, Berry A. The laryngeal mask airway for dental surgery—a review. *Aust Dent J* 1995;40:10–14.

Donlon JV Jr. Anesthesia for eye, ear, nose, and throat surgery. In: Miller RD, ed. *Anesthesia,* 6th ed. New York: Churchill Livingstone, 2005: 2173–2198.

Ferrari LR, Vassallo SA. Anesthesia for otorhinolaryngology procedures and anesthesia for ophthalmology. In: Coté CJ, Todres ID, Ryan JF, Goudzousian N, eds. *A practice of anesthesia for infants and children,* 3rd ed. Philadelphia: WB Saunders, 2001:461–492.

Litman RS. Anesthesia for pediatric ophthalmologic surgery. In: Litman RS, ed. *Pediatric anesthesia the requisite in anesthesiology.* Philadelphia: Elsevier Mosby, 2004:267–274.

Litman RS, Samadi DS, Tobias JD. Anesthesia for pediatric ENT surgery. In: Litman RS, ed. *Pediatric anesthesia the requisite in anesthesiology.* Philadelphia: Elsevier Mosby, 2004:236–251.

McGoldrick KE, ed. *Anesthesia for ophthalmic and otolaryngologic surgery.* Philadelphia: WB Saunders, 1992.

Rampil IJ. Anesthesia for laser surgery. In: Miller RD, ed. *Anesthesia,* 6th ed. New York: Churchill Livingstone, 2005:2573–2587.

Supkis DE, Dougherty TB, Nguyen DT, et al. Anesthetic management of the patient undergoing head and neck cancer surgery. *Int Anesthesiol Clin* 1998;36: 21–29.

Troll GF. Regional ophthalmic anesthesia: safe techniques and avoidance of complications. *J Clin Anesth* 1995;7:163–172.

Anesthesia for Urologic Surgery

Ross Blank and William R. Kimball

I. **Anesthesia for specific urologic procedures**

A. **Cystoscopy and ureteroscopy** are performed to diagnose and treat lesions of the lower (urethra, prostate, bladder) and upper (ureter, kidney) urinary tracts.

  1. Warmed irrigation fluids are used to improve visualization and to remove blood, tissue, and stone fragments.

    a. **Electrolyte solutions,** such as normal saline and lactated Ringer's, are isotonic and do not cause hemolysis upon intravascular absorption. Because of ionization, they cannot safely be used for procedures involving electrocautery.

    b. **Sterile water** has optimal visibility and is nonconductive. However, intravascular absorption can cause hemolysis and hyponatremia/hypoosmolality.

    c. **Nonelectrolyte solutions** of glycine, sorbitol, and mannitol have good visibility and are nonconductive. Near isotonicity minimizes hemolysis, although large volume absorption may cause hyponatremia (without significant hypoosmolality).

  2. **Anesthesia**

    a. Depending on the patient and procedure, anesthesia for cystoscopy/ureteroscopy can range from topical lubrication alone to monitored anesthesia care to regional and/or general anesthesia. Placement of a rigid cystoscope (particularly in males) and distention of the bladder and ureters can be quite stimulating. However, postoperative pain is minimal.

    b. If regional anesthesia is used, a T-6 level is required for upper tract instrumentation, whereas a T-10 level is adequate for lower-tract surgery.

    c. General anesthesia can be effected with a variety of short-acting intravenous (IV) and inhaled anesthetics. Transient muscle relaxation may be required if manipulation of bladder lesions located near the obturator nerves causes involuntary leg movement.

    d. Lithotomy position is most common.

B. **Transurethral resection of the prostate (TURP)** is performed in older males to treat urinary obstruction due to benign prostatic hypertrophy. This procedure uses a modified cystoscope (resectoscope) with a wire loop connected to an electrocautery unit for resection of tissue and coagulation of bleeding vessels.

  1. During surgery, large prostatic venous sinuses are opened, which allows irrigant to be absorbed. The quantity of fluid absorbed depends on the following factors:

    a. Irrigant hydrostatic pressure, proportional to the height of the irrigant above the patient.

b. Surgical technique: duration of surgery, irrigation flow rate, and cystoscope size

c. Number and size of venous sinuses opened (influenced by prostate size).

d. Peripheral venous pressure (lower pressure favors increased absorption).

2. **Anesthesia**

a. If general anesthesia is used, it is essential to prevent coughing or patient movement, which can cause increased bleeding or bladder/prostatic capsule perforation. Positive pressure ventilation may decrease irrigant absorption by raising venous pressure.

b. Advantages of regional anesthesia may include an atonic bladder (improved surgical visualization) and elimination of bladder spasms (more rapid hemostasis postoperatively). In addition, awake patients may report symptoms that allow earlier detection of the TURP syndrome or bladder perforation.

c. Spinal anesthesia can be achieved with a hyperbaric solution of local anesthetic with or without opioid, providing adequate anesthesia with minimal hemodynamic effects. Some authors recommend a T-10 level because of possible pain from bladder distention. Lower venous pressures associated with neuraxial blockade may reduce bleeding but increase irrigant absorption.

d. Methods for monitoring fluid absorption intraoperatively include volumetric fluid balance, gravimetric weighing, and measurement of breath ethanol when a known amount of ethanol is added to the irrigating fluid.

3. **Complications**

a. **TURP syndrome** refers to a collection of neurologic and cardiovascular symptoms and signs caused by excessive irrigant absorption. It may appear early (direct intravascular absorption) or after several hours (absorption from retroperitoneal and perivesicular spaces). Similar concerns apply to hysteroscopic procedures in gynecology.

   (1) **Central nervous system** changes include nausea, agitation, confusion, visual changes, seizures, and coma. These effects are likely multifactorial and have been attributed to hyponatremia/hypoosmolality leading to cerebral edema, hyperglycinemia/hyperammonemia (glycine is hepatically metabolized to ammonia) associated with glycine solutions, and concomitant sedating medications.

   (2) Cardiovascular findings include hyper-/hypotension, bradycardia, dysrhythmias, pulmonary edema, and cardiac arrest, which are likely secondary to pronounced fluid shifts and associated electrolyte disturbances. Hypervolemia initially occurs with fluid absorption, followed by rapid redistribution of the irrigant to the interstitium.

   (3) The surgeon should be notified, the procedure completed as quickly as possible, and hemodynamic instability treated. There is disagreement in the literature about the most appropriate therapy. Fluid restriction and diuresis with furosemide have been advocated to treat volume overload, reserving hypertonic saline for severe symptoms or hyponatremia (serum sodium <120 mmol/L). Others suggest that the diuretic strategy may exacerbate intravascular volume depletion and hyponatremia and recommend early use of hypertonic saline (with slow correction of hyponatremia to minimize the risk of central pontine myelinolysis), reserving diuresis for acute pulmonary edema. In any case, therapy should be guided by regular measurements of serum sodium and osmolality.

b. Bladder perforation

(1) Extraperitoneal perforation is more common and manifests as suprapubic fullness, abdominal spasm, or pain in the suprapubic, inguinal, or periumbilical regions.

(2) Intraperitoneal perforation presents as upper abdominal pain or referred pain from the diaphragm to the shoulder; this may result in hypertension, tachycardia, and abdominal distention, followed by hypotension and cardiovascular collapse.

c. Bacteremia is likely due to absorption of bacteria through prostatic venous sinuses, commonly associated with indwelling urinary catheters or with subclinical/partially treated prostatitis.

d. Blood loss and coagulopathy. Assessing blood loss is extremely difficult during TURP because of massive dilution by irrigant.

(1) Continuous postoperative bleeding may result from dilutional thrombocytopenia, disseminated intravascular coagulation, or the release of fibrinolytic enzymes from the prostate.

(2) Hemodynamic responses to blood loss may be masked by hypervolemia from irrigant absorption.

4. Alternatives to TURP include medical management (alpha blockers, hormonal therapies) and newer minimally invasive techniques including laser ablation, microwave thermotherapy, and prostatic stents. Although such procedures have not been compared with TURP in large prospective trials, they have been advocated for patients whose comorbidities place them at heightened risk for surgical or anesthetic complications.

C. Open prostatectomies are performed for resection of large prostatic masses or, more commonly, tumors.

1. Anesthesia

a. These operations may be performed safely under general, general/epidural, epidural, or spinal anesthesia. Several small-scale prospective randomized trials have compared general with epidural techniques and have found modest benefits of epidural anesthesia in reducing operative blood loss, reducing postoperative pain, and hastening recovery of bowel function, while other studies have shown little difference in outcomes. However, any benefits must be weighed against the observation that experienced surgeons routinely perform prostatectomies under general anesthesia with minimal blood loss, pain well-controlled by intraoperative opioid and postoperative nonsteroidal anti-inflammatory drug analgesia, and short hospital stays with discharge as early as postoperative day 1.

    b. Diagnostic dyes may be used during the procedure to demonstrate the integrity of the reconstructed urinary tract.

        (1) Methylene blue 1% (1 mL) bolus may lead to hypotension. It may also cause transient erroneous decreases in pulse oximetry readings (SaO_2) to as low as 65%, lasting 10 to 70 seconds.

        (2) Indigo carmine 0.8% (5 mL), an alpha-agonist, may cause hypertension.

    c. Urine output measurements are interrupted during mobilization of the prostatic urethra.

  2. Complications generally are related to blood loss, including hypothermia, anemia, and coagulopathy. Large-bore IV access is recommended.

D. Nephrectomy is performed for neoplasm, transplantation, chronic infection, trauma, and severe cystic or calculous disease.

  1. Patients undergoing nephrectomy for renal cell carcinoma require preoperative staging. If the tumor extends into the inferior vena cava (IVC) or right atrium, two potential complications need to be considered:

    a. The tumor may partially or fully occlude the IVC, leading to poor venous return and hypotension. Full resection of tumor may necessitate temporary clamping of the IVC, with attendant exacerbation of decreased venous return requiring vasopressor support. Intraoperative transesophageal echocardiogram can be used to monitor such tumor thrombus.

    b. Tumor fragments may embolize to the pulmonary circulation. Consequently, pulmonary artery catheterization and some central venous access approaches are risky if catheter placement dislodges tumor in the IVC or right atrium. **Cardiopulmonary bypass** may be used to minimize the risk of pulmonary emboli intraoperatively.

  2. Anesthesia

    a. The patient is positioned supine for a transabdominal approach or in the lateral decubitus position for a retroperitoneal approach. In the lateral position, a kidney rest and table flexion are often used to improve exposure. Hypotension can be produced by the kidney rest position, likely due to IVC compression.

    b. A thoracoabdominal incision may be required for larger or upper pole tumors.

    c. Combined general/epidural anesthesia is commonly used to maximize postoperative analgesia with an upper abdominal or thoracoabdominal incision.

    d. Large-bore IV access with or without arterial line is required as blood loss can be massive because of the size and vascularity of the tumor.

E. Radical cystectomy with or without ileal/colonic conduit is performed for invasive bladder tumors. Other patients with pelvic malignancies, neurogenic bladder dysfunction, chronic lower urinary tract obstruction, or postradiation bladder dysfunction may require an ileal or colonic urinary diverting procedure.

1. **Anesthesia**
   a. Large-bore IV access is imperative as significant blood loss may occur.
   b. Arterial or central venous access may be indicated as large volume shifts occur while the ureters are disconnected.
   c. Combined general/epidural anesthesia should be considered.

F. **Orchidopexy, orchiectomy, and urogenital plastic surgery procedures** are performed to treat congenital deformities, neoplasms, and impotence. Patients with torsion of the testicle may require emergency reduction and orchidopexy to prevent ischemia. A T-9 sensory level is required of regional anesthesia.

G. **Laparoscopic techniques** increasingly are being used to perform traditionally open procedures including prostatectomy, nephrectomy, cystectomy, pyeloplasty, and stone extraction. Traditional laparoscopic ports are used with some procedures requiring a limited incision for hand assistance. Robotic systems may be used to control the camera. Laparoscopic prostatectomies in particular are promoted for their minimal invasiveness and comparable clinical outcomes, although they have not been compared with open procedures in randomized controlled trials and long-term follow-up is lacking. Anesthetic considerations are similar to those for laparoscopic procedures in general surgery or gynecology. Retroperitoneal insufflation of carbon dioxide may be associated with increased systemic absorption compared with intraperitoneal insufflation, although reports are conflicting.

H. **Renal transplantation** is performed for patients with end-stage renal disease. The recipients commonly have hypertension and/or diabetes mellitus and are at increased risk for coronary artery disease and congestive heart failure. Attention must also be paid to the electrolyte and acid-base abnormalities, anemia, and platelet dysfunction commonly seen in uremic patients. Preoperative dialysis, if possible, can improve potassium and acid-base abnormalities.

1. **Anesthesia**
   a. IV access may be difficult and placement in extremities with fistulas or shunts should be avoided; the benefits of additional invasive monitors (arterial or central venous lines) should be weighed against the risks of catheter-related sepsis in immunosuppressed patients.
   b. Medications with primarily renal metabolism should be avoided or decreased in dose.
   c. Patients may have delayed gastric emptying from diabetes, uremia, and preoperative opioids.
   d. Hyperkalemia may contraindicate succinylcholine.
   e. Regional anesthesia may be contraindicated by coagulopathy.
   f. Normal saline may be preferred to lactated Ringer's when hyperkalemia is present.
   g. Graft function depends on adequate intravascular volume before and after vascular anastomosis to maintain perfusion to the transplanted kidney. Useful intravascular volume expanders include crystalloid, albumin, and mannitol.

h. Intraoperative hypotension may compromise renal perfusion and should be treated promptly by addressing mechanical factors such as IVC compression or treating hypovolemia with additional volume. If pharmacologic support is necessary, inotropes (dopamine, dobutamine) are preferred to alpha-agonists (phenylephrine, norepinephrine), which may raise systemic blood pressure but decrease renal blood flow via vasoconstriction. In cases of marked acidemia, sodium bicarbonate may improve hemodynamics.

i. Urine output provides an immediate gauge of renal function, which may be affected by hypovolemia, acute rejection, or patency of the anastomoses. Both mannitol and furosemide may be requested to promote diuresis after anastomosis.

II. Extracorporeal shock wave lithotripsy (ESWL)

A. ESWL focuses acoustic shock waves at urinary stones. At interfaces between materials of differing density, such as between soft tissue and stones, reflections of these acoustic waves set up complex patterns of internal echoes resulting in stresses that cause stones to fracture. While early-generation lithotripters required patient immersion into water baths, current models allow positioning on an operating table and have smaller cutaneous "shock entry" zones.

B. Anesthesia

1. The patient is generally positioned supine but may be prone depending on the precise location of the stone(s). Lithotomy position may be necessary for cystoscopy or stent placement.

2. Monitored anesthesia care is usually adequate with newer lithotripters, as they cause much less pain than first-generation devices. Adequate pain control can generally be achieved with IV short-acting opioids (i.e., remifentanil, alfentanil) with additional sedation titrated to patient comfort. Many other strategies have been used successfully including neuraxial blockade and general anesthesia.

3. Adequate IV hydration with occasional diuretic supplementation may aid passage of stone fragments.

4. Absolute contraindications are pregnancy, untreated infections or bleeding diatheses, and abdominal pacemakers. Relative contraindications are pacemakers/ICDs, abdominal aortic or renal artery aneurysms, orthopedic prostheses, and morbid obesity.

C. Complications

1. Ureteral colic soon after the procedure may manifest as nausea, vomiting, or bradycardia.

2. Hematuria is common and treated with hydration and diuretics.

3. Cardiac dysrhythmias such as bradycardia, premature atrial contractions, and premature ventricular contractions occur secondary to mechanical strains on the cardiac conduction system during the procedure. If premature ventricular contractions are frequent or symptomatic, they may be minimized by synchronization of the shock waves to the cardiac cycle.

4. Renal (subcapsular) hematoma may result from collateral damage to renal vasculature, especially in hypertensive patients.

5. Hypertension occurs primarily in patients who have autonomic dysreflexia.

6. Severe pulmonary or intestinal damage is rare and occurs if the shock waves are inadvertently applied to the lung or intestines, as may occur with a patient movement during treatment.

III. **Patients with spinal cord pathology**

A. Spinal cord injury frequently causes urinary retention, which promotes urinary tract infections, nephrolithiasis, and vesicoureteric reflux. Urologic procedures are a common reason for patients with chronic spinal cord injury to present to the operating room.

B. **Autonomic dysreflexia** is a condition manifested by acute onset of sympathetic hyperreactivity to certain stimuli below the cord lesion in patients with lesions generally at or above the T-6 to T-7 level. The syndrome may appear at any time from a few months to many years after the injury.

1. Common findings include hypertension (potentially severe), headache, diaphoresis, flushing or pallor, and bradycardia.

2. Common precipitants include visceral stimulation, most commonly bladder distension, although urinary tract infection, fecal impaction, uterine contraction, bowel distention, and other intra-abdominal and cutaneous stimuli have been reported.

3. Pathophysiology is thought to involve disorganized connections between afferent neurons and sympathetic neurons at the level of the injury that lead to inappropriate sympathetic responses unmitigated by descending inhibition.

4. Treatment of autonomic dysreflexia includes removal of the inciting stimulus, increasing anesthetic depth, and pharmacologic treatment of persistent hypertension with rapidly acting agents such as sublingual nifedipine or IV nitroglycerin or nitroprusside.

5. Neuraxial anesthesia has the advantage of blocking both limbs of the reflex arc and thereby preventing autonomic dysreflexia. However, determining the level of anesthesia by cutaneous testing is difficult with a preexisting complete sensory deficit. For short procedures, spinal may be preferable to epidural anesthesia because of more reliable block without spared segments; saddle block may be sufficient for many urologic procedures.

SUGGESTED READING

Conacher ID, et al. Anaesthesia for laparoscopic urological surgery. *Br J Anaesth* 2004;93(6):859–864.

Gottschalk A, et al. Preemptive epidural analgesia and recovery from radical prostatectomy: a randomized controlled trial. *JAMA* 1998;279(14):1076–1082.

Gravenstein D. Extracorporeal shock wave lithotripsy and percutaneous nephrolithotomy. *Anesthesiol Clin North Am* 2000;18(4):953–971.

Hahn RG. Fluid absorption in endoscopic surgery. *Br J Anaesth* 2006;96(1):8–20.

Hambly PR, Martin B. Anaesthesia for chronic spinal cord lesions. *Anaesthesia* 1998;53:273–289.

Sprung J, et al. Anesthesia for kidney transplant surgery. *Anesthesiol Clin North Am* 2000;18(4):919–951.

Streich B, et al. Increased carbon dioxide absorption during retroperitoneal laparoscopy. *Br J Anaesth* 2003;91(6):793–796.

Trabulsi EJ, Guillonneau B. Laparoscopic radical prostatectomy. *J Urol* 2005;173:1072–1079.

Whalley DG. Anesthesia for radical prostatectomy, cystectomy, nephrectomy, pheochromocytoma, and laparoscopic procedures. *Anesthesiol Clin North Am* 2000;18(4):899–917.

Yokoyama M, et al. Haemodynamic effects of the lateral decubitus and the kidney rest lateral decubitus position during anaesthesia. *Br J Anaesth* 2000;84(6): 753–757.

27

Anesthesia for Geriatric Patients

Zhongcong Xie and Jill Lanahan

I. **Physiology changes associated with aging**
   A. **Cardiovascular**
      1. **Arteries stiffen with age,** leading to faster propagation and reflection of the pulse pressure waveform. The reflected waveform augments the pressure at the aortic root. With increasing age, the reflected energy arrives progressively earlier in the cardiac cycle, shifting from early diastole to late systole. Thus, aging causes decreased diastolic and increased systolic pressure (and pulse pressure) and leads to ventricular thickening and prolonged ejection.
      2. **Slower myocardial relaxation and ventricular hypertrophy** lead to late diastolic filling and diastolic dysfunction. Atrial contraction is important to maintain late filling.
      3. **Reduced venous capacitance** decreases the "vascular reserve volume" available to buffer hemorrhage.
      4. **Reduced baroreceptor reflexes** result from increased sympathetic tone, decreased parasympathetic tone, decreased baroreceptor sensitivity, and decreased responsiveness to β-adrenergic stimulation. Thus, hypotension occurs frequently with changes in volume, position, anesthetic depth, and regional anesthetic-induced sympathetic blockade.
      5. **Maximal heart rate decreases with age while stroke volume remains constant,** but end-diastolic volume increases and ejection fraction decreases.
      6. **Maximal oxygen consumption decreases** because of reductions in arteriovenous oxygen tension difference and cardiac output.
   B. **Respiratory**
      1. **Parenchymal changes.** Approximately 30% of alveolar wall tissue is lost between ages 20 and 80, diminishing elastic recoil and parenchymal traction that maintain airway patency. The loss produces the following:
         a. **Increased residual volume, closing volume, and functional residual capacity;** decreased vital capacity and forced expiratory volume in first second.
         b. **Progressive mismatching of ventilation to perfusion,** with an age-dependent decrease in arterial oxygen tension.
         c. **Increased physiologic dead space** and reduced diffusing capacity.
      2. **Chest wall changes:** multiple factors lead to a stiffer chest wall, while respiratory muscle mass decreases.
      3. **Depressed ventilatory response** to hypoxia and hypercarbia.
      4. **Decreased protective airway reflexes** increase aspiration risk.
   C. **Central nervous system**
      1. Progressive loss of neurons and decreased neurotransmitter

activity contribute to **decreased anesthetic requirements** for all agents.

    2. Cerebral autoregulatory responses to blood pressure, CO_2, and O_2 are maintained.

D. Renal

    1. **Serum creatinine remains stable** with advancing age because age-associated decreases of creatinine clearance are offset by reduced creatinine production from skeletal muscle. A normal creatinine level in the elderly should not be interpreted as an absence of renal impairment. For example, a healthy 80-year-old patient is expected to have half the creatinine clearance of a 20-year-old patient, even though they may have similar serum creatinine levels.

    2. Progressive atrophy of renal parenchyma and sclerosis of vascular structures lead to **diminished renal blood flow and glomerular filtration rate.**

    3. Reduced ability to correct alterations in electrolyte concentrations, intravascular volume, and free water.

    4. **Reduced glomerular filtration rate** leads to delayed renal drug excretion.

E. Hepatic

    1. Decreased liver mass as well as portal and hepatic blood flows result in reduced hepatic drug clearance.

    2. Cytochrome P-450 activity decreases with aging.

    3. Phase 1 (oxidation and reduction) and phase 2 (conjugation) reactions may be depressed with aging.

F. Body composition and thermoregulation

    1. Basal metabolism and heat production decrease because of skeletal muscle atrophy and variable replacement with adipose tissue.

    2. The propensity for hypothermia increases because of blunted central thermoregulation and body compositional changes.

    3. Decreases in muscle mass and total body water, coupled with increases in body fat, reduce the volume of distribution of water-soluble drugs and increase it for lipid-soluble drugs.

II. Pharmacology changes associated with aging

  A. Pharmacokinetics changes in elderly

    1. **Protein binding of anesthetic drugs is reduced** because of decreased quantity of circulating serum protein—e.g., albumin. Pharmacological effects are therefore potentiated.

    2. Reduction in blood volume, an increase in percentage of body fat, and a decrease in hepatic and renal function result in prolonged drug elimination anesthetic effects.

  B. Pharmacodynamic changes in elderly

    1. The brain is more sensitive to drugs in the elderly. There is a reduction in neuronal density, cerebral blood flow, and oxygen consumption that results in an **age-related reduction in inhalation and intravenous anesthetic requirements.**

    2. Drug sensitivity varies with the type of drug. Responses to specific drugs are difficult to predict and may vary widely in the elderly. For example, catecholamines require higher doses for equivalent effects, and benzodiazepines exert greater effects in the elderly.

3. The rate of adverse drug reaction increases with age and with the number of drugs administered.

III. **Anesthesia consideration for elderly patients**
   A. **Preoperative evaluation**
      1. Age-related coexisting disease is a major predictor for perioperative mortality and serious morbidity. Age-related coexisiting disease increases elderly patients' risks for perioperative
         a. Myocardial infarction
         b. Congestive heart failure
         c. Delirium
         d. Stroke
         e. Aspiration and pneumonia
         f. Sepsis
         g. Adverse drug reactions
         h. Falls
         i. Pressure sores
      2. Age alone is a minor predictor for perioperative complications.
      3. **Assessment of health and functional status.** A detailed history and physical examination is required, with emphasis on physical condition, ambulation, activities of daily living, preoperative living situation, and preexisting disabilities.
      4. **Preoperative testing. Testing should be based on coexisting disease and recommended guidelines (see Chapter 1). Recommended testing in elderly patients includes** electrocardiogram, chest radiograph, complete blood count, electrolyte panel that includes blood urea nitrogen, creatinine, potassium (especially if the patient is receiving a diuretic), and glucose.
   B. **Intraoperative management**
      1. **Major risk factors** for serious adverse perioperative events in the elderly include emergency surgery, operative site within a major body cavity, vascular surgery, and poor American Society of Anesthesiologists physical status.
      2. No significant difference in perioperative complications can be attributed to any specific anesthetic agent or to regional versus general anesthesia.
      3. In general, the elderly have reduced functional reserves of all organ systems and a diminished therapeutic index of anesthetic interventions. The therapeutic diminution is highly variable and unpredictable because of environmental effects, physical deconditioning, and undiagnosed diseases. Diminished functional reserves may be manifest only under severe stress, such as that of surgery. Thus, vigilance and preparation for contingencies are essential in conducting anesthesia for the elderly.

IV. **Anesthesia care for patients with aging-related diseases**
   A. **Disorders of the central nervous system**
      1. **Delirium** is "a transient potentially reversible disorder of cognition and attention characterized by an acute onset and a fluctuating course."
         a. Risk factors include dementia, use of psychoactive drugs, hip fractures and electrolyte abnormalities.
         b. Common causes include acute infection, hypoxemia, hypotension, use of psychoactive drugs, and stroke.

    c. **Pathophysiology.** The most frequently proposed explanations are decreased cholinergic activity and increased anticholinergic activity.

    d. Treatment focuses on treating any underlying disorder, encouraging interaction with family members, encouraging normal sleep-wake cycles, and avoiding restraints, if possible. Haloperidol and benzodiazepines are commonly used pharmacotherapies.

2. **Dementia** is a persistent impairment of cognitive and emotional abilities that interferes with activities of daily living.

    a. Alzheimer disease is the most common cause of dementia in the elderly and affects 30% to 50% of people by age 85.

        (1) Pathogenesis is thought to be related to the aberrant production and deposition of Aβ peptide, the dominant component of neuritic plaques.

        (2) The pathologic hallmarks of the disease include neurofibrillary tangles, neuritic plaques, neuronal thread protein, and marked cortical atrophy with ventricular enlargement.

        (3) The current treatment is with cholinesterase inhibitors such as tacrine, donepezil, and rivastigmine.

        (4) Anesthetic considerations include avoiding preoperative sedation and avoiding centrally acting anticholinergic agents. Hypoxia and hypocapnia should also be avoided in patients with Alzheimer disease.

    b. Other causes of dementia include Pick disease, vascular dementia, Parkinson disease, normal pressure hydrocephalus, and Creutzfeldt-Jakob disease.

3. **Parkinson disease** is characterized by diminished facial expression, stooped posture, slowness of voluntary movement, shuffling gait, and "pill rolling" tremor.

    a. **Pathogenesis.** Degeneration of dopaminergic neurons of the substantia nigra, which project to the striatum, and a reduction in striatal dopamine content result in the clinical manifestations of tremor, rigidity, bradykinesia, and impairment of postural and righting reflexes.

    b. **Pharyngeal and laryngeal muscle dysfunction may increase the risk for aspiration.**

    c. About 10% to 15% of patients with Parkinson disease develop dementia.

    d. Treatment is directed at controlling symptoms and includes anticholinergics, levodopa, and dopamine agonists such as bromocriptine and pergolide.

    e. Anesthetic considerations.

        (1) Antiparkinsonian medications should be continued perioperatively because of the short half-life of levodopa.

        (2) Phenothiazines, butyrophenones, and metoclopramide should be avoided as they may exacerbate symptoms as a consequence of their antidopaminergic activity.

        (3) Anticholinergics and antihistamines may be used for acute exacerbations.

    (4)   Patients with pharyngeal/laryngeal muscle involvement should receive a rapid sequence induction with cricoid pressure.

    (5)   Response to nondepolarizing muscle relaxants is normal. Hyperkalemia has been reported in a Parkinson patient who received succinylcholine.

    (6)   Hemodynamic instability may occur with induction of anesthesia, especially in patients receiving long-term levodopa therapy. Invasive arterial blood pressure monitoring may be warranted. Direct-acting vasopressors (e.g., phenylephrine) should be used to treat hypotension.

    (7)   Cardiac irritability may increase the risk for dysrhythmias. Ketamine and local anesthetics with epinephrine should be used cautiously.

B. Visual impairment in the elderly

    1. Cataracts are opacities of the crystalline lens that may affect visual acuity, contrast sensitivity, and light perception.

        a.   The prevalence of cataracts approaches 100% in patients 90 years old.

        b.   Cataract surgery is the most commonly performed surgery in elderly patients and is the only effective therapy for cataracts.

        c.   Anesthesia for cataract surgery can be general or regional (retrobulbar block, see Chapter 25).

    2. Glaucoma is an optic neuropathy with peripheral vision loss occurring before loss of central vision. It is characterized by an acute (narrow-angle) or chronic (usually open-angle) increase in intraocular pressure.

        a.   Treatments include beta-blockers (decrease aqueous production by the ciliary bodies), miotic eye drops (constrict the pupils to enhance aqueous outflow), carbonic anhydrase inhibitors (decrease aqueous production from the ciliary bodies), and synthetic prostaglandin (decreases intraocular pressure).

        b.   Use of anticholinergic drugs as a preoperative medication or in combination with anticholinesterases to reverse neuromuscular blockade is acceptable because these drugs do not result in significant pupillary dilation.

        c.   **Scopolamine should be avoided** as it may cause a significant increase in the diameter of the pupil.

        d.   Use of succinylcholine may cause a transient increase in intraocular pressure.

    3. Macular degeneration is the deterioration of the central portion of the retina with preservation of peripheral vision. Cigarette smoking is a risk factor for macular degeneration.

    4. Retinal detachment is separation between the photoreceptors and retinal pigment epithelium with accumulation of fluid or blood in the potential space. **Nitrous oxide should be avoided** as the gas may diffuse into any air bubbles within the globe.

C. Cervical spine changes associated with aging

    1. Extension and flexion of the neck are diminished.

    2. Loss of flexibility and extensibility of the cervical spine increases the distance from the posterior portion of the cricoid ring to

the anterior portion of the vertebral body. It may be difficult to apply effective cricoid pressure.
3. Direct laryngoscopy may be more difficult in elderly patients, and fiberoptic tracheal intubation may be indicated when neck mobility is severely limited.
D. **Hip fractures are a major cause of disability, functional impairment, and death in the elderly.**
1. **Risk factors** include osteoporosis, gait disturbances, physical inactivity, and poor general health.
2. The choice of anesthesia has not been shown to affect postoperative morbidity and mortality.
E. **Dehydration**
1. **Types of dehydration**
a. Isotonic—the balanced loss of sodium and water, as in fasting, diarrhea, vomiting.
b. Hypertonic—water losses exceed sodium losses, as in fever.
c. Hypotonic—sodium losses exceed water losses, as in diuretic use.
2. **Diagnosis of dehydration** may be difficult because symptoms may be vague or absent in the elderly. Indicators include the following:
a. Poor skin turgor.
b. High urine specific gravity.
c. Orthostatic hypotension or orthostatic increase in heart rate.
d. Blood urea nitrogen:creatinine ratio >25.
3. **Treatment of dehydration**
a. Fluid requirement in the elderly is about **30 mL/kg/day** and may be replaced orally (by sports replacement drinks or the equivalent) or parenterally.
b. Patients should be monitored carefully for signs and symptoms of volume overload.
F. **Malnutrition**
1. **Incidence** of malnutrition is **20% to 40%** of elderly inpatients.
2. **Predisposing factors** of malnutrition are congestive heart failure, chronic obstructive pulmonary disease, and cancer.
3. **Indicators of malnutrition** include weight loss, low body mass index, nutrient-related disorder (e.g., anemia), and albumin <3.5 g/dL.

SUGGESTED READING

Cook DJ. *Geriatric anesthesia.* www.americangeriatrics.org, 2004.

Gibbs J, Cull W, Henderson W, Daley J, Hur K, Khuri SF. Preoperative serum albumin level as a predictor of operative mortality and morbidity: results from the National VA Surgical Risk Study. *Arch Surg* 1999;134:36–42.

O'Hara DA, Duff A, Berlin JA, et al. The effect of anesthetic technique on postoperative outcomes in hip fracture repair. *Anesthesiology* 2000;84:450–455.

Pedersen T, Eliasen K, Henriksen E. A prospective study of mortality associated with anaesthesia and surgery: risk indicators of mortality in hospital. *Acta Anaesthesiol Scand* 1990;34:176–182.

Stoelting RK, Dierdorf SF. Diseases associated with aging. In: *Anesthesia and co-existing Disease,* 4th ed. New York: Churchill Livingstone, 2002:739–756.

Williamson J, Chopin JM. Adverse reactions to prescribed drugs in the elderly: a multicentre investigation. *Age Ageing* 1980;9:73–80.

28

Anesthesia for Surgical Emergencies in the Neonate

Jesse D. Roberts Jr., Ion Hobai, and
Jonathan H. Cronin

I. **Development**
   A. **Organogenesis** is virtually complete after the 12th gestational week
   B. **Respiratory development**
      1. **Anatomic**
         a. **The lungs** begin as a bud on the embryonic gut in the fourth week of gestation. Failure of separation of the lung bud from the gut later results in the formation of a **tracheoesophageal fistula (TEF).**
         b. **The diaphragm** forms during the 10th week of gestation, dividing the abdominal and thoracic cavities.
            (1) If the diaphragm is not completely formed when the midgut reenters the abdomen from the umbilical pouch, the abdominal contents can enter the thorax.
            (2) The presence of abdominal contents within the thorax is associated with arrested lung growth.
            (3) The lungs from patients with **congenital diaphragmatic hernia** have a decreased number of arterioles in the hypoplastic lung. In addition, the pulmonary arteries of both lungs are abnormally thick and reactive, resulting in increased pulmonary vascular resistance.
      2. **Physiologic**
         a. **Lung development** is generally insufficient for survival at less than the 23rd week of gestation.
         b. Secretion of **surfactant,** which reduces alveolar wall surface tension and promotes alveolar aeration, is inadequate until the last month of gestation.
            (1) Birth before 32 weeks gestation is associated with **respiratory distress syndrome (RDS).**
            (2) Because glucose metabolism affects lung maturation, babies from mothers with diabetes may have RDS if born later in gestation.
            (3) Antenatal treatment with steroids is associated with a decrease in the incidence of RDS in premature newborns.
         c. After birth, the onset of breathing is stimulated by hypoxemia, hypercarbia, tactile stimulation, and a decrease in plasma prostaglandin E_2. After aeration and distension of the lung, the pulmonary vascular resistance decreases, and pulmonary blood flow increases nearly 10-fold. Failure of the reduction of pulmonary vascular resistance after birth is associated with extrapulmonary shunting of blood

and severe hypoxemia and is called **persistent pulmonary hypertension in the newborn (PPHN).**

C. **Cardiovascular development**
1. **Anatomic**
   a. The primitive **cardiac tube** forms during the first month of gestation and consists of the sinoatrium, the primitive ventricle, the bulbus cordis (primitive right ventricle), and the truncus (primitive main pulmonary artery). During the second month of gestation, a heart with two parallel pumping systems develops out of this initially tubular system. During this process, various structures divide and migrate. Failure of structural maturation at this stage of development causes numerous cardiac malformations. For example:
      (1) Failure of division of the sinoatrium into the two atria results in a single atrium. Improper closure results in an **atrial septal defect.**
      (2) Failure of migration of the ventricular septum and atrioventricular valve between the primitive ventricle and the bulbus cordis results in a **double-outlet left ventricle** (single ventricle). Minor migrational defects result in a **ventriculoseptal defect.**
      (3) Failure of division of the truncus into the pulmonary artery and the aorta results in **truncus arteriosus.**
   b. The aortic arch system initially consists of six pairs of arches.
      (1) The sixth arches produce the pulmonary arteries. The **ductus arteriosus** develops from the distal portion of the right sixth arch. Although the left proximal sixth arch usually degenerates, it can persist and form an aberrant left ductus arteriosus.
      (2) Failure of regression of various portions of the aorta and arch system can result in aberrant vessels. For example, failure of regression causes a **double aortic arch.** Regression of the left-sided but not the right-sided arches can result in a right-sided aortic arch.
2. **Physiologic**
   a. **Fetal circulation:** After the 12th week, the circulatory system is in its final form. Oxygenated blood from the placenta passes through the umbilical vein and the ductus venosus and returns to the heart. Subsequently, most of the blood bypasses the pulmonary circulation by passing right to left through the foramen ovale and the ductus arteriosus into the aorta.
   b. **At birth,** umbilical placental circulation ceases with the clamping of the umbilical cord. The blood flow through the ductus venosus decreases. The ductus venosus closes in 3 to 7 days. The decrease in venous return causes reduced right atrial pressure and functional closure of the foramen ovale. At the same time, the gas exchange is transferred from the placenta to the newly ventilated lungs. Pulmonary resistance decreases as the postnatal pulmonary circulation is established, and systemic resistance increases because the high-capacitance placental circulation has been removed. With increasing Pao_2, constriction

of the ductus arteriosus occurs. Cessation of ductus arteriosus blood flow often occurs within several hours.

D. Body composition

1. **Extracellular fluid** (ECF) decreases as the fetus grows. ECF is 90% of total body weight at 28 weeks, 80% at 36 weeks, and 75% at term.

2. After birth, a physiologic diuresis occurs, with the term infant losing 5% to10% of ECF in the first few days of life. Premature infants may lose up to 15% of ECF.

3. Before 32 weeks of gestation, the **neonatal kidney is immature** and less able to concentrate urine or handle solute loads. Renal tubular function improves with postnatal age.

II. General assessment

A. History

1. In collecting the **neonate's history,** it is important to include information about antenatal events. Fetal growth and development are affected by **maternal disorders,** including hypertension, diabetes, and drug, cigarette, and alcohol use. Polyhydramnios, abnormal α-fetoprotein, maternal infections, and premature labor are often associated with neonatal problems.

2. **Perinatal history** also includes gestational age, time of onset of labor and rupture of membranes, use of tocolytics and fetal monitors, signs of fetal distress, type of anesthesia used at and the mode of the newborn's delivery (spontaneous, forceps or vacuum assisted, or cesarean), condition of the infant at delivery, Apgar scores, and immediate resuscitation steps required. Also inquire about and ensure that vitamin K and ocular antibiotic ointment were given after birth.

B. Physical examination

1. A complete, systematic evaluation is needed. No assumptions should be made about the development, location, or function of organ systems. An abnormality in one system may be associated with abnormalities in another.

2. **Vital signs** provide a useful physiologic screen of organ function. If a cardiac abnormality is suspected, an electrocardiogram (ECG) and four extremity blood pressure measurements are required. In addition, an echocardiogram and pediatric cardiology consultation should be considered. Normal vital signs are summarized in Table 28.1.

3. **The Apgar score** reflects the degree of intrapartum stress as well as the effectiveness of initial resuscitation (Table 28.2). Points are awarded for each of the five criteria, with the maximum score being 10. Although the Apgar score at 1 minute

Table 28.1. Normal vital signs

Vital Sign	Term	Preterm
Pulse (beats/min)	80–120	120–160
Respiration (breaths/min)	30–40	50–70
Blood pressure (mm Hg)	60–90/40–60	40–60/20–40
Temperature (°C)	37.5 (rectal)	37.5

Table 28.2. Apgar scores

Sign	Score		
	0	1	2
Heart rate	Absent	<100/min	>100/min
Respiratory effort	Absent	Irregular	Good, crying
Muscle tone	Limp	Some flexion	Active motion
Reflex irritability	Absent	Grimace	Cough or sneeze
Color	Blue	Acrocyanosis	Completely pink

correlates with intrauterine conditions, the 5- and 10-minute Apgar scores correlate best with neonatal outcome.

4. **Gestational age** influences care, management, and survival potential of the neonate. An infant is considered preterm if the gestational age is less than 37 weeks, term if it is 37 to 41 weeks, and postterm if the gestational age is more than 42 weeks. Although the date of conception and ultrasound examination can be used to predict gestational age, a physical examination and Dubowitz scoring to determine gestational age should be performed. **The Dubowitz scoring system** involves evaluation of physical characteristics of the skin, external genitalia, ears, breasts, and neuromuscular behavior to assess gestational age.

5. **Weight determination.** Infants who are **small for gestational age** often have had intrauterine growth retardation. This may be the result of chromosomal defects, maternal hypertension, chronic placental insufficiency, maternal cigarette or drug use, or congenital infection. These infants have a high incidence of hypoglycemia, hypocalcemia, and polycythemia. Infants who are **large for gestational age** (LGA) may have mothers with diabetes. In the immediate postnatal period, LGA newborns should be evaluated for hypoglycemia and polycythemia.

6. **Respiratory.** Signs of respiratory distress include tachypnea, grunting, nasal flaring, intercostal retractions, rales, rhonchi, asymmetry of breath sounds, and apneic periods. **Pulse oximetry** is used to screen the levels of systemic oxygenation in neonates.

7. **Cardiovascular.** Central cyanosis and capillary refill should be assessed. Distal pulses should be palpated, noting whether they are bounding. A delay between brachial and femoral pulses is suggestive of **coarctation of the aorta.** Note the character and location of murmurs and splitting of the second heart sound. During the first 48 hours, murmurs may appear as intracardiac pressure gradients change, or they may disappear as the ductus arteriosus closes.

8. **Gastrointestinal.** A scaphoid abdomen suggests **diaphragmatic hernia.** A normal umbilical cord has two arteries and one vein. Note the location and patency of the anus; the size of the liver, spleen, and kidney by palpation; and the presence of hernias or abdominal masses.

9. **Neurologic.** A thorough examination includes evaluation of motor activity, strength, symmetry, tone, and newborn reflexes

(Moro, tonic neck, grasp, suck, and stepping reflexes). Full-term newborns should have an up-going Babinski reflex and brisk deep tendon reflexes.

10. **Genitourinary.** The gonads may be differentiated or ambiguous, and the testes should be palpable. The location of the urethra should be determined, remembering that hypospadias precludes a circumcision.

11. **Musculoskeletal.** Any deformities, unusual posturing, or asymmetric limb movement should be noted, and the hips should be examined for possible dislocation. Clavicles may be fractured during a difficult delivery.

12. **Craniofacial.** One should determine head circumference, the location and size of the fontanelles, and the presence of hematoma or caput. Observing nasal gas flow despite occluding each naris will rule out choanal atresia.

C. **Laboratory studies.** Routine laboratory studies may include an initial hematocrit and serum glucose. Additional studies should be guided by the individual problem. For example, blood type and Coombs determination may be indicated in infants at risk for hyperbilirubinemia. Special considerations for newborns are as follows.

D. **Fluids.**
   1. **Volume** varies with birth weight.
      a. Less than 1.0 kg, use 100 mL/kg/day.
      b. 1.0 to 1.5 kg, use 90–80 mL/kg/day.
      c. 1.5 to 2.5 kg, use 80 mL/kg/day.
      d. Greater than 2.5 kg, use 60 mL/kg/day.
   2. **Isosmolar solutions** should be used.
      a. **Electrolyte supplementation** is not required within the first day of life for maintenance fluids in full-term infants. For premature infants, check the electrolytes at 8 to 12 hours of life and consider adjusting the fluid infusion rate and/or adding electrolytes as the results indicate.
      b. **Dextrose** (5% to 10%) in water (D/W) may be used for babies under 1.0 kg and 10% D/W may be used for those weighing more than 1.0 kg.
   3. Additional fluids may be required **for insensible water loss.**
      a. Fluid requirements increase with lower birth weight and with phototherapy and radiant warmer use.
      b. These losses must be replaced as well as those from pathologic causes (e.g., omphalocele, gastroschisis, neural tube defect). The electrolyte composition of the replacement fluid should match that of what is lost.
      c. Infants who are mechanically ventilated absorb free water from their respiratory system.
   4. Several signs will determine the adequacy of fluid infusions.
      a. Urine output at 0.5 mL/kg/hour.
      b. Only a 1% loss in body weight per day for the first 10 days of life.
      c. Stable hemodynamics and good perfusion.

E. **Electrolytes.**
   1. The usual electrolyte requirements after the first 12 to 24 hours of life are as follows:

    a. Na^+, 2 to 4 mEq/kg/day.
    b. K^+, 1 to 2 mEq/kg/day.
    c. Ca^{+2}, 150 to 220 mEq/kg/day.
  2. The frequency of laboratory tests for serum electrolyte levels will be determined by the rate of insensible losses.

F. Glucose. Supplemental glucose should be given after birth to keep blood glucose levels between 40 and 125 mg/dL.

  1. In most infants 10% D/W at maintenance fluid rates will provide adequate glucose. This infusion rate provides the 5 to 8 mg/kg/minute of glucose required for basal metabolism.

  2. Infants with hyperinsulinism or intrauterine growth retardation can require higher glucose infusion rates as high as 12 to 15 mg/kg/minute.

  3. In peripheral intravenous lines, up to 12.5% D/W may be infused; 15% to 20% D/W may be infused via central lines.

  4. Hypoglycemia (glucose ≤40 mg/dL) is treated with a bolus of glucose and increased glucose infusion rate.

    a. Glucose at 200 mg/kg intravenously (IV) is given over a minute (for example, 10% D/W at 2 mL/kg).

    b. The glucose infusion rate is increased from the current level or started at 8 mg/kg/min IV.

    c. Serial blood tests are necessary to determine the effectiveness of the increased glucose.

G. Nutrition. The gastrointestinal tract is functional after 28 weeks of gestation but is of limited capacity. Requirements vary with each neonate.

  1. Calories. Requirements are 100 to 130 kcal/kg/day.

  2. Protein. Requirements are 2 to 4 g/kg/day.

  3. Fat. Initiate at 1 g/kg/day and increase as tolerated so that the fat provides 40% of the calories.

  4. Vitamins A, B, D, E, C, and K should be provided.

  5. Iron. Requirements are 2 to 4 mg/kg/day of elemental iron. The adequacy of iron supplementation can be assessed by measuring the hemoglobin or hematocrit and the reticulocyte count.

  6. Minerals. Calcium, phosphate, magnesium, zinc, copper, manganese, and iron need to be replaced.

  7. Enteral feedings. A formula that simulates human milk with a high whey-to-casein ratio is preferred. Preterm infants often have lactose intolerance, for which nonlactose or low-lactose formulas are available. Infants less than 32 weeks gestation often have poor suck and swallow reflexes and require gavage feedings. With all premature infants or ill neonates, small feedings with a slowly advancing schedule should be used.

  8. Parenteral feeding. When needed, parenteral nutrition should be started as soon as possible to promote positive nitrogen balance and growth. The infant should be followed closely to adjust the solutions to the infant's needs and to identify signs of toxicity from hyperalimentation. Usual studies include serum glucose, electrolytes, osmolality, liver function tests, blood urea nitrogen, creatinine, lipid levels, and platelet count.

III. Common neonatal problems
  A. Respiratory disorders
    1. Differential diagnosis. Many diseases have the same signs and symptoms as pulmonary parenchymal disease and should

be considered when evaluating an infant with respiratory distress.

   a. **Airway obstruction.** Choanal atresia, vocal cord palsy, laryngomalacia, tracheal stenosis, and obstruction of the trachea by external masses (e.g., cystic hygroma, hemangioma, and vascular ring).

   b. **Developmental anomalies.** Tracheoesophageal fistula, congenital diaphragmatic hernia, congenital emphysema, and lung cysts.

   c. **Nonpulmonary.** Cyanotic heart disease, persistent pulmonary hypertension of the newborn, congestive heart failure, and metabolic disturbances (e.g., acidosis).

2. **Laboratory studies** for an infant in respiratory distress should include an arterial blood gas, pre- and postductal oxygen saturation (determined by pulse oximetry), hemoglobin or hematocrit, 12-lead ECG, and chest x-ray. Should these be abnormal, it would be important to consider obtaining a blood gas measurement while the patient breathes at an F_{IO_2} (fraction of inspired oxygen) of 1.0, an echocardiogram, and cardiology consultation to help evaluate potential congenital heart disease.

3. **Apnea**
   a. **Etiology**
      (1) **Central apnea** is due to immaturity or depression of the respiratory center (e.g., narcotics). It is related to the degree of prematurity and is exacerbated by metabolic disturbances, such as hypoglycemia, hypocalcemia, hypothermia, hyperthermia, and sepsis. Central apnea is often treated with **methylxanthines** such as theophylline and caffeine.

      (2) **Obstructive apnea** is caused by inconsistent maintenance of a patent airway and may be associated with incomplete maturation and poor coordination of upper airway musculature. This form of apnea may respond to changes in head position, insertion of an oral or nasal airway, or placing the infant in a prone position. Occasionally, administration of **continuous positive airway pressure** (CPAP) or a high-flow oxygen nasal cannula may be beneficial.

      (3) **Mixed apnea** represents a combination of both central and obstructive apnea.

   b. **Postoperative apnea in the neonate**
      (1) Apnea may be associated with anesthesia in formerly preterm infants. Although it has been associated with general anesthesia, some reports of apnea have been associated with local anesthesia.

      (2) If it is not possible to delay elective surgery, it is prudent to use **postoperative apnea monitoring** in neonates who undergo anesthesia at less than 45 weeks postconception.

4. **Respiratory distress syndrome**
   a. **Pathophysiology.** RDS (formerly referred to as hyaline membrane disease) results from physiologic surfactant deficiency. This causes decreased lung compliance, alveolar instability, progressive atelectasis, and hypoxemia resulting from intrapulmonary shunting of deoxygenated blood.

b. **Infants at risk** for RDS include those born prematurely or from diabetic mothers. Infants at risk may be identified prenatally by amniocentesis and evaluation of the amniotic fluid phospholipid profile. Lung maturity is associated with a lecithin-to-sphingomyelin ratio greater than 2, saturated phosphatidylcholine level greater than 500 μg/dL, or presence of phosphatidylglycerol in the specimen.

c. **Glucocorticoid (betamethasone) treatment** of the mother at least 2 days before delivery decreases the incidence and severity of RDS. Only one full course of a glucocorticoid treatment regimen during a pregnancy is necessary.

d. **Clinical features** include tachypnea, nasal flaring, grunting, and retractions. Cyanosis appears shortly after birth. Because of the intrapulmonary shunt, the infants remain hypoxemic despite breathing at high FIO_2.

e. The **chest x-ray** will show low lung volumes. A "ground-glass" pattern of the lung fields and air bronchograms may also be evident.

f. **Initial treatment** includes warmed, humidified oxygen administered by hood. The FIO_2 should be adjusted to maintain the PaO_2 between 50 and 80 mm Hg (SaO_2 less than 96%). If an FIO_2 greater than 60% is required to keep the patient oxygenated, **nasal CPAP** can be administered. With more severe disease, or if the nasal CPAP is poorly tolerated, intubation and ventilation with positive end-expiratory pressure may be required. Endotracheally administered exogenous **surfactant** decreases the severity, morbidity, and mortality of the disease. **High frequency oscillatory ventilation** (HFOV) decreases the incidence of air leaks and chronic lung disease in infants with severe RDS.

g. **Broad-spectrum antibiotics** are often begun after appropriate cultures are obtained, because the clinical signs and chest x-ray (CXR) of patients with RDS are indistinguishable from pneumonia.

h. In more mature newborns, RDS may be self-limited; clinical improvement after 2 to 3 days may be associated with a spontaneous diuresis. In extremely premature newborns, RDS may progress to chronic lung disease .

i. The **morbidity and mortality** of patients with RDS are directly related to the degree of prematurity, perinatal resuscitation, and the coexistence of other problems (e.g., patent ductus arteriosus, infection). **Pneumothoraces** and **pulmonary interstitial emphysema** may complicate the recovery and may be associated with the evolution to chronic lung disease.

5. **Chronic lung disease (CLD)**

a. **Etiology.** CLD, formally referred to as **bronchopulmonary dysplasia,** is defined as the continued need for respiratory support with oxygen therapy or mechanical ventilation beyond 36 weeks postconceptual age. CLD usually follows severe RDS and is associated with oxygen toxicity, chronic inflammation, and mechanical injury in the lung. CLD can be worsened by the presence of a patent ductus arteriosus. However, in some premature infants, CLD occurs in the absence of significant lung injury. Recent studies suggest that the evolution of CLD is associated with lung injury-induced up-regulation of transforming growth factor β signaling.

b. Clinical features include retractions, rales, and areas of lung hyper- and underinflation. Because of nonhomogenous ventilation, an intrapulmonary shunt may produce hypoxemia and hypercarbia in patients with CLD. Hypoxia and hypercarbia may also be associated with bronchospasm in many patients with severe CLD. Many patients with severe CLD have growth failure and require high-caloric feeds.

c. Treatment consists of supportive respiratory care, aggressive nutrition, and diuretic therapy. Because the patients with CLD may have lung segments with long time constants, a ventilatory pattern with low respiratory rates and increased inspiratory and expiratory time may decrease gas trapping and improve gas exchange. In addition, **bronchodilator therapy** may be life-saving in patients with CLD and bronchospasm. Systemic or inhaled steroids sometimes are used to treat patients with chronic lung disease. However, because of adverse long-term neurodevelopmental outcomes observed in infants treated with systemic steroids, this therapy is no longer recommended.

d. Prognosis varies with the severity of the disease. Of severely affected infants, 20% die within the first year. Most infants are generally asymptomatic by 2 years of age but still have evidence of increased pulmonary reactivity. It is rare for infants to have signs and symptoms of CLD beyond 5 to 8 years of age.

6. Pneumothorax

a. Etiology. Pneumothorax can occur in mechanically ventilated newborns. In addition, nonventilated otherwise-normal full-term infants can also have spontaneous pneumothoraces. The incidence is 2% in patients born by cesarean deliveries, 10% in patients with meconium staining, and 5% to 10% in RDS.

b. Clinical features. The diagnosis should be considered in any neonate with respiratory distress or in the ventilated infant with an acute deterioration in clinical condition (e.g., sudden cyanosis and hypotension). Occasionally, asymmetric chest movement with ventilation and asymmetric breath sounds may be appreciated. An endobronchial intubation should be ruled out.

c. Laboratory studies. Transillumination of the chest with a strong light usually will show a hyperlucent hemithorax. A chest x-ray will confirm the diagnosis.

d. Treatment

(1) In otherwise stable and well-oxygenated infants with minimal respiratory distress, a nitrogen washout by breathing a high concentration of oxygen may cause resolution of the pneumothorax and may be the only therapy required. However, data to support this mode of therapy are minimal and should be weighed

against newer ones suggesting that hyperoxia is associated with end-organ injury.

(2) In the **unstable infant,** immediate aspiration of the pleural space with an IV catheter should be performed. Reaccumulation of air after aspiration warrants placement of a chest tube.

7. **Meconium aspiration syndrome**

   a. **Meconium staining of amniotic fluid** occurs in 14% of all births and may be associated with fetal distress and asphyxia.

   b. To **decrease the effects of aspiration,** it is prudent to intubate and suction the airways of infants with meconium-stained fluid who are born with depressed respirations.

   c. **Meconium aspiration** may produce lung airspace disease by mechanical obstruction of the airways and pneumonitis. Complete obstruction of the airways by meconium results in distal atelectasis. Partial obstruction of the airway may produce overinflation of distal air spaces by a ball-valve effect, leading to pneumothorax. The bile in meconium may cause chemical pneumonitis and airway edema.

   d. **Meconium aspiration syndrome** has also been associated with PPHN (see section III.B.5).

   e. **Respiratory support** for meconium aspiration is dependent on the etiology of the poor gas exchange. Obstruction of airways with meconium may require mechanical ventilation with long expiratory times to decrease gas trapping. Pneumothorax is treated by placement of a chest tube. Sometimes high-frequency oscillatory ventilation is useful to recruit closed lung segments and improve gas exchange. Alkalosis and **inhaled nitric oxide** have been useful to decrease pulmonary vasoconstriction in patients with meconium aspiration. Exogenous **surfactant** has also been observed to be beneficial as meconium inhibits endogenous surfactant activity.

8. **Congenital diaphragmatic hernia (CDH)**

   a. **CDH** occurs in 1 in 5,000 live births. It has a high mortality, with 50% not surviving infancy. Seventy percent of the defects occur on the left.

   b. **Clinical features.** The defect is often detected during the prenatal ultrasound. At birth, a scaphoid abdomen can be observed, and breath sounds are absent on the involved side. Rarely, bowel sounds are heard in the affected hemithorax. Although the clinical spectrum may vary and is probably related to the degree of lung hypoplasia, patients often exhibit severe respiratory distress in the immediate postnatal period.

   c. The **diagnosis** is confirmed by chest x-ray. The intestine and stomach are often observed in the thorax.

   d. **Treatment** consists of respiratory and cardiovascular support as indicated. To decrease air entry into the stomach and intestines, patients are often intubated in the delivery room and mechanically ventilated. Insufflation of the stomach and intestines is minimized by intubating the patients while they are spontaneously breathing. However, if the patients are apneic, ventilation with bag and mask should be accomplished with minimal airway pressures. Continuous gastric suction also decreases air insufflation. Treatment is often geared toward decreasing pulmonary vascular resistance and facilitating CO_2 elimination. Conventional ventilation or HFOV is used. Ventilation with inhaled NO has been observed to decrease pulmonary vasoconstriction and cyanosis in some patients. The main causes of mortality are respiratory insufficiency and PPHN (see section III.B.5). Pneumothorax in the unaffected lung can occur and is often the cause of death during resuscitation. Hypotension and shock are often seen. They can be secondary to prolonged systemic hypoxemia, cardiac impairment caused by shifting of the mediastinal contents by the hernia, and gastrointestinal fluid losses.

   e. **Surgical repair** involves replacing the abdominal contents and repairing the diaphragm. In the past, this was performed urgently in the critically ill infant. Many patients are now first stabilized with medical and ventilatory treatment and **extracorporeal membrane oxygenation** (ECMO) before surgery (see section III.B.5.d.5).

   f. **Anesthetic considerations**

     (1) **Decompression of the gut** with continuous nasogastric suction.

     (2) Although **spontaneous ventilation** may prevent gastric inflation and lung compression, ventilator support is often needed. Nevertheless, using the lowest effective inflating pressures reduces the risk of pneumothorax in the normal lung on the side opposite the hernia.

     (3) **Nitrous oxide** is avoided because it may distend the gut and compromise lung function.

     (4) **An arterial catheter** is indicated for the frequent assessment of acid-base balance, oxygenation, and ventilation. Sodium bicarbonate and hyperventilation are used to treat metabolic and respiratory acidosis, respectively. In addition, alkalosis and inhaled nitric oxide might decrease pulmonary vasoconstriction.

     (5) Muscle relaxation, narcotics, and oxygen therapy are often used during anesthesia.

     (6) **Body temperature** is maintained with warming lights, a fluid warmer, and a warming mattress.

B. Cardiovascular disorders

  1. **Laboratory studies.** In the infant with signs and symptoms of cardiovascular disease, relevant studies include an arterial blood gas, pre- and postductal oxygen saturations, determination of arterial blood gas tension during inhalation of pure oxygen ("**hyperoxia test**"), hemoglobin or hematocrit, chest x-ray, and ECG. Echocardiography is frequently performed to detect potential structural heart lesions.

  2. **Patent ductus arteriosus (PDA)**

   a. **Clinical features.** PDA is commonly seen in the premature infant and is characterized by a murmur at the left sternal border radiating to the back, bounding pulses, widened pulse pressure, evidence of increased pulmonary blood flow by CXR, and excessive weight gain. In some cases, cardiac dysfunction associated with a PDA may decrease systemic blood pressure, peripheral perfusion, and urine output and may be associated with metabolic acidosis.

b. Although **early treatment** of a PDA consists of fluid restriction and diuretic therapy, it is important to maintain systemic perfusion. If the degree of shunt through the ductus arteriosus is significant, and renal and platelet function are adequate, pharmacologic closure of the ductus with **indomethacin** may be attempted. **Surgical closure** of a PDA is used for the infant for whom indomethacin has not closed the ductus or for those with decreased renal or platelet function (contraindications to indomethacin). In addition, surgery is often indicated for those with decreased systemic oxygenation because of intrapulmonary shunt associated with the open ductus arteriosus.

3. Cyanosis

a. **Etiology.** There are many causes of cyanosis, including diffusion abnormalities in the lung, intracardiac and extracardiac shunts, and polycythemia. These need to be considered when evaluating an infant with cyanosis. Additional causes of lung diffusion abnormalities are described above.

b. **Cardiac lesions** may cause systemic hypoxemia by decreasing pulmonary blood flow or causing a mixture of systemic and pulmonary venous blood via shunts.

c. In the fetus and newborn, the **ductus arteriosus may permit pulmonary blood flow** in patients with transposition of the great arteries, pulmonic stenosis or atresia, tetralogy of Fallot, or ventricular hypoplasia. Most of these infants become symptomatic as the ductus arteriosus closes at 2 to 3 days of life. If a ductus-dependent lesion exists, prevention of ductal closure is critical to maintain pulmonary blood flow. This may be accomplished with a **prostaglandin E_1** infusion. Side effects include apnea, hypotension, and seizure activity.

d. Many patients with **septal defects** may be asymptomatic during the fetal and neonatal period. However, with increased pulmonary vascular resistance, right to left shunting of blood may produce systemic hypoxemia. Later in life, with decreased pulmonary vascular resistance, increased pulmonary blood flow may cause pulmonary vascular disease and pulmonary hypertension.

e. A CXR and a hyperoxia test can confirm the diagnosis of an intracardiac shunt. The CXR may reveal decreased pulmonary blood flow. The PaO_2 remains below 150 mm Hg when an infant breathes 100% oxygen. An echocardiogram is invaluable in determining the etiology of the intracardiac shunt.

4. Dysrhythmias

a. **Supraventricular tachycardia** (SVT) is the most frequent dysrhythmia seen in neonates. This may be self-limited and well tolerated, but if hypotension or hemoglobin desaturation occurs, treatment may be required.

    b. **Treatment** consists of vagal maneuvers such as nasopharyngeal stimulation or placement of cold on the face. Massage of the eye should be avoided, as this may lead to disruption of the lens in neonates. **Adenosine** and **esophageal pacing** also are useful for acute management of SVT.

    c. Digoxin will usually convert paroxysmal atrial tachycardia to sinus rhythm; maintenance therapy for 1 year is sometimes indicated. **Beta blockers** and **quinidine** are second-line medications.

    d. Electrocardioversion is indicated if the patient is hemodynamically unstable.

5. **Persistent pulmonary hypertension of the newborn**

    a. **Pathophysiology.** PPHN, previously referred to as persistent fetal circulation, is manifested by an increase in pulmonary vascular resistance with resulting pulmonary arterial hypertension, right-to-left shunting across the foramen ovale and the ductus arteriosus, and profound cyanosis.

    b. **Etiology.** It is suspected that many newborns with PPHN have abnormal pulmonary artery reactivity and structure. Although many infants with PPHN may have asphyxia, meconium aspiration, bacterial pneumonia, or sepsis, the role of these in causing the disease is unknown.

    c. **Clinical features.** Newborns with PPHN have severe systemic hypoxemia unrelieved by breathing at high FIO_2. They may have shunt evidenced by higher oxygen saturations in the upper versus lower extremities. ECG may reveal right ventricular hypertrophy; CXR may show decreased pulmonary vascular markings. Echocardiography may show shunting of blood at the level of the PDA and/or PFO.

    d. **Treatment** of PPHN

        (1) **Endotracheal intubation and mechanical ventilation at high FIO_2.** Treatment with narcotics (e.g., fentanyl 1 to 2 μg/kg/hour) and muscle relaxation will often facilitate ventilation.

        (2) Induced respiratory and/or metabolic alkalosis.

        (3) Aggressive **blood pressure support** with vasopressors and, if indicated, fluids.

        (4) In many patients, **inhaled nitric oxide** rapidly decreases pulmonary vasoconstriction and extrapulmonary shunt and increases systemic oxygenation without causing systemic hypotension. Inhaled NO alleviates hypoxemia in babies with PPHN and decreases the need for ECMO.

        (5) **ECMO** may be life-saving for some patients with PPHN refractory to ventilatory and medical therapy.

            (a) The **ECMO circuit** consists of tubing, a reservoir, pump, membrane oxygenator, and heat exchanger. To prevent clotting, the patient is treated with heparin. Because of platelet consumption during ECMO, platelet infusions are often required.

      (b)   **Access.** General anesthesia is required for the cannulation that is required for the establishment of ECMO. In some patients, a **venoarterial** ECMO is facilitated by cannulation of the right common carotid artery and the right internal jugular vein or the femoral artery and vein. In other patients, **venovenous** ECMO is performed with a single double-lumen catheter placed in the right ventricle via a central vein.

      (c)   **Morbidity** may be related to ECMO. Heparin treatment can cause intracranial hemorrhage and bleeding from other sites. Right-sided cerebral injuries (focal left-sided seizures, left hemiparesis, and progressive right cerebral atrophy) are thought secondary to cannulation and ligation of the right internal carotid artery.

      (d)   Because of the potential risks of ECMO, it is reserved for patients with severe systemic hypoxemia. In addition, most infants with intraventricular hemorrhage are excluded because of their unacceptable risk of hemorrhage extension while being treated with heparin. Also excluded are infants with multiple congenital anomalies, severe neurologic impairment, or cyanotic congenital heart disease. It is often technically difficult to obtain adequate ECMO circuit flows to increase systemic oxygenation in preterm infants.

C. Hematologic disorders

  1. **Hemolytic disease of the newborn (erythroblastosis fetalis)**

     a. **Isoimmune hemolytic anemia** in the fetus is caused by the passage of maternal antibody against fetal erythrocytes transplacentally into the fetus. Only IgG can cross the placenta.

     b. **Rh hemolytic disease** is usually caused by the anti-D antibody but can also be caused by antibodies to minor antigens including Kell, Duffy, Kidd, and Ss antigens. The absence of D antigen makes one Rh negative. A mother can be sensitized to fetal antigens by leakage of fetal blood into the maternal circulation during pregnancy, delivery, abortion, or amniocentesis. To prevent sensitization, an unsensitized Rh-negative mother is given **anti-D immune globulin** during pregnancy and after delivery. Once a mother is sensitized, immune prophylaxis is of no value. Even if treated with immune globulin, a mother can still be sensitized during pregnancy if a large fetomaternal transfusion occurs.

     c. **ABO hemolytic disease** can occur without maternal sensitization, because a mother with group O blood has naturally occurring anti-A and anti-B antibodies in her circulation. These are usually IgM antibodies, but some may be IgG. This disease tends to be milder than Rh disease, with little or no anemia, mild indirect hyperbilirubinemia, and rare need for exchange transfusion.

    d. An **indirect Coombs test** on maternal blood can detect the presence of IgG antibodies.

    e. A **direct Coombs test** on the infant's blood can detect cells already coated with antibody, thus indicating a risk for hemolysis.

    f. **Hemolysis** occurs when antibody crosses the placenta and attaches to the corresponding antigen on fetal erythrocytes. Hepatosplenomegaly results from increased hematopoiesis triggered by hemolysis.

    g. **Clinical features.** Physical examination may reveal hepatosplenomegaly, edema, pallor, or jaundice.

    h. **Laboratory studies** often reveal anemia, thrombocytopenia, a positive direct Coombs test, indirect hyperbilirubinemia, hypoglycemia, hypoalbuminemia, and an elevated reticulocyte count that increases proportionally with the severity of the disease. Serial hematocrit and indirect bilirubin levels should be followed.

    i. **Treatment** consists of **phototherapy.** An exchange transfusion may be required if the level of bilirubin is very high or the rate of rise of bilirubin exceeds 1 mg/dL/hour.

2. **Hydrops fetalis**

    a. **Hydrops fetalis** is defined as excessive accumulation of fluid by the fetus and can range from mild peripheral edema to massive anasarca.

    b. **Etiologies.** Hydrops can be seen in hemolytic disease and is thought to be due to increased capillary permeability secondary to anemia. Other etiologies of hydrops include anemias (e.g., fetomaternal hemorrhage, donor twin-twin transfusion), cardiac arrhythmias (e.g., complete heart block, supraventricular tachycardia), congenital heart disease, vascular or lymphatic malformation (e.g., hemangioma of the liver, cystic hygroma), or infection (e.g., viral, toxoplasmosis, syphilis).

    c. **Treatment.** The main goals of therapy include prevention of intrauterine or extrauterine death from anemia and hypoxia, restoration of intravascular volume, and avoidance of neurotoxicity from hyperbilirubinemia.

        (1) Survival of the unborn infant may be improved by in utero transfusion via the umbilical vein.

        (2) Care of the liveborn infant should include correction of hypovolemia and acidosis as well as potential exchange transfusion.

        (3) Late complications include anemia, mild graft-versus-host reactions, inspissated bile syndrome (characterized by persistent icterus with elevated direct and indirect bilirubin), and portal vein thrombosis (as a complication of umbilical vein catheterization).

D. **Gastrointestinal disorders**

    1. **Hyperbilirubinemia**

        a. **Pathophysiology.** Bilirubin is formed from the breakdown of heme, then bound to albumin, transported to the liver (where it is conjugated with glucuronate), and delivered to the intestine in bile. In the intestine, it is either deconjugated by intestinal bacteria and reabsorbed or it is converted to excretory urobilinogen.

b. Etiology. Hyperbilirubinemia results from overproduction (e.g., hemolysis, absorption of sequestered blood, polycythemia), underconjugation (e.g., immature or damaged liver), or underexcretion (e.g., biliary atresia). It is often seen in sepsis, asphyxia, and metabolic disorders (e.g., hypothyroidism, hypoglycemia, galactosemia) as well as in healthy newborns and breast-fed infants.

c. Toxic effects. Unconjugated (indirect) bilirubin is lipid soluble and is capable of entering the central nervous system. Toxic levels result in bilirubin staining and necrosis of neurons. This process, known as **bilirubin encephalopathy** or **kernicterus,** may have clinical symptoms ranging from mild lethargy and fever to convulsions. Infants with respiratory distress, sepsis, metabolic acidosis, hypoglycemia, hypoalbuminemia, or severe hemolytic disease are at risk for kernicterus. Survivors evaluated in childhood are found to have neurologic sequelae ranging from diminished cognitive function to mental retardation and choreoathetoid cerebral palsy.

d. Physiologic jaundice results from increased red cell turnover and an immature hepatic conjugation system. It occurs in 60% of term newborns, and peak bilirubin levels occur by day 2 to 4 of life. Premature infants have an increased incidence (80%) and later bilirubin peak (day 5 to 7).

e. Breast milk jaundice develops gradually, occurring in the second or third week of life, with peak bilirubin levels of 15 to 25 mg/dL, which may persist for 2 to 3 months. Other causes should be excluded before making this diagnosis. Interrupting nursing for a few days results in a marked decrease in serum levels, at which time nursing can be restarted. This is a benign type of jaundice without adverse sequelae.

f. Laboratory studies include total and direct bilirubin, direct Coombs test, reticulocyte count, blood smear for red cell morphology, electrolytes, blood urea nitrogen, creatinine, and appropriate cultures if sepsis is suspected. Because hyperbilirubinemia may be the presenting sign of a urinary tract infection, urinalysis and urine cultures should be considered.

g. Treatment

(1) Management of physiologic or mild hemolytic jaundice consists of monitoring serial bilirubin levels and starting early feeding to reduce enterohepatic cycling of bilirubin.

(2) Phototherapy is used if moderate indirect bilirubin levels or an accelerated rate of rise is noted (e.g., indirect bilirubin level greater than 5 in a full-term infant on day 1 of life). Light therapy of 420- to 470-nm wavelength results in photoisomerization of bilirubin, making it water soluble. Eyes must be shielded to prevent retinal damage.

(3) For severe hyperbilirubinemia, **exchange transfusion** is indicated (e.g., indirect bilirubin >25 mg/dL in a full-term infant).

2. **Esophageal atresia and TEF**

   a. Esophageal atresia is usually associated with TEF. The location of the fistula is variable in these patients.

   b. **Pathophysiology.** The proximal blind esophageal pouch has a small capacity, resulting in overflow aspiration. This leads to the classic clinical triad of coughing, choking, and cyanosis. Occasionally, drooling requiring frequent suctioning may be the only early symptom.

   c. The **diagnosis** is confirmed by the inability to pass a nasogastric tube into the stomach. A CXR with air or water-soluble contrast agent will confirm the existence of esophageal atresia.

   d. **Medical treatment** is directed at reducing aspiration. Neonates should be kept NPO. A nasogastric tube is placed on continuous low suction and the head of the bed is elevated. Aspiration pneumonia should be treated with antibiotics and oxygen as required. Endotracheal intubation and ventilation may be required for severe pneumonia. However, ventilation may be difficult when a tracheoesophageal fistula exists.

   e. **Surgical treatment** depends on the stability of the infant. In newborns with severe pneumonia, it is often prudent to delay surgery until the lungs improve. Nevertheless, if required to decompress the stomach, a gastrostomy tube may be placed under local anesthesia. In stable patients, definitive repair of the esophagus and fistula may occur.

   f. **Anesthesia.** It is critical, and sometimes difficult, to establish an airway in patients with a TEF. Surgeons should be readily available during the induction should emergent decompression of the stomach be required. The patient should be fully monitored; a precordial chest piece should be placed over the left thorax. If the patient has a gastrostomy tube, it should be placed to water seal. An inhalation induction or awake intubation should be performed. To facilitate placement of the tip of the endotracheal tube between the fistula and the carina, the tube first may be placed into the right mainstem bronchus. The tube then may be withdrawn slowly until breath sounds are heard over the left thorax. Decreased breath sounds and insufflation of the stomach or gas exiting from the gastrostomy tube suggest that the end of the endotracheal tube is above the fistula and that it should be advanced. Once the tube is in a good location, then it is critical to secure it in place. We often assign one person to monitor the location of the tube throughout the surgery.

   g. **Intraoperative management.** Inhalation anesthesia with spontaneous ventilation should be maintained until a gastrostomy is performed. Positive pressure ventilation should be attempted before a muscle relaxant is administered.

3. **Duodenal atresia**

   a. **Clinical features.** Duodenal atresia usually presents with bile-stained emesis, upper abdominal distention, and increased volume of gastric aspirates. It is associated with trisomy 21 and may coexist with other intestinal malformations.

b. An **abdominal x-ray** often reveals a **"double bubble,"** representing air in the stomach and upper duodenum.

c. **Treatment** consists of avoiding oral feeds, use of nasogastric suction, ensuring adequate hydration, and managing electrolytes. Anesthesia consists of awake or rapid sequence intubation, avoidance of nitrous oxide, and, often, the use of muscle relaxants.

4. Pyloric stenosis

a. Although usually presenting in the second or third week of life, pyloric stenosis may present in the immediate newborn period.

b. **Clinical features** include persistent nonbilious emesis and a metabolic alkalosis from loss of hydrochloric acid because of prolonged gastric suctioning. With protracted vomiting, the patient may present with metabolic acidosis and shock. An abdominal mass consisting of the hypertrophic pylorus or "olive" is often palpable.

c. An **abdominal x-ray** usually shows gastric dilatation. The diagnosis is confirmed by abdominal ultrasound or by barium swallow.

d. **Treatment** consists of rehydration, correction of metabolic alkalosis, and nasogastric drainage before surgical repair.

e. **Intraoperative management.** It is critical to empty the stomach before induction. Often the patient's nasogastric tube is blocked with barium or other matter. We will often replace the nasogastric tube with a fresh one and suction the patient while they are supine, lateral, and prone before induction. A rapid-sequence or awake intubation may be performed. Inhalation anesthetics or muscle relaxants can be used as needed. The neonate should be fully awake and breathing adequately before removing the endotracheal tube.

5. Omphalocele and gastroschisis

a. An **omphalocele** is caused by failure of the migration of the intestine into the abdomen and subsequent closure of the abdominal wall at 6 to 8 weeks gestation. The viscera remain outside the abdominal cavity where they are covered with intact peritoneum. Omphaloceles may be associated with genetic abnormalities, cardiac lesions, extrophy of the bladder, and Beckwith–Wiedeman syndrome.

b. **Gastroschisis** occurs later in fetal life (12 to 18 weeks gestation) from interruption of the omphalomesenteric artery. The resulting paraumbilical defect allows exposure of the bowel to the intrauterine environment without peritoneal coverage; bowel loops are often edematous and covered with an inflammatory exudate.

c. **Medical stabilization** includes nasogastric drainage, IV hydration, and protection of the viscera before surgical repair. If the peritoneal sac is intact, the omphalocele should be covered with sterile, warm, saline-soaked gauze to decrease heat and water loss and the risk of infection. If the sac has ruptured or if the infant has gastroschisis, warm saline-soaked gauze should be used to wrap the exposed viscera; the infant should then be wrapped in warm sterile towels before surgical repair.

6. **Necrotizing enterocolitis** (NEC)

   a. **NEC** is an acquired intestinal necrosis that appears in the absence of functional (e.g., Hirschsprung disease) or anatomic (e.g., malrotation) lesions. It occurs predominantly (90%) in premature infants and may be endemic or epidemic. It usually develops during the first few weeks of life, almost always after the institution of enteral feedings. Mortality may be as high as 40%. Clinical studies suggest that feeding with breast milk protects against NEC.

   b. **Pathogenesis** is unclear but involves critical stress of an immature gut by ischemic, infectious, or immunologic insults. Enteral feedings seem to potentiate mucosal injury.

   c. **Clinical features** include abdominal distention, ileus, increase in gastric aspirates, abdominal wall erythema, or bloody stool. The infant may demonstrate temperature instability, lethargy, respiratory and circulatory instability, oliguria, and bleeding diathesis.

   d. **Laboratory studies** should include an abdominal x-ray (which may show **pneumatosis intestinalis,** fixed loops of bowel, portal air, or free intraperitoneal air), complete blood count (revealing leukocytosis, leukopenia, thrombocytopenia), arterial blood gases (demonstrating acidosis), stool guaiac (often showing occult blood), and stool Clinitest (showing evidence of carbohydrate malabsorption). Because the differential diagnosis includes sepsis, cultures of blood, urine, and stool should also be obtained. If the patient is stable and disseminated intravascular coagulation is not evident, cerebrospinal fluid (CSF) should be obtained by lumbar puncture for Gram stain and culture.

   e. **Treatment.** When necrotizing enterocolitis is suspected, enteral feedings are discontinued, and the stomach is decompressed with a nasogastric tube. Oral feeds are withheld for at least 10 to 14 days and the patient is supported with parenteral feedings. Broad-spectrum antibiotics (ampicillin, an aminoglycoside, and, if perforation is suspected, metronidazole) are administered empirically.

   f. **Surgical consultation** is indicated, although laparotomy is usually reserved for intestinal perforation, a fixed loop on serial abdominal x-rays, or persistent metabolic acidosis.

7. **Volvulus**

   a. **Volvulus** may occur as a primary lesion or, more commonly, as the result of intestinal malrotation. If present in utero, intestinal necrosis may be present at birth, and immediate resection is indicated.

   b. **Clinical features** may include abdominal distention, bilious emesis, and signs of sepsis or shock.

   c. **The diagnosis** of malrotation is made by upper gastrointestinal and small bowel follow-through examination, which demonstrates an abnormally positioned ligament of Treitz.

   d. **Treatment** involves volume resuscitation, placement of a nasogastric tube, and surgical repair.

e. **Intraoperative management.** After evacuation of the stomach, a rapid sequence induction should be performed and anesthesia maintained with inhalation or IV anesthetics as tolerated. Nitrous oxide should be avoided. Oxygen should be diluted with air to minimize the risk of pulmonary or ocular toxicity.

E. Neurologic disorders

1. Seizures

a. **Seizures** may be generalized, focal, or subtle.

b. **Etiologies** include birth trauma, intracranial hemorrhage, postasphyxial encephalopathy, metabolic disturbances (hypoglycemia or hypocalcemia), drug withdrawal, and infections.

c. **Laboratory evaluation**

(1) Initial evaluation includes electrolytes, glucose, calcium, magnesium, and arterial blood gas and pH determination. If a metabolic disease is suspected, serum/urine amino acids and urine for organic acids should be obtained.

(2) Complete blood count with differential, platelet count, and the appropriate cultures, including CSF.

(3) Appropriate neuroimaging may include cranial ultrasound, computed tomography (CT) scan, and/or magnetic resonance imaging (MRI). T2 diffusion-weighted MRI images are helpful in identifying hypoxic-ischemic areas of the brain.

(4) Electroencephalogram before and after pyridoxine administration.

d. **Treatment** includes supportive care. It is critical to ensure that the patient maintains adequate oxygenation. In addition, it is important to correct underlying problems (e.g., hypoglycemia, hypocalcemia). Anticonvulsants are started, and, if indicated, a test dose of pyridoxine is administered.

e. **Anticonvulsants**

(1) Acute medical treatments include the following:

(a) **Benzodiazepine** (e.g., lorazepam 0.1 to 0.3 mg/kg IV).

(b) **Phenobarbital,** 20 mg/kg IV load over 10 minutes; maintenance dose of 2.5 mg/kg twice daily to maintain a serum level of 20 to 40 μg/mL.

(c) **Fosphenytoin,** 15 to 20 mg/kg IV load over 15 minutes; maintenance dose of 2.5 mg/kg twice daily to maintain a therapeutic level of 15 to 30 μg/mL.

(2) Chronic treatment for neonatal seizures is usually with phenobarbital.

2. Intracranial hemorrhage

a. **Intraventricular hemorrhage** occurs in more than 30% of infants with birth weights below 1,500 g. Subdural and subarachnoid hemorrhages are much less common.

b. **Clinical features.** Intraventricular hemorrhage is often asymptomatic, although it may present with unexplained lethargy, apnea, or seizures. On examination, the head circumference is increased and the fontanelle may be bulging.

c. **Laboratory studies.** Laboratory examination may show anemia and acidosis. Diagnosis is made by cranial ultrasound or CT scan.

d. **Grading of intraventricular hemorrhage**
   (1) **Grade I.** Subependymal bleeding only.
   (2) **Grade II.** Intraventricular bleeding without dilatation of ventricles.
   (3) **Grade III.** Intraventricular bleeding with dilatation of ventricles.
   (4) **Grade IV.** Grade III with intraparenchymal blood.

e. The **major complication** of intraventricular hemorrhage is CSF obstruction resulting in posthemorrhagic **hydrocephalus.** This is followed by measuring daily head circumferences and by serial cranial ultrasounds. Intraventricular shunting is often required.

f. Hypertonic agents (e.g., 25% dextrose in water) that had previously been advocated in the treatment of hypoglycemia have been implicated in the etiology of intraventricular hemorrhage and should be avoided.

3. **Retinopathy of prematurity (ROP)**
   a. **Etiologies**
      (1) **The risk of ROP** is increased in premature neonates requiring oxygen therapy. ROP is seen in infants with birth weights less than 1,700 g, with an 80% incidence in infants weighing less than 1,000 g. To decrease the incidence of ROP, **hyperoxia should be avoided.**
      (2) Factors other than hyperoxic exposure and prematurity may produce ROP, as it has been demonstrated in full-term infants, infants with cyanotic heart disease, stillborn infants, and infants with no hyperoxic exposure as well as in a single eye. Factors that may increase risk include anemia, infection, intracranial hemorrhage, acidosis, and PDA.

   b. **Pathophysiology.** ROP begins in the temporal peripheral retina, which is the last part of the retina to vascularize. An elevated ridge demarcating vascularized and nonvascularized retina is initially seen. **Fibrovascular proliferation** from this border extends posteriorly, and, in 90% of patients, gradual resolution occurs from this stage. These patients may develop strabismus, amblyopia, myopia, or peripheral retinal detachment in later life.

   c. In 10% of patients, fibrovascularization extends into the vitreous, resulting in vitreous hemorrhage, peripheral retinal scarring, temporal dragging of the disk and macula, and partial retinal detachment. In severe disease, extensive fibrovascular proliferation can result in a retrolental white mass (leukokoria), complete retinal detachment, and loss of vision.

   d. All infants at risk are examined with indirect ophthalmoscopy after 1 month at 32 weeks corrected gestational age. If ROP is identified, the infant is reexamined at

2-week intervals until spontaneous resolution occurs. New cases of ROP do not occur after 3 months of age.

e. **Treatment** for severe manifestations of ROP has included photocoagulation, diathermy, cryotherapy, and vitrectomy.

F. Infectious diseases

1. Environment

a. **Neonates are particularly vulnerable to infection.** They have decreased cellular and humoral immune defense systems and are at increased risk for colonization and nosocomial infection.

b. **Prevention.** Infectious transmission may be reduced by using separate equipment and isolettes for each infant, by hand washing before and after each contact, and by wearing cover gowns.

2. Risk factors for infection.
Prolonged rupture of membranes is associated with a high incidence of amnionitis and subsequent ascending bacterial and viral infection in the neonate. Maternal fever, maternal leukocytosis, and fetal tachycardia are also associated with neonatal infection.

3. Laboratory studies
include complete blood count with differential and blood cultures. A lumbar puncture for culture and analysis of CSF may be indicated. If appropriate, viral cultures should be obtained.

4. Neonatal sepsis

a. Organisms responsible for infections soon after birth are usually acquired in utero or during birth. These can include group B β-hemolytic streptococcus, *Escherichia coli, Listeria,* and herpes. Later-onset infections may be caused by *Staphylococcus aureus, Staphylococcus epidermidis, Enterobacter cloacae,* enterococcus, and *Pseudomonas aeruginosa.*

b. **The clinical features of sepsis** include respiratory failure, seizures, and shock. Subtle signs, including respiratory distress, apnea, irritability, and poor feeding, are often seen first and warrant evaluation.

c. **Laboratory studies** should include blood, urine, and CSF cultures; complete blood count with platelet count; urinalysis; and chest x-ray.

d. **Antibiotic coverage** with ampicillin and an aminoglycoside is begun and continued for 48 to 72 hours. If cultures are positive, treatment should continue as indicated by the severity and location of infection. Aminoglycoside serum levels should be monitored and dosages adjusted to prevent toxicity.

SUGGESTED READING

American Academy of Pediatrics. Postnatal corticosteroids to treat or prevent chronic lung disease in preterm infants. *Pediatrics* 2002;109:330–338.

Bartlett RH, et al. Extracorporeal circulation in neonatal respiratory failure: a prospective randomized study. *Pediatrics* 1985;76:479–487.

Cronin JH. High frequency ventilator therapy for newborns. *J Intensive Care Med* 1994;9:71–85.

Dennery PA, et al. Neonatal hyperbilirubinemia. *N Engl J Med* 2001;344:581–590.

Findlay RD, et al. Surfactant replacement therapy for meconium aspiration therapy. *Pediatrics* 1996;97:48–52.

Friedman S, et al. Prenatal and postnatal steroid therapy and child neurodevelopment. *Clin Perinatol* 2004;31:529–544.

Gersony W, Peckham G, Ellison R. Effects of indomethacin in premature infants with patent ductus arteriosus: results of a national collaborative study. *J Pediatr* 1983;102:895–906.

Gregory G. Life-threatening apnea in the ex-premie. *Anaesthesia* 1983;59:495–498.

Hammerman C, Aramburo MJ. Prolonged indomethacin therapy for the prevention of recurrences of patent ductus arteriosus. *J Pediatr* 1990;117:771–776.

Kurth CD, et al. Postoperative apnea in premature infants. *Anesthesiology* 1987;66:483–488.

Liu LMP, et al. Life threatening apnea in infants recovering from anesthesia. *Anesthesiology* 1983;59:506–510.

Murphy BP, et al. Impaired cerebral cortical gray matter growth after treatment with dexamethasone for neonatal chronic lung disease. *Pediatrics* 2001;107:217–221.

O'Rourke PP, et al. Extracorporeal membrane oxygenation and conventional medical therapy in neonates with persistent pulmonary hypertension of the newborn: a prospective randomized therapy. *Pediatrics* 1989;84:957–963.

Roberts JD Jr, Shaul P. Persistent pulmonary hypertension of the newborn: recent advances in diagnosis and treatment. *Ped Clin North Am* 1993;40:983–1004.

Roberts JD Jr, et al. Inhaled nitric oxide in persistent pulmonary hypertension. *N Engl J Med* 1997;336:605–610.

Roberts JD Jr, et al. Nitric oxide inhalation decreases pulmonary artery remodeling in the injured lungs of rat pups. *Circ Res* 2000;87:140–145.

Roberts JD Jr, Cronin J, Todres ID. Neonatal emergencies. In: Cote C, Todres ID, Goudsouzian N, and Ryan J, eds. *A practice of anesthesia for infants and children,* 3rd ed. Philadelphia: Saunders, 2001.

Rudolph AM, Yuan S. Response of the pulmonary vasculature to hypoxia and H(super +) ion concentration changes. *J Clin Invest* 1966;45:399–411.

Shannon DC, et al. Prevention of apnea and bradycardia in low-birthweight infants. *Pediatrics* 1975;55:589–594.

Soll RF, et al. Multicenter trial of single dose Survanta for prevention of respiratory distress syndrome (RDS). *Pediatrics* 1990;85:1092–1102.

Spitzer AR. *Intensive care of the fetus and neonate,* 2nd ed. Philadelphia: Elsevier Saunders, 2005.

Steward DJ. Preterm infants are more prone to complications following minor surgery than are term infants. *Anesthesiology* 1982;56:304–306.

Taeusch HW, et al. *Avery's diseases of the newborn,* 8th ed. Philadelphia: Elsevier Saunders, 2005.

29

Anesthesia for Pediatric Surgery

Susan A. Vassallo and Hemanth A. Baboolal

I. **Anatomy and physiology**
   A. **Upper airway**
      1. **Neonates are obligate nose breathers** because of weak oropharyngeal muscles. Their nares are relatively narrow, and a significant fraction of the work of breathing is needed to overcome nasal resistance. Occlusion of the nares by bilateral choanal atresia or tenacious secretions can cause complete airway obstruction. Placement of an oral airway, a laryngeal mask airway, or an endotracheal tube may be necessary to reestablish airway patency during sedation or anesthesia.
      2. **Infants have a relatively large tongue,** which makes mask ventilation and laryngoscopy challenging. The tongue can easily obstruct the airway if excessive submandibular pressure is applied during mask ventilation.
      3. **Infants and children have a more cephalad glottis** (C-3 vertebral level in premature infants, C-4 in infants, C-5 in adults) and **a narrow, long, angulated epiglottis,** which can make laryngoscopy difficult.
      4. In infants and young children, **the narrowest part of the airway is at the cricoid cartilage,** rather than at the glottis (as in adults). An endotracheal tube that passes through the cords may still be too large distally.
      5. **Deciduous teeth** erupt within the first year and are shed between ages 6 and 13 years. To avoid dislodging a loose tooth, it is safest to open the mandible directly, without introducing a finger or appliance into the oral cavity. Loose teeth should be documented on the preoperative evaluation. In some instances, unstable teeth should be removed before laryngoscopy. Parents and patients should be informed of this possibility in advance.
      6. **Airway resistance** in infants and children can be increased dramatically by subtle changes in an already small-caliber system. Even a small amount of edema can significantly increase airway resistance and cause airway compromise.
   B. **Pulmonary system**
      1. Neonates have **high metabolic rates,** resulting in an elevated oxygen consumption (6 to 9 mL/kg/minute) compared with adults (3 mL/kg/minute).
      2. **Neonatal lungs have high closing volumes,** which fall within the lower range of their normal tidal volume. Below closing volume, alveolar collapse and shunting occur.
      3. To meet the higher oxygen demand, infants have a **higher respiratory rate and minute ventilation.** An infant's functional residual capacity (FRC) is nearly equivalent to that of an adult (FRC of an infant, 25 mL/kg; adult, 40 mL/kg). Their higher minute ventilation to FRC ratio results in rapid inhalational

515

induction. The tidal volume for infants and adults is equivalent (7 mL/kg).

4. **Anatomic shunts** including patent ductus arteriosus and patent foramen ovale may develop significant right-to-left flow with increases in pulmonary artery pressure (e.g., hypoxia, acidosis, or high positive airway pressure).

5. The characteristics of the infant's pulmonary system contribute to **rapid desaturation during apnea.** Profound desaturation can occur when an infant coughs or strains and alveoli collapse. Treatment may require deepening anesthesia with intravenous (IV) drugs or using neuromuscular relaxants.

6. The **diaphragm** is the infant's major muscle of ventilation. Compared with the adult diaphragm, the newborn has only half the number of Type I, slow-twitch, high-oxidative muscle fibers essential for sustained increased respiratory effort. Thus, the infant's diaphragm fatigues earlier than the adult's. By 2 years of age, the infant's diaphragm has attained mature levels of Type I fibers.

7. The **pliable rib cage** (compliant chest wall) of an infant cannot maintain negative intrathoracic pressure easily. This diminishes the efficacy of the infant's attempts to increase ventilation.

8. An infant's **dead space** is 2 to 2.5 mL/kg, equivalent to an adult's.

9. Infants' high baseline minute ventilation limits their ability to increase their ventilatory effort further. End-tidal CO_2 concentrations should be followed if spontaneous ventilation is permitted under anesthesia; assisted or controlled ventilation may be necessary.

10. **Alveolar maturation** occurs by 8 to 10 years of age when alveoli number and size reach adult ranges.

11. **Retinopathy of prematurity** (see Chapter 28, section III.E.3).

12. **Apnea and bradycardia** after general anesthesia occur with increased frequency in infants who are premature and in infants who have anemia, sepsis, hypothermia, central nervous system disease, hypoglycemia, hypothermia, or other metabolic derangements. These patients should have cardiorespiratory monitoring for a minimum of 24 hours postoperatively. Such infants are not candidates for ambulatory day surgery. The guidelines for discharge vary among institutions. Most hospitals agree that infants who are less than 45 to 55 weeks postconceptual age are monitored postoperatively. Any full-term infant who displays apnea after general anesthesia is also monitored.

C. **Cardiovascular system**

1. **Heart rate** and **blood pressure** vary with age and should be maintained at age-appropriate levels perioperatively (Tables 29.1 and 29.2).

2. **Cardiac output** is 180 to 240 mL/kg/minute in newborns, which is two to three times that of adults. This higher cardiac output is necessary to meet the higher metabolic oxygen consumption demands.

Table 29.1. Age dependence of typical respiratory parameters

Variable	Newborn	1 Year	3 Years	5 Years	Adult
Respirations (breaths/minute)	40–60	20–30	Gradual decrease to 18–25	18–25	12–20
Tidal volume (mL)	15	80	110	250	500
FRC (mL/kg)	25		35		40
Minute ventilation (L/minute)	1	1.8	2.5	5.5	6.5
Hematocrit (%)	47–60	33.42			40–50
Arterial pH	7.30–7.40	7.35–7.45			—
$PaCO_2$ (mm Hg)	30–35	30–40			—
PaO_2 (mm Hg)	60–90	80–100			—

FRC, functional residual capacity.

Table 29.2. Cardiovascular variables

	Blood Pressure (mm Hg)		
Age	Heart Rate (Beats/min)	Systolic	Diastolic
Preterm neonate	120–180	45–60	30
Term neonate	100–180	55–70	40
1 Year	100–140	70–100	60
3 Years	84–115	75–110	70
5 Years	84–100	80–120	70

3. The **ventricles** are less compliant and have a relatively smaller contractile muscle mass in newborns and infants. The ability to increase contractility is limited; increases in cardiac output occur by increasing heart rate rather than stroke volume. Bradycardia is the most deleterious dysrhythmia in infants, and hypoxemia is a frequent cause of bradycardia in infants and children.

D. **Fluid and electrolyte balance**
   1. The **glomerular filtration rate** at birth is 15% to 30% of the normal adult value. Adult value is reached by 1 year of age. Renal clearance of drugs and their metabolites is diminished during the first year of life.
   2. Neonates have an intact renin-angiotensin aldosterone pathway, but the distal tubules resorb less sodium in response to aldosterone. Thus, newborns are "obligate sodium losers," and IV fluids should contain sodium.
   3. The **total body water** in the preterm infant is 90% of body weight. In term infants, it is 80%; at 6 to 12 months, it is 60%. This increased percentage of total body water affects drug volumes of distribution. The dosages of some drugs (e.g., thiopental, propofol, succinylcholine, pancuronium, and rocuronium) are 20% to 30% greater than the equally effective dose for adults.

E. **Hematologic system**
   1. Normal values for hematocrit are listed in Table 29.1. The nadir of physiologic anemia is at 3 months of age, and the hematocrit may reach as low as 28% in an otherwise healthy infant. Premature infants may demonstrate a decrease in hemoglobin concentration as early as 4 to 6 weeks of age.
   2. At birth, **fetal hemoglobin** (HbF) predominates, but β-chain synthesis shifts to the adult type (HbA) by 3 to 4 months of age. Fetal hemoglobin has a higher affinity for oxygen (the oxyhemoglobin dissociation curve is shifted to the left), but this is not clinically significant.
   3. See section VII.B for calculations of blood volume and red cell mass.

F. **Hepatobiliary system**
   1. **Liver enzyme systems,** particularly those involved in phase-II (conjugation) reactions, are immature in the infant. Drugs

metabolized by the P-450 system may have prolonged elimination times.

2. **Jaundice** is common in neonates and can be physiologic or have pathologic causes.

3. **Hyperbilirubinemia** and displacement of bilirubin from albumin by drugs can result in kernicterus. Premature infants develop kernicterus at lower levels of bilirubin than do term infants (see Chapter 28, section III.D.1).

4. **Plasma levels of albumin** are lower at birth and this results in decreased protein binding of some drugs, and higher free drug concentration.

G. Endocrine system

1. **Newborns,** particularly premature babies and those small for gestational age, have decreased glycogen stores and are more susceptible to **hypoglycemia.** Infants of diabetic mothers have high insulin levels because of prolonged exposure to elevated maternal serum glucose levels and are prone to hypoglycemia. Infants who fall into these groups may have dextrose requirements as high as 5 to 15 mg/kg/minute. Normal glucose concentrations in the full-term infant are greater than or equal to 45 mg/dL (2.5 mmol/L).

2. **Hypocalcemia** is common in infants who are premature, small for gestational age, asphyxiated, offspring of diabetic mothers, or who have received transfusions with citrated blood or fresh-frozen plasma. Serum calcium concentration should be monitored in these patients and calcium chloride administered if the ionized calcium is less than 4.0 mg/dL (1.0 mmol/L).

H. Temperature regulation

1. Compared with adults, infants and children have a greater surface area to body weight ratio, which increases loss of body heat.

2. Infants have significantly less muscle mass and cannot compensate for cold by shivering or adjust their behavior to avoid the cold.

3. Infants respond to cold stress by increasing norepinephrine production, which enhances metabolism of brown fat. Norepinephrine also produces pulmonary and peripheral vasoconstriction, which can lead to right-to-left shunting, hypoxemia, and metabolic acidosis. Sick and preterm infants have limited stores of brown fat and therefore are more susceptible to cold. Strategies to prevent cold stress are discussed in section IV.C.

II. The preanesthetic visit. General principles of the preanesthetic visit are discussed in Chapter 1. The preoperative visit is an excellent opportunity to address the concerns of the child and parents. At least 90% of preoperative visits occur in an outpatient setting.

A. History should include the following:

1. Maternal health during gestation, including alcohol or drug use, smoking, diabetes, and viral infections.

2. Prenatal tests (e.g., ultrasound and amniocentesis).

3. Gestational age and weight.

4. Events during labor and delivery, including Apgar scores and length of hospital stay.

5. Hospitalizations/emergency room visits.

6. Congenital, chromosomal, metabolic anomalies or syndromes.

7. Recent upper respiratory infections, tracheobronchitis, "croup," reactive airway disease (asthma), exposure to communicable diseases, cyanotic episodes, or history of snoring.

8. Sleeping position (prone, side, or supine).

9. Growth history.

10. Vomiting, gastroesophageal reflux.

11. Siblings' health.

12. Parents who smoke.

13. Past surgical and anesthetic history.

14. Allergies (environmental, drugs, food, and latex).

15. Bleeding tendencies.

B. **Physical examination** should include the following:

1. General appearance, including alertness, color, tone, congenital anomalies, head size and shape, activity level, and social interaction.

2. Vital signs, height, and weight.

3. Loose teeth, craniofacial anomalies, or large tonsils that could complicate airway management.

4. Signs of upper respiratory infection and/or reactive airways disease. Excessive secretions may predispose patients to laryngospasm and bronchospasm during induction and emergence of anesthesia.

5. Heart murmurs, which may indicate flow through anatomic shunts.

6. Potential vascular access sites.

7. Strength, developmental milestones, activity level, and motor and verbal skills.

C. **Laboratory data** appropriate for the child's illness and proposed surgery should be obtained. Most centers agree that a "routine hematocrit" is unnecessary for healthy children. If indicated, laboratory tests can often be obtained after induction of general anesthesia (e.g., blood bank sample).

III. Premedication and fasting guidelines

A. **Premedication**

1. Children have a range of social development. Their behavior may be influenced by experiences they have had at home, in day care or school, and during previous hospitalizations. Honesty about procedures and associated pain is essential to maintaining the trust of children regardless of their level of development.

2. Infants less than 10 months old generally tolerate short periods of separation from parents and usually do not require premedication.

3. Children 10 months to 5 years of age cling to their parents and may require sedation before the induction of anesthesia (see section V.B).

4. Older children generally respond well to information and reassurance. Parental and patient anxiety may be reduced by having parents accompany children to the operating room. An especially anxious child may benefit from premedication. **Midazolam,** 0.5 mg/kg orally (PO), or **diazepam,** 0.2 to 0.3 mg/kg PO, given 15 to 20 minutes before surgery, is frequently used; it causes sedation with minimal respiratory

Table 29.3. Fasting guidelines (hours)

Age (Months)	Milk/Solids	Clear Liquid
≤36	6	2
>36	8	2

Note: Water and apple juice are examples of clear liquids. Breast milk is considered a solid.

---

depression. **Chloral hydrate** (25 to 50 mg/kg PO or rectally) is a drug used by pediatricians and radiologists for sedation during procedures. It causes minimal respiratory depression but may need to be repeated.

5. Premedication with intramuscular (IM) **anticholinergics** is not recommended. If vagolytic drugs are indicated, they are usually administered IV at the time of induction of anesthesia.

6. In the presence of **gastroesophageal reflux, ranitidine** (2 to 4 mg/kg PO, 2 mg/kg IV) along with **metoclopramide** (0.1 mg/kg) can be administered 2 hours before surgery to increase gastric pH and reduce gastric volume.

7. Children receiving medications for medical problems such as reactive airways disease, seizures, or hypertension should continue to take these medications preoperatively.

B. **Premedication and fasting guidelines**

1. Milk, breast milk, formula, and solid foods should be restricted as outlined in Table 29.3.

2. The **last feeding** should consist of clear fluids or sugar water. Studies document that there is no increased risk of aspiration if clear fluids are offered up to 2 hours preoperatively. This policy decreases the chance of preoperative dehydration and hypoglycemia and contributes to a smooth induction and stable operative course. We recommend that patients receive clear fluids until 2 hours before surgery is scheduled. Oral intake is then restricted (see Table 29.3).

3. If schedule delays occur, clear fluids may be given. Some patients may need to have an IV started for hydration.

IV. **Preparation of the operating room**

A. **Anesthetic circuit**

1. The **semiclosed circuit** normally used in adults has some disadvantages if used in very small infants:

   a. The inspiratory and expiratory valves increase resistance during spontaneous ventilation.

   b. The large volume of the absorber system acts as a reservoir for anesthetic agents.

   c. The tubing has a large compression volume.

2. The **nonrebreathing, open circuit (Mapleson D)** solves these problems (see Chapter 9). **Rebreathing** is prevented by using fresh gas flows 2.0 to 2.5 times the minute ventilation to wash out carbon dioxide. Capnography is essential in recognizing rebreathing (inspired $CO_2 >0$) and avoiding excessive hyperventilation. This circuit is useful for very small

infants who are allowed to breathe spontaneously and during transport.

3. A passive heat and moisture exchanger may be used with either circuit.

4. The **reservoir bag volume** should be at least as large as the child"s vital capacity but small enough so that a comfortable squeeze does not overinflate the chest. General guidelines for bag volumes are as follows: newborns, 500-mL bag; 1 to 3 years, 1,000-mL bag; and more than 3 years, 2,000-mL bag.

5. For most infants and children, the semi-closed-circuit-absorber system can be used with a smaller reservoir bag and a pediatric breathing circuit with small-caliber tubing (circle system).

B. **Airway equipment**

1. A **mask** with minimal dead space should be chosen. A clear plastic type is preferred because the lips (for color) and mouth (for secretions and vomitus) can be visualized.

2. The appropriate size of **oral airway** can be estimated by holding the airway in position next to the child's face. The tip of the oral airway should reach to the angle of the mandible.

3. **Laryngoscopy**

   a. A **narrow handle** is preferred because it has a more natural feel when using a smaller blade.

   b. A **straight blade** (Miller or Wis-Hipple) is recommended for children less than 2 years old. The smaller flange and long tapered tip of the straight blade provide better visualization of the larynx and manipulation of the epiglottis in the confined spaces of a small oral cavity.

   c. **Curved blades** are generally used for patients more than 5 years old.

   d. **Guidelines for laryngoscope blade sizes** (Table 29.4):

4. **Endotracheal tubes.** Traditionally, uncuffed tubes were used for children under 6 to 7 years of age (5.5-mm inner diameter endotracheal tube or smaller). Today, the risk of tracheal stenosis is minimal with modern low-pressure cuffs, and cuffed tubes may be used when indicated (e.g.,

Table 29.4. Guidelines for choice of laryngoscope blades

Age	Blade
Premature and neonate	Miller 0
Infant up to 6–8 mo	Miller 0–1
9 months to 2 yr	Miller 1
	Wis-Hipple 1.5
2 to 5 yr	Macintosh 1
	Miller 1–1.5
Child over 5 yr	Macintosh 2
	Miller 2
Adolescent to adult	Macintosh 3
	Miller 2

Table 29.5. Guidelines for endotracheal tube sizes

Age	Size (mm Internal Diameter)
Premature newborn	2.5–3.0
Full-term newborn	3.0
6–12 mo	3.5
12–20 mo	4.0
2 yr	4.5
Over 2 yr	$4 + [$age (years)$/4]$
6 yr	5.5
10 yr	6.5

Note: Tube length at mouth (cm) = [10 + age (years)] /2.

tonsillectomy or proximal bowel obstruction). Care must be taken not to overinflate the cuff and to realize that N_2O can diffuse into the cuff. At the time of intubation, endotracheal tubes that are one size larger and smaller than the estimated size should be available. Special techniques of endotracheal intubation are discussed in section VI. Table 29.5 provides guidelines for endotracheal tube sizes.

C. Temperature control
   1. The **operating room should be warmed** to between 80°F and 90°F before the child's arrival and a heating blanket placed on the operating room table. Infants should be kept covered with a blanket and a hat.
   2. **A servocontrolled radiant warmer** will keep infants warm during the induction of anesthesia and positioning. Skin temperature should be measured and should not exceed 39°C.
   3. **Passive heat and moisture exchangers** can be used for most routine cases. Some practitioners prefer to actively heat and humidify inspired gases during prolonged surgery.
   4. Fluids, blood products, and irrigation solutions should be warmed.

D. Monitoring
   1. In addition to standard monitoring (Chapter 10), a **precordial or esophageal stethoscope** provides information about heart and respiratory function.
   2. **Blood pressure**
      a. A blood pressure cuff should cover at least two-thirds of the upper arm but not encroach on the axilla or antecubital space.
      b. The cuff can be placed on the leg if the arms are inaccessible (e.g., cast present).
   3. **Pulse oximetry** is important, not only because of the rapid rate of desaturation in infants and small children, but also in avoiding unnecessary hyperoxic conditions in premature infants.
   4. Observed **end-tidal carbon dioxide measurements** usually will be lower than expected when a nonrebreathing circuit is

used, because exhaled gas will be diluted with high flows of fresh gases.

5. **Temperature** should always be monitored. In small infants esophageal, rectal, or axillary probes are acceptable. Once the drapes are placed, the warming blanket and room temperature should be adjusted so that children (especially small infants) do not become hyperthermic.

6. **Urine output** is an excellent reflection of volume status in children. In newborns, 0.5 mL/kg/hour is adequate; for infants over 1 month of age, 1.0 mL/kg/hour usually indicates adequate renal perfusion.

E. **IV setup and supplies**

1. For children less than 10 kg, a control chamber (burette) should be used to prevent inadvertent overhydration.

2. For older children, a pediatric infusion set is used where 60 drops equal 1 mL.

3. Extension tubing with a short T-piece connection is used so that injection ports are not draped out of reach. Drugs should be administered as close to the IV insertion site as possible to avoid excessive administration of flush solution.

4. Extra care should be taken to purge IV tubing of air, because it is possible for infants to shunt right to left through a patent foramen ovale. An air filter should be used in infants and children with known intracardiac shunts.

V. **Induction techniques**

A. **Infants less than 8 months old** can be transported to the operating room without sedation; anesthesia can then be induced by an inhalation technique (see section V.C). The vessel-rich organs are proportionately larger and the muscle and fat groups are smaller in neonates than in adults, affecting uptake and distribution of inhalation agents (see Chapter 11).

B. **Sedation options for children 8 months to 6 years old** include the following:

1. **Oral midazolam,** 0.5 to 1.0 mg/kg, dissolved in sweet syrup, usually produces sedation within 20 minute, although the time to onset of action can be quite variable. Patients often remain awake but sedated, and, generally, they will have no recall of leaving their parents or of induction of anesthesia.

2. **Ketamine,** 5 mg/kg given orally produces sedation within 10 to 15 minute and is synergistic with midazolam. Emergence time may be prolonged. This may be partially avoided by inserting an orogastric tube and emptying the stomach after induction.

3. **Oral transmucosal fentanyl** (Actiq, 5 to 15 μg/kg) provides both sedation and analgesia. Because respiratory depression can occur, an anesthetist must be immediately available when fentanyl is given.

4. Rectal methohexital (Brevital), 25 to 30 mg/kg in a 10% solution dissolved in sterile water can be administered via a syringe fitted with soft plastic tubing into the distal 2 cm of the rectum. Peak effect is at 10 to 15 minute; resuscitation equipment and an anesthetist should be available when giving this drug.

5. **Pulse oximetry** is used routinely once a patient is sedated.

C. Inhalation induction

1. This is the most common approach for pediatric patients, except when a rapid sequence IV induction is indicated.

2. An **"excitement stage"** of anesthesia often is encountered during inhalation induction. Therefore, noise and activity in the operating room should be minimized. This stage should be explained to parents if they will be present during induction.

3. **Techniques**

   a. **Children 8 months to 5 years old** may be anesthetized after premedication. The face mask is held near, but not touching, the child's face, and low flow rates (1 to 3 L/min) of oxygen and nitrous oxide are begun. The concentration of volatile agent (sevoflurane or halothane) is gradually increased in 0.5% increments. When the eyelid reflex disappears, the mask can be applied to the child's face and the jaw gently lifted.

   b. A **slow inhalation induction** may be used in cooperative toddlers and older children who have not been premedicated. Children are shown how to breathe through a clear anesthetic mask. Oxygen and N_2O are given via face mask, and then a volatile anesthetic is gradually added to the mixture. An engaging story incorporating breathing instructions can be very useful.

   c. A **"single-breath induction"** may be accomplished with a few breaths of a mixture of a volatile anesthetic with nitrous oxide.

      (1) Loss of consciousness can be achieved with a single vital capacity breath of 4% halothane or 8% sevoflurane and 70% N_2O-O_2. Sevoflurane has gained in popularity, due to less myocardial depression and bradycardia during induction than halothane. Desflurane, a very pungent volatile anesthetic, is not recommended for inhalation induction.

      (2) The circuit is prefilled with 70% N_2O-O_2 and 7% to 8% sevoflurane or 4% to 5% halothane. The end of the circuit should be occluded with a plug or another reservoir bag and the pop-off valve left open to minimize nonscavenged anesthetic spillage.

      (3) Painting the mask with flavor extracts may increase acceptance by children.

      (4) The child is instructed to take a deep breath (vital capacity) of room air, blow it all out (forced expiration), and then hold his or her breath. At this point, the anesthetist gently places the mask on the patient's face. The child then takes a deep inspiration of the anesthetic mixture and again holds his or her breath. This sequence is repeated for four or five breaths.

      (5) Most children will be anesthetized within 60 seconds; a few children will need longer.

   d. Children can become frightened, uncooperative, and even combative during an inhalation induction. Should this occur, it is imperative to have a backup plan, such as an IM injection of a sedative or hypnotic.

D. Intramuscular induction. For the extremely uncooperative or developmentally delayed child, anesthesia may be induced with ketamine (4 to 8 mg/kg IM), which takes effect in 3 to 5 minutes. Atropine (0.02 mg/kg IM) or glycopyrrolate (0.01 mg/kg IM) should be mixed with the ketamine to prevent excessive salivation. Midazolam, 0.2 to 0.5 mg/kg IM, may also be given to reduce the chance of emergence delirium.

E. IV induction

1. **For children more than 8 years old:** Often, older children may prefer an IV technique rather than a mask. Anesthesia can be induced with propofol (3 to 4 mg/kg) or thiopental (4 to 6 mg/kg).

2. IV induction at this age is often preferable to a mask induction because many older children do not like the smell of volatile anesthetics. Local anesthesia before IV placement can be achieved with subcutaneous injection of lidocaine 1%. Alternatively (or additionally), **EMLA cream** (a eutectic mixture of 2.5% lidocaine and 2.5% prilocaine) or LMX cream (lidocaine 4%) can be applied to the skin approximately 45 min before IV placement. EMLA cream is also useful to reduce the pain of accessing a Portacath.

F. Children with "full stomachs"

1. For **rapid sequence induction,** in general, the same principles apply to infants and children as for adults. In addition:

   a. **Atropine** (0.02 mg/kg) may be given IV to prevent bradycardia, especially if succinylcholine will be given.

   b. Children require larger doses of thiopental (4 to 6 mg/kg), propofol (3 to 4 mg/kg), and succinylcholine (1.5 to 2.0 mg/kg) because of a larger volume of distribution for these drugs.

   c. Infants with gastric distention (pyloric stenosis) should have their stomachs decompressed by an orogastric tube before induction of anesthesia. This gastric tube should again be suctioned before the trachea is extubated.

   d. **Ranitidine** (2 to 4 mg/kg) can be given to decrease gastric volume and increase gastric pH: **Ondansetron, (0.15 mg/kg) can be given for postoperative nausea and vomiting prophylaxis.**

   e. **Metoclopramide** should not be given if gastric outlet or bowel obstruction is suspected.

2. **An awake laryngoscopy and intubation** is an option for the moribund infant or an infant with a grossly abnormal airway (e.g., a severe craniofacial anomaly) and a "full stomach."

3. **A cuffed endotracheal tube** should be considered for a child with a full stomach. This option minimizes the need for replacing an uncuffed tube that proves too small. The cuff volume can be adjusted to ensure an appropriate air leak.

VI. Endotracheal intubation

A. Oral approach

1. Older children are placed in the "sniffing" position using a blanket. Infants and small children have large occiputs, and a small towel placed under the scapulae is more helpful.

2. During laryngoscopy, the tip of the blade is used to elevate the epiglottis. If this technique does not provide a good view of the glottis, the laryngoscope blade may be placed in the vallecula even with a straight blade.

3. The distance from the glottis to the carina is about 4 cm in a term neonate. Pediatric endotracheal tubes have a single black line located 2 cm from the tip and a double black line at 3 cm; these markings should be observed while the tube is passed beyond the vocal cords.

4. If resistance is met during intubation, a half-size smaller tube should be tried.

5. After intubation, the chest should be examined for bilateral equal expansion and the lungs auscultated for equal breath sounds. There should be a leak around an uncuffed tube when 15- to 20-cm H_2O positive pressure is applied. If the leak is present at less than 10 cm H_2O pressure, the endotracheal tube should be changed to the next larger size. Capnography should demonstrate consistently appropriate end-tidal CO_2 values.

6. The chest should be auscultated after every change in head or body position to verify equal bilateral breath sounds. Extension of the head can result in extubation, while flexion can result in tube advancement into either main-stem bronchus.

7. Endotracheal tubes should be securely taped and the numerical marking on the tube closest to the gingiva noted; migration of the endotracheal tube will be apparent from any change in this relation.

8. The **laryngeal mask airway** (see Chapter 13, section IV) has revolutionized pediatric anesthesia. It has replaced the mask airway for simple cases (e.g., herniorrhaphy) and the endotracheal tube for many procedures (e.g., magnetic resonance imaging or computed tomography scan).

B. **Nasal approach**
   1. This method is generally similar to that for adults (see Chapter 13).
   2. The cephalad position of the infant larynx makes unaided intubation difficult; Magill forceps frequently are needed to guide the tip of the tube through the vocal cords.
   3. Nasal intubation should be performed only when specifically indicated (e.g., oral surgery) because of the risk of epistaxis from enlarged adenoids.

C. **Apneic infants** will become hypoxemic within 30 to 45 seconds, even after preoxygenation. If bradycardia, cyanosis, or desaturation occurs, intubation attempts should cease immediately and 100% oxygen administered until the oxygen saturation improves.

D. **Muscle relaxants**
   1. **Muscle relaxants** often are used to facilitate endotracheal intubation. Muscle relaxants may be contraindicated in infants and children with abnormal airway anatomy.
   2. The use of **halothane and succinylcholine** together during induction is associated with an increased incidence of masseter spasm. This drug combination is rarely used in current practice; instead, nondepolarizing relaxants are generally selected unless rapid sequence induction is specifically indicated.

3. **Succinylcholine** can produce bradycardia, which may be exaggerated with repeated doses. If atropine has not been administered before the first dose of succinylcholine, it should be given before the second dose. The use of succinylcholine in children with occult myopathies may result in life-threatening hyperkalemia manifesting as wide-complex bradycardia, ventricular tachycardia, ventricular fibrillation, or asystole. A history of mild muscle weakness or failure to attain age-appropriate physical milestones may be absent, as the Duchenne and Becker types of muscular dystrophy may not be apparent until the child is 4 years of age. Any suspicion of muscle weakness, particularly in male infants, should warrant a preoperative creatine kinase level. Hence the FDA "black box" warning that "Succinylcholine in children should be reserved for emergency intubation or instances where immediate securing of the airway is necessary, e.g., laryngospasm, difficult airway, full stomach." Succinylcholine should not be given to children with a close family history of malignant hyperthermia (see Chapter 18, section XVII).

4. **Rocuronium** (0.6 to 1.2 mg/kg) and **mivacurium** (0.20 to 0.25 mg/kg) have a quick onset of action. In most cases, these drugs have replaced succinylcholine when a rapid sequence induction is mandated.

5. Routine neuromuscular relaxation can be achieved with **cisatracurium** (0.1 to 0.2 mg/kg) for intubation.

6. For very long cases (e.g., craniotomy, cardiac surgery), **pancuronium** (0.1 mg/kg) is an option. Reversal of neuromuscular blockade with **neostigmine** (0.05 to 0.06 mg/kg) and an anticholinergic drug (e.g., atropine or glycopyrrolate) should occur if the twitch monitor or clinical exam suggests weakness.

VII. **Fluid management.** The following calculations may be used to estimate fluid requirements for infants and children. Other reflections of volume status, including blood pressure, heart rate, urine output, central venous pressure, and osmolarity may guide further adjustments.

A. **Maintenance fluid requirements**
   1. Administer 4 mL/kg/hour for the first 10 kg of body weight (100 mL/kg per day), 2 mL/kg/hour for the second 10 kg (50 mL/kg per day), and then add 1 mL/kg/hour for more than 20 kg (25 mL/kg per day). For example, maintenance fluids for a 25-kg child would be ([4 × 10] + [2 × 10] + [1 × 5]) = 65 mL/hour.
   2. The usual solution for replacement of fluid deficits and ongoing losses in the healthy child is **lactated Ringer's solution.** A second solution of 5% dextrose frequently is used in the perioperative period for premature infants, septic neonates, infants of diabetic mothers, and those receiving total parenteral nutrition. These patients should have blood glucose levels measured periodically.

B. **Estimated blood volume (EBV) and blood losses**
   1. **EBV** is 95 mL/kg in premature neonates, 90 mL/kg in full-term neonates, 80 mL/kg in infants up to 1 year old, and 70 mL/kg thereafter.

2. **Estimated red cell mass (ERCM)**
ERCM = EBV × patient hematocrit/100.
3. **Acceptable red cell loss (ARCL)**
ARCL = ERCM − ERCM$_{acceptable}$,
which is the ERCM at the lowest acceptable hematocrit.
4. **Acceptable blood loss (ABL)**
ABL = ARCL × 3.
   a. If the amount of the blood loss is less than one-third of the ABL, it can be replaced with lactated Ringer's solution.
   b. If the amount of blood loss is greater than one-third of the total ABL, one should consider replacement with colloid (e.g., 5% albumin).
   c. If the amount of blood loss is greater than ABL, replace with packed red blood cells and an equal amount of colloid. Fresh-frozen plasma and platelet transfusions should be guided by results of coagulation tests, estimates of the present and anticipated blood losses, and adequacy of clot formation in the wound.
   d. For infants and young children, blood loss should be measured using small suction containers and by weighing sponges. Because it is sometimes difficult to measure small-volume blood losses precisely in young children, monitoring of hematocrit will help avoid unnecessary transfusions and also alert the anesthetist to the need for blood transfusion.
   e. The **"acceptable hematocrit"** is no longer considered to be 30%. Each patient is evaluated with respect to the need for red blood cell transfusion. A healthy child with normal cardiac function can compensate for acute anemia by increasing cardiac output. A debilitated child, confronting sepsis, chemotherapy, or massive surgery, may require a higher hematocrit.
C. **Estimated fluid deficit** = (maintenance fluid per hour) × hours since the last oral intake. The entire estimated fluid deficit is replaced during all major cases; the first half is administered during the first hour, and the remaining deficit is infused over the next 1 to 2 hours.
D. **Third-space losses** may require up to an additional 10 mL/kg/hour of lactated Ringer's solution or normal saline if there is extensive exposure of the intestine or a significant ileus.
VIII. **Emergence and postanesthesia care**
A. **Extubation**
1. **Laryngospasm** may occur during emergence, especially during the critical period of excitement.
2. In most cases, the trachea is extubated after emergence from anesthesia. Coughing is not a sign that the child is ready for extubation. Instead, children should demonstrate purposeful activity (e.g., reaching for the endotracheal tube) or eye opening before extubation. In the infant, hip flexion and strong grimaces are useful indications of awakening.
3. Alternatively, the trachea may be extubated while the patient is still anesthetized deeply. This can be done in operations such as inguinal herniorrhaphy where coughing on emergence is undesirable or in patients with reactive airways

disease. A "deep" extubation would not be appropriate for a child with an abnormal airway or one who has eaten recently.

B. **During transport** to the postanesthesia care unit (PACU), the child's color and ventilatory pattern should be continuously monitored. Supplemental oxygen is administered if indicated (e.g., the child with anemia or pulmonary disease).

C. **In the PACU,** early reunion of the child and parents is desirable.

IX. Specific pediatric anesthesia problems

A. The compromised airway

1. **Etiologies**

   a. Congenital abnormalities (e.g., choanal atresia, Pierre Robin syndrome, tracheal stenosis, or laryngeal web).

   b. Inflammation (e.g., tracheobronchitis or "croup," epiglottitis, pharyngeal abscess).

   c. Foreign bodies in the trachea or esophagus.

   d. Neoplasms (e.g., congenital hemangioma, cystic hygroma, or thoracic lymphadenopathy).

   e. Trauma.

2. **Initial management**

   a. Administer 100% oxygen by face mask.

   b. Keep the child as calm as possible. Evaluation should be efficient, because it may increase agitation and cause further airway compromise. Parents are invaluable in their ability to pacify their children and should remain with them as long as feasible.

   c. An anesthetist must be present during transport to the operating room. Oxygen, a resuscitation bag and mask, laryngoscope, atropine, succinylcholine, drugs suitable for sedation and hypnosis, appropriate endotracheal tubes and laryngeal mask airways, oral airways, and pulse oximetry must be available.

3. **Induction of anesthesia**

   a. **Minimize manipulation of the patient.** A precordial stethoscope and pulse oximeter are adequate monitors during the initial induction of anesthesia.

   b. The child may remain in a **semisitting position,** with the parents present if indicated. A **gradual inhalation induction** with either sevoflurane or halothane is the next step (see section V.C.3). Airway obstruction and poor air exchange will prolong induction.

   c. Parents are asked to leave when the child becomes unconscious, and an IV is started. If indicated, atropine may be given at this time.

   d. **Patients with croup** may benefit from gentle application of continuous positive airway pressure, but any positive pressure can cause acute airway obstruction in patients with epiglottitis or a foreign body.

   e. The **oral endotracheal tube** should have a stylet and be at least one size smaller than the predicted size. If postoperative ventilation is anticipated (e.g., epiglottitis), a cuffed endotracheal tube may be indicated.

   f. At this point, patients usually are hypercarbic (PetCO$_2$ between 50 and 60 mm Hg), but generally this is well tolerated provided they are not also hypoxemic.

Bradycardia is an indication of hypoxemia and requires immediate establishment of a patent airway.

g. Perform laryngoscopy only when the child is deeply anesthetized. The decision to give a muscle relaxant depends on the situation. A muscle relaxant facilitates intubation and obviates the need for deep anesthesia in certain circumstances. In other cases, muscle relaxation may further compromise the airway. In general, orotracheal intubation should be accomplished before any further airway procedures are attempted. **Bronchoscopy** is indicated before intubation in cases of large upper airway foreign bodies or friable subglottic tumors (e.g., hemangioma).

h. **A nasal tube** may be more appropriate for illnesses that require several days of intubation (e.g., epiglottitis). An orotracheal tube may be changed to a nasotracheal tube at the end of the procedure, provided the oral intubation was easily accomplished. Never jeopardize a secure oral endotracheal tube for the sake of changing it to a nasal endotracheal tube.

i. Children should be sedated during transport to the intensive care unit; a combination of a narcotic and a benzodiazepine or propofol infusion is effective. Propofol is not approved in the United States for prolonged sedation of pediatric intensive care patients. Breathing may be spontaneous or assisted during the immediate postoperative period.

4. **Management of the inhaled foreign body (FB)**

a. Foreign body aspiration usually occurs between 7 months and 4 years of age. About 75% of foreign bodies lodge in the proximal airway (larynx, trachea, right/left mainstem bronchus). Most deaths occur at the time of aspiration, and the mortality in most series is zero if the child reaches the hospital alive.

b. Choking and wheezing following a witnessed aspiration event is the most common **presentation.** The triad of coughing, wheezing, and reduced breath sounds is present in only 50% of cases. Chest x-ray may show radio-opaque objects, postobstructive emphysema, or a localized pneumonia but has a false-negative rate of 40%.

c. **Management** is prompt rigid bronchoscopy regardless of chest x-ray findings. It is vital to communicate with the bronchoscopist before and during the procedure. An emergency tracheotomy and thoracotomy kit should be prepared. There are two approaches to the anesthetic: spontaneous ventilation and controlled ventilation.

d. **Spontaneous ventilation:** After good preoxygenation and IV atropine or glycopyrrolate, an inhalational induction is performed in 100% oxygen. Sevoflurane is preferred to halothane because of the lack of sensitization of the heart to endogenous catecholamines. Spontaneous ventilation is maintained. Once an adequate depth is achieved, the vocal cords and subglottic space are sprayed with topical lidocaine (2% in school-age children, 1% for small infants). The trachea is then intubated with a ventilating bronchoscope. A sufficient depth of anesthesia is required to prevent moving and coughing. Consider a small dose of muscle relaxant just before removal of the FB through the vocal cords. The stomach is then suctioned and the patient is allowed to emerge breathing through either a mask or an endotracheal tube placed after FB removal. Advantages of this technique are better air flow distribution and ventilation-perfusion matching, uninterrupted ventilation, and being able to immediately assess ventilatory mechanics after FB removal. Disadvantages are the risks of patient movement, coughing, laryngospasm, and prolonged emergence.

e. **Controlled ventilation:** Anesthesia is commenced with a rapid sequence induction using propofol and succinylcholine. Maintenance is achieved with a propofol/remifentanil infusion, and muscle relaxation is achieved with a short-acting agent such as mivacurium (bolus or infusion). The trachea is intubated with a ventilating bronchoscope, and ventilation is performed in concert with the bronchoscopists' interventions. When the bronchoscope is in place, ventilation is achieved with high inspiratory pressures, and long expiratory times are necessary to prevent barotrauma. Emergence is achieved in a manner similar to the spontaneous ventilation technique. The advantages of controlled ventilation are rapid control of the airway, no patient movement, and lower anesthetic requirements. However ventilation is intermittently interrupted, and there are risks of displacing the FB distally and of possible barotrauma with ball-valve hyperinflation.

f. A large retrospective study showed that **ventilatory technique** did not affect the success of foreign body removal or influence adverse outcomes (hypoxia, hypercarbia, bradycardia, hypotension).

B. **Recent upper respiratory infection.** Infants and children can have 6 to 10 upper respiratory infections each year. It is important to balance the severity of symptoms with the urgency of surgery. Wheezing, fever, and cough are signs of lower respiratory inflammation and are associated with an increased risk of perioperative airway complications. Conversely, myringotomy and ear tube placement may relieve the rhinorrhea associated with chronic otitis media.

C. **Intra-abdominal malformations** include pyloric stenosis, gastroschisis, omphalocele, atresia of the small intestine, and volvulus (see Chapter 28).

1. **Gastrointestinal emergencies** frequently produce marked dehydration and electrolyte abnormalities. Repair of pyloric stenosis should be delayed until intravascular volume is restored and the hypokalemic, hypochloremic, metabolic alkalosis is corrected. The situation is more urgent with other diagnoses (e.g., duodenal atresia), and rehydration can be continued intraoperatively.

2. **Abdominal distention** in infants and young children rapidly causes respiratory compromise, so nasogastric drainage is

mandatory. Even so, a few moribund infants may require endotracheal intubation before the induction of anesthesia.

3. Children with less severe physiologic disturbances and only mild or moderate distention can undergo a rapid sequence induction of anesthesia.

4. A severely dehydrated and septic child may require additional monitoring (e.g., arterial line, central venous line, and urinary catheter).

5. Volatile anesthetics are appropriate for the previously healthy infant undergoing a simple operation (such as pyloromyotomy). In the case of an extremely ill child (e.g., perforated viscous), the anesthetic management should include an O_2-air mixture and drugs causing minimal myocardial depression. Opioids (morphine 0.1 to 0.2 mg/kg IV; fentanyl 1 to 2 (g/kg IV; or meperidine, 1 to 2 mg/kg IV), benzodiazepines, and neuromuscular relaxants are usually better tolerated than volatile anesthetics. Nitrous oxide should be avoided because it may add to abdominal distention.

6. **Fluid and heat losses.** When the bowel is exposed and manipulated, third-space losses may be excessive and remarkable fluid volumes may be necessary. Even when using all possible warming strategies, heat loss may be unavoidable.

7. Postoperative ventilatory support is often indicated until abdominal distention is diminished, hypothermia resolves, and fluid requirements decrease.

D. Thoracic emergencies
1. **Tracheoesophageal fistula.** See Chapter 28.
2. **Congenital diaphragmatic hernia.** See Chapter 28.

E. Congenital heart disease. See Chapters 2, 23, and 28.

F. Head and neck procedures
1. Strabismus repair. See Chapter 25.
2. Tonsillectomy, adenoidectomy, and emergency surgery in the child with bleeding tonsils. See Chapter 25.

X. Regional anesthesia for pediatric patients has gained acceptance because of a better understanding of the pharmacokinetics and pharmacodynamics of local anesthetics in infants and children and the availability of specifically designed equipment.

A. Pharmacology of local anesthetics
1. **Protein binding** of local anesthetics is decreased in neonates because of decreased levels of serum albumin. Free drug concentration may be increased, especially for bupivacaine.

2. **Plasma cholinesterase activity** may be decreased in infants less than 6 months old, which theoretically diminishes clearance of amino esters.

3. **Hepatic microsomal enzyme systems** are immature in the neonate and this will decrease the clearance of amino amides.

4. **The increased volume of distribution** in the infant and child acts to decrease free local anesthetic concentrations in the blood.

5. **Systemic toxicity** is the most frequent complication of regional anesthetics, and doses should be carefully calculated on a weight basis. The risk of accumulation of free drug after repeated doses of local anesthetics is increased in infants and children.

B. Spinal anesthesia

1. Indications

   a. Premature infants less than 60 weeks postconceptual age and infants with a history of apnea and bradycardia, bronchopulmonary dysplasia, or need for long-term ventilatory support are at increased risk for apnea and cardiovascular instability after general anesthesia. Spinal anesthesia may decrease the likelihood of these postoperative anesthetic complications. These infants still require a minimum of 24 hours of cardiorespiratory monitoring postoperatively, regardless of the anesthetic technique. Sedation during spinal anesthesia may negate all these potential benefits.

   b. Children at risk for malignant hyperthermia.

   c. Children with chronic airways disease such as reactive airway disease or cystic fibrosis.

   d. Cooperative older children and adolescents with full stomachs undergoing peripheral emergency surgery (e.g., fractured ankle).

2. Anatomy. See Chapter 16.

3. Technique

   a. The procedure may be performed with the patient in the lateral decubitus or sitting position. Premature infants and neonates are positioned in the sitting position to limit rostral spread of drug. The head is supported upright to prevent upper airway obstruction. A 22-gauge, 1.5-inch spinal needle is used for infants, because cerebrospinal fluid flow is very slow. In children older than 2 years, a 25-gauge needle is preferable.

   b. An IV should be started before spinal anesthesia and the patient should be monitored throughout the procedure. Maintaining normothermia is essential, especially for premature infants and neonates. The infant should remain supine after placement of the spinal anesthetic; the Trendelenburg position should be avoided because this may move the drug cephalad in the subarachnoid space.

4. Drugs and dosage

   a. Hyperbaric solutions of bupivacaine or tetracaine are used most frequently.

   b. The dosage requirements are increased and the duration of action is decreased in infants.

   c. **Recommended dosages** (for a T-6 spinal level)

   (1) **Bupivacaine,** 0.75% in 8.25% dextrose, 0.3 mg/kg in both infants and children.

   (2) **Tetracaine,** 1%, combined with an equal volume of 10% dextrose, 0.8 to 1.0 mg/kg in the infant, and 0.25 to 0.5 mg/kg in the child. This dose is large compared with adult dosage, but it is necessary in infants.

   d. **Duration of surgical anesthesia** averages 90 minutes with tetracaine and less with bupivacaine. The duration of the block may be prolonged by adding epinephrine, 10 μg/kg (up to 0.2 mg), or phenylephrine, 75 μg/kg (up to 2 mg).

5. **Complications and contraindications**
   a. **The anesthetic level** recedes much more quickly in children than in adults. If the block wears off, supplemental sedation must be used cautiously, especially in premature infants and neonates. If subarachnoid anesthesia is inadequate, it is best to initiate general anesthesia before positioning.
   b. **Hypotension** is rare in children less than 7 to 10 years old, perhaps because resting sympathetic vascular tone is lower than in adults. A high spinal anesthetic may be heralded only by mottled skin or apnea and bradycardia.
   c. **Contraindications** are similar to those in adults, with particular attention to congenital anatomic defects of the central nervous system and a history of intraventricular hemorrhage.

C. **Caudal and lumbar epidural anesthesia**
   1. **Indications.** These techniques are useful in combination with general anesthesia for minor and major procedures of the thorax, abdomen, pelvis, bladder, and lower extremities, particularly when significant postoperative pain is anticipated (e.g., orthopedic surgery).
   2. **Anatomy** is outlined in Chapter 16. Note that the dural sac ends at the level of the S-3 vertebra in the neonate; care is required to avoid dural puncture during placement of the caudal needle.
   3. **Technique** is outlined in Chapter 16.
      a. Most caudal and lumbar epidural anesthetics are placed after induction of general anesthesia.
      b. **Caudal anesthesia** may be administered as a single injection of local anesthetic through a 1.5-inch, short-bevel needle placed into the caudal epidural space. This technique is ideally suited for short procedures with mild to moderate postoperative pain such as inguinal herniorrhaphy, orchiopexy, and circumcision. For longer procedures or prolonged postoperative analgesia, a catheter may be advanced from the sacral epidural space. Intermittent boluses or a continuous infusion of local anesthetic with or without an opioid may be used. In infants, 22-gauge caudal catheters are placed through 20-gauge, 40- to 50-mm Tuohy needles; older children require 20-gauge catheters placed through 17- or 18-gauge, 90- to 100-mm Tuohy needles.
      c. **Caudal catheters** can be advanced to lumbar or thoracic levels in young children because the epidural space is not yet extensively vascularized. The recommended levels are T-6 to T-9 vertebral level for thoracic surgery (e.g., pectus excavatum repair), T-10 to T-12 vertebral level for abdominal surgery (e.g., Nissen fundoplication or bowel resections), and L-3 to L-4 vertebral level for pelvic procedures. Usually these catheters advance easily; resistance may indicate malpositioning. If necessary, confirmation of catheter placement can be done with contrast dye and fluoroscopy. While easy to place, compared with a lumbar catheter, the caudal catheter has a greater potential to become contaminated

from stool. Also, the catheter may become dislodged postoperatively.

d. **Epidural catheters** may be placed via lumbar or thoracic approaches. The distance from the skin to the epidural space is short (1 to 2 cm) in children, and, again, care must be taken to avoid dural puncture. Loss of resistance is usually accomplished with the aid of saline rather than air. In older children, 18-gauge Tuohy needles and 20-gauge catheters are used. Thoracic catheters are useful for pectus excavation repair or thoracotomy. Placement of a thoracic epidural catheter in anesthetized children depends on the practitioner's skills and experience. Some might argue that this method may cause inadvertent injury, while others believe that an awake 7-year-old cannot reliably remain still during this procedure.

4. **Drugs and doses**

a. In **single-dose caudal anesthesia,** a long duration of sensory blockade with minimal motor blockade is desirable. Bupivacaine, 0.125% to 0.25% with epinephrine, is administered according to the formula of 0.06 mL of local anesthetic per kg per segment, where the number of segments is counted from the S-5 spinal level to the desired level of analgesia. A simple alternative dosing scheme is to administer 0.125% bupivacaine with epinephrine at a dose of 1 mL/kg. Increasing the concentration of bupivacaine above 0.25% does not appear to improve analgesia. Dosages of bupivacaine up to 3.5 mg/kg result in plasma levels in infants and children below the toxic range determined for adults. Ropivacaine and levobupivacaine have been successfully used in caudal anesthesia in concentrations of 0.125% and 0.25% at doses of 1 mL/kg for minor elective surgery. There appears to be no or minimal motor block at these concentrations that have equal efficacy.

b. The addition of adjunct drugs may prolong postoperative analgesia. The addition of **clonidine** 1 to 2 μg/kg to 0.25% bupivacaine prolongs duration of analgesia by 2 to 3 hours. It may cause increased sedation postoperatively and should be avoided in babies at risk of apnea (neonates and ex-preterm infants). The use of preservative–free racemic **ketamine** [or the $S +$ enantiomer], prolongs analgesic duration significantly more than clonidine. At a dose of 1 mg/kg, $S +$ ketamine appears to have no cardiorespiratory, sedative, emetic, or behavioral side effects. Ketamine is synergistic with clonidine (1 μg/kg).

c. **Caudal or epidural catheter anesthesia**

(1) **Intermittent bolus dosing.** Initially, 1% lidocaine, 0.5 mL/kg, followed by 0.5% lidocaine, 0.5 mL/kg every hour as needed, or initially, 0.25% to 0.5% bupivacaine, 0.5 mL/kg, followed by 0.25% bupivacaine, 0.25 mL/kg every 1.5 to 2.0 hours as needed, is recommended.

(2) **Continuous infusion.** An initial loading dose of 0.04 mL/kg per segment of 0.1% bupivacaine with or without fentanyl, 3 μg/ml in infants and children younger than 7 years and 0.02 mL/kg per segment for children older than 7 years, is recommended. An infusion of 0.1% bupivacaine with or without fentanyl, 3 μg/ml at 0.1 mL/kg/hour, is started immediately after the bolus. The infusion rate may be increased to 0.3 mL/kg/hour as needed, with the total hourly dose of fentanyl not to exceed 1 μg/kg/hour. Infants younger than 1 year generally do not receive fentanyl in the epidural infusion, unless they are in a closely monitored setting (see Chapter 37, section III.E).

   d. Postoperative analgesia may be provided by infusion through the caudal or epidural catheter. Generally, an infusion of 0.1% bupivacaine with fentanyl, 3 μg/ml at 0.1 to 0.3 mL/kg/hour, will provide good analgesia without motor blockade. However, some patients benefit from omission of local anesthetic from the infusion, and fentanyl, 0.5 to 1.0 μg/kg/hour can be used in these patients. Infants younger than 1 year old, as noted above, usually do not receive epidural opioids because of concern about postoperative respiratory depression. These infants receive an infusion of 0.1% bupivacaine, 0.1 to 0.3 mL/kg/hour.

   5. Contraindications are the same as for spinal anesthesia (see section X.B.5).

   6. Complications of epidural and caudal anesthesia are discussed in Chapter 16.

D. Brachial plexus blocks (for upper extremity surgery), **penile blocks** (for circumcision), and **ilio-inguinal blocks** (for inguinal herniorrhaphy) are particularly useful regional techniques in the pediatric population. See the texts by Gregory and Dalen for additional details (Suggested Readings).

XI. Current issues in pediatric anesthesia

A. Postanesthesia excitation

   1. Sevoflurane has essentially replaced halothane as the volatile agent of choice during inhalational inductions. Sevoflurane has rapid, smooth induction characteristics; lacks adverse cardiovascular effects; and has low solubility. However, anesthesia maintained with sevoflurane is associated with a higher **risk** of postanesthesia excitation (incidence of 27% to 67%) compared with halothane (5% to 30%).

   2. Etiology of the excitation is unclear. It occurs independently of good analgesia and is present even after regional anesthesia and nonsurgical procedures such as magnetic resonance imaging scanning. While rapid emergence is thought to be a factor, excitation is not observed after propofol or remifentanil-based anesthesia.

   3. Postanesthesia excitation **presents** soon after emergence and may occur even if the child arrives asleep in the PACU. It is characterized by crying, thrashing, inconsolability, combativeness, restlessness, and confusion for up to 30 minutes unaffected by parental presence on emergence. **Risk factors** include maintenance with low-solubility agents (sevoflurane, desflurane), young age (<6 years of age), preoperative anxiety, and temperament (children with separation anxiety and those prone to temper tantrums). During this phase there is a risk of patient injury, loss of venous access, parental distress, and disruption of the PACU environment. It appears to be a time-limited phenomenon, and there is no evidence for negative behavioral changes in the first 30 days after surgery.

4. **Preemptive strategies** have included pre/intraoperative midazolam, intraoperative opioids, α_2 agonists, and small doses of propofol on emergence. A common practice supported by anecdotal evidence is to switch to isoflurane after induction or to change to a propofol-based anesthetic. Randomized trials have shown that IV clonidine (2 μg/kg), dexmedetomidine (0.3 μg/kg), and fentanyl (2 μg/kg) have been effective in preventing excitation.

5. **Treatment strategies** include IV fentanyl (1 μg/kg), supportive measures, minimizing external stimuli, and preventing injury with padded rails. Reversible causes of excitation such as ventilatory issues, electrolyte abnormalities, hypovolemia, and pain should be ruled out before assuming a residual volatile effect.

B. **Propofol infusion syndrome**
1. Propofol has been a popular drug for **off-license sedation** in the PICU owing to its record of safety in the operating room, lack of accumulation, and rapid recovery after discontinuation. However, the recognition of propofol infusion syndrome (PRIS), an uncommon but usually fatal condition described in critically ill children, has changed sedation practice in the PICU.

2. PRIS is **characterized** by progressive metabolic acidosis; rhabdomyolysis; lipemia; bradydysrhythmias (occasionally tachydysrhythmias); and cardiac, renal, and hepatic dysfunction usually leading to death.

3. **Biochemical abnormalities** are consistent with a disruption of fatty acid oxidation and impaired mitochondrial electron transport, resulting in the buildup of toxic intermediates of fatty acid metabolism and impaired cellular respiration. Typical serum findings include raised lactate, creatinine, creatinine kinase, troponin I, myoglobin, transaminases, and acylcarnitines (which may serve as an early marker).

4. **Risk factors** include critically ill intubated, ventilated children with upper respiratory tract infections or acute central nervous system disease/injury receiving high propofol infusion rates (>4 mg/kg/hour) for prolonged infusion periods (although PRIS may occur much earlier) and receiving inadequate carbohydrate intake (<6 mg/kg/minute).

5. **Treatment** involves early institution of charcoal hemoperfusion or continuous veno-veno hemofiltration. Pressors and pacing appear ineffective without instituting these measures, and stopping the infusion alone does not halt the clinical progression.

C. **Dexmedetomidine applications**
1. Dexmedetomidine, the dextro isomer of the benzyl imidazole medetomidine, is an α_2 **agonist** that is 8 to 10 times more specific than clonidine and is approved by the FDA for short-term sedation in adult ICU patients. It has a mean

elimination half-life of 1.5 to 3 hours, is metabolized extensively by the liver, and is excreted renally. It has anxiolytic, sedative, and analgesic **properties.** In the pediatric population, it has been successfully used for sedation during mechanical ventilation, during noninvasive radiological procedures, and in refractory postoperative pain.

2. The usual **dose** is a load of 0.5 to 1 μg/kg over 10 minutes followed by an infusion of 0.5 to 1 μg/kg/hour. It may cause clinically insignificant decreases in mean arterial pressure and heart rate and minor effects on ventilation in spontaneously breathing patients. It has been used to reduce emergence agitation at a dose of 0.5 μg/kg, but it may then cause slightly increased times to emergence and extubation.

SUGGESTED READING

Behrman RE, Kliegman RM, Jenson HB. *Nelson textbook of pediatrics,* 17th ed. Philadelphia: WB Saunders, 2005.

Cloherty JP, Stark AR. *Manual of neonatal care,* 4th ed. Philadelphia: Lippincott Williams & Wilkins, 1998.

Coté CJ, Ryan JF, Goudsouzian NG. *A practice of anesthesia for infants and children,* 3rd ed. Philadelphia: WB Saunders, 2000.

Dalens B, Khandwala R. *Regional anesthesia in infants, children, and adolescents.* Baltimore: Williams & Wilkins, 1995.

Dorsch J, Dorsch S. The Mapleson breathing systems. In: *Understanding anesthesia equipment,* 4th ed. Baltimore: Williams & Wilkins, 1999:207–227.

Greeley WJ. *Pediatric anesthesia.* New York: Churchill Livingstone, 1999.

Gregory GA. *Pediatric anesthesia,* 4th ed. New York: Churchill Livingstone, 2001.

Miller RD, ed. *Anesthesia,* 6th ed. New York: Elsevier-Churchill Livingstone, 2005.

Motoyama EK, Davis PJ. *Smith's anesthesia for infants and children,* 6th ed. St. Louis: Mosby–Year Book, 1996.

O'Neill JA, Rowe MI, Grosfeld J, et al. *Pediatric surgery,* 5th ed. St. Louis: Mosby–Year Book, 1998.

Siberry GK, Iannone R, Childs B. *The Harriet Lane handbook: a manual for pediatric house officers,* 17th ed. St. Louis: Mosby–Year Book, 2005.

30

Anesthesia for Obstetrics and Gynecology

Ritu Kapoor, Jeannie C. Min, and Lisa Leffert

I. **Maternal physiology in pregnancy (Table 30.1)**
   A. **Respiratory system**
      1. **Capillary engorgement of the mucosa** occurring throughout the respiratory tract begins early in the first trimester and increases throughout pregnancy. As a result a 6.0- to 6.5-mm (inner diameter) endotracheal tube is recommended for intubation to decrease the possibility of airway trauma. **Airway edema** may worsen during labor and make intubation more difficult. Nasotracheal intubation can cause epistaxis and thus is avoided in pregnant women.
      2. **Elevation of the diaphragm** secondary to the gravid uterus affects maternal lung volumes. Most notably, there is a 20% decrease in maternal functional residual capacity. Also during pregnancy, minute ventilation is increased to meet the higher oxygen requirements of the mother and fetus.
   B. **Cardiovascular system**
      1. **Cardiac output increases 50%** with pregnancy. During labor, contractions of the engorged uterus provide a 300- to 500-mL autotransfusion into the maternal circulation, leading to a further increase in cardiac output. Cardiac output becomes highest immediately postpartum and can reach 80% to 100% above the prelabor value. Blood pressure is not increased in normal pregnancy because of decreased peripheral vascular resistance.
      2. After 20 weeks gestation, the gravid uterus may **obstruct the aorta and inferior vena cava** of the patient, especially when she is supine. This may decrease venous return and result in signs and symptoms of maternal hypotension and decreased uteroplacental blood flow. Left uterine displacement is used to minimize aortocaval compression when the patient is supine.
   C. **Hematology**
      1. **Blood volume increases** markedly throughout the course of pregnancy. Because the plasma volume increases more than red cell volume increases, a relative dilutional anemia occurs.
      2. The pregnant patient is **hypercoagulable** throughout gestation. The concentration of most coagulation factors increases in pregnancy as does platelet activation and consumption. This hypercoagulable state helps to limit blood loss at delivery. Normal blood loss is about 500 mL for vaginal delivery and 1,000 mL for cesarean section.
   D. **Nervous system**
      1. The **minimum alveolar concentration** for inhalational anesthetics is decreased up to 40% during pregnancy. The

Table 30.1. Physiologic changes associated with pregnancy

System	Parameters	Changes
Respiratory	*Capacities/volume*	
	Total lung capacity	−5%
	Vital capacity	No change
	Functional residual capacity	−20%
	Inspiratory reserve volume	+5%
	Expiratory reserve volume	−20%
	Residual volume	−15
	Closing capacity	No change
	Tidal volume	+45%
	Mechanics	
	FEV_1	No change
	FEV_1/FVC	No change
	Minute ventilation	+45%
	Alveolar ventilation	+45%
	Blood gases	
	$PaCO_2$	−10%
	PaO_2	+5–10%
	pH	No change
	HCO_3^-	Decrease
	Oxygen consumption	+20%
	P50 at term	30 mm Hg
Cardiovascular	Cardiac output	+50%
	Stroke volume	+25%
	Heart rate	+20–25%
	Systematic vascular resistance	−20%
Hematology	Blood volume	+45%
	Plasma volume	+55%
	Red blood cell volume	+25%
	Coagulation factors	
	Factors VII, VIII, IX, X, XII, fibrinogen	Increase
	Prothrombin	No change
	Factors XI, XIII	Decrease
	Platelet count	No change or decrease
	Total protein (albumin, globulin)	Decrease
Central nervous system	MAC	Decrease
	Local anesthetic requirement	Decrease
Gastrointestinal	*Gastric emptying*	
	First trimester	No change
	Second trimester	No change
	Third trimester	No change
	Labor	Decrease
	Postpartum (18 h)	No change

(continued)

Table 30.1. *Continued.*

System	Parameters	Changes
	Barrier pressure	
	First, second, third trimester, labor	Decrease
Hepatic	AST, ALT, LDH, bilirubin	Increase
	Alkaline phosphatase	Increase
Renal	Glomerular filtration rate	+50%
	Renal plasma flow	+75%

etiology is unclear but may be related to alterations of hormone and endorphin concentrations during pregnancy, resulting in increased pain threshold or pregnancy-induced analgesia.

2. The pregnant patient requires **less local anesthetic** to produce the same degree of epidural and spinal anesthesia than a nonpregnant patient. Reasons for this include the following:

    a. **Distension of epidural veins** during pregnancy was historically thought to decrease the dose requirement of local anesthetics for **epidural anesthesia** in addition to the presence of enhanced neural susceptibility. However, because this distension is compensated by a decrease in cerebrospinal fluid (CSF), the extravascular epidural volume does not change. Thus, mechanical distension of the epidural veins actually may not affect the spread of local anesthetics for **epidural anesthesia.** However, because there is a reduction of spinal CSF volume during the second and third trimesters of pregnancy, there may be an enhancement of local anesthetic spread and a reduction of segmental dose requirement for **spinal anesthesia.**

    b. **Low CSF protein** increases the unbound fraction of local anesthetic, resulting in a greater proportion of free active drug.

    c. **Elevated CSF pH** increases the unionized fraction of the local anesthetic.

    d. The **biochemical changes** of pregnancy may increase sensitivity to local anesthetics. The need for 30% less local anesthetic for subarachnoid anesthesia has also been noted. In the case of epidural anesthesia, local anesthetic dose requirements appear to be decreased in pregnant versus nonpregnant patients when small doses are given, but they are unchanged when large doses are given.

3. Because of increased intra-abdominal pressure, **the epidural veins become distended,** making a bloody tap during placement of an epidural catheter more common.

4. During pregnancy, the role of **the sympathetic nervous system (SNS) increases.** The parturient is highly dependent on the SNS for hemodynamic control, which reflects the

significant decrease in blood pressure seen after regional anesthesia. The role of the SNS returns to normal by 36 to 48 hours postpartum.

E. **Gastrointestinal system.** The gravid uterus causes a shift in the position of the stomach, resulting in gastric reflux and heartburn in most pregnant patients. Although gastric emptying is not delayed during most of pregnancy, it is delayed during labor. Thus, the pregnant patient should be considered at increased risk for aspiration. If general anesthesia is planned, a nonparticulate antacid should be given routinely; a histamine (H_2) blocker and metoclopramide should be considered; and a rapid sequence induction should be performed. The exact time during pregnancy when a woman becomes at risk for aspiration is controversial. Barrier pressure, which is the difference between intragastric pressure and the tone of the lower esophageal high-pressure zone, is decreased as early as the first trimester. In general, any patient in her third trimester or with symptoms of esophagitis during pregnancy should have a rapid sequence induction.

F. **Renal system.** Renal plasma flow and glomerular filtration may increase up to 50%, leading to increased creatinine clearance and a decrease in normal blood urea nitrogen and creatinine levels.

G. **Musculoskeletal.** Exaggeration of the normal lumbar lordosis secondary to the enlarging uterus can cause stretching of the lateral femoral cutaneous nerve. This can produce a sensory loss over the anterolateral thigh or meralgia parasthetica. Carpal tunnel syndrome and a widening of the pubic symphysis are thought to be secondary to an increase in the hormone relaxin during pregnancy.

II. **Labor and delivery**
   A. **Labor** can be divided into three stages.
      1. The **first stage** begins with the onset of regular contractions and ends with full cervical dilation. It is divided into a slow latent phase and a rapidly progressive active phase, which is characterized by accelerated cervical dilation.
      2. The **second stage** extends from full cervical dilation to delivery of the infant.
      3. The **third stage** begins with delivery of the infant and ends with delivery of the placenta.
   B. **Pain** during the early first part of labor is primarily caused by uterine contractions and cervical dilation. Nerve fibers that transmit pain during the early first part of labor enter the spinal cord from T-10 to L-1. In late first-stage and early second-stage labor, pain is due to perineal stretching and travels through the S-2 to S-4 segments via the pudendal nerve.
   C. **Physiologic changes during labor** tend to accentuate many of the changes already present during pregnancy. Oxygen uptake, which may increase 20% in a normal pregnancy, may increase an additional 60% during painful uterine contractions.
   D. **Electronic fetal heart rate monitoring** consists of evaluating fetal heart patterns that may be associated with reassuring or worrisome neonatal outcomes. Normal fetal heart rate (FHR) ranges from 120 to 160 beats per minute. Monitoring the response of the FHR to uterine contractions can alert physicians to possible distress. Fetal tachycardia may signify fetal asphyxia, maternal fever, chorioamnionitis, or maternally administered drugs. Fetal

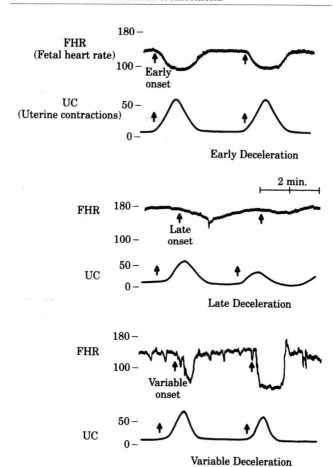

Figure 30.1. Patterns of periodic FHR decelerations in relation to uterine contractions (UC).

bradycardia is generally secondary to hypoxia; however, central nervous system depressants can also cause a decrease in FHR. The American College of Obstetrics and Gynecology recommends using intermittent auscultation or continuous fetal heart monitoring (Fig. 30.1).

1. **Early decelerations** occur concomitantly with uterine contractions, provide a mirror image of the contraction, and are 20 beats per minute or less below the baseline FHR. They are thought to be caused by an increase in fetal vagal tone, perhaps from compression of the fetal head, and do not require intervention.

2. **Late decelerations** occur 10 to 30 seconds after the onset of uterine contractions and resolve 10 to 30 seconds after

the contraction has ended. These are caused by a decrease in uterine blood flow during the contraction, leading to fetal hypoxia. Late decelerations are cause for alarm. When associated with loss of normal baseline "beat-to-beat" variability, they may be indicative of direct fetal myocardial hypoxia. Vigorous efforts should be made to eliminate late decelerations by correcting maternal hypotension, ensuring the adequacy of left uterine displacement, and administering oxygen by face mask to the mother. If these interventions fail to eliminate late decelerations, delivery of the fetus may be necessary.

3. **Variable decelerations** are variable in duration and appearance from one contraction to the next and are usually associated with umbilical cord compression and decreased umbilical blood flow. They may be associated with fetal compromise when severe (a heart rate below 70 for more than 60 seconds) and when prolonged for periods greater than 30 min. Vigorous efforts should be made to correct these as well.

4. **Fetal scalp blood pH monitoring** is used to determine the degree of fetal acidosis from asphyxia when abnormal fetal heart rate patterns cannot be corrected or their significance is unclear. In general, if the pH is above 7.25, the fetus will be vigorous at birth. A pH below 7.20 suggests that the fetus is acidotic and requires immediate delivery. If the pH is in the range of 7.20 to 7.25, close FHR monitoring and repeated scalp blood sampling are recommended.

III. **Medications commonly used for labor and delivery**

A. **Vasopressors.** Warning symptoms of maternal hypotension include lightheadedness, nausea, difficulty breathing, and diaphoresis. Maternal hypotension can result from aortocaval compression, peripartum hemorrhage, or regional anesthesia. Regional anesthesia that produces a sympathetic blockade decreases systemic vascular resistance and may lead to uteroplacental insufficiency. An ideal vasopressor for obstetric anesthesia is one that increases maternal blood pressure without decreasing uteroplacental blood flow.

1. **Ephedrine** stimulates both α- and β-adrenergic receptors. It thus provides cardiac stimulation with a subsequent increase in peripheral and uterine blood flow. Ephedrine has traditionally been the drug of choice for treatment of maternal hypotension.

2. **Pure α-adrenergic agents** such as phenylephrine traditionally have been thought to increase maternal blood pressure at the expense of uteroplacental flow. However, recent evidence suggests that, with regard to the treatment of maternal hypotension, there is no difference between phenylephrine and ephedrine. With respect to the incidence of fetal acidosis, studies have shown that there is either no difference between phenylephrine and ephedrine or that the incidence may be increased in mothers who are treated with ephedrine. Hence, phenylephrine may be safely used to treat maternal hypotension. More potent vasoconstrictors such as norepinephrine and epinephrine should be reserved for cases of severe maternal hypotension where volume resuscitation and ephedrine and phenylephrine are ineffective.

B. Oxytocics are agents that stimulate uterine contractions.
1. **Indications**
   a. To induce or augment labor.
   b. To control postpartum bleeding and uterine atony.
   c. To induce therapeutic abortion.
2. The most frequently used drugs include the synthetic posterior pituitary hormone, **oxytocin** (Pitocin); the ergot alkaloids, **ergonovine** (Ergotrate) and **methylergonovine** (Methergine); and **prostaglandin 15-methyl $F_{2\alpha}$** (Hemabate).
   a. **Oxytocin** acts on the uterine smooth muscle to stimulate the frequency and force of contractions. The cardiovascular side effects of oxytocin include vasodilation, hypotension (with greater decrease in diastolic blood pressure), tachycardia, and arrhythmias. In high doses, oxytocin may have an antidiuretic effect and produce water intoxication, cerebral edema, and subsequent convulsions in the presence of overzealous intravenous (IV) hydration. Pitocin routinely is diluted and is given by continuous IV infusion.
   b. **Ergot alkaloids** in small doses increase the force and frequency of uterine contractions, which are followed by normal uterine relaxation. At higher doses, contractions are more intense and prolonged; resting tonus is increased; and tetanic contractions occur. For these reasons, the use of ergot alkaloids is restricted to control postpartum bleeding in the third stage of labor. Cardiovascular side effects include vasoconstriction and hypertension augmented in the presence of vasopressors. Intramuscular (IM) administration is recommended because IV injection has been associated with severe hypertension, convulsions, stroke, retinal detachment, and pulmonary edema. Ergot alkaloids should be avoided or used with caution in patients with peripheral vascular disease, hypertension, and coronary artery disease.
   c. **Prostaglandin 15-methyl $F_{2\alpha}$** has become the third line of therapy, following oxytocin and ergot alkaloids, to achieve tetanic uterine contraction as treatment for uterine atony. Transient hypertension, severe bronchoconstriction, and increased pulmonary vascular resistance have been reported after its use. Caution must be used in patients with a history of asthma. The usual dose is 250 μg IM or intramyometrially, not more frequently than every 15 minutes, with a total maximum dose of 2 mg.

C. Tocolytics are used to delay or stop premature labor. They are used for fetuses with gestational ages between 20 and 34 weeks. Cervical dilation of less than 4 cm and cervical effacement of less than 80% are associated with a greater likelihood of terminating premature labor.
1. **Indications**
   a. To delay or prevent premature labor.
   b. To slow or arrest labor while initiating other therapeutic measures (e.g., betamethasone to mature fetal lungs).
   c. Allow transfer from a community hospital to a tertiary care center with a neonatal intensive care unit.

2. **Contraindications**
   a. Chorioamnionitis.
   b. Fetal distress.
   c. Intrauterine fetal demise.
   d. Severe chronic or pregnancy-induced hypertension.
   e. Severe hemorrhage.
3. **Specific drugs**
   a. **Selective β_2-adrenergic agonists** such as terbutaline are used to inhibit preterm labor. It produces myometrial inhibition by directly relaxing uterine smooth muscle. β_2 stimulation also produces maternal bronchodilation, vasodilation, and tachycardia. Metabolic effects include hyperglycemia, hypokalemia, hyperinsulinemia, and metabolic (lactic) acidosis. Pulmonary edema (secondary to increased antidiuretic activity) and chest pain may develop but usually only after 24 hours of therapy. Before beginning treatment with a β_2-adrenergic agonist, a baseline electrocardiogram should be considered and preexisting hyperglycemia should be corrected.
   b. **Magnesium sulfate** is used for the treatment of preeclampsia and is also a tocolytic agent. Magnesium sulfate has infrequent cardiovascular side effects and thus is widely used for tocolysis. However, patients should be monitored closely for pulmonary edema and signs of neurotoxicity due to hypermagnesemia. The exact mechanism of action is uncertain, although competition with Ca^{2+} appears to play a role.
   c. **Indomethacin** and **calcium channel blockers** are occasionally used for their tocolytic properties.
IV. **Placental transfer of drugs**
   A. **Placental transport of anesthetics** occurs primarily by passive diffusion. Drugs with a high diffusion constant more readily cross placental membranes. Factors that promote rapid diffusion include the following:
      1. Low molecular weight (<600 daltons).
      2. High lipid solubility.
      3. Low degree of ionization.
      4. Low protein binding.
   B. Most of the agents used to produce anesthesia readily cross the placenta because they are of low molecular weight, high lipid solubility, relatively nonionized, and minimally protein bound.
   C. **Muscle relaxants** are water soluble, are ionized, have high molecular weights, and therefore tend not to cross the placenta.
   D. Damage to the placenta, as occurs with hypertension, preeclampsia, and diabetes may lead to the loss of placental capillary integrity and the nonselective transfer of materials across the placenta. Once materials are across the placenta, fetal acidosis and low pH can cause trapping of ionized drugs.
V. **Anesthesia for labor and vaginal delivery**
   A. **Natural childbirth.** Many women choose to undergo labor and delivery without the use of analgesics. However, it remains prudent to have prior knowledge of a patient's significant past medical problems in case there is a need for an emergency cesarean delivery.
   B. **Supplemental medication.** Systemic medications can be used to relieve pain and anxiety during labor and delivery. There is

no ideal medication because they all cross the placenta and may depress the fetus. The most commonly used drugs are opioids such as **meperidine** and **oxymorphone** and agonist–antagonist agents such as **butorphanol** and **nalbuphine. Sedatives** such as midazolam, hydroxyzine, or promethazine may be used in low doses if needed. Larger doses have been associated with newborn hypotonia and impaired thermal regulation.

C. **Epidural blockade** can provide analgesia through labor and delivery as well as provide anesthesia for cesarean section. Epidural analgesia usually is initiated when active labor has been achieved. In the past, it was thought that the administration of epidural analgesia could minimally slow the progress of labor so that oxytocins may be necessary. However, a recent study suggests that women with neuraxial analgesia (i.e., combined spinal-epidural) instituted early in labor have more effective analgesia and a shorter first stage of labor than women treated with systemic opioid analgesia. This study also showed that early intrathecal opioid analgesia, compared with systemic opioid analgesia, did not significantly increase the rate of cesarean sections.

1. **Advantages**
   a. The need for systemic pain medications that may produce neonatal depression is decreased.
   b. Reducing pain will decrease endogenous catecholamine secretion and may improve uteroplacental perfusion.
   c. Reducing pain may reduce hyperventilation during contractions and minimize the decrease of uteroplacental perfusion that results from alkalosis.
   d. The mother is awake and able to participate in labor and delivery.
   e. The epidural can be used to provide anesthesia for cesarean section.
   f. Compared with general anesthesia, there is a lower risk of pulmonary aspiration.

2. **Disadvantages**
   a. Hypotension is common and can produce uteroplacental insufficiency.
   b. Toxic reactions to local anesthetic agents are possible.
   c. Postdural puncture headache is possible.
   d. Unexpected high block is possible.

3. **Contraindications**
   a. Patient refusal.
   b. Coagulation disorder (e.g., in abruption or preeclampsia).
   c. Infection at the site of catheter placement.
   d. Hypovolemia.
   e. Increased intracranial pressure due to an intracranial lesion with mass effect.

4. **Technique**
   a. A large-bore IV catheter should be placed, and at least 500 to 1,000 mL of crystalloid (preferably warmed) should be infused before placement of the epidural. Volume expansion may help minimize hypotension secondary to peripheral vasodilation.
   b. A 30-mL dose of a nonparticulate antacid should be administered before beginning epidural placement.

    c. Vital signs and fetal heart rate should be recorded at the beginning, at the end, and at regular intervals throughout epidural placement.

    d. Patients may be in the lateral decubitus or sitting position for lumbar catheter placement. Avoidance of the sitting position in patients being treated with magnesium for preeclampsia may be beneficial.

5. Anesthetics

    a. **A test dose** of 3 mL of 1.5% lidocaine with 1:200,000 epinephrine or 0.25% bupivacaine with 1:200,000 epinephrine should be given to test for subarachnoid or intravascular placement. If the patient has preeclampsia, a test dose without epinephrine may be chosen to prevent severe hypertension if the drug is injected intravascularly.

    b. For analgesia during labor, the goal is to provide relief from pain without producing significant motor block-ade. The more concentrated local anesthetics such as 2% lidocaine with epinephrine or 3% 2-chloroprocaine tend to produce more motor blockade and should be reserved for cesarean sections. Epidural 0.75% bupivacaine is no longer approved for use in obstetric anesthesia secondary to case reports of cardiac arrest in the obstetric popula-tion. A mixture of a dilute, long-acting local anesthetic such as 0.08% or 0.125% bupivacaine or ropivacaine with added narcotic is most commonly used for labor epidurals. Our current practice is to use 0.08% bupiva-caine and fentanyl at 2 μg/mL. After the 3-mL test dose of 1.5% lidocaine with epinephrine, a bolus of 15 to 18 mL of this mixture is administered in divided doses, followed by a continuous infusion at a rate of 12 to 15 mL/hour. Onset of analgesia is usually within 5 min-utes, and continues to build for 15 to 20 minutes. As labor progresses, it is common to adjust the rate of infu-sion or to bolus with more concentrated local anesthetic or opioid. In particular, as the fetal head descends, the patient may complain of rectal pressure; fentanyl, 50 to 100 μg, diluted and given into the epidural is often ef-fective.

    c. Whenever a bolus dose is administered via epidural, blood pressure should be monitored every few minutes for the next 20 to 30 minutes, and then every 15 minutes thereafter. Hypotension may be treated with ephedrine, 5 to 10 mg IV, repeated as necessary. Cautious adminis-tration is recommended for patients with preeclampsia.

    d. **Patient-controlled epidural analgesia (PCEA).** Studies comparing PCEA with continuous epidural infusions have reported reduced drug dose in the PCEA group and no difference in pain and sedation scores between the two groups. PCEA has been associated with greater patient satisfaction and autonomy.

6. Complications

    a. **Neurologic complications.** The most common neuro-logic complication is **postdural puncture headache.** A dural puncture with an epidural needle is likely to pro-duce headache because of the large (17-gauge) needle.

The incidence of headache in parturients with a "wet-tap" is 55 % to 80%. Bed rest, hydration, and analgesics are the initial treatments of choice. Caffeine preparations have proved to be of some help, although nursing mothers may prefer to avoid caffeine ingestion. If 24 to 48 hours of conservative measures fail or if the headache is severe, it is best treated with an epidural blood patch. Studies suggest that up to 75% of patients can have symptomatic relief after an initial blood patch. Those who do not have relief after the initial blood patch may benefit from a second blood patch.

    b. Intravascular injection most often is heralded by agitation, visual disturbances, tinnitus, and convulsions and may lead to loss of consciousness. If any of these symptoms is noted, the injection should be discontinued and immediate attention should be given to airway management. The patient should be given 100% oxygen by mask. Endotracheal intubation and hyperventilatation may be necessary to ensure fetal oxygenation and to offset metabolic acidosis. If seizures ensue, they may be terminated with thiopental or propofol and/or a benzodiazepine. If cardiovascular collapse occurs, immediate cardiopulmonary resuscitation and cesarean delivery should be undertaken. Maintenance of left uterine displacement is absolutely vital during this time.

    c. Total spinal anesthesia. Subdural or intrathecal injection of local anesthetic intended for the epidural space may produce a high or total spinal anesthesia. Nausea, hypotension, and unconsciousness may be followed by respiratory and cardiac arrest if appropriate interventions are not undertaken. Should a total spinal anesthesia occur, the patient should be placed in the supine position with left uterine displacement. The patient's lungs should be ventilated with 100% oxygen as cricoid pressure is applied followed by intubation of the trachea. Hypotension secondary to the total spinal anesthesia should be treated with fluids and vasopressors.

D. Spinal or subarachnoid anesthesia may be used. "Saddle block" with anesthetic doses of local anesthetic produces a motor blockade that can interfere with delivery. It can be useful as a last-minute anesthetic for a forceps delivery, for postpartum repair of vaginal or perineal lacerations, or for removal of retained placenta. For labor analgesia, it has become popular to use a subarachnoid injection of a small dose of short-acting, lipophilic opioid such as fentanyl 25 μg, with or without a small dose of local anesthetic such as 2.5 to 3 mg of bupivacaine. Analgesia, especially early in labor, is usually achieved within 5 minutes and lasts for 1.5 to 2 hours.

E. Combined spinal-epidural analgesia has become more common as the use of intrathecal injections for labor has increased, particularly very early in labor or very close to delivery. With this technique, the epidural space is located by using the standard 3.5-inch epidural needle, and a 4-inch spinal needle is passed through the epidural needle into the subarachnoid space. After intrathecal drug injection, the spinal needle is removed, and the epidural catheter is introduced as usual. When additional analgesia becomes necessary, the epidural catheter is tested, and epidural analgesia is achieved in the standard fashion. Labor spinals have been associated with fetal bradycardia soon after placement but have not been shown to increase the incidence of emergency cesarean sections.

VI. **Anesthesia for cesarean section.** The most frequent indications for cesarean delivery are failure to progress, fetal distress, cephalopelvic disproportion, and prior uterine surgery or cesarean section. Anesthetic choice will depend on the urgency of the procedure and the condition of mother and fetus.

A. **Regional anesthesia**

1. **Spinal anesthesia** is a simple, rapid, and reliable technique to provide anesthesia for cesarean delivery if no contraindications exist. The patient is hydrated and then given metoclopramide and a nonparticulate antacid. At our institution, 1.6 mL of hyperbaric bupivacaine (0.75% bupivacaine mixed with 8.25% dextrose) is commonly used to attain a T4 sensory level. Lidocaine spinals are no longer recommended secondary to reports of increased incidence of transient radicular irritation. Addition of fentanyl 10 to 25 μg to the local anesthetic may decrease visceral discomfort. Subarachnoid morphine, 0.1 to 0.25 mg, may be mixed with the local anesthetic for postoperative analgesia. If it is used, a protocol should be established to monitor delayed respiratory depression and for the treatment of aggravating minor side effects such as pruritus.

2. **Epidural anesthesia** is an alternative for patients who are having elective cesarean sections. The dose of anesthetic can be titrated to effect and repeated as necessary. For elective cesarean section, 2% lidocaine with epinephrine may be used. The addition of fentanyl, 50 to 100 μg, to the epidural is helpful in reducing the discomfort of uterine manipulation. An epidural can be used effectively for an emergency cesarean delivery in a patient who already has a catheter in place for labor analgesia. An incremental bolus dose of 15 to 20 mL of 3% 2-chloroprocaine or 2% lidocaine with epinephrine is commonly used. For rapid onset, sodium bicarbonate, 1 mL for each 10 mL of 2-chloroprocaine or lidocaine, can be added. Morphine, 3 mg, may be added after the umbilical cord is clamped to provide postoperative analgesia. As in the case of spinal analgesia, if morphine is administered in the epidural space, a protocol also should be established for monitoring delayed respiratory depression and for the treatment of aggravating minor side effects.

3. **Combined spinal-epidural analgesia** has also become popular to use for cesarean sections. Most commonly, combined spinal-epidural analgesia is used for repeat cesarean sections or for patients who have had prior abdominal surgery, necessitating increased surgical time.

B. **General anesthesia** is the technique of choice for emergency cesarean sections when regional anesthesia is refused or contraindicated or when substantial hemorrhage is anticipated.

1. **Advantages**

a. Rapid induction allows surgery to be started immediately.

    b. Optimal control of the airway and ventilation is achieved.

    c. There is decreased incidence of hypotension in the hypovolemic patient.

2. Disadvantages

    a. The inability to intubate the trachea remains a major cause of maternal morbidity and mortality. A recent study from Europe, which defined a failed intubation as one not being accomplished with a single dose of succinylcholine, suggests that the incidence of failed intubations in the obstetric population may be close to 1 in 238 intubations.

    b. The risk of aspiration is increased.

    c. General anesthetics may cause fetal depression.

    d. Awareness under anesthesia is possible for emergent cesarean section.

3. Technique

    a. Thirty milliliters of a nonparticulate antacid is administered before induction. If time permits, metoclopramide, 10 mg, and cimetidine, 300 mg, or ranitidine, 50 mg, may be given IV. A large-bore IV catheter and standard monitoring are used. The patient is positioned supine with left uterine displacement.

    b. The patient is preoxygenated with 100% oxygen for 3 min if time allows or takes five or six deep breaths if time is limited. The obstetricians should prepare and drape the abdomen while the anesthesiologist preoxygenates the patient.

    c. A rapid sequence intubation with cricoid pressure is performed with propofol, 2 to 2.5 mg/kg (reduce doses for hypovolemic or bleeding patients), and succinylcholine, 1.0 to 1.5 mg/kg, IV. Etomidate or ketamine may be used in cases of maternal hypovolemia.

    d. Until delivery, a 50% mixture of nitrous oxide and oxygen is used with isoflurane or sevoflurane. After recovery from succinylcholine, a nondepolarizing muscle relaxant such as cisatracurium is administered. Pseudocholinesterase activity may decrease up to 30% during pregnancy. However, increased volume of distribution of succinylcholine during pregnancy compensates for the decrease in pseudocholinesterase activity. Thus, recovery from succinylcholine ultimately is not prolonged during pregnancy. Hyperventilation should be avoided because of its adverse effects on uterine blood flow.

    e. Oxytocin (Pitocin) (10 to 20 units/L) is added to the IV infusion and administered after delivery of the placenta to stimulate uterine contraction.

    f. Volatile anesthetics may be used (doses should be decreased to <0.5 minimum alveolar concentration once the baby is delivered) for maintenance of anesthesia, recognizing that they may decrease uterine tone. Alternatively, once the cord is clamped, a balanced technique with nitrous oxide, opioid, and relaxant may be chosen.

    g. An orogastric tube is passed to empty the stomach. Extubation is performed when the patient is fully awake.

VII. Preeclampsia and eclampsia

A. Preeclampsia is defined as the development of hypertension with proteinuria after 20 weeks of gestation. It occurs in approximately 7% of all pregnancies. If seizures occur, the condition is known as **eclampsia,** which has an incidence of about 0.3%. Preeclampsia is most often seen in young nulliparous women but also is associated with hydatidiform mole, multiple pregnancy, diabetes, and Rh incompatibility. Genetic contributions from both parents are important determinants of the predisposition and development of preeclampsia. Mild preeclampsia is characterized by hypertension with a systolic blood pressure greater than 140 mm Hg or a diastolic blood pressure greater than 90 mm Hg in a patient who had a prepregnant normal blood pressure. Mild preeclampsia is also associated with proteinuria of greater than 300 mg over 24 hours. **Severe preeclampsia** is characterized by the addition of one or more of the following:

   1. Two measured blood pressures with a systolic blood pressure greater than or equal to 160 mm Hg and diastolic blood pressure greater than or equal to 110 mm Hg less than 6 hours apart during a time when the patient is on bed rest.

   2. Proteinuria greater than 5 g in 24 hours.

   3. Urine output of less than 500 mL over 24 hours.

   4. Visual or other neurologic disturbances.

   5. Pulmonary edema.

   6. Impaired liver function.

   7. Thrombocytopenia.

   8. The acronym **HELLP** stands for hemolysis, elevated liver enzymes, and low platelets. It is considered one of the most serious forms of preeclampsia.

B. The pathophysiology of preeclampsia is thought to be related to immunological-mediated endothelial dysfunction. It is associated with high circulating levels of renin, angiotensin, aldosterone, and catecholamines, which can produce generalized vasoconstriction and endothelial damage. Fluid shifts can result in edema, hypoxemia, and hemoconcentration. Renal blood flow, glomerular filtration rate, and urine output may also be reduced. Disseminated intravascular coagulation (DIC) is rare in the absence of other inciting causes, but coagulation abnormalities such as thrombocytopenia, increased fibrin split products, and a slightly prolonged partial thromboplastin time may occur. Hyperreflexia occurs, and central nervous system irritability often increases.

C. Management. Definitive treatment involves prompt delivery of the fetus. Symptoms usually abate within 48 hours of delivery. Until then, treatment of hypertension, intravascular volume depletion, and coagulation abnormalities and prevention or termination of seizures are high priorities.

   1. Hypertension

      a. Hydralazine is a commonly used vasodilator because it decreases systemic vascular resistance by preferentially affecting arterioles.

      b. Labetalol is a very useful alternative because of its α- and β-adrenergic blocking effects.

      c. Sodium nitroprusside or **nitroglycerin** may be used for treating a hypertensive crisis or the acute increases of blood pressure associated with laryngoscopy.

Table 30.2. Systemic effects of magnesium

Plasma Level of Magnesium (mEq/L)	Systemic Effect
4–8	Therapeutic range
5–10	Electrocardiographic changes ↑PR interval, ↑QRS
10–15	↓DTRs Respiratory depression
15–20	Respiratory arrest SA and AV conduction defects
>20	Cardiac arrest

AV, atrioventricular; DTR, deep tendon reflex; PR, pulse rate; QRS, principal deflection in electrocardiogram; SA, sinoatrial.

2. **Fluid management.** Intravascular depletion should be corrected with crystalloid. If needed, aggressive fluid resuscitation may be guided by measuring central venous pressure. A pulmonary artery catheter is rarely placed but may be beneficial in preeclamptic patients with coexisting cardiopulmonary disease.

3. **Coagulation abnormalities.** The patient's coagulation status should be assessed, especially in severe preeclampsia. Administration of platelets, fresh-frozen plasma, and red cells may be necessary.

4. **Magnesium sulfate** is a mild vasodilator and central nervous system depressant. By relaxing the myometrium, it also causes an increase in uteroplacental blood flow. It may also cause postpartum uterine atony, especially when oxytocin has been used to augment a long labor. Magnesium may cross the placenta, resulting in muscle weakness or apnea in the neonate. IV calcium may counteract this weakness in both mother and newborn, but calcium may simultaneously antagonize the anticonvulsant effect of magnesium in the mother. Of note, magnesium increases the sensitivity to both depolarizing and nondepolarizing muscle relaxants. After an initial IV-loading dose of 4 to 6 g over 20 minutes, a continuous infusion of 1 to 2 g/hour is used to maintain therapeutic blood levels of 4 to 8 mEq/L. Systemic effects of magnesium are presented in Table 30.2.

D. **Anesthesia**

1. **Epidural anesthesia** is recommended for cesarean delivery in the preeclamptic patient with hypovolemia. Epidural analgesia early in labor may help to reduce circulating levels of maternal catecholamines, thus improving uteroplacental perfusion.

2. **Spinal anesthesia** has not been recommended in the past for patients with severe preeclampsia because of concern that the rapid onset of sympathectomy would precipitate maternal hypotension. However, neonatal assessment and maternal morbidity outcomes have not been found to be different among spinal, epidural, and general anesthetic techniques in these patients.

3. **General anesthesia** is used for emergency cesarean deliveries if the patient has a coagulopathy or if there are other contraindications to regional anesthesia. These patients are prone to periglottic edema, making rapid-sequence induction particularly difficult. The hemodynamic response to intubation may be blunted by administration of labetalol, 10 mg IV. Systemic and pulmonary hypertension increases the incidence of stroke and pulmonary edema. The sensitizing effects of magnesium on muscle relaxants must also be considered.

VIII. **Peripartum hemorrhage is the major cause of maternal mortality.**
   A. **Antepartum hemorrhage** is most commonly due to placenta previa or placental abruption.
      1. **Placenta previa** occurs when the placenta is implanted at or very near the cervical opening. Bleeding is usually painless and can vary from minimal spotting to massive hemorrhage. Placenta previa in a patient with a previous cesarean section has a higher incidence of abnormal placental attachment **(placenta accreta).** The incidence of gravid hysterectomy is higher in this population. If the patient is not actively bleeding and is euvolemic, spinal or epidural anesthesia may be performed. Pelvic examination in patients with placenta previa is typically avoided. Ultrasound usually allows for accurate identification of placenta previa. However, if the source of vaginal bleeding needs to be confirmed through vaginal examination, a "double set-up" should be used. A "double set-up" consists of the following:
         a. Transfer patient to the operating room (OR).
         b. Administer 30 mL of a nonparticulate antacid.
         c. Place a large-bore (14- or 16-gauge) IV with a pump set.
         d. Blood (two to four units) in the OR.
         e. Abdomen prepared and draped by the obstetricians.
         f. All preparations for general anesthesia available.
         g. Available assistance.
      2. **Placental abruption** is the premature separation of the normally implanted placenta before birth. Bleeding is usually painful and may be either visible with obvious bleeding from the vagina or concealed behind the placenta within the uterus. Abruption is the most common cause of DIC in pregnancy. Anesthetic management is essentially the same as for placenta previa except that coagulation studies ideally are checked before initiating regional anesthesia. Regional anesthesia should be used only in cases of mild abruption when there is no fetal distress, hypovolemia, or coagulopathy. Consumption of coagulation factors and activation of the fibrinolytic system occur frequently and should be treated with blood products as needed.
   B. **Intrapartum hemorrhage**
      1. **Uterine rupture** can occur at any point during labor and delivery and is associated with the following:
         a. Separation of a prior uterine scar or traumatic rupture such as during a difficult forceps application.
         b. History of previous difficult deliveries.
         c. Rapid, spontaneous, tumultuous labor.
         d. Prolonged labor in association with excessive oxytocin stimulation.

2. **Vaginal birth after cesarean section (VBAC).** Certain patients who have had prior cesarean section may have a trial of labor, attempting to have a vaginal birth after cesarean section. The concern is for possible uterine rupture at the site of a prior incision. In general, patients with a singleton fetus in vertex presentation, prior low transverse uterine incisions, who do not require prostaglandin cervical ripening, and are with no other maternal risk factors, are the best candidates for VBAC. Oxytocin augmentation is not a contraindication for VBAC, but close maternal and fetal monitoring is advised. It is safe to use regional techniques in these patients. The most common signs of uterine rupture are changes in uterine tone and contraction pattern, variations in fetal heart rate, and persistent maternal pain between contractions. If uterine rupture occurs, a functioning epidural provides a means for establishing a quick, safe anesthetic for surgical intervention. If uterine rupture causes massive hemorrhage, anesthetic management is the same as for any actively bleeding, acutely hypovolemic patient.

3. **Vasa previa** is a condition in which the fetal umbilical cord passes in front of the presenting part of the fetus. The vessels of the umbilical cord are vulnerable to trauma during vaginal examination or during artificial rupture of membranes. Because bleeding is from the fetal circulation in this circumstance, the fetus is at great risk and immediate delivery is warranted.

C. **Postpartum hemorrhage**

1. **Retained placenta** occurs in up to 1% of all vaginal deliveries. It usually requires manual exploration of the uterus and is facilitated by an epidural or spinal block. If additional uterine relaxation is necessary and bleeding has not been excessive, nitroglycerin in 50- to 100-μg IV boluses will effectively relax the uterus. Small doses of ketamine or an inhalation anesthetic may be used if a regional anesthetic is not in place. If bleeding has been excessive and the patient is hypovolemic, a regional block may be contraindicated secondary to hypotension. General anesthesia with a potent volatile inhalation agent and a rapid sequence induction may be necessary. As soon as the uterus is relaxed sufficiently to allow extraction, the volatile anesthetic should be discontinued to prevent uterine atony and further bleeding.

2. **Uterine atony** occurs in up to 2% to 5% of patients. Infusion of crystalloid, colloid, and blood products should be used as needed. Pharmacologic therapy involves IV oxytocin to cause uterine contraction. If this fails, the ergot preparation methergine, 0.2 mg IM, should be administered. If uterine contraction is still not adequate, then 15-methyl prostaglandin $F_{2\alpha}$ should be given IM or injected directly into the uterus by the obstetrician. If these measures fail, then emergency hysterectomy or internal iliac artery ligation may be necessary.

3. **Laceration of the vagina, cervix, or perineum** is a common cause of postpartum hemorrhage. Bleeding may be insidious and difficult to estimate.

4. **Uterine inversion** is a very rare cause of postpartum hemorrhage. This represents a true obstetric emergency because the patient can exsanguinate rapidly. General anesthesia is often required to produce immediate uterine relaxation in the face of rapidly developing hypovolemia. Help should be summoned immediately.

IX. Amniotic fluid embolism

A. **Pathophysiology.** Amniotic fluid embolism occurs in 1:20,000 to 1:30,000 deliveries, and most cases are fatal. As many as 10% of all maternal deaths result from amniotic fluid embolism. The pathogenesis of this disorder may involve a tear through the amnion or chorion (opening uterine or endocervical veins) and pressure sufficient to force the fluid into the venous circulation.

B. **Clinical features** include respiratory distress with pulmonary edema, cyanosis, and possible pulmonary hypertension; shock, coagulopathy, and hemorrhage (from DIC); and altered mental status, which may be characterized by seizures and coma.

C. **Laboratory studies.** The diagnosis may be supported by the presence of fetal squamous cells, lanugo hair, vernix, or mucin in the buffy coat of heparinized maternal blood sampled from a pulmonary artery catheter. These signs are not always present and are not pathognomonic. Diagnostic workup includes arterial blood gas tensions and pH, coagulation studies, chest radiograph, and electrocardiogram.

D. **Treatment** is supportive and consists of cardiopulmonary resuscitation and immediate delivery of the fetus. Endotracheal intubation and ventilatory support using increased oxygen concentrations and positive end-expiratory pressure may be necessary. Diuretics are used to treat the pulmonary edema, and transfusions of blood products may be necessary to correct hematologic derangements.

X. Anesthesia for nonobstetric surgery during pregnancy

A. Approximately 0.75% to 2% of women undergo nonobstetric surgery during pregnancy. The objectives in the anesthetic management of these procedures include the following:

1. **Maternal safety.** The anesthetic plan must take into consideration that physiologic changes of pregnancy begin in the first trimester.

2. **Fetal safety.** If possible, surgery should be avoided during the period of organogenesis during the first trimester. Optimally, all elective surgical procedures should be postponed until after delivery. Nonelective surgical procedures should be performed in the second trimester if feasible. In general, efforts should be made to prevent preterm labor, maintain uteroplacental blood flow, and avoid teratogenic substances. No anesthetic agent has been proven to be teratogenic in humans, although nitrous oxide and diazepam have been shown to be possibly teratogenic in certain situations in animals.

B. **Procedures directly related to pregnancy**

1. **Ectopic pregnancy** results when the fertilized ovum implants abnormally outside the endometrial lining of the uterus. Ruptured ectopic pregnancy is the leading cause of first-trimester maternal death. It is considered a surgical emergency and usually requires an emergent laparoscopy or laparotomy. It is prudent to volume resuscitate these patients and to

have blood products available before the induction of anesthesia.

2. **Abortion or miscarriage** refers to the loss of pregnancy before 20 weeks gestation or at a fetal weight less than 500 g. An **inevitable abortion** refers to cervical dilation or rupture of membranes without expulsion of products of conception. A **complete abortion** refers to spontaneous expulsion of products of conception. An **incomplete abortion** refers to a partial expulsion of products of conception. A **missed abortion** refers to unrecognized fetal demise. A dilation and evacuation are indicated in incomplete abortions and in missed abortions. Monitored anesthesia care, spinal, epidural, or general anesthesia can be used after careful assessment of the patient to evaluate fasting (NPO) status, volume status, and presence of DIC and sepsis.

3. **Surgeries for incompetent cervix** include the Shirodkar cerclage and the McDonald cerclage. Both are placed transvaginally during the first or the second trimester, either prophylactically or emergently with the onset of cervical change. Regional anesthesia (spinal preferred over epidural) is usually the anesthetic of choice.

4. **Anesthesia for postpartum sterilization.** Many patients and obstetricians prefer to schedule tubal ligation during the immediate postpartum period.
   a. **Advantages**
      (1) The enlarged uterus brings the fallopian tubes up out of the pelvis, so the surgery can be done through a small laparotomy incision.
      (2) A second hospital visit is avoided, which is an advantage with respect to cost, convenience, and childcare, compared with laparoscopic tubal ligation done at 6 weeks postpartum.
      (3) The chance that the patient will experience an undesired pregnancy while awaiting sterilization is greatly minimized.
   b. **Disadvantages**
      (1) Physiologic changes of pregnancy may not fully return to prepregnant status until 6 weeks postpartum. In particular, gastric emptying slows during labor and after administration of opioids. It is not clear how soon after delivery gastric emptying returns to baseline.
      (2) Tubal ligation is an elective procedure with effective alternatives available.
   c. **Recommendations.** Patients who request tubal ligation but refuse regional anesthesia should be considered for laparoscopic tubal ligation at least 6 weeks postpartum. If the patient has a functioning labor epidural and if the patient and her infant are both stable, the patient is kept NPO after delivery and the procedure is performed as soon as personnel and the labor floor resources allow. In some cases, the labor epidural catheter may have become dislodged and may be nonfunctional. If no effect is seen after a test dose of 3 to 5 mL of bicarbonated 2% lidocaine, the catheter is removed. Another epidural

catheter is placed or a spinal anesthetic is administered. If the patient does not have an epidural for labor, she is generally kept NPO for 8 hours, and her procedure is then performed under spinal anesthesia. Particularly for spinal anesthesia, these postpartum patients when compared with pregnant patients will likely require a higher dose of local anesthetic to attain the same level of anesthesia. Under regional anesthesia, a T4-6 sensory level, comparable to that for cesarean section, is required for patient comfort.

C. **Procedures incidental to pregnancy**

1. **Postpone elective surgery** until 6 weeks postpartum (when the physiologic changes of pregnancy have returned to normal). Elective surgical procedures are relatively contraindicated in pregnancy. If a surgical procedure has to be performed, the second trimester is considered to be a preferable time.

2. **Consult with an obstetrician** preoperatively for all but the most minor surgical procedures.

3. **Use regional techniques when possible,** especially spinal anesthesia, to minimize fetal exposure to local anesthetic and to decrease the risk of maternal aspiration and failed intubation.

4. Depending on the operative site and the fetal gestation, **continuous fetal heart rate monitoring** may be used perioperatively. Communication with the obstetrician is important for interpretation of fetal heart rate tracings.

5. **A uterine tocodynamometer** should be used to detect preterm labor, especially in the postoperative period.

XI. **Cardiopulmonary resuscitation during pregnancy**

A. **Cardiac arrest during pregnancy** is rare. When it occurs, resuscitation is more difficult and less successful than in nonpregnant individuals for several reasons.

1. After approximately 24 weeks gestation, **aortocaval compression** by the gravid uterus impedes venous return so that closed chest compressions may be ineffective.

2. The increased oxygen demands of pregnancy make hypoxia more likely even with adequate perfusion.

3. Enlarged breasts and upward displacement of abdominal contents make effective closed chest compressions more difficult.

B. **Recommendations** when cardiac arrest occurs:

1. **Immediately** secure the airway.

2. **Maintain left uterine displacement** in the case of cardiac arrest after 24 weeks gestation and in the immediate postpartum period.

3. **Immediately page a neonatologist** for likely imminent delivery of a depressed, possibly preterm infant.

4. **Consider cesarean section** to alleviate aortocaval compression and to increase the chance of survival of both mother and fetus if resuscitative measures are unsuccessful by 4 minutes.

5. **Utilize standard advanced cardiac life support protocols,** using the usual recommended drugs, doses, and countershocks.

6. **Consider open-chest cardiac massage** if perfusion is inadequate.

7. **Consider institution of cardiopulmonary bypass** in cases of bupivacaine toxicity or massive pulmonary embolus.

XII. **Anesthesia for gynecologic surgery**
   A. **Laparoscopy**
   1. Laparoscopy requires **pneumoperitoneum,** occasionally extreme Trendelenburg positioning, and the use of electrocoagulation during sterilization procedures.
   2. **Insufflation** of the peritoneal cavity with carbon dioxide often causes an elevation of the partial pressure of arterial carbon dioxide. Hypercarbia results from decreased pulmonary compliance, decreased functional residual capacity, and absorption of the carbon dioxide used for pneumoperitoneum. Excess carbon dioxide may be eliminated with controlled ventilation 1.5 times the basal requirements. Gas insufflation at pressures of 20 to 25 cm H_2O may produce increases in abdominal pressure, central redistribution of blood volume, and changes in central venous pressure. Pressures greater than 30 to 40 cm H_2O may produce a decrease in central venous pressure and cardiac output by decreasing right heart filling.
   3. **Techniques.** General anesthesia is most commonly used for laparoscopic procedures. Spinal or epidural techniques generally are not well tolerated because of the increased ventilatory load associated with pneumoperitoneum, unless insufflation is less than 2 L.
   B. **Abdominal procedures** (see Chapter 20). Most of these procedures are performed through a low abdominal incision, and a regional or general anesthetic is appropriate. Although the patient may experience discomfort from peritoneal stimulation, the addition of epidural or intrathecal fentanyl to regional anesthesia may be helpful. However, a steep Trendelenburg position commonly used for pelvic surgery may not be tolerated for very long in an awake patient; thus, general anesthesia may be used in this case. In addition, general anesthesia usually is chosen for extensive pelvic and abdominal procedures with large blood loss and fluid shifts.
   C. **Vaginal procedures.** Although both regional and general anesthetics may be used, regional techniques are more common. When placing the regional anesthetic, the sitting position will promote adequate sacral analgesia. Some procedures require an extreme Trendelenburg with lithotomy position. This may impair ventilation, necessitating general anesthesia. Also, major transvaginal procedures may be associated with large occult blood losses.

XIII. **Anesthesia for assisted reproductive techniques**
   A. **In vitro fertilization and embryo transfer** have become increasingly popular for treating infertility. Hormone manipulation is used to stimulate the maturation of multiple ovarian follicles. Preovulatory oocytes are then harvested and combined with semen, and the resulting embryos are transferred into the uterine cavity. Ultrasonically guided follicle aspiration is the most commonly used method for oocyte retrieval. The procedure involves puncture and aspiration of follicles using real-time ultrasound through a transvaginal approach.
   1. **Local infiltration** of the posteriolateral vaginal fornix, combined with small doses of sedatives and narcotics, have been used successfully. This technique may be inadequate if the

surgeons desire an immobile patient to maximize oocyte retrieval.

2. **Spinal anesthesia** can provide excellent operating conditions. Some centers avoid spinal anesthesia because of the risk of postdural puncture headache and possible prolonged recovery. The incidence of postdural puncture headache is less than 1%, and the need for an epidural blood patch is very low with the use of small-gauge, pencil-point needles such as a 24-g Sprotte needle or a 25-g Whitacre needle. Commonly, either hyperbaric 0.75% bupivacaine or hyperbaric 1.5% mepivacaine is used for the spinal anesthetic. Intrathecal fentanyl, 10 to 25 μg, may be added to decrease the pain of peritoneal stimulation.

3. **General anesthesia** may be used for oocyte retrieval. The effects of inhalation anesthetics on cell division and implantation are incompletely understood. All inhalational anesthetics can interfere with some stages of reproductive physiology *in vitro*. In particular, nitrous oxide inhibits methionine synthetase activity and could affect DNA synthesis. However, there is no convincing evidence that any of the commonly used inhalational anesthetics adversely affect pregnancy and live-birth rates for in vitro fertilization procedures. General anesthesia with a benzodiazepine, opioid, and propofol appears to be a safe alternative to inhalational anesthesia for oocyte retrieval.

B. **Gamete intrafallopian transfer** begins with transvaginal oocyte retrieval. If oocytes are confirmed in the laboratory, laparoscopy is performed immediately. The oocytes along with washed sperm are injected into the fallopian tube. Thus, fertilization is in vivo and requires a normal fallopian tube for success. Although regional anesthesia is possible, this laparoscopic procedure requires immobility and thus general anesthesia is usually chosen.

SUGGESTED READING

Birnbach DJ, Ostheimer GW. *Ostheimer's manual of obstetric anesthesia,* 3rd ed. New York: Churchill Livingstone, 2000.

Briggs GG, Freeman RK, Yaffe SJ. *Drugs in pregnancy and lactation: a reference guide to fetal and neonatal risk,* 6th ed. Philadelphia: Lippincott Williams & Wilkins, 2001.

Chestnut DH. *Obstetric anesthesia: principles and practice,* 3rd ed. St. Louis: Mosby–Year Book, 2004.

Cunningham FG, Gant NF, Leveno LJ, et al. *Williams obstetrics,* 21st ed. New York: McGraw-Hill, 2001.

Datta S. *Anesthetic and obstetric management of high risk pregnancy,* 2nd ed. St. Louis: Mosby–Year Book, 1996.

Datta S. *The obstetric anesthesia handbook,* 3rd ed. Philadelphia: Hanley & Belfus, 2000.

Duffy PJ, Crosby ET. The epidural blood patch: resolving the controversies. *Can J Anesth* 1999;46:878–886.

Hughes SC, Levinson G, Rosen MA. *Shnider and Levinson's anesthesia for obstetrics,* 4th ed. Philadelphia: Lippincott Williams & Wilkins, 2002.

Martin RW. Amniotic fluid embolism. *Clin Obstet Gynecol* 1996;39:101–106.

Ngan Kee WD, Khaw KS, Ma ML. Patient-controlled epidural analgesia after caesarean section using meperidine. *Can J Anaesth* 1997;44:702–706.

Pian-Smith MCM, Leffert L eds. *Obstetric anesthesia.* New York: PocketMedicine.com, Inc., 2005.

Rahman K, Jenkins JG. Failed tracheal intubation in obstetrics: no more frequent but still managed badly. *Anaesthesia* 2005;60(8):821.

Santos AC, O'Gorman DA, Finster M. Obstetric anesthesia. In: Barash PG, Cullen BF, Stoelting RK, eds. *Clinical anesthesia*, 4th ed. Philadelphia: Lippincott Williams & Wilkins, 2001:1141–1170.

Wong C, et al. The risk of cesarean delivery with neuraxial analgesia given early versus late in labor. *NEJM* 2005;352:655–665.

Ambulatory Anesthesia

Sissela Park and Lisa Warren

I. Patient selection

A. The **volume of patients** receiving ambulatory anesthesia and surgical care exceeds the number of inpatient procedures. There is a continual shift of formerly inpatient procedures to the outpatient surgicenter and surgeon's office. Outpatient surgery is now routinely performed on many American Society of Anesthesiologists (ASA) class III and IV patients who are stable medically as well as on ASA I and II patients. Recent studies have documented the safety of this practice. Admissions and complications correlate with type of procedure, duration of surgery, use of general anesthesia, and patient age, rather than ASA classification.

B. Patients inappropriate for outpatient surgery
   1. **Pediatric**
      a. **Formerly premature infants** of less than 46 weeks postconceptual age, even if healthy, have an increased risk of postanesthetic apnea. Regardless of the type of anesthesia, these infants should be admitted for a day of postoperative apnea monitoring.
      b. **Infants with respiratory disease** such as severe bronchopulmonary dysplasia, apnea, or bronchospasm.
      c. **Infants with cardiovascular disease** such as congestive heart failure or hemodynamically significant congenital heart anomalies.
      d. **Children with fever, cough, sore throat, coryza,** or other signs of recent onset or worsening upper respiratory infection.
   2. **Adult**
      a. Patients expected to have **major blood loss** or undergoing major surgery.
      b. **ASA III and IV patients who require complex or extended monitoring** or postoperative treatment.
      c. **Morbidly obese patients** with significant respiratory disease, including sleep apnea.
      d. Patients with a need for **complex pain management.**
      e. **Patients with significant fever, wheezing, nasal congestion, cough,** or other symptoms of a recent upper respiratory infection.

II. Patient preparation

A. **Preoperative testing.** The need for preoperative testing is minimal in healthy patients. Preoperative testing should be based on the patient's medical condition and the planned surgical procedure (see Chapter 1).

B. **Prehospital instructions**
   1. Patients are instructed (by either the physician's office or the preadmission area) as to the time of expected arrival,

appropriate clothing, diet restrictions, duration of surgery, and the need for escort home.

2. **Current diet guidelines.** Current recommendations are taken from the recent ASA Task Force on preoperative fasting. Intake of clear liquids until 2 hours and solids until 8 hours preoperatively has been accepted and found to be safe.

3. **Medications.** Patients should be instructed to continue their cardiovascular, asthma, pain, anxiety, anticonvulsant, and antihypertensive medications until the time of surgery. Warfarin (Coumadin) should be stopped several days before surgery to allow the prothrombin time to return to normal. Diuretics are usually withheld on the morning of surgery. An accepted regimen for diabetic patients is to withhold regular insulin the morning of surgery and give half the usual dose of long-acting insulin such as neutral-protamine-Hagedorn insulin. If the patient is traveling alone or over a long distance, the insulin may be given on arrival coincident with an intravenous (IV) infusion of glucose.

4. **Preanesthetic visit.** For healthy ambulatory patients, an evaluation by an anesthesiologist is usually performed immediately before the planned procedure. When a patient has a potentially serious problem or a complex medical condition, a consultation with an anesthesiologist should be arranged in advance. The consultation occurs in a preadmission testing clinic where patients are seen before their inpatient procedures. A standard history and physical examination are performed with special attention to the heart, lungs, and airway, and any significant new problems are explored (e.g., symptoms of an upper respiratory infection or unexplained chest pain). Time of last oral intake is confirmed and compliance with preoperative medications is determined. Any required preoperative laboratory tests are also performed at this time. The anesthetic plan is discussed, and informed consent is obtained.

III. **Anesthetic management**
A. **Premedication**
1. **Anxiolytics.** Reassurance and rapport with the patient usually are all that are required. If necessary, **midazolam** (Versed), 1 to 2 mg IV may be administered.

2. **Aspiration prophylaxis.** Patients with extreme anxiety, morbid obesity, diabetic gastroparesis, symptomatic hiatal hernias, or other conditions causing esophageal reflux are at higher risk of pulmonary aspiration of gastric contents. They should be premedicated with one or more of the following:
   a. **Nonparticulate antacids** (Bicitra), 30 mL by mouth (PO), just before the procedure.
   b. **Histamine (H_2)-receptor antagonist** such as ranitidine, 150 mg PO, preferably the night before and the morning of surgery, or 50 mg IV before surgery.
   c. **Metoclopramide,** 10 mg PO or IV before surgery. Metoclopramide may be most useful to increase gastric emptying in patients with diabetic gastroparesis.

3. **Opioids.** Fentanyl, 50 to 100 μg IV, may be given, especially if preoperative pain is present. Nurse supervision

and oxygen saturation monitoring should be employed after administration of IV sedatives or opioids in the preinduction area.

B. Intravenous access. An IV catheter is started, frequently in an antecubital vein to diminish the pain associated with injection of propofol.

C. Standard monitoring is used (see Chapter 10). In addition, a bispectral index monitor (Aspect Medical Systems, Newton, MA) often is used during general anesthesia to allow more accurate titration of hypnotic agents and speed recovery in the ambulatory patient.

D. General anesthesia

1. **Induction. Propofol** is used most commonly for induction in adults because of its short duration, depression of pharyngeal reflexes, and reduced incidence of postoperative emesis compared with barbiturates. **Lidocaine,** 20 mg, may be added to each 200 mg of propofol to decrease the pain associated with injection into small veins. Small doses of alfentanil or fentanyl may be added or given before the propofol to reduce the induction dose. **Sevoflurane** may be used for mask induction in children and adults

2. **Airway management.** The choice of using a face mask, a laryngeal mask, or tracheal intubation is discussed in Chapters 13 and 14. Succinylcholine or mivacurium is used to facilitate intubation for short procedures. Pretreatment with small doses of a nondepolarizing muscle relaxant may minimize the myalgias that follow succinylcholine administration. For longer procedures, an intubating dose of a short-acting nondepolarizing agent (cisatracurium) is used.

3. **Maintenance.** Volatile anesthetics (e.g., isoflurane, desflurane, or sevoflurane), with or without nitrous oxide, are commonly used with total gas flow rates of less than 1 L/minute (2 L/minute for sevoflurane) after the first 10 to 15 minutes to reduce wastage. Propofol and alfentanil or remifentanil infusions are also used in conjunction with nitrous oxide. Supplemental local anesthesia provided by the surgeon early in the procedure reduces general anesthetic requirements and provides early postoperative analgesia and greater efficiency for recovery services.

E. Regional anesthesia

1. The ideal outpatient technique involves the use of agents with rapid onset to minimize case delay and short duration to facilitate quick recovery and discharge. Patient selection is important, because the benefits of regional anesthesia will be negated if heavy sedation is required. Performing peripheral nerve blocks in a separate designated area well in advance of the scheduled surgery time will decrease time in the operating room (OR) waiting for onset of anesthesia. Separate areas for regional blocks should be fully equipped with standard monitoring and resuscitative devices in the event that complications occur.

2. **Specific blocks**

a. **Spinal anesthesia**

(1) **Subarachnoid anesthesia** is a fast, reliable technique providing adequate conditions for lower abdominal,

groin, pelvic, perineal, and lower extremity surgery. The duration can be adjusted by appropriate selection of local anesthetic.

- **(2)** **Mepivacaine, lidocaine, and bupivacaine** are used most commonly in ambulatory surgery (see Chapter 15).
- **(3)** **Complications**
    - **(a)** **Postdural puncture headache (PDPH)** occurs in 5% to 10% of outpatients. Patients under 40 years of age and women are at greater risk. Informed consent should include discussion of the risk of PDPH and treatment options. Routine use of a 24- to 27-gauge Sprotte needle has reduced the incidence of spinal headaches.
    - **(b)** **Urinary retention.** Men are at greater risk of delayed return of bladder tone and subsequent urinary retention. Catheterization may be required, and persistent inability to void may be an indication for admission. Reducing intraoperative IV fluids to a minimum may help avoid the problem.
    - **(c)** **Transient radicular irritation** and neurologic symptoms occurring with the use of lidocaine preparations have led some anesthetists to use exclusively low-dose bupivacaine or mepivacaine for spinal anesthesia.

b. **Epidural anesthesia** can be used to reduce the risk of PDPH. Common use is predicated on the ability to initiate the block in a separate area to reduce the time between operations. When used with a catheter, it provides regional anesthesia for appropriate procedures of uncertain duration.

c. **Peripheral nerve blocks** (see Chapter 17).

- **(1)** **IV regional for hand or forearm surgery.** The advantages include simplicity, rapid onset, high reliability, and early recovery and discharge. In the average patient, 50 mL of 0.5% lidocaine without epinephrine is used. The addition of **clonidine** (1 μg/kg) to the lidocaine has been shown to significantly enhance the duration of analgesia in the postoperative period. Disadvantages include a maximum case time of approximately 1.5 hours because of the need for an inflated tourniquet, lack of postoperative analgesia, and risk of local anesthetic toxicity if the tourniquets fail within the first few minutes after injection.
- **(2)** **Brachial plexus blockade** for upper extremity surgery usually is indicated when patients prefer regional anesthesia as an alternative to general anesthesia and when their medical condition increases the risks associated with general anesthesia. For shoulder surgery, the **parascalene** or **interscalene block** is used to provide anesthesia to the upper extremity above the midhumeral line. For elbow or hand

surgery, an **axillary** or **infraclavicular block** is most effective.

- (3) **Paravertebral block** for breast surgery or inguinal herniorrhaphy may provide excellent analgesia and a useful alternative anesthetic when avoidance of general anesthesia is preferred.
- (4) **Lower extremity anesthesia** using femoral or sciatic nerve blocks is not performed as frequently because of the requirement for early ambulation and discharge. **Popliteal** and **ankle blocks,** however, can provide an excellent alternative for the ambulatory patient wishing to avoid general anesthesia.

    d. **Indwelling peripheral nerve catheters.** In appropriately selected patients, continuous peripheral nerve blockade facilitated by placement of an indwelling catheter with infusion pump may provide superior analgesia in the postoperative period and minimize the usage of and complications associated with parenteral opioids. Adequate patient education and contact must occur to safely manage analgesia, complications (catheter migration, local anesthetic toxicity), and catheter removal.

- F. **Monitored anesthesia care.** For some patients with complex medical problems whose operations would ordinarily be done under local anesthesia, an anesthetist may be asked to monitor the patient and provide medications, usually sedatives or opioids, supplemental to the local anesthesia provided by the surgeon. Standard monitoring should be used, and the anesthetist should be prepared to administer general anesthesia if the local anesthesia plus sedation is not sufficient.

IV. Postoperative care

- A. **Postanesthesia care unit (PACU) admission.** Patients usually are admitted from the OR to a phase I PACU. Some patients who are awake after minor procedures may be ready for a phase II recovery area directly from the OR. Indications for this accelerated recovery process are being developed. Currently, the standard recovery protocol for outpatients receiving general anesthesia is a criteria-driven progression from the OR to the PACU and then to the phase II PACU, followed by discharge to home when they have met the discharge criteria. If the criteria used to discharge patients from the PACU are met in the OR, it is usually appropriate to "fast track" the patient, bypassing the PACU and transferring the patient directly to the phase II PACU. For patients to bypass the phase I PACU, they must be awake and oriented, have stable vital signs, have no nausea or vomiting, have minimal pain or discomfort, and be able to sit up without assistance. If these criteria are met, the anesthetist assists the patient into a reclining lounge chair and transfers the patient to the phase II PACU.

- B. **Pain.** If the patient has pain on admission to the PACU, IV supplementation with an opioid, usually fentanyl or meperidine, is administered. When awake, the patient is usually given oral acetaminophen (Tylenol, 975 mg), oxycodone (Percocet, one or two tablets), or ibuprofen (Motrin, 600 mg).

- C. **Nausea and vomiting.** Predisposing factors include a previous history of vomiting after anesthesia, female gender, a history of motion sickness, use of perioperative opioids, pelvic procedures in young females, gastric distension, and severe postoperative pain. **Ondansetron,** 4 mg IV, may be given if a history of severe nausea and vomiting is elicited preoperatively. Transdermal scopolamine, Haldol (1 mg IV), and IV dexamethasone are other drugs that can be used to treat postoperative nausea and vomiting.

D. **Discharge criteria.** Criteria for final discharge from the recovery areas include an operative site without hematoma or excessive bleeding, stable vital signs, ambulation, ability to urinate after spinal anesthesia, the ability to take PO, the absence of nausea and vomiting, and adequate pain control. Discharge instructions are reviewed with the patient by the surgeon or nurse in the recovery areas.

E. **Unanticipated admission.** The unanticipated admission rate after outpatient surgery is about 1%. Nausea, vomiting, pain, and operative site bleeding are the most common causes. Extended stay or inpatient facilities should be available for those patients who cannot be discharged after a reasonable stay in the PACU areas.

SUGGESTED READING

American Society of Anesthesiologists Task Force on Preoperative Fasting. Report by the American Society of Anesthesiologists Task Force on Preoperative Fasting. Practice guidelines for preoperative fasting and the use of pharmacologic agents to reduce the risk of pulmonary aspiration: application to healthy patients undergoing elective procedures. *Anesthesiology* 1999;90:896–905.

American Society of Anesthesiologists. *ASA guidelines for ambulatory anesthesia and surgery.* Park Ridge, IL: ASA. Amended by ASA House of Delegates, October 15, 2003.

Apfelbaum JL. Bypassing PACU: a cost-saving measure. *Can J Anaesth* 1998;45: R91–R94.

Auroy Y, Benhamou D, Bargues L, et al. Major complications of regional anesthesia in France: the SOS regional anesthesia hotline service. *Anesthesiology* 2002;97:1274–1280.

Bryson GL, Chung F, Finegan BA, et al. Patient selection in ambulatory anesthesia—an evidence-based review: part I. *Can J Anesth* 2004;51:768–781.

Bryson GL, Chung F, Cox RG, et al. Patient selection in ambulatory anesthesia—an evidence-based review: part II. *Can J Anesth* 2004;51:782–794.

Buckenmaier CC, Steele SM, Nielsen KC, et al. Paravertebral somatic nerve blocks for breast surgery in a patient with hypertrophic obstructive cardiomyopathy. *Can J Anesth* 2002;49:571–574.

Cameron D, Gan TJ. Management of postoperative nausea and vomiting in ambulatory surgery. *Anesthesiol Clin North Am* 2003;21:347–365.

Ilfeld BM, Enneking FK. Continuous peripheral nerve blocks at home: a review. *Anesth Analg* 2005;100:1822–1833.

Joshi GP. Inhalational techniques in ambulatory anesthesia. *Anesthesiol Clin North Am* 2003;21:263–272.

Liu SS, Strodtbeck WM, Richman JM, Wu CL. A comparison of regional versus general anesthesia for ambulatory anesthesia: a meta-analysis of randomized controlled trials. *Anesth Analg* 2005;101:1634–1642.

Mayfield, J. BIS Monitoring reduces phase 1 PACU admissions in an ambulatory surgical unit. *Anesthesiology* 1999;91:3A:A28.

McGrath B, Chung F. Postoperative recovery and discharge. *Anesthesiol Clin North Am* 2003;21:367–386.

Mulroy MF, McDonald SB. Regional anesthesia for outpatient surgery. *Anesthesiol Clin North Am* 2003;21:289–303.

Pasternak LR. Preoperative screening for ambulatory patients. *Anesthesiol Clin North Am* 2003;21:229–242.

Richman JM, Liu SS, Courpas G, et al. Does continuous peripheral nerve block provide superior pain control to opioids? A meta-analysis. *Anesth Analg* 2006;102:248–257.

Tesniere A, Servin F. Intravenous techniques in ambulatory anesthesia. *Anesthesiol Clin North Am* 2003;21:273–288.

Vaghadia H. Spinal anesthesia for outpatients: controversies and new techniques. *Can J Anaesth* 1998;45[Suppl 5 Part 2]:R64–R70.

32

Anesthesia Outside of the Operating Room

John J. A. Marota

I. **General considerations.** For all patients requiring general anesthesia or monitored anesthesia care in locations remote from the operating room, the same principles and requirements for anesthesia equipment, monitoring standards, and patient preparation outlined in Chapters 9, 10, and 14, respectively, should be met.

   A. **Required equipment in remote locations.** The anesthetist must determine that all standards are met before an anesthetic is initiated.

      1. A **central supply of oxygen and suction** is a minimum requirement. Two independent supplies of oxygen and suction (patient use and **waste gas scavenging**) are required at an anesthetizing location. In addition, a **full reserve tank of oxygen** must be available for each case. For locations that do not have a central supply of nitrous oxide, a reserve tank is available on the machine. Adequate **lighting and electrical power outlets** are required. A source of medical grade compressed air is desirable in cases (e.g., embolization) where nitrous oxide is not used but not mandatory.

      2. **Functioning anesthesia machine** appropriate for the anesthetic. Extra-long gas supply hoses may necessary; anesthesia breathing circuit tubing may require extensions to reach the patient.

      3. **Anesthesia supply cart** should be readily available that contains appropriate supplies and drugs necessary for provision of anesthesia.

      4. **Resuscitation equipment**: defibrillator, medications, and self-inflating hand resuscitator bag for transport must be immediately available.

   B. **Workspace area and patient access** often are limited.

      1. Areas outside the operating room where anesthesia is performed should be designated as "approved anesthetizing locations" by the hospital.

      2. A direct means of communication is necessary in case of emergency.

      3. Monitoring must be adapted if the anesthetist cannot remain in the room (e.g., during irradiation); viewing the patient by window or closed-circuit television may be necessary. Anticipate and provide for necessary monitoring during transport.

      4. Patient positioning may be difficult in confined spaces of magnetic resonance imaging (MRI) and computed tomography (CT) scanners. Additional padding may be necessary to prevent injury from compression of soft tissues during prolonged procedures.

5. Imaging often requires that anesthetized patients repeatedly move significant distances. Adequate lengths of ventilation, intravenous (IV), and monitoring cables are necessary; a "test move" of full excursion of patient movement is helpful before the procedure begins.

6. Anesthetists should take appropriate precautions to minimize radiation exposure to themselves during procedures.

C. **Conscious sedation versus monitored anesthesia care**

1. Specially trained nurses provide sedation for most patients requiring invasive procedures outside of the operating room. **Conscious sedation** is defined as a medically controlled state of depressed consciousness that allows protective reflexes to be maintained and retains the patient's ability to maintain a patent airway and to respond appropriately to physical and verbal stimulation. American Society of Anesthesiologists (ASA), Joint Commission on Accreditation of Healthcare Organizations, and state agencies (licensing boards) have set guidelines for provision of conscious sedation by nonanesthesiologists and nonphysicians.

2. An anesthesiologist is required to provide sedation for any patient in which **airway management** is considered complex (mask ventilation perceived as difficult or impossible or potentially difficult intubation) or if **significant comorbid pathology** exists (such as ASA Physical Status Class III and IV) that would require medical management by a physician.

II. **Contrast media**

A. **Ionic and nonionic contrast media** are administered IV and intra-arterially to supplement imaging; complexed gadolinium may be administered for both MRI and x-ray-based imaging. Hyperosmolar media are used rarely.

B. **Acute contrast media reactions.** Serious or fatal reactions are rare but unpredictable and not dose related. They are considered anaphylactoid because they possess features of anaphylaxis but are IgE negative in most instances.

1. Risk factors include history of previous adverse reaction, asthma, hay fever allergy requiring medical therapy, concurrent use of β-blockers or interleukin 2.

2. Symptoms develop within 5 to 30 minutes of exposure; present as generalized skin reactions, airway obstruction, angioedema, and cardiovascular collapse.

3. Treatment of acute reactions is supportive. Generalized anaphylactoid reactions should be treated with immediate administration of corticosteroids, H1 and H2 blockers. Oxygen, epinephrine, β_2-agonists, and intubation may be necessary to treat bronchospasm and laryngeal edema; support circulation with IV fluids and pressors.

4. Routine prophylaxis with prednisolone 30 mg or methylprednisolone 32 mg orally 12 and 2 hours before exposure; ranitidine 50 mg and diphenhydramine 50 mg orally may be indicated. Corticosteroids given less than 6 hours before contrast medium are not effective. For emergency procedures in high-risk patients, pretreat with 50 mg of diphenhydramine IV and 200 mg of hydrocortisone IV immediately and every 4 hours until the procedure is completed.

C. In patients with **compromised renal function,** *N*-acetylcysteine is often administered before and after procedures to reduce the incidence of **contrast-induced nephropathy.** Recently, periprocedural hydration with crystalloid or sodium bicarbonate has been advocated as equally effective.

III. **Anesthesia for CT**

A. **CT scans** are usually performed without general anesthesia. Children and uncooperative adults (e.g., head-injured patients) may require sedation or general anesthesia to minimize motion artifacts; if so, standard monitors as outlined in Chapter 10 are required. Capnography is useful to provide evidence of ventilation during sedation; fitting a side-stream sampling tube to nasal cannula or oxygen facemask provides qualitative assessment of ventilation.

B. **Adults**: small IV doses of a benzodiazepine, a narcotic, or a short-acting hypnotic (e.g., propofol) are useful for sedation; continuous infusions should be titrated to effect.

C. **Infants and children** less than 3 months of age may not need sedation; most children, however, will require some level of sedation or general anesthesia.

1. **Laryngeal mask airway (LMA)** or **endotracheal intubation** may be necessary to maintain a patent airway during deep sedation or general anesthesia.

2. Sedation

a. **Chloral hydrate** (30 to 50 mg/kg orally or per rectum [PR] administered 30 to 60 minutes before the procedure) is an adequate mild sedative for children. This drug may be safely administered by non-anesthesia personnel in sedating doses because it is not associated with respiratory depression or loss of airway. The "failure" rate, as defined by movement during imaging, is 15%.

b. **Methohexital, PR** (25 to 30 mg/kg), has more rapid onset (5 to 10 minutes) than chloral hydrate and lasts approximately 30 minutes. It is useful for the induction of general anesthesia; however, effects may vary because absorption is unpredictable. Because deep sedation or general anesthesia may occur, only an anesthetist should administer methohexital with appropriate monitoring and provisions to secure the airway. The drug is not appropriate in patients at risk of reflux of gastric contents.

D. **General anesthesia** using either IV or inhalational agents may be required. The airway may be maintained with LMA or endotracheal intubation as necessary.

IV. **Anesthesia for MRI**

A. The physical environment of the MRI suite presents several challenges for anesthetizing a patient.

1. The long narrow bore of the magnet in which the patient reclines does not allow ready access to or viewing of the patient during imaging. Scanners are located in shielded rooms that contain the magnetic field and shield against radiofrequency noise that produces image artifacts.

2. The high **magnetic field** is present at all times and exerts a force on all ferromagnetic materials (e.g., steel gas tanks, batteries). **Ferromagnetic objects brought near the magnetic field can be forcibly pulled toward the magnet,**

potentially injuring people or equipment in their path.
The static field and magnetic gradients generated during scanning can interfere with mechanical components (solenoids) in automated noninvasive blood pressure monitors, ventilators, and infusion pumps; specialized compatible equipment is necessary. Standard stethoscopes and batteries within laryngoscopes are ferromagnetic; only plastic stethoscopes and magnet-compatible laryngoscopes may be used in the magnet area. Credit cards, watches, and pagers must be left outside the scanning room.

3. **Radiofrequency signals** are generated during scanning; these may disturb electronic monitoring devices and produce artifacts. The noise generated by scanning makes it difficult to hear breath and heart sounds.

4. **Metallic implants (joint prostheses, aneurysm clips) or implanted devices (pacemakers, implantable cardioverter defibrillators [ICDs], insulin infusion pumps)** potentially may be dislodged, dysfunction, or suffer permanent damage by the magnetic field and scanning. Heating may occur from radiofrequency signals generated during scanning. Patients with implanted pacemakers, ICDs, or pulmonary artery catheters ***may not*** have MRI scans. Cerebral aneurysm clips are not considered an absolute contraindication to MRI; it is important, however, to identify the type of clip present to determine MR compatibility. Not all clips are compatible. Each MRI site carries a list of medical devices designated MRI compatible by the U.S. Food and Drug Administration (FDA). Because medical devices may be upgraded or altered by a manufacturer without notifying the FDA, MRI centers should, in addition, contact the manufacturer if questions arise about specific devices.

B. Duration of an MRI scan varies. Immobility is required only during the actual scanning, 3 to 12 minutes at a time. General anesthesia with either LMA or endotracheal intubation is necessary for most infants and children. General anesthesia can be induced in the magnet area; compatible laryngoscopes are commercially available. Alternatively, induction can be performed in an area out of the magnetic field and the anesthetized patient can be moved into the scanner. Maintenance of anesthesia is provided with specially modified anesthesia machines that contain only nonferrous metal. The patient ***must*** be removed from the magnetic field if cardiopulmonary resuscitation is required.

C. **Monitors** must be safe for the patient, function within the magnetic field, and have a minimal effect on imaging. Specialized compatible monitoring equipment is available that can remain in the magnetic field and communicate to a "slave" monitor outside the shielded magnet area.

1. The standard electrocardiogram (ECG) is subject to interference during scanning.

2. Scanning interferes with standard **pulse oximeters,** which may interfere with image acquisition. Specialized "MRI-compatible" devices are available; sensors work by fiberoptic cables.

3. Temperature probes are not used because of the potential for cutaneous burns.

4. Visualize patients during scanning via a shielded window.
5. Electrical currents induced in coiled cables during scanning can burn patients; cables should be kept as straight as possible to minimize this risk.

V. **Anesthesia for neuroradiologic procedures.** Anesthetic management may be necessary for diagnostic procedures (angiography, balloon test occlusion) or during therapeutic interventions (embolization, cerebral vasospasm, vertebroplasty/kyphoplasty). Patient access after start of the procedure may be limited to the left arm and leg.

A. **Endovascular embolization** is performed to treat ruptured as well as unruptured cerebral aneurysms, to interrupt blood supply to intra- and extracranial arteriovenous fistulas and malformations, vascular tumors, and bleeding vessels in the nose or pharynx.

1. **Embolization** requires access to the vascular tree, commonly via the femoral artery, and advancement of a small catheter into the aneurysm or blood vessels supplying the area of pathology. Once position is confirmed by angiography, the vascular occlusive material (detachable metal coils, glue, or small particles) is deployed via the catheter.

2. **Anesthetic goals** include provision of a still field during placement of the micro-catheter and deployment of the occlusive material, stable hemodynamics, and rapid recovery after the procedure to test neurologic function. This often necessitates light general anesthesia to provide amnesia during paralysis. Anesthesia can be accomplished with IV techniques (propofol, muscle relaxant, and narcotics) and supplemented with low doses of volatile anesthetics. Nitrous oxide is avoided to minimize consequences of inadvertent arterial air emboli. These procedures are relatively painless with little stimulation.

3. Hyperosmolar contrast dyes produce a brisk diuresis requiring urinary catheterization and IV fluid administration.

4. Invasive arterial blood pressure monitoring via a radial artery is often necessary to control hemodynamics; alternatively, blood pressure may be transduced from the femoral artery sheath placed during the procedure.

5. **Hypertension** should be avoided, because it may increase the risk of hemorrhage or aneurysm rupture. Vasoactive drugs such as phenylephrine should be used with great caution in patients with unprotected cerebral aneurysms. β-Blockers, calcium channel blockers, hydralazine, nitroglycerin, and sodium nitroprusside may be useful to treat hypertension.

6. Procedures may be lengthy and place the patient at risk for untoward embolic events. Patients often require **anticoagulation** (heparin or argatroban) to minimize propagation of thrombus from the embolization coils or microcatheters; anticoagulation is monitored by activated clotting time. Eptifibitide (**Integrilin**) may be administered by bolus and infusion to minimize platelet aggregation.

7. Intraprocedural complications include rupture of the aneurysm or arteriovenous fistulas and malformations, dissection or rupture of a blood vessel, and inadvertent occlusion of a blood vessel. If intracranial hemorrhage is suspected, immediate placement of a ventriculostomy may be

necessary to drain cerebrospinal fluid (CSF) emergently to reduce intracranial pressure (ICP). Unlike intraoperative aneurysm rupture in open procedures (Chapter 24), there is no significant blood loss because the cranium is closed. Persistent elevation of ICP may require hyperventilation, diuresis, or barbiturate coma. Immediate CT scan may be necessary to determine the extent of hemorrhage and need for emergency surgery to decompress the brain.

B. **Embolization for control of epistaxis and extracranial vascular lesions** presents potential problems of hemorrhage, hemodynamic instability, large amounts of blood in the airway, and aspiration. Typed and cross-matched blood should be available; large-bore IV access may be necessary if acute hemorrhage is a potential. Endotracheal intubation may be required for airway control and difficult if the pathology involves the airway or face.

C. **Balloon test occlusion** of the carotid artery or other major blood vessel is performed to determine whether permanent obstruction of the vessel will lead to neurologic deficit. Occlusion is performed endovascularly by temporary inflation of a balloon in the vessel to completely obstruct blood flow; if no deficit is apparent on neurologic exam, hypotension is induced and maintained for 20 to 30 minutes to elicit signs of ischemia. Often, cerebral blood flow is evaluated during the hypotensive period by IV injection of a positron emission tomography (PET) isotope; PET scan is obtained after the procedure. With any deterioration in neurologic function, the balloon is immediately deflated and blood pressure is returned to normal. While sedation is appropriate during initial angiography and placement of the balloon, **a completely awake, nonsedated patient is necessary for neurologic testing during occlusion**; short-acting agents are preferred. **Hypotension is induced with rapidly reversible agents** (nitroprusside or nitroglycerine). The tachycardic response (which may increase blood pressure) to induced hypotension may be offset by administering β-blockers. Emergency airway management including endotracheal intubation may be required if seizures or loss of the airway occurs during test occlusion.

D. **Cerebral and spinal angiography** are painless diagnostic procedures. Only children or adults who are uncooperative because of dementia or delirium require general anesthesia for angiography. Adult patients requiring general anesthesia for intracranial angiography may have depressed mental status because of elevated ICP, encephalopathy, recent stroke, or intracerebral hemorrhage; meticulous attention to hemodynamics may require invasive blood pressure monitoring. Catheterization of the bladder is indicated because of diuresis from the contrast agent. Spinal angiography requires several hours for each vessel supplying the spinal cord to be identified and the angiogram to be performed. The duration of the procedure may need to be limited based on the upper limit of contrast agent dosing. Patients are anesthetized for comfort; invasive hemodynamic monitoring is not usually necessary.

E. **Vertebroplasty and kyphoplasty** are performed to treat painful vertebral body fractures that occur most commonly from osteoporosis, particularly in elderly women. The procedure is performed in the prone position; percutaneously, a stylet is driven through the pedicle into the fractured vertebral body. Bone cement is then deposited under pressure via the stylet. Multiple levels can be performed at one sitting and often stylets are placed bilaterally at each level. In kyphoplasty, a balloon is inflated with contrast agent in the vertebral body to create a void for cement and reform height lost from fracture; cement is then deposited in the void. Either monitored anesthesia care or general anesthesia is appropriate. Sedation can be accomplished with diphenhydramine (25 to 50 mg IV), promethazine (5 to 25 mg IV), or benzodiazepines (midazolam 1 to 2 mg IV). Injection of cement can be painful and narcotic analgesia may be necessary. Patients remain supine for several hours afterward to permit the cement to harden completely.

F. Thrombolysis of acute stroke is an emergency procedure performed to restore blood flow to cerebral vessels occluded by thrombus in patients with symptoms of acute ischemic stroke. Intravenous thrombolytic therapy with tissue plasminogen activator (tPA) may be initiated in patients with symptoms of ≤3 hours duration. Intra-arterial infusion of tPA directly at the site of thrombus requires angiography and is recommended in basilar artery occlusions and for acute ischemic strokes in patients with symptoms up to 6 hours duration. Angioplasty of atherosclerotic plaque or placement of an intra-arterial stent may be used to supplement thrombolytic therapy to maintain patency of the occluded vessel. General anesthetic with endotracheal intubation is preferred for angiography and invasive therapeutic interventions. History and physical exam may be limited because of time constraints; often consent is obtained by a neurologist or interventional radiologist. Arterial catheterization for hemodynamic monitoring is accomplished after start of the procedure to save time. Patients are anticoagulated after recannulization; antiplatelet aggregation therapy may be necessary with IV **eptifibitide (Integrilin).**

G. Cerebral vasospasm is a common and potentially devastating late complication of subarachnoid hemorrhage. Patients may require angiography and local **intra-arterial infusion** of vasodilating drugs (**papavarine, nicardipine, or milrinone**) or even angioplasty to increase the diameter of segments of cerebral blood vessels that are critically constricted. Medical management includes **hypervolemia, hemodilution, and hypertension** to increase blood flow through stenotic segments of feeding vessels; patients are often on large doses of vasopressors (phenylephrine, norepinephrine, or vasopressin) to induce hypertension. ICP may be elevated from brain edema secondary to initial injury or evolving ischemic strokes.

1. **ICP monitoring** is necessary during the procedure because intracranial hypertension is common and ICP may increase with therapy. Intraventricular catheter is preferable because it permits drainage of CSF to treat increased ICP; "Camino" bolt is adequate for monitoring but CSF cannot be withdrawn.

2. Anesthetic goals are to optimize cerebral perfusion **by maintaining systemic hypertension and intracranial normotension,** maintain a hyperdynamic cardiovascular state, and provide a rapidly reversible general anesthetic so that neurologic exam can be assessed immediately after intervention.

Patients may require postprocedure mechanical ventilation to control ICP. If ICP is not increased, light general anesthesia may be accomplished with a low concentration of volatile anesthetics supplemented with narcotics and paralysis. Alternatively, propofol infusion may be necessary to control ICP. Paralysis and mechanical ventilation are necessary to control partial pressure of carbon dioxide.

3. ICP may rise and blood pressure may fall dramatically with intra-arterial infusions of **papavarine** and **nicardipine.** Increased dosages of vasopressors or supplementation with cardiac inotropes (ephedrine 5 to 25 mg IV) may be necessary.

4. Because hyperglycemia may worsen consequences of cerebral ischemia, patients may be receiving insulin infusion with 5% dextrose in normal saline to maintain tight control of glucose.

5. Patients are often febrile. Normothermia can be maintained with surface cooling; hyperthermia may worsen consequences of cerebral ischemia.

H. **Trigeminal neuralgia.** Percutaneous neurolysis of trigeminal ganglion and/or terminal nerves is effective therapy for management of chronic pain. Patients frequently also suffer from multiple sclerosis. Placement of a lesioning electrode is performed in the awake patient to best define areas for ablation; neurologic examination and evaluation require an awake and fully cooperative patient. Narcotics are avoided because pain is the symptom evaluated; narcotic analgesics can blunt sensory neurologic exam to distinguish painful from nonpainful stimulation. Brief periods of general anesthesia are necessary for placement of the electrode in the trigeminal ganglion via foramen ovale and actual ablation because this may be excruciatingly painful. Standard monitoring is used, and unconsciousness is produced with methohexital 1% (0.5 to 1.0 mg/kg IV) or propofol (1 to 2 mg/kg IV). Proper position of the needle is confirmed by fluoroscopy and brief electrical stimulation to reproduce the sensory distribution of the patient's area of pain. Neurolytic techniques include injection of alcohol, or, most commonly, radiofrequency lesion ablation. Hypertension is common during lesioning and may require invasive blood pressure monitoring in some patients and treatment with esmolol, labetalol, nitroglycerin, or nitroprusside. Bradycardia and asystole may occur by stimulation of the oculocardiac reflex; hemodynamically significant reactions may require treatment with atropine or glycopyrrolate or chest compressions. Mask ventilation may be difficult when the electrode is in place.

VI. **Anesthesia for vascular, thoracic, and gastrointestinal/genitourinary radiology procedures.**

A. **Transjugular intrahepatic portosystemic shunt** is used to decompress the portal system in patients with decompensated portal hypertension. It is a less invasive technique that may replace open portocaval and splenorenal shunts. Patients may have advanced liver disease, actively bleeding esophageal varices, massive ascites, and severely compromised liver function. Hepatorenal syndrome may cause oliguria.

1. After cannulation of the right internal jugular, a trochar is directed into a hepatic vein and passed through liver parenchyma to enter a portal vein and create a connection for egress of portal blood into systemic circulation; the conduit

is dilated and patency is maintained with a stent. Portal vein may be visualized fluoroscopically with retrograde insufflation of carbon dioxide gas via the hepatic vein.

2. Monitored anesthesia care with standard monitors may be sufficient in some patients but light general anesthesia is common because of the procedure length and discomfort.

3. Patients with bleeding or ascites should be considered to have full stomachs and receive a rapid sequence induction. It is preferable to perform paracentesis to drain ascites before induction of general anesthesia to avoid consequences of sympathectomy on rapid decompression of the portal system.

4. No anesthetic technique is superior. Liver failure patients are often hyperdynamic with low systemic vascular resistance because of arteriovenous fistulas in the lung and liver (Chapter 5).

5. Patients with actively bleeding varices may be treated with continuous infusion of octreotide to reduce mesenteric blood flow.

B. **Percutaneous lung biopsy** under CT guidance is a relatively painless procedure amenable to light conscious sedation. Standard monitoring usually is sufficient. The patient is usually prone and must remain immobile during needle placement and biopsy. Pneumothorax is a potential complication; patients receive a chest x-ray after recovery to rule out significant pneumothorax.

C. **Percutaneous insertion of gastrostomy, nephrostomy, cholecysto-, or choledochostomy tubes** rarely requires general anesthesia. Comorbid conditions may require aggressive medical management during procedures necessitating the presence of an anesthesiologist. Procedures are performed under fluoroscopy or CT.

VII. **Anesthesia for cyclotron therapy and radiation therapy**

A. **Proton-beam radiation therapy** is used to treat arteriovenous malformations, pituitary tumors, and retinoblastomas. Irradiation is painless, but targeting and exact positioning may take several hours during which the patient's head must remain in a fixed position. To achieve this, the head is placed in a stereotactic frame locked to the positioning device.

1. **In adults,** placement of small pins or screws in the skull can be performed under local anesthesia with 2% lidocaine with epinephrine. If "ear bars" are used, a satisfactory ear block can be performed by subcutaneous injection of 3 mL of 2% lidocaine with epinephrine in the outer ear canal. Sedation is usually not recommended because patient cooperation is required.

2. **For children,** a general anesthetic is usually administered. The procedure typically is performed daily for about 4 weeks; a propofol induction (3 mg/kg IV) and maintenance infusion (approximately 75 μg/kg/minute) through an implanted Broviac or Hickman catheter is a suitable technique. Spontaneous ventilation should be permitted whenever possible. The patient's head is placed in a sniffing position and a plaster mold is formed that maintains the head in the correct position for treatment. Supplemental oxygen can be provided by nasal prongs or a facemask. LMA is considered if a natural airway cannot be maintained. Standard monitoring is used

and patients are monitored and viewed via closed-circuit television because the anesthetist must leave the room during the brief period of radiation.

B. **Anesthesia for radiation therapy.** Children receiving radiation therapy often require general anesthesia.

1. Typical treatment course is three or four times a week for 4 weeks. It is desirable to choose an anesthetic that allows rapid recovery with minimal risk of nausea and vomiting.

2. The first radiation procedure may be time-consuming (1 to several hours) because measurements must be performed and molds made of the patient. Subsequent treatments are typically less than 30 minutes.

3. Many patients have indwelling venous access for chemotherapy. An IV induction and maintenance with propofol infusion is a suitable technique. Intramuscular injection of a combination of midazolam, glycopyrrolate, and ketamine may be useful in children with difficult venous access.

VIII. **Electroconvulsive therapy (ECT)** is used to treat major depression in patients who have not responded to medications, are debilitated by serious side effects, or are acutely suicidal. Patients who suffer from delusions, hallucinations, or profound psychomotor retardation are less responsive to medication, and thus early ECT is preferred for them as well. Usually a series of 6 to 12 treatments over 2 to 4 weeks is required for a clinical response.

A. **Physiologic effects of ECT**

1. The electrical stimulus produces a grand mal seizure consisting of a tonic phase lasting 10 to 15 seconds, followed by a clonic phase lasting 30 to 50 seconds.

2. An initial vagal discharge may result in bradycardia and mild hypotension. Subsequent sympathetic nervous system activation produces hypertension and tachycardia, which can persist for 5 to 10 minutes. ECG changes are common and may include pulse-rate interval prolongation, increased QT interval, T-wave inversions, and atrial or ventricular arrhythmias.

3. Increased cerebral blood flow and metabolic rate lead to increased ICP. Increased intraocular and intragastric pressure may occur.

B. **Anesthetic goals**

1. Provide amnesia and a rapid return to consciousness.

2. Prevent damage from tonic-clonic contracture (e.g., long-bone fractures).

3. Control hemodynamic response.

4. Avoid interference with initiation and duration of induced seizure.

C. The one absolute contraindication to ECT is **intracranial hypertension** (elevated ICP). **Relative contraindications** include presence of an intracranial mass lesion (with normal ICP), intracranial aneurysm, recent myocardial infarction, angina, congestive heart failure, untreated glaucoma, major bone fractures, thrombophlebitis, pregnancy, and retinal detachment. Patients on maintenance treatment with benzodiazepines or lithium should discontinue these treatments before ECT; benzodiazepines are anticonvulsants that may abolish or attenuate the seizure; lithium is associated with post-ECT confusion and delirium.

D. **Anesthetic management**
1. Sedative premedication is not indicated and may prolong emergence. Anticholinergic drugs are indicated only in patients prone to bradycardia. Ondansetron may be useful in patients with a history of nausea and vomiting.
2. A small-gauge IV cannula is placed for drug administration; standard monitors (ECG, pulse oximetry, and noninvasive blood pressure) are applied.
3. The patient is preoxygenated with 100% oxygen; anesthesia is induced with methohexital (0.5 to 1.0 mg/kg IV) and succinylcholine (0.5 to 1.0 mg/kg IV). Patients are ventilated with 100% oxygen via mask and Ambu bag. Mivacurium can be used in patients with contraindications to succinylcholine. Pretreatment with labetalol (10 to 50 mg IV) or esmolol (40 to 80 mg IV) blunts the hypertensive response in patients with hypertension or coronary artery disease.
4. Other anesthetic induction agents may be used; however, thiopental and midazolam raise seizure threshold and may prolong emergence and propofol reduces seizure duration. Ketorolac may decrease muscle pains after ECT.
5. Rolled gauze pads placed bilaterally as bite blocks protect gums and lips from biting from electrical stimulus and subsequent seizure.
6. Nature and duration of induced seizures can be monitored by electroencephalogram or by "isolated arm" technique. With the latter, inflation of a blood pressure cuff interrupts blood supply to one arm before injecting muscle relaxant; seizure activity is apparent in the isolated arm.
7. Patients are ventilated with oxygen by facemask until spontaneous ventilation resumes. They are then placed in a lateral decubitus position and monitored in a recovery area until awake and alert. Agitated delirium from tardive seizures may occur after ECT and can be treated with small doses of propofol or benzodiazepine.
8. Patients with underlying medical conditions may require special attention:
   a. Patients with gastroesophageal reflux may require aspiration prophylaxis and rapid sequence intubation.
   b. Patients with severe cardiac dysfunction may require invasive monitoring.
   c. Patients with intracranial mass lesions may require invasive blood pressure monitoring for tight hemodynamic control; hyperventilation before inducing a seizure may reduce the ICP response.
   d. Pregnant patients may require endotracheal intubation, fetal monitoring, and left uterine displacement.
9. Rarely, an induced seizure will not terminate spontaneously. Ventilation with 100% oxygen is continued, and seizure is terminated within 3 minutes with propofol (20 to 50 mg IV) or benzodiazepines.
E. **Psychiatric drug interactions.** Patients requiring ECT may be treated with psychotropic drugs that have potent side effects and interactions with anesthetic drugs.
1. **Tricyclic antidepressants** (e.g., amitriptyline, nortriptyline, desipramine, imipramine, and doxepin) potentiate effects

of norepinephrine and serotonin by preventing reuptake. Adverse effects include postural hypotension, sedation, dry mouth, urinary retention, and tachycardia. Anesthesia and ECT-induced ECG changes (including prolonged PR interval, widened QRS complex, and T-wave changes) are relatively common in patients receiving tricyclic antidepressants.

2. **Monoamine oxidase inhibitors (MAOIs)** (e.g., phenelzine and isocarboxazid) increase availability of norepinephrine at postsynaptic receptors; orthostatic hypotension and severe hypertension may occur. Tyramine, present in certain foods, may produce a hypertensive crisis in patients taking MAOIs. Although it has been recommended that MAOI therapy be discontinued at least 10 days before elective surgery, the risk of severe depression outweighs the risks of continuing the drug. **Important interactions** between MAOIs and anesthetics include exaggerated hypotension during spinal anesthesia and severe hypertension with indirectly acting vasopressors (ephedrine). Administration of **meperidine** (and meperidine derivatives) to patients receiving MAOIs has been associated with a syndrome of serotonin excess characterized by severe hemodynamic instability, respiratory depression, malignant hyperpyrexia, seizures, coma, and death.

3. **Selective serotonin reuptake inhibitors** (e.g., fluoxetine, sertraline, fluvoxamine, and paroxetine) are associated with only mild adverse effects. There are no known significant interactions with anesthetic drugs.

IX. **Upper and lower endoscopy** and interventional procedures including endoscopic retrograde cholangiopancreatography (**ERCP**) and percutaneous endoscopic gastrostomy tube placement (**PEG**) can be performed successfully in adults with minimal sedation; uncooperative patients or those with significant comorbid pathology may require the care of an anesthesiologist. Children often require general anesthesia. Procedures are not painful and stimulation is limited to the procedure itself. Upper endoscopy, ERCP, or PEG requires endotracheal intubation to maintain an adequate airway; colonoscopy is performed in the decubitus position and may be performed with an LMA if appropriate. Patients often have active reflux necessitating rapid sequence induction and intubation.

SUGGESTED READING

Albers GW, et al. Antithrombotic and thrombolytic therapy for ischemic stroke; the seventh ACCP conference on antithrombotic and thrombolytic therapy. *Chest* 2004;126:483–512.

Coté CJ. Anesthesia outside the operating room. In: Coté CJ, Todres ID, Goudsouzian NG, Ryan JF, eds. A practice of anesthesia for infants and children, 3rd ed. Philadelphia:WB Saunders, 2001:571–583.

Ding Z, White PF. Anesthesia for electroconvulsive therapy. *Anesth Analg.* 2002;94:1351–1364.

Dolenc TJ, et al. Electroconvulsive therapy in patients taking monoamine oxidase inhibitors. *J ECT.* 2004;20:258–261.

Gilbertson LI, ed. Conscious sedation. *Int Anesthesiol Clin* 1999;37:1–129.

Jorgensen NH, et al. ASA monitoring standards and magnetic resonance imaging. *Anesth Analg* 1994;79:1141–1147.

Merten GJ, et al. Prevention of contrast-induced nephropathy with sodium bicarbonate: a randomized controlled trial. *JAMA* 2004;19:2328–2334.

Morcos SK. Acute serious and fatal reactions to contrast media: our current understanding. *Br J Radiol* 2005;78:686–693.

Oudemans-van Straaten HM. Strategies to prevent contrast nephropathy. *Minerva Cardioangiol* 2005;53:445–463.

Russell, GB. Alternate-site anesthesia: the expanding world of anesthesia outside the operating room. *Curr Opin Anaesthesiol* 1998;11:411.

Schubert A, Deogaonkar A, Lotto M, Niezgoda J, Luciano M. Anesthesia for minimally invasive cranial and spinal surgery. *Neurosurg Anesthesiol* 2006;18:47–56.

Young WL, Pile-Spellman J. Anesthetic considerations for interventional neuroradiology. *Anesthesiology* 1994;80:427–456.

Anesthesia for Trauma and Burns

Ala Nozari and Keith Baker

I. **Initial evaluation of the trauma patient.** Rapid assessment of injuries and institution of resuscitative measures are particularly important in trauma patients. Life-threatening injuries should be identified immediately and treatment measures initiated simultaneously, based on Airway, Breathing, Circulation, Disability/neurological function, and Environmental priorities. Assume that all patients have a cervical spine injury, have a full stomach, and are hypovolemic until proven otherwise.

A. **Airway**

1. Airway assessment should include inspection for foreign bodies; facial, laryngeal, and tracheal fractures (palpable fracture, subcutaneous emphysema); and expanding cervical hematomas. Remove all secretions, blood, vomitus, and any existing foreign bodies (e.g., dentures or teeth).

2. **Minimize movement of the cervical spine during airway manipulation.** If immobilizing devices must be removed temporarily, an assistant should keep the head in a neutral position with manual in-line immobilization.

3. A definitive airway should be established if there is any doubt about the patient's ability to maintain airway integrity. With blunt or penetrating injuries to the neck, endotracheal intubation may worsen a laryngeal or bronchial injury. Functional suction equipment should always be immediately available, as trauma patients may vomit and aspirate.

   a. **The awake patient.** Depending on injuries, the patient's ability to cooperate, and stability of the patient, several options are available (see Chapter 13):

      (1) Awake nasal or orotracheal intubation with the use of a laryngoscope or fiberoptic bronchoscope.

      (2) Blind nasal intubation of the spontaneously breathing patient.

      (3) Rapid sequence intubation. This is our most common approach to the airway.

      (4) Awake tracheostomy, a rare option.

   b. **The combative patient.** A rapid-sequence orotracheal intubation is often the most expedient approach provided there are no problems precluding neuromuscular blockade. Hypoxemia must always be excluded in an agitated patient. Blind nasal intubation may be attempted; however, sedating these patients to control their agitation may lead to further airway compromise.

   c. **The unconscious patient.** Orotracheal intubation is usually the safest and most expeditious approach.

   d. If the patient arrives with an esophageal obturator airway or esophageal gastric tube airway, perform **endotracheal**

intubation before removing these devices, because vomiting frequently occurs with their removal.

4. **The intubated patient.** Verify the position of an endotracheal tube by auscultation for breath sounds bilaterally and by detecting exhaled or end-tidal CO_2. Secure the endotracheal tube and ensure adequate ventilation and oxygenation.

B. **Breathing.** Adequate function of the lungs, diaphragm, and chest wall should be evaluated rapidly. Supplemental oxygen should be provided to all trauma patients, either by a mask or via the endotracheal tube.

1. Assess the chest wall excursion and auscultate the lungs to ensure adequate gas exchange. Visual inspection and palpation may rapidly detect injuries such as a pneumothorax.

2. Tension pneumothorax, massive hemothorax, and pulmonary contusion are three common conditions that may acutely impair ventilation and should always be identified. Positive-pressure ventilation may worsen a tension pneumothorax and can rapidly lead to cardiovascular collapse.

3. The trauma patient's breathing and gas exchange should be reevaluated after intubation or initiation of positive-pressure ventilation and periodically after the initial assessment.

C. **Circulation**

1. **Hemodynamics** are initially assessed by palpating pulses and measuring the blood pressure. Skin color and level of consciousness are helpful in evaluating the circulatory status within seconds.

2. **Intravenous (IV) access.** Check IV lines already in place to ensure that they function well. At least two large (minimum 16-gauge) catheters should be placed. These lines should be placed above the level of the diaphragm in patients with injuries of the abdomen (and with the potential for major venous disruption). IV access below the level of the diaphragm is helpful when obstruction or disruption of the superior vena cava, innominate, or subclavian vein is suspected.

3. **Peripheral venous cannulation failure.** In this event, percutaneous subclavian or femoral vein cannulation should be carried out. Although the internal and external jugular veins remain options, access to these structures is frequently hindered by immobilization of the head and neck for a suspected cervical spine injury. If these approaches prove unsuccessful, **surgical cutdowns** should be performed. The saphenous vein at the ankle and the antecubital venous system are acceptable options.

4. **Volume resuscitation** begins immediately with the establishment of venous access. Hemodynamic response to initial volume replacement may be used to direct continued volume resuscitation.

   a. Hemodynamics will improve in most hypovolemic trauma patients after rapid administration of warmed crystalloid (1 to 3 L of Ringer's lactate solution in adults or at 20 mL/kg for pediatric patients). If possible, defer blood replacement until cross-matched units are available.

   b. Patients who do not respond to rapid infusion of crystalloid are candidates for transfusion of type-specific, non–cross-matched blood as soon as it is available (this should be available with 15 minutes of the patient's arrival.) and a search for other causes of circulatory collapse (tension pneumothorax, tamponade, hypoxia, myocardial dysfunction, esophageal intubation, etc.) should be performed.

c. Low-titer, type O-negative, non–cross-matched blood may be lifesaving if the patient remains moribund despite rapid infusion of crystalloid and before type-specific blood becomes available.

d. There is no proven advantage of colloids (e.g., albumin, hetastarch, and gelatin products) during the acute phase of trauma resuscitation. The use of currently available dextrans is restricted in the management of hemorrhagic shock because of potential coagulopathy.

5. **Vasopressor infusions** should not substitute for adequate volume replacement during initial resuscitation. Vasopressors may be necessary as a temporizing measure if perfusion pressure is clearly inadequate during ongoing volume resuscitation.

6. **Limited or hypotensive resuscitation** is a controversial approach to the hypotensive penetrating trauma patient with **uncontrolled** hemorrhage. The approach limits the systolic blood pressure to <100 mm Hg while the surgical team gains rapid control of the bleeding source. Once the bleeding site is controlled, normotensive, normovolemic resuscitation is carried out. Head trauma is a clear contraindication to this approach.

D. **Disability/neurologic evaluation.** A brief neurologic examination yields useful information in assessing cerebral perfusion or oxygenation and can provide a simple and quick means of predicting a patient's outcome.

1. The level of consciousness can be described by the AVPU method (A = **a**lert, V = responds to **v**erbal stimuli, P = responds only to **p**ainful stimuli, U = **u**nresponsive to all stimuli) but a more detailed and quantitative assessment with the Glasgow coma score (best motor response, verbal response, and eye opening) is preferable.

2. An altered level of consciousness dictates immediate reevaluation of the patient's oxygenation and circulation, even though it can be of central nervous system origin (trauma or intoxication).

3. Neurologic deterioration can rapidly occur in trauma patients and necessitates frequent neurologic reevaluation.

E. **Environmental control.** Trauma patients are often hypothermic upon arrival at the hospital and require aggressive efforts to maintain body heat.

1. External warming devices should be applied, IV fluids should be warmed before infusion, and a warm environment should be maintained.

2. Controversy still exists regarding the role of mild hypothermia (>34°C) in the management of shock or traumatic head injury.

F. **Diagnostic studies**

1. **Laboratory studies** include blood type and cross-matching, complete blood count, platelet count, prothrombin time, activated partial thromboplastin time, electrolytes, glucose, blood urea nitrogen, creatinine, urinalysis, and, if indicated, toxicologic screening.

2. **Radiographic studies** should include a lateral cervical spine film, a chest radiograph (CXR), and an anteroposterior view of the pelvis on all patients with blunt trauma. At the minimum, obtain a CXR in all patients with penetrating injuries of the trunk. Additional studies include thoracic, lumbar, and sacral spine films and chest and abdominal computed tomography (CT) studies.

   a. **Lateral radiographs of the cervical spine** must include the C-7–T-1 interface and must be of sufficient quality to delineate the structures of interest (i.e., soft tissues and bones).

   b. If the patient's clinical condition allows time for additional studies, obtain **open-mouth odontoid and anteroposterior views of the neck** (standard trauma cervical-spine series).

   c. If the clinical evaluation demonstrates a patient with significant neck pain and tenderness but no evidence of fracture or dislocation on the plain radiographs, CT and magnetic resonance imaging may help delineate an occult injury.

3. Obtain a **12-lead electrocardiogram (ECG)** on all major trauma patients to help evaluate the presence of myocardial injury (e.g., contusion, tamponade, ischemia, and arrhythmia).

G. **Monitoring** is dictated by the severity of the patient's injuries and preexisting medical problems.

   1. **An arterial line** may prove useful in patients with hemodynamic instability or respiratory failure.

   2. **A central venous pressure line** may be required to assess volume status and administer vasoactive drugs.

   3. A **pulmonary artery catheter** may be helpful in patients with ventricular dysfunction, severe coronary artery disease, valvular heart disease, or multiple organ system involvement. Placement is planned according to the time available and the clinical status of the patient.

II. **Specific injuries**

A. **Intracranial and spinal cord trauma** (see Chapter 24).

B. **Facial trauma.** Considerable force is required to produce facial fractures. Accordingly, these injuries often are associated with other injuries such as intracranial and spinal cord trauma, thoracic injury, myocardial contusion, and intra-abdominal bleeding. Brisk oral or nasal bleeding, broken teeth, vomitus, or tongue or pharyngeal injury may occlude the airway and complicate airway management. Trismus may be associated with these injuries and should be assessed before induction of anesthesia. Emergency cricothyroidotomy or tracheostomy may be lifesaving.

   1. **Maxillary fractures** are grouped by the **LeFort classification** (Fig. 33.1).

      a. **Type I (transverse or horizontal).** The body of the maxilla is separated from the base of the skull above the level of the palate and below the level of the zygomatic process.

      b. **Type II (pyramidal).** Vertical fractures through the facial aspects of the maxilla extend upward through the nasal and ethmoid bones.

      c. **Type III (craniofacial dysjunction).** Fractures extend through the frontozygomatic suture lines bilaterally, across

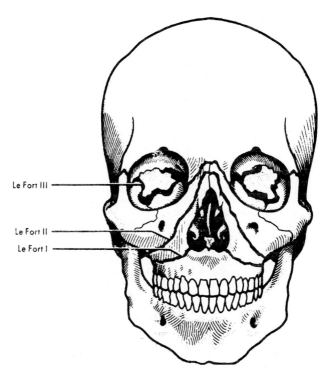

Figure 33.1. The LeFort classification. (From Rosen P, et al., eds.
Emergency medicine: Concepts and clinical practice, **2nd ed. St. Louis: Mosby, 1988:407.)**

the orbits, and through the base of the nose and the ethmoid region.

d. **Le Fort and related fractures** are frequently associated with skull fractures and **cerebrospinal fluid rhinorrhea.** Nasotracheal intubation and placement of nasogastric tubes are relatively contraindicated under these circumstances. Elective nasal intubation (or tracheostomy) may be necessary, however, before operative repair.

e. In the presence of rhinorrhea, positive pressure mask ventilation can potentially cause pneumocephalus.

2. Mandibular fractures

a. Malocclusion, limitation of mandibular movement, loose or missing teeth, sublingual hematoma, and swelling at the fracture site complicate airway management.

b. **Posterior displacement of the tongue** producing airway obstruction is associated with bilateral condylar or parasymphyseal fractures of the mandible. Simple forward traction on the tongue often provides relief.

c. Reestablishment of normal occlusion may necessitate intermaxillary fixation, which can also be combined with rigid fixation. Awake nasotracheal intubation is recommended if the nose has not been severely traumatized.

3. **Ocular trauma** usually requires general anesthesia for repair. Special considerations for open-eye injuries are discussed in Chapter 25, section I.C.1.

4. **Anesthetic management.** Most displaced facial fractures require general anesthesia for repair. Although children usually require general anesthesia, many soft-tissue injuries can be treated with local anesthesia. Maintenance of a patent airway is the principal concern, and induction may require awake nasotracheal intubation, fiberoptic laryngoscopy, or tracheostomy under local anesthesia.

C. **Neck trauma** may cause cervical spine injury, esophageal tears, major vascular injuries, and airway injuries. Airway injuries may present with obstruction, subcutaneous emphysema, hemoptysis, dysphonia, or hypoxemia.

1. **"Clothesline"** injuries occur from direct trauma to the upper airway and can result in the avulsion of the larynx from the trachea and separation between the cricoid cartilage and the first tracheal ring. These injuries do not always present with an open neck wound. Additional injuries include laryngotracheal transection, laryngeal fractures, and vascular injury.

2. Blunt injury over the carotid arteries may result in intimal disruption and dissection, even in the absence of initial symptoms. Angiography or ultrasonography may be required to exclude these injuries.

3. Initial management of **penetrating trauma** includes direct compression of involved vessels to control hemorrhage and prevent air embolism.

4. Associated **thoracic injuries,** such as pneumothorax and hemorrhage from injury to the great vessels, may occur with lower-neck injuries.

5. **Anesthetic management**
   a. **Securing the airway** is the most important issue in these patients. A coordinated approach among members of the trauma team is necessary. A surgical airway or direct intubation of an open airway defect can be lifesaving. Anesthesia induction via spontaneous ventilation of a potent inhalational agent can be useful in the presence of airway disruption.
   b. **Great vessel injuries** in the neck may necessitate lower extremity IV access.

D. **Chest trauma** can involve injuries to the trachea or larynx, heart, great vessels, thoracic duct, esophagus, lung, or diaphragm.

1. **Rib fractures** are a common feature of major thoracic trauma and mandate assessment for pneumothorax by CXR. First-rib fractures should alert the clinician to the potential for associated internal injuries. Multiple rib fractures most commonly involve ribs 7 to 10 and often accompany lacerations of the spleen or liver.

2. The hypoxemia and respiratory failure that accompany **flail chest** and other major chest injuries are indicative of underlying pulmonary contusion. IV fluids should be

administered judiciously, as the injured lung is sensitive to fluid overload.

3. The presence of **subcutaneous emphysema** may indicate the presence of a pneumothorax or laryngeal, tracheobronchial, or esophageal trauma. Pneumothorax and hemothorax may lead to respiratory and cardiovascular collapse. If these conditions are present or highly suspected, chest tubes should be placed under local anesthesia before induction of general anesthesia. Avoid central line insertion (particularly by the subclavian route) on the side opposite an injury because of the potential consequence of bilateral pneumothorax. Avoid the ipsilateral side if a concomitant major venous injury is suspected.

4. **Traumatic diaphragmatic injury** can present as an elevated diaphragm, gastric dilatation, loculated pneumothorax, or subpulmonic hematoma. An upper gastrointestinal contrast study should be considered if the diagnosis is not clear.

5. **Anesthetic management**
   a. Patients with significant chest injuries almost always require general anesthesia.
   b. The necessity for mechanical ventilation may extend into the postoperative period.
   c. Avoid nitrous oxide when a pneumothorax is suspected and a chest tube has not yet been placed. Airway pressures must be closely monitored during positive-pressure ventilation.
   d. Isolate a lung that is hemorrhaging into the airways before blood floods the uninjured side. Double-lumen endotracheal tube placement, main-stem intubation, or endobronchial blockade may be lifesaving under these circumstances (see Chapter 21).
   e. Regional anesthesia (i.e., intercostal nerve blockade or thoracic epidural anesthesia) may be useful for multiple painful rib fractures. Adequate pain relief can reduce chest wall splinting, regional hypoventilation, and progressive hypoxemia.

E. **Cardiac and major vascular trauma**
1. **Blunt cardiac injury** can result in myocardial muscle contusion, chamber rupture, or valvular disruption.
2. **Cardiac trauma** may be associated with a fractured sternum, hemothorax, pericardial tamponade, myocardial dysfunction, valvular dysfunction, and ECG changes (persistent sinus tachycardia, multiple premature ventricular contractions and other dysrhythmias, bundle branch block, nonspecific ST-segment and T-wave changes, and overt ischemia).
   a. **Beck's triad** of distended neck veins, muffled heart sounds, and hypotension is present in only 30% of patients with pericardial tamponade, and pulsus paradoxus is even less reliable. The diagnostic test of choice is cardiac ultrasound.
   b. **Pericardiocentesis** may be used to stabilize the patient until surgical repair can be performed. A subxiphoid pericardial window is preferably performed in the operating room.
3. A widened mediastinal profile and lack of clarity of the aortic knob on the CXR mandate **emergency angiography** to rule out traumatic aortic rupture. High-resolution CT and

transesophageal echocardiography also are used to diagnose aortic dissection. Potentially salvageable patients with aortic rupture often have an incomplete laceration near the ligamentum arteriosum. An intact adventitial layer or contained hematoma prevents immediate death.

4. **The subclavian artery** is subject to injury with hyperextension of the neck and shoulder.

5. **Anesthetic management**

   a. These patients are often **severely hypovolemic** and may have compromised cardiac function. Cardiopulmonary bypass may be required for certain repairs.

   b. Etomidate and ketamine are good choices for induction, but use of the latter must be weighed against its risk in patients with concomitant head injury.

   c. Cross-matched type-specific blood or O-negative blood should be available before induction. Inotropic and vasopressor agents should be immediately available to treat severe hypotension.

F. **Abdominal trauma**

1. In stable patients without peritonitis, **penetrating abdominal wounds** (with the exception of gunshot wounds) are initially evaluated by local wound exploration. If the exploration is equivocal, diagnostic peritoneal lavage, abdominal ultrasound, or an abdominal CT scan may be performed.

2. All patients with **gunshot wounds of the abdomen** are surgically explored.

3. With **impalement injuries** (e.g., stab wounds or falls onto sharp objects), the penetrating object, if still present in the wound, will usually be removed in the operating room after anesthesia has been induced and the patient stabilized. Removal in an uncontrolled environment may result in exsanguination.

4. **Blunt trauma** may result in intra-abdominal or retroperitoneal bleeding.

   a. The **spleen** is the most frequently injured abdominal organ in blunt trauma. Signs and symptoms include abdominal or referred shoulder pain, abdominal rigidity, a falling hematocrit, or hypotension. Minor splenic hematomas are often managed nonoperatively, but grade IV (active bleeding) and V (shattered/avulsed spleen) injuries require splenectomy.

   b. The **liver** frequently fractures with blunt abdominal trauma. Minor injuries are managed nonoperatively unless other injuries mandate laparotomy. Thus, liver injuries that require operation are often complex with large blood loss and high mortality. Manual compression can temporarily control bleeding and allow time for volume resuscitation. Perihepatic packing with reexploration is sometimes considered for patients with severe injuries.

G. **Genitourinary trauma**

1. All multiple trauma patients should have a **Foley catheter** placed. If pelvic or perineal injury has occurred, as evidenced by blood at the urethral meatus, a perineal hematoma, or a high-riding prostate, retrograde urethrography should be performed before urethral catheterization.

2. All patients with penetrating abdominal or back injuries and those with significant hematuria after blunt trauma should have a radiographic **kidney-ureter-bladder** examination and undergo **IV pyelography or** contrast-enhanced CT.
3. Eighty-five percent of renal injuries can be managed nonoperatively, but patients with refractory hypotension should go directly to the operating room for exploration.
   a. **Ureteral laceration** is managed by surgical intervention after locating the disruption by retrograde urography.
   b. **Bladder** contusions may be treated nonoperatively, but rupture usually requires exploration.
   c. The inability of the patient to void or clinical signs of injury indicates **injury to the urethra** (see section II.G.1). Diagnostic urethrography should precede treatment with suprapubic cystostomy for urinary diversion and control of hemorrhage. Most disruptions can undergo delayed repair.

H. **Peripheral vascular trauma**
   1. Check **peripheral pulses** in all extremities during the evaluation of trauma patients. Arteriography can be used when doubt exists.
   2. **Anesthetic management** should focus on the recognition of hypovolemia secondary to uncontrolled hemorrhage. Repair of injuries in stable patients may be amenable to regional anesthetic techniques.

I. **Orthopedic trauma**
   1. All **fractures or dislocations** that compromise nerve or vascular function may constitute surgical emergencies (e.g., radial nerve injury with humeral shaft fractures and aseptic necrosis of the femoral head with hip dislocation) and must be reduced immediately. It is important to document the neurovascular examination immediately before anesthesia and upon awakening.
   2. **Upper extremity**
      a. Severe **depression or hyperabduction of the shoulder girdle** can stretch or tear the brachial plexus. Horner syndrome may present with damage to the cervical sympathetic chain.
      b. When the shoulder is struck hard from the side, the medial end of the clavicle may be dislocated upward or retrosternally. Pressure on the trachea in a retrosternal dislocation may cause life-threatening airway compromise.
      c. Dislocation of the glenohumeral joint can cause axillary nerve injury.
      d. **Fractures of the humeral shaft,** especially the middle or distal part, are frequently associated with radial nerve injury.
      e. Neurovascular compromise of the forearm can occur with **fracture or dislocation of the elbow.** Peripheral ischemia is often complicated by edema of the anterior compartment with risk for nerve and muscle necrosis. Fasciotomy may be indicated.
      f. Median nerve compression is possible with **fractures at the wrist** or with carpal dislocation and may require division of the transverse carpal ligament.

3. **Pelvis**
   a. Patients who have sustained pelvic injuries can be divided into one of three major categories:
      (1) **Exsanguinating hemorrhage** from external bleeding in open fractures or from retroperitoneal hematoma in closed fractures (0.5% to 1.0%). These patients almost always present with either severe hypotension or cardiac arrest and rarely respond to resuscitative measures.
      (2) **Hemodynamically stable** with a relatively uncomplicated course (75%). Urgent or elective surgery for repair of bony and ligamentous pelvic disruptions may be required.
      (3) An **intermediate group** in critical condition with various degrees of overall injury, hemorrhage, and hemodynamic instability (25%).
   b. **Initial management** for these injuries may include the application of a compressive binder for "open book" fractures, pelvic angiography (with or without therapeutic embolization to control hemorrhage), and external pelvic fixation.
   c. Pelvic fractures without major disruption, such as type I anterior posterior compression (APC) injury or type I lateral compression injury, can be treated with bed rest and delayed open reduction and internal fixation (ORIF). More complex injuries such as APC II (widened sacroiliac joint with hemorrhagic and vascular consequences) require acute external fixation with delayed conversion to internal fixation, acute ORIF, or arterial embolization.
   d. **Fat embolism** can occur with pelvic and major long-bone fractures (see Chapter 18, section XV.C).
   e. **Crush injuries** may be associated with **myoglobinuria.** Early reversal of hypovolemia and alkalinization of the urine may help prevent acute renal failure.

4. **Lower extremity**
   a. Fractures of the **tibia and fibula,** the most common major skeletal injuries, can be associated with neurovascular trauma.
   b. With a fracture of the **femur,** blood loss can be much greater than is evident from superficial inspection.
   c. **Hip fractures** are common in the elderly, whose clinical picture is often dominated by other complicating medical illnesses. Traction is used initially for pain relief, but most fractures require open reduction and internal fixation to ensure adequate healing and function and to avoid the complications of prolonged immobilization.
   d. Regional, general anesthesia, and combined techniques can be considered for patients with isolated lower-extremity injuries.

5. **Extremity reimplantation**
   a. **Indications.** In general, these procedures are performed on the upper extremities and only in patients who are otherwise stable. An amputated arm, hand, or digit will not be reimplanted if it has sustained a severe crush injury or has been raggedly torn from major nerves and blood

vessels. Reimplantations may be extremely lengthy procedures, occasionally in excess of 24 hours.

    b. Anesthetic management

      (1) General anesthesia is usually chosen because of the long duration of these procedures. A combined technique will reduce anesthetic requirements and provide for postoperative analgesia (especially with catheter placements, rather than single-dose brachial plexus blocks), and the resulting sympathectomy may improve blood flow.

      (2) During general anesthesia, the head and pressure points must be evaluated every 1 to 2 hours to avoid pressure-induced injury (e.g., scalp ulceration and hair loss). Low-pressure mattresses and padded sponge blocks should be used to minimize pressure on susceptible peripheral nerves (e.g., ulnar, sciatic, peroneal, or sural). The endotracheal tube cuff pressure should be periodically assessed, because nitrous oxide will diffuse into the cuff and increase the pressure on the tracheal mucosa.

      (3) Patients should be kept warm and adequately hydrated. Avoid hyperventilation or the use of vasoconstrictors.

      (4) Consider invasive hemodynamic monitoring for optimization of the perfusion pressure and for prolonged cases. If a noninvasive blood pressure cuff is used, it should be rotated among multiple sites. The need for anticoagulation is determined intraoperatively.

      (5) Blood loss can be vastly underestimated. Blood samples should be sent periodically to assess hemoglobin levels.

III. The pediatric trauma patient

  A. General considerations

    1. A clear understanding of the salient anatomic and physiologic differences among adults, children, and infants as well as a working knowledge of the specific anesthetic considerations for this patient population is required (see Chapters 28 and 29).

    2. Blunt trauma, usually from falls or motor vehicle accidents, predominates in children. Multiple injuries are the rule rather than the exception, but diagnosis is often more difficult because of the child's inability to provide an accurate history.

  B. Specific considerations

    1. Although the pediatric trauma patient frequently presents with significant blood loss, initially the **vital signs** may be minimally altered. **Reliance on vital signs alone may seriously underestimate the severity of injury.**

    2. Orotracheal intubation with protection of the cervical spine is the preferred method of obtaining airway control. Nasotracheal intubation is **not** recommended in children under the age of 12 years. **Surgical cricothyroidotomy** is rarely performed in the infant or small child because of technical difficulties. If airway control and ventilation cannot be accomplished, needle cricothyroidotomy is an appropriate temporary approach for oxygenation.

3. **Intraosseous infusion** is an acceptable procedure for critically injured pediatric patients in whom venous access cannot be established (see Chapter 29).

4. The small child who is **hypothermic** may be refractory to therapy for shock. During initial evaluation and management, overhead heaters or thermal blankets will be needed to maintain body temperature.

IV. **The pregnant trauma patient**
   A. **General considerations**
      1. Pregnancy must always be suspected in any female trauma patient of childbearing age (see Chapter 30 for management of the pregnant patient).
      2. Because the fetus depends on its mother for its oxygen requirements, an **uninterrupted supply of oxygenated blood** must be provided to the fetus at all times. The uterus remains an intrapelvic organ until the 12th week of gestation and reaches the umbilicus by 20 weeks. **Compression of the vena cava by the gravid uterus** after 20 weeks of gestation reduces venous return to the heart, thereby decreasing cardiac output and exacerbating shock. The pregnant patient should be transported and evaluated with left uterine displacement.
      3. Although diagnostic irradiation poses a risk to the fetus, necessary radiographic studies should always be obtained.
      4. If the amniotic fluid gains access to the intravascular space, it can be a source of amniotic fluid embolism and disseminated intravascular coagulation.
      5. Fetomaternal hemorrhage in an Rh-negative patient should warrant Rh-immunoglobulin therapy.
   B. **Treatment**
      1. If the mother's condition is stable, the status of the fetus and the extent of uterine injury will determine further management. Consultation with the patient's obstetrician is advisable.
      2. A potentially viable fetus that shows no signs of distress should be monitored by external ultrasound. Because premature labor is always a possibility in these patients, an external tocotransducer must be used to detect the onset of contractions. Initiate tocolytic therapy if premature labor develops.
      3. When a viable fetus shows signs of distress despite successful resuscitative measures, a cesarean delivery must be performed expeditiously. A nonviable fetus may be managed conservatively in utero to optimize maternal oxygenation and circulation.
      4. Primary repair of all maternal wounds should be attempted in a critically injured mother carrying a viable gestation, even at the expense of fetal distress.

V. **Major burn injuries**
   A. **Physiologic implications of burn injury**
      1. **Deep thermal injury** destroys skin, the body's barrier to the external environment. Skin plays a vital role in thermal regulation, fluid and electrolyte homeostasis, and protection against bacterial infection. Significant heat and protein loss, massive fluid shifts, and infections all commonly occur in patients with severe thermal injuries. In major burns, circulating mediators trigger a systemic response, characterized by systemic inflammation, hypermetabolism, and immune suppression. There is also diffuse alteration in the permeability of cell

membranes to sodium, resulting in generalized cellular swelling. Microvascular injury results from local damage by heat and from the release of vasoactive substances from the burned tissue. Therefore, edema occurs in both burned and unburned tissues.

a. **Cardiovascular effects**

   (1) Alterations in microvascular permeability result in a trans-capillary fluid flux and significant tissue edema 12 to 24 hours after a thermal injury. Large amounts of water, electrolytes, and proteins are lost into the extravascular space leading to intravascular fluid depletion and hypovolemic shock (burn shock).

   (2) Circulating humoral factors and reduced responsiveness to endogenous catecholamines initially result in *decreased* cardiac output. Systemic vascular resistance is also increased, coincident with the decrease in cardiac output. The magnitude of these pathophysiologic changes depends on the size and the depth of the burn injury.

   (3) The cardiovascular response 24 to 48 hours after successful resuscitation of a major burn is characterized by an *increase* in cardiac output and *reduced* systemic vascular resistance, consistent with the pathophysiology of the systemic inflammatory response syndrome.

b. A **hypermetabolic state** develops 3 to 5 days after the burn injury. For major burn injuries, the estimated caloric need is 1.5 to 1.7 times the calculated basal metabolic rate and the protein need is near 2.5 g/kg/day. Early initiation of enteral feeding may decrease muscle catabolism and reduce bacterial translocation through the intestinal mucosa. Ambient temperature should be kept within the thermoneutral range to avoid cooling and a further increase in the metabolic rate.

c. Capillary leakage results in **hemoconcentration** immediately after injury. Despite apparent adequate fluid resuscitation, the hematocrit level often remains increased during the first 48 hours after injury. Bleeding from wounds and a shortened erythrocyte half-life, however, can result in anemia.

d. Microaggregation of the platelets in the skin and smoke-damaged lung and aggressive volume resuscitation result in early **thrombocytopenia** after major burns. Thrombotic and fibrinolytic mechanisms are activated and disseminated intravascular coagulation may complicate the course of a massive burn injury. A decrease in antithrombin III, protein C, and protein S levels can increase the thrombogenicity of these patients later in their clinical course and theoretically can cause venous thrombosis and pulmonary embolism.

e. **Acute renal failure** is not uncommon in patients with major burn injury and is associated with high mortality. Decreased renal blood flow secondary to hypovolemia and decreased cardiac output, as well as increased levels of catecholamines, aldosterone, and vasopressin, can contribute to renal failure. Other mechanisms include nephrotoxic effects of drugs, rhabdomyolysis, hemolysis, and sepsis (see Chapter 4, section III).

 f. **Gastrointestinal function** is diminished immediately after burn injury, secondary to the development of gastric and intestinal ileus. The stomach should be adequately vented with a nasogastric tube because of the danger of pulmonary aspiration of gastric contents.

  (1) **Curling's ulcers (mucosal erosion)** will occur at variable times after major burns and may lead to gastric hemorrhage or perforation. These ulcers seem to be more common in children than in adults. Therapy consists of antacids and histamine (H_2) receptor antagonists.

  (2) **Other gastrointestinal complications of burns** include esophagitis, tracheoesophageal fistula (from prolonged intubation and the presence of a nasogastric tube), hepatic dysfunction, pancreatitis, acalculous cholecystitis, and mesenteric artery thrombosis.

 g. **Infection** of burned areas delays healing and prevents successful skin grafting. Bacterial invasion of underlying tissue may result in septicemia. Common organisms involved are staphylococci, beta-hemolytic streptococci, and Gram-negative rods such as *Pseudomonas* and *Klebsiella* sp. Local treatment with topical antimicrobials and early skin grafting are important measures to reduce risk of infection.

 h. **Muscle acetylcholine receptors** proliferate at the burn site and at sites distant from the burn injury. An increase in acetylcholine receptors is usually associated with resistance to nondepolarizing neuromuscular blocking agents and increased sensitivity to depolarizing muscle relaxants.

2. In **electrical burns,** current creates thermal energy that destroys tissue, particularly tissues with high resistance such as skin and bone. Exposure to high voltage can result in compartment syndromes, fractures of long bones and the axial spine, myocardial injury, and rhabdomyolysis with subsequent renal injury.

3. In **chemical burns,** the degree of injury depends on the chemical, its concentration, duration of contact, and the penetrability and resistance of the tissues involved. Some substances producing chemical burns, such as phosphorus, are absorbed systemically, producing significant and often life-threatening injury. Hydrofluoric acid exposure will cause severe hypocalcemia and requires close monitoring of serum calcium levels. Subeschar injection of calcium gluconate and emergent wound excision may be indicated.

B. **Classification of burn injury**

 1. Burns are classified according to the total body surface area (TBSA) burned, depth of burn, and the presence or absence of inhalational injury

 2. **The extent of a burn** (TBSA) is calculated by using a Lund-Browder or other burn diagram.

  a. The **rule of nines** guides estimation (Fig. 33.2).

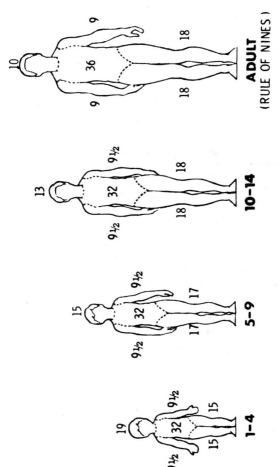

Figure 33.2. Rule of nines (Lung and Browder chart). (Modified from Ryan JF, et al., eds. *A practice of anesthesia for infants and children.* Philadelphia: WB Saunders, 1986:230.)

(1) **Adults:** The head and each upper extremity represent 9% TBSA. The anterior trunk, posterior trunk, and each lower extremity represent 18% TBSA.

(2) **Infants and children:** Because of the different proportions of body surface area relative to patient age, reference must be made to the proper burn chart when calculating percent TBSA to avoid significant errors (see Fig. 33.2).

b. Another practical method to estimate percent TBSA is that the area of the patient's hand will cover about 1% TBSA.

3. The **depth of the burn** determines therapy (i.e., conservative management versus excision and grafting). Burn depth is difficult to determine visually; however, there are some useful guidelines.

a. The area under a **partial-thickness burn** should have normal or increased sensitivity to pain and temperature and should blanch with pressure.

b. A **full-thickness burn** will be anesthetic and will not blanch with pressure.

C. **Initial evaluation of the burn patient**

1. **Airway and breathing**

a. Brief exposure of the epiglottis or larynx to either dry air at 300°C or steam at 100°C leads to massive edema and rapid airway obstruction. Chemical products of combustion such as ammonia, sulfur oxide, and chlorine dissolve in the tracheobronchial tree, forming acids and irritating the mucous membrane of the respiratory tract.

b. In general, it is better to tracheally intubate the burn patient early rather than late. Intubation should always be performed before airway edema occurs. Continued swelling and distortion of the soft tissues will progress at a rapid rate, rendering intubation difficult if not impossible.

c. **Circumferential full-thickness burns** of the thorax will decrease chest wall compliance, which can lead to hypoxemia and respiratory failure. Emergency escharotomies may be required.

d. **Smoke inhalation injury** may occur during a fire within a closed space or when heated noxious vapors are inhaled.

(1) An inhalation injury should be suspected in the presence of burns of the head or neck; singed nasal hairs; swelling of the mucosa of the nose, mouth, lips, or throat; a brassy cough; or carbonaceous sputum. Both the upper airway and pulmonary parenchyma may be affected.

(2) **Chemical products** of combustion combine with water in the respiratory tract to form strong acids and alkali (see C1), causing bronchospasm, edema, and mucous membrane ulceration. Inhalation of gases such as phosgene and sulfuric acid can damage the alveolar membrane and cause partial or complete airway obstruction. Aldehydes such as acrolein impair ciliary function and damage mucosal surfaces.

(3) Combustion of polyurethane-containing products (e.g., insulation and wall paneling) releases

hydrogen cyanide, which causes tissue asphyxia by inhibiting cytochrome-oxidase activity. Patients may present with an anion gap metabolic acidosis and an elevated mixed venous Po_2. Plasma lactate levels correlate with the cyanide levels. Treatment is supportive but can include administration of sodium nitrite (300 mg IV over more than 5 minutes in a volume of 100 mL of 5% dextrose) and sodium thiosulfate (12.5 g) and, in severe cases, inhaled amyl nitrite.

- **(4)** **Carbon monoxide** binds hemoglobin, displacing oxygen and shifting the oxyhemoglobin curve to the left. Tissue hypoxia ensues.
    - **(a)** All burned patients, especially those burned within a closed space, may have sustained some degree of tissue hypoxia with their thermal injury. Oxygen administration should begin at the scene.
    - **(b)** Because oxyhemoglobin and carboxyhemoglobin (CO) absorb light at the same wavelength, conventional pulse oximetry cannot be used as an indicator of CO poisoning. Diagnosis is made on clinical suspicion and the level of arterial or venous carboxyhemoglobin, measured spectrophotometrically with a CO-oximeter.
    - **(c)** The half-life of carboxyhemoglobin is inversely related to the inspired oxygen concentration (Fio_2); it is 5 to 6 hours when breathing room air but 30 to 60 minutes when breathing 100% oxygen.
    - **(d)** Treatment is supportive and consists of supplemental oxygen until the carbon monoxide is eliminated. Hyperbaric oxygen should be considered in comatose patients and in those with severe carbon monoxide poisoning.
    - **(e)** **Indirect respiratory injury** and pulmonary edema may occur in burn patients without an inhalational injury. Mechanisms involved include the effect of burn wound mediators on the lung, decreased plasma oncotic pressure, and complications of burn therapy.

2. Cardiovascular resuscitation
- **a.** **Fluid replacement** consists of crystalloid, usually Ringer's lactate, with or without the addition of colloid. Standard protocols for fluid replacement use body weight in kilograms and percent TBSA burned.
    - **(1)** **Parkland formula** (most commonly used at the Massachusetts General Hospital): 4.0 mL of Ringer's lactate per kg per % TBSA burn per 24 hours (see section V.C.2.b below).
    - **(2)** **Brooke formula:** 1.5 mL of crystalloid per kg per % TBSA burn per 24 hours plus 0.5 mL of colloid per kg per % TBSA burn per 24 hours plus 2,000 mL of 5% dextrose in water per 24 hours (see section V.C.2.b. below).

    b. Half the calculated fluid deficit is administered during the first 8 hours postburn and the remainder is administered over the next 16 hours. The patient's daily maintenance fluid requirements are given concurrently.

    c. The endpoints of fluid therapy are hemodynamic stability and maintenance of an adequate urine output. In extensive burns, fluid management is adjusted according to appropriate invasive monitors and laboratory studies.

D. Management of the burn wound

    1. Early excision and grafting of burned areas is a widely accepted procedure and appears to decrease mortality. Patients may be brought to the operating room in the acute phase of injury, with hemodynamic instability and respiratory dysfunction. Special emphasis should be placed on correcting acid-base and electrolyte disturbances and coagulopathy. Blood loss during wound excision and grafting can be massive. Adequate colloid and blood products should be ordered in advance. IV access should be adequate for resuscitation.

    2. Topical agents are used to minimize the colonization of healing wounds. Common topical agents include the following:

       a. Silver nitrate. Methemoglobinemia is a rare complication.

       b. Mafenide acetate, a carbonic anhydrase inhibitor, may cause metabolic acidosis if absorbed.

       c. Silver sulfadiazine. Leukopenia is the main disadvantage but reverses with discontinuation.

    3. The incidence of **sepsis** may be reduced by using temporary biologic dressings, which may be allografts (cadaver skin or amnion) or xenografts (porcine). Artificial skin (e.g., Integra) bioengineered from collagen and cultured epidermis can be used when a conventional autograft is not available.

    4. The use of **systemic antibiotics** is limited to treatment of documented systemic infection (as opposed to colonization) and as prophylaxis before surgical procedures.

E. Anesthetic considerations

    1. Burns are a form of trauma; thus, the airway, breathing, and circulation should be initially assessed (see section I.A to I.E). The patient's age, preexisting disease, and the extent of burn injury provide an index of the patient's likely physiologic condition. Altered pharmacokinetics, drug tolerance, difficult IV access, and anatomic derangements of the airway (neck scar or mouth contracture) are main considerations.

    2. Airway. Obtaining an adequate mask fit may be difficult because of edema in the early phases of burn injury or because of scars and contractures later on. The same processes can render endotracheal intubation extremely difficult in burn patients.

    3. Monitoring and IV access

       a. Often IV access will still be in place from the initial resuscitation. Large-bore IVs are mandatory to allow for massive fluid replacement.

       b. In massive burns, ECG electrodes may be placed directly on debrided tissue. Alternatively, needle electrodes can be used.

       c. Arterial lines are indispensable for continuous blood pressure monitoring and frequent blood sampling. The cannulation site will depend on the availability of unburned areas. If all appropriate sites are burned, the line may have to be placed through the burn wound after the area has been prepared in a sterile fashion.

    d. **Central venous pressure lines** are useful both for monitoring central pressures and as central access for drug infusions.

    e. A **pulmonary artery catheter** may be required for management of patients with myocardial dysfunction, persistent oliguria or hypotension, or sepsis.

4. Muscle relaxants

    a. **Depolarizing agents** (succinylcholine) are generally safe in the immediate hours after thermal injury. They become dangerous after the initial 12 to 24 hours, because they can produce profound hyperkalemia and cardiac arrest.

    b. **Nondepolarizing relaxants** are used when muscle relaxation is required. Burn patients show a "resistance" to these drugs (i.e., diminished response to conventional doses, see above), in some cases requiring three- to five-fold greater doses than nonburn patients.

5. Anesthetics

    a. There is no single preferred agent or combination of agents; however, **ketamine** and **etomidate** may have advantages in patients with an uncertain volume status.

    b. These patients may have **greatly increased opioid requirements** due to tolerance and an increase in the apparent volume of distribution for drugs. It is important to provide adequate analgesia, which may necessitate massive doses of narcotics.

6. Temperature regulation. The most comfortable body temperature for a burn patient is about 100°F (38°C). In the burn intensive care unit, patients are cared for in warmed, humidified rooms. Every effort should be made to maintain normothermia during transport and surgery. The operating room, IV fluids, and blood products should be warmed and inspired gases heated and humidified. Pediatric patients should be placed under a radiant heat source and on a warming blanket whenever possible.

7. Immunosuppression. The immune system is suppressed for weeks to months after burn injury, and the wound itself serves as an excellent medium for bacterial growth. Every attempt should be made to practice aseptic technique when handling patients, suctioning airways, and inserting intravascular lines.

8. Postanesthetic care. It is important to maintain normothermia while transporting patients back to the intensive care unit because shivering results in vasoconstriction and could contribute to graft loss. Supplemental oxygen should be given until patients are fully recovered from anesthesia. Severe pain is common and patient responses vary, necessitating individual titration of analgesics and frequent reassessment of the effect.

SUGGESTED READING

American College of Surgeons. *Advanced trauma life support (ATLS) student. Manual,* 7th ed. Chicago: American College of Surgeons, 2004.

Bickell WH, Wall MJ Jr, Pepe PE, et al. Immediate versus delayed fluid resuscitation for hypotensive patients with penetrating torso injuries. *N Engl J Med* 1994;331:1105–1109.

MacLennan N, Heimbach DM, Cullen BF. Anesthesia for major thermal injury. *Anesthesiology* 1998;89:749–770.

Martyn JA, Richtsfeld M. Succinylcholine-induced hyperkalemia in acquired pathologic states: etiologic factors and molecular mechanisms. *Anesthesiology* 2006;104:158–169.

Watson D. ABC of major trauma. Management of the upper airway. *BMJ* 1990;300:1388–1391.

34

Transfusion Therapy

Rae M. Allain and Jonathan E. Charnin

I. **Indications for transfusion therapy.** Blood component transfusion usually is performed because of decreased production; increased utilization, destruction, or loss; or dysfunction of a specific blood component (red cells, platelets, or coagulation factors).

A. **Anemia**

1. **Red cell mass.** The main reason for transfusing red cells is to maintain oxygen-carrying capacity to the tissues, a primary determinant of which is the hemoglobin (Hb) level. **For healthy individuals** or **individuals with chronic anemia** can usually tolerate Hb levels of 6.5 to 8 g/dL, assuming normal intravascular volume. In the past, it was common practice to maintain the perioperative Hb greater than 10 g/dL. However, the use of a "restrictive transfusion practice," aiming for Hb of 7 to 9 g/dL, is safe and may reduce the risk of death compared with transfusing toward a higher (10 to 12 g/dL) Hb goal. The reason for reduced mortality in the restrictively transfused group has not been clearly delineated, but the effects of allogeneic transfusion on diminished immune function have been substantiated in animal and human studies (see section VIII.D). For **patients with coronary artery disease,** the risk of myocardial ischemia due to anemia has resulted in most practitioners transfusing to a higher (9 to 10 g/dL) Hb level. Studies to support this practice, however, are lacking and those that exist have produced contradictory results. A recent study of medical patients with acute coronary syndromes also found a higher mortality rate attributable to red cell transfusion in otherwise stable patients with a hematocrit (Hct) >25%. In conclusion, the recent scientific evidence and consensus opinion of experts supports perioperative red cell transfusion directed at individual physiologic need, taking into account the risks and benefits of transfusion, rather than seeking arbitrary Hb or Hct goals.

2. If a patient is anemic preoperatively, the etiology should be clarified. It may be secondary to decreased production (marrow suppression or nutritional deficiencies), increased loss (hemorrhage), or destruction (hemolysis).

3. **Estimating blood volumes**

a. **Intraoperative blood transfusion** depends on red cell loss. This can be roughly estimated by measuring blood in suction canisters, weighing sponges, and checking blood loss in the drapes.

b. **Estimated allowable blood loss** (EABL) can be calculated as follows:

$$EABL = [(Hct_{starting} - Hct_{allowable}) \times BV] /$$
$$[(Hct_{starting} + Hct_{allowable})/2]$$

Blood volume (BV) in an adult is approximately 7% of lean body mass. This may be calculated as approximately 70 mL/kg of body weight in a normal adult man and approximately 65 mL/kg of body weight in a normal adult woman (see Chapter 29, section VII.B for pediatric considerations).

c. **Estimating the volume of blood to transfuse** can be calculated as follows:

$$\text{Volume to transfuse} = [(\text{Hct}_{desired} - \text{Hct}_{present}) \times \text{BV}]/\text{Hct}_{transfused\,blood}$$

A unit of packed red blood cells has a Hct of 70% to 85% using the Adsol preservative.

B. **Thrombocytopenia.** Thrombocytopenia is due to either decreased bone marrow production (e.g., chemotherapy, tumor infiltration, or alcoholism) or increased utilization or destruction (e.g., hypersplenism, idiopathic thrombocytopenia purpura, DIC, or drug effects). It is also seen with the dilution and loss associated with massive blood transfusion (see section IX.A.1). Spontaneous bleeding is unusual with platelet counts above 20,000/mm^3. Platelet counts above 50,000/mm^3 are preferable for surgical hemostasis.

C. **Coagulopathy.** Bleeding associated with documented factor deficiencies or prolonged clotting studies (prothrombin time and partial thromboplastin time) mandates replacement therapy to maintain normal coagulation function. See sections II and IX for a discussion of coagulopathy.

II. **Coagulation studies.** The most important clue to a clinically significant bleeding disorder in an otherwise healthy patient remains the history. Prior surgical bleeding, gingival bleeding, easy bruising, epistaxis, or menorrhagia should raise concern. Many tests are available to assess the coagulation system. However, the clinician must remember that the coagulation system is a complex interplay of platelets and coagulation factors. No single test measures the integrity of the entire coagulation system.

A. **Activated partial thromboplastin time (aPTT)** is performed by adding particulate matter to a blood sample to activate the intrinsic coagulation system. Normal values for the PTT are 22 to 34 seconds, varying according to the reagent and instruments used by the specific laboratory. The aPTT assesses factors in the intrinsic (XI, XII, VIII, IX, and contact factors) and the common (II, V, X, and fibrinogen) coagulation pathways. The test is sensitive to decreased amounts of coagulation factors and is elevated in patients on heparin therapy. The aPTT will be abnormal in patients who have hemophilia or a circulating anticoagulant present (e.g., lupus anticoagulant or antibodies to factor VIII). The clinician should remember that an abnormal aPTT does not necessarily correlate with clinical bleeding. Aggressive correction of an abnormal aPTT in surgical patients is not always indicated, unless the patient is actively bleeding.

B. **Prothrombin time (PT)** is a measure of factors of the extrinsic (VII and tissue factor) and common (see above) coagulation pathways and is measured by adding tissue factor to a blood sample. While both PT and aPTT are affected by levels of factors V and

X, prothrombin, and fibrinogen, the PT is specifically sensitive to deficiencies of factor VII. The PT is normal in deficiencies of factors VIII, IX, XI, XII, prekallikrein, and high-molecular-weight kininogen.

C. The **INR (international normalized ratio)** is a means of standardizing PT values to allow comparisons among different laboratories or at different times. It is the ratio of patient's PT to the control PT value that would be obtained if international reference reagents had been used to perform the test. Before development of the INR, differences in thromboplastin reagent activity prevented meaningful comparisons of PT values. Now, oral anticoagulation therapy may be guided by a target INR value that is independent of laboratory variability of the PT. For example, an INR of 2.0 to 3.0 is recommended for prophylaxis against thromboembolism in atrial fibrillation.

D. **Bleeding time** reflects the interaction of platelets with the vessel endothelium, which leads to formation of an initial clot. The test suffers from numerous shortcomings: 1) performance requires adherence to a standardized protocol; 2) results are technician dependent and poorly reproducible; 3) results do not correlate to clinical hemostasis in the perioperative setting. For these reasons, the bleeding time is not recommended for assessment of perioperative coagulation status and the test is no longer used or available in many institutions.

E. **Activated clotting time** (ACT) is a modified whole-blood clotting time in which diatomaceous earth is added to a blood sample to activate the intrinsic clotting system. The ACT is the time until clot formation. A normal ACT is 90 to 130 seconds, depending on the instrument used. The ACT is a relatively easy and expedient test to perform and is useful in monitoring heparin therapy in the operating room (see Chapter 23).

F. **D-dimer and fibrin split products.** When fibrinolysis occurs, plasmin degrades both fibrin and fibrinogen. Fibrin-split products reflect degradation of both fibrinogen and fibrin. D-dimer measurements, which reflect degradation of cross-linked fibrin, are more specific for primary fibrinolysis and **disseminated intravascular coagulation (DIC)**. The test is performed by mixing antibody-coated latex beads with patient plasma in serial dilutions. An elevated titer of D-dimer is common in patients with DIC but may also be seen with deep venous thrombosis, liver disease, or after recent surgery (within 48 hours). Fibrin fragments can interfere with normal coagulation by impairing platelet function and the normal formation of fibrin clot.

G. **Thromboelastography.** Thromboelastography (TEG), is available in some centers for clinical use, often as a point-of-care test. TEG is performed by placing a small aliquot of blood into a heated oscillating cup into which is suspended a pin on a torsion wire. Clot formation in the oscillating cup generates torque on the pin, and the torque is measured and converted to an electrical signal. The signal is recorded by a computer, creating a characteristic trace (Fig. 34.1) that may be analyzed for abnormalities of clot formation. By measuring clot formation and visco-elastic clot strength, TEG provides information about the adequacy of clotting factors, fibrin levels, and platelets.

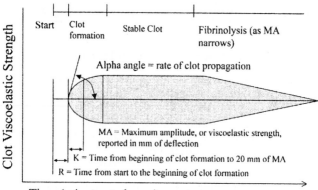

Figure 34.1.

III. **Blood typing and cross-matching**
   A. **Donor and recipient blood** is typed using the red cell surface
      ABO and Rh systems and screened for antibodies to other cell
      antigens. "Direct" cross-matching involves directly mixing the pa-
      tient's plasma with the donor's red cells to establish that hemolysis
      does not occur from any undetected antibodies. An individual's
      red cells have either A, B, AB, or no surface antigens. If the pa-
      tient's red cells are lacking either surface antigen A or B, then
      antibodies will be produced against it. A person who is type B
      will have anti-A antibodies in the serum, and a type O individual
      (having neither A nor B surface antigens) will have circulating
      anti-A and anti-B antibodies. Consequently, a person who is type
      AB will not have antibodies to either A or B and can receive red
      blood cells from any blood type. Type O blood has neither A nor
      B surface antigens and can donate blood cells to any other type
      (universal red cell donor; Table 34.1).
   B. **Rh-surface antigens** are either present (Rh-positive) or absent
      (Rh-negative). Individuals who are Rh-negative will develop an-
      tibodies to the Rh factor when exposed to Rh-positive blood. This

Table 34.1.   Transfusion compatibility

Recipient Blood Type	RBC Donor	FFP Donor
AB	AB, A, B, or O	AB
A	A or O	A or AB
B	B or O	B or AB
O	O	A, B, AB or O
Rh+	Rh+ or Rh+	Rh+ or Rh−
Rh−	Rh−	Rh+ or Rh−

is not a problem with the initial exposure, but with subsequent exposures hemolysis will occur due to the circulating antibodies. This can be a particular problem during pregnancy. The anti-Rh antibodies are IgG and freely cross the placenta. Rh-negative mothers who have developed Rh antibodies will transmit these antibodies to the fetus. If the fetus is Rh-positive, massive hemolysis will occur. **RHO-immune globulin,** an Rh-blocking antibody, prevents the Rh-negative patient from developing anti-Rh antibodies. It should be administered to Rh-negative individuals who receive Rh-positive blood and to Rh-negative mothers delivering Rh-positive babies (some fetal maternal blood mixing occurs at delivery). The recommended dose is 300 μg intramuscularly for every 15 mL of Rh-positive blood transfused.

C. **If an emergency blood transfusion is needed,** type-specific (ABO) red cells usually can be obtained within minutes if the patient's blood type is known. If type-specific blood is unavailable, type O Rh-negative red cells should be transfused (type O+ blood can be used emergently in males). Type-specific blood should be substituted as soon as possible to minimize the amount of type O plasma (containing anti-A and anti-B antibodies) transfused.

IV. **Blood component therapy**

A. **General considerations**

1. One unit of **packed red blood cells** (PRBCs; Hct about 70%, volume about 250 mL) usually will increase the Hct by 2% to 3% or the Hb by 1 g/dL in an euvolemic adult once equilibration has taken place. PRBCs must be ABO compatible to the recipient.

2. One unit of **platelets** increases the platelet count by 5,000 to 10,000/mm^3. A usual platelet transfusion is 1 unit per 10 kg of body weight. If thrombocytopenia is caused by increased destruction (due to development of antiplatelet antibodies) or if platelets are dysfunctional, platelet transfusions will be less efficacious. Transfusion of ABO-compatible platelets is not obligatory, although they may provide a better post-transfusion platelet count. Single-donor or HLA-matched platelets may be required for patients with a refractory response to platelet transfusion. A unit of single-donor platelets provides the equivalent of approximately six random-donor units of platelets.

3. **Fresh-frozen plasma** (FFP), in a dose of 10 to 15 mL/kg, generally will increase plasma coagulation factors to 30% of normal, the minimal level necessary for hemostasis (excepting fibrinogen where 50% of the normal 200 to 400 mg/dL is required). Fibrinogen levels increase by 1 mg/dL per milliliter of plasma transfused. Acute reversal of warfarin is often achieved with only 5 to 8 mL/kg of FFP, although the PT may remain modestly prolonged. FFP transfusions must be ABO compatible (see Table 34.1).

4. **Cryoprecipitate** is prepared from FFP and contains concentrated factor VIII, factor XIII, fibrinogen, von Willebrand factor, and fibronectin. Indications for cryoprecipitate include hypofibrinogenemia, von Willebrand disease, hemophilia A (when factor VIII is unavailable), and preparation of fibrin glue. Dosage is 1 unit per 7 to 10 kg, which will raise the plasma fibrinogen by about 50 mg/dL in a

patient without massive bleeding. ABO compatibility is not mandatory for cryoprecipitate transfusion.

B. **Technical considerations**

1. **Compatible infusions.** Blood products should not be infused with 5% dextrose solutions, because they cause hemolysis, or with lactated Ringer's, which contains calcium and may induce clot formation. Normal saline (0.9%) solution, albumin (5%), and FFP are compatible with red blood cells.

2. **Blood filters.** Standard blood filters (170 to 200 μm) remove debris and should be used for all blood components.

   a. **Leukocyte reduction is achieved by filtration, either in the blood bank or at the bedside.** Microaggregate filters (20 to 50 μm), which should not be used for platelets, remove 70% to 90% of leukocytes. Third-generation or adhesion filters remove more than 99.9% of leukocytes via a combination of filtration and adhesion of white blood cells. These filters are recommended for use in patients with a history of febrile, nonhemolytic transfusion reactions; for prevention of alloimmunization to foreign leukocyte antigens (e.g., in the oncologic patient expected to require multiple platelet transfusions); or to prevent cytomegalovirus (CMV) transmission in organ transplant recipients. Other potential but as yet unproved benefits of leukocyte reduction include a diminished immunomodulatory effect of allogeneic transfusion; reduced transmission of bacterial, viral, or prion diseases; prevention of transfusion-related acute lung injury; and decreased incidence of graft-versus-host disease. Several countries have implemented universal leukoreduction of transfused cellular blood products. The proposed benefits and cost-efficiency of universal leukoreduction is a matter of significant controversy within transfusion medicine and is not mandatory in the United States at this time.

   b. Manufacturer recommendations for specific bedside blood filters should be followed with respect to the component to be filtered and the number of units administered per filter.

   c. Severe **hypotensive reactions** associated with use of bedside leukocyte reduction filters have been reported. The pathophysiology may involve activation of bradykinin by the leukocyte filter, and the hypotensive effect may be exaggerated in patients taking ACE-inhibitors. When this reaction occurs, the transfusion should be stopped and the blood pressure supported. These interventions usually result in rapid resolution of hypotension. Products that are leukoreduced in the blood bank may carry a lower risk of this hypotensive reaction as bradykinin is rapidly metabolized in stored blood.

C. **Blood substitutes.** Despite years of research intent upon finding a blood substitute capable of oxygen transport, none provides general clinical usefulness at this time. Fluosol-DA, a synthetic perfluorocarbon capable of carrying oxygen, has been tested in humans but offers limited applicability of oxygen transport in vivo. Free hemoglobin solutions are under investigation, but none is clinically available at this time. Limiting problems include short plasma half-lives (about 8 hours) and hypertension with administration.

V. **Plasma substitutes.** Various colloid products are available commercially. Their main limitations are their cost, potential allergic reactions, and their effects on coagulation.

   A. **Albumin** is available as either an isotonic 5% or a hypertonic 20% or 25% solution. Albumin has an intravascular half-life of 10 to 15 days.

   B. **Dextran** 70 and dextran 40 are high–molecular-weight polysaccharides. Dextran 70, having a higher molecular weight, is not filtered by the kidney. The dextrans have relatively short half-lives (2 to 8 hours) and are either excreted or metabolized. Decreased platelet adhesiveness and depressed von Willebrand factor (vWf) levels are side effects of dextrans commonly seen at dosages greater than 1.5 g/kg. Anaphylactoid reactions have been seen in approximately 1% of patients. These reactions can be avoided by pretreating with dextran 1 (20 mL IV), a hapten that binds the patient's dextran-binding antibodies, although this product is not currently available in the United States.

   C. **Hydroxyethyl starch** (hetastarch) is manufactured from amylopectin. After infusion, hydroxyethyl starch undergoes both renal excretion and tissue redistribution, including storage in the reticuloendothelial cells of the liver for many weeks. Metabolic degradation occurs by serum amylase; this process can cause an increase in serum amylase for several days, which may confuse the diagnosis of pancreatitis. Hetastarch's effects on coagulation include decreased fibrinogen, vWf, and factor VIII levels as well as decreased platelet function. Doses from 500 to 1,500 mL per day for a 70-kg person are well tolerated. Anaphylactoid reactions are rare.

VI. **Pharmacologic therapy**

   A. **Erythropoietin** increases red blood cell mass by stimulating proliferation and development of the erythroid precursor cells. It can be used before elective surgery to increase red blood cell (RBC) production. A higher preoperative Hct has been shown to allow increased autologous red blood cell donation. Results about erythropoietin's ability to diminish allogeneic blood exposure perioperatively have been mixed, with baseline mildly anemic patients seeming to gain the greatest benefit. Preoperative erythropoietin treatment should be accompanied by supplemental iron administration. Several dosing regimens for preoperative erythropoietin are used, including 300 IU/kg subcutaneously (SC) daily for 15 days beginning 10 days before surgery or 600 IU/kg SC weekly for 3 weeks before surgery.

   B. **Desmopressin** (DDAVP) is an antidiuretic hormone that is known to be helpful in patients with mild hemophilia A and in some patients with von Willebrand disease. Desmopressin increases endothelial cell release of vWf, factor VIII, and plasminogen activator. Desmopressin is also useful for patients with platelet defects associated with uremia. The dosage of desmopressin is 0.3 μg/kg. Tachyphylaxis may occur if dosing is greater than every 48 hours. The intravenous (IV) dose should be given slowly, because hypotension or hypertension may result.

C. The **lysine analogues,** aminocaproic acid and tranexamic acid, inhibit fibrinolysis, the endogenous process by which fibrin clot is broken down. They act by displacing plasminogen from fibrin, diminishing plasminogen conversion to plasmin, and preventing plasmin from binding to fibrinogen or fibrin monomers. The uses of aminocaproic acid include prophylaxis for dental surgery in hemophiliacs, reduction of bleeding in prostatic surgery, and reduction of hemorrhage in cases of excessive fibrinolysis. Because cardiopulmonary bypass has been shown to initiate fibrinolysis, aminocaproic acid has been used during cardiac surgery to decrease postoperative chest tube drainage. The drug's efficacy at diminishing blood transfusion has been demonstrated only when the transfusion trigger was low (Hb approximately 7 g/dL). Theoretic risks of thrombosis with aminocaproic acid have not been demonstrated clinically; nevertheless, the drug is contraindicated in DIC. Dosage in adults is 5 g IV load over 1 hour followed by 1 to 2 g per hour IV infusion.

D. **Aprotinin** is a serine protease inhibitor shown to be effective in diminishing blood loss after cardiopulmonary bypass. In a dose-dependent fashion, aprotinin inhibits trypsin, plasmin, and kallikrein. In addition, aprotinin protects the glycoprotein Ib receptor on platelets during cardiopulmonary bypass, thereby preserving platelet adhesive capability. The drug also has anti-inflammatory and antioxidant effects. Of note, celite ACTs are artificially prolonged following heparinization of patients receiving aprotinin. To maintain appropriate heparin anticoagulation for cardiopulmonary bypass, kaolin-activated ACTs should be performed or heparin should be administered by a fixed-dose regimen. Complications of aprotinin treatment include potential anaphylactic reaction. The incidence is approximately 0.3%, but it rises with repeat exposure; an initial test dose of 1 mL administered IV is recommended. Aprotinin may increase serum creatinine levels, but this appears to be reversible and dose related. For cardiac surgery, "high-dose" aprotinin consists of 2 million kallikrein inactivation units (KIU) IV load after induction of anesthesia and 500,000 KIU per hour IV infusion through completion of surgery; another 2 million KIU is added to the cardiopulmonary bypass pump prime. "Low-dose" aprotinin is one-half this regimen. Advantages of low-dose therapy may be preserved blood conservation with potentially less renal toxicity, but this remains controversial. The precise role for intraoperative aprotinin therapy continues to be defined. It has an established role in patients undergoing cardiac procedures at high risk for hemorrhagic complications. It has also been used to decrease bleeding and transfusion requirements in patients undergoing prostatectomy, total hip replacement, and liver resection or transplantation. Risks of thrombosis with aprotinin remain unclear. One large study on cardiac patients showed no increased risk of myocardial infarction, but a higher early graft occlusion rate when aprotinin was used.

VII. **Conservation and salvage techniques**

A. **Autologous donation** usually begins 6 weeks before surgery and can greatly reduce the amount of homologous blood transfused. The length of the predonation period is limited by the length of time that blood can be stored, currently 42 days unless the blood is frozen. Current blood bank guidelines require a predonation Hb of at least 11 g/dL, donations no more frequently than every 3 days, and no donations in the 72 hours before surgery. Most patients tolerate autologous donation without complication. Patients with severe aortic stenosis or unstable angina are not candidates for autologous donation. Patients donating autologous blood should receive supplemental iron because depleted iron stores frequently limit RBC recovery. Recombinant erythropoietin treatment (see section VI.A) also may be considered. Because a risk of transfusion reaction exists due to clerical error, autologous blood should not be transfused unless a transfusion is clinically indicated.

B. Normovolemic hemodilution. Preoperative or intraoperative hemodilution entails phlebotomizing a patient of 1 or more units of fresh whole blood while replacing the lost volume with either colloid or crystalloid. By using normovolemic hemodilution before intraoperative blood loss, fresh autologous blood is available for later reinfusion after surgical blood loss is complete. Also, any blood shed after hemodilution will constitute more plasma loss and less red cell loss. Hemodilution may also be helpful in situations in which platelet function is altered intraoperatively (e.g., cardiopulmonary bypass), because the phlebotomized blood has normal platelets and clotting factors when reinfused. Obviously, if surgical blood loss is extreme, the fresh autologous blood should be transfused before any homologous blood. It should also be remembered that the autologous blood has a Hct similar to the patient's preoperative Hct, as opposed to a unit of packed red blood cells, which has a Hct of approximately 70%. While hemodilution alone may not eliminate the need for homologous transfusion, when used in combination with preoperative autologous donation, it may decrease the need for homologous units. Unless the preoperative Hct is high, the patient can tolerate a low target Hct, and the expected blood loss is large, nomovolemic hemodilution will only modestly diminish the need for homologous transfusion.

C. Intraoperative autotransfusion (cell saver) utilizes blood collected from the surgical field by a double-lumen suction device. As the shed blood is suctioned from the surgical field into one lumen, it is mixed with an anticoagulant (citrate-phosphate-dextrose or heparin) solution from the other lumen to prevent clotting of the blood in the filtered collecting reservoir. The blood then undergoes a series of steps of filtering, centrifuging, and washing designed to remove debris, plasma, free Hb, and anticoagulant. The final product is a collection bag of red blood cells having a Hct of 50% to 70%, which is ready for reinfusion immediately after about 3 minutes of processing time. Blood collected via intraoperative autotransfusion is deficient in plasma, clotting factors, and platelets. The technique is generally restricted to clean surgical fields and nononcologic procedures because of risks of reinfusing bacteria or tumor cells into patients.

VIII. Complications of blood transfusion therapy
   A. Transfusion reactions
   1. Acute hemolytic transfusion reactions occur when ABO-incompatible blood is transfused, resulting in recipient antibodies attaching to donor RBC antigens and forming an

Table 34.2.   Approach to suspected acute hemolytic transfusion reaction

1. *Stop the transfusion.*
2. Quickly check for error in patient identity or donor unit.
3. Send donor unit and newly obtained blood sample to blood bank for recross match.
4. Treat hypotension with fluids and vasopressors as necessary.
5. If transfusion is required, use type O-negative PRBC and type AB FFP as necessary.
6. Support renal function: first, administer fluids to correct hypovolemia and second, administer diuretics (furosemide ± mannitol) to maintain brisk urine output.
7. Monitor for signs of DIC clinically and with appropriate laboratory studies; treat supportively (see section IX.B).
8. Send patient blood sample for direct antiglobulin (Coombs) test, free hemoglobin, haptoglobin; send urine for hemoglobin.

DIC, disseminated intravascular coagulation; FFP, fresh-frozen plasma; PRBC, packed red blood cells.

antigen–antibody complex. This antigen–antibody complex activates complement, resulting in intravascular RBC lysis with release of RBC stroma and free hemoglobin. Immune system activation also results in bradykinin release (leading to hypotension) and mast cell activation (causing serotonin and histamine release). The net result may be shock, renal failure due to hemoglobin precipitation in renal tubules, and DIC (see section IX.B). Many signs and symptoms of an acute hemolytic transfusion reaction appear immediately and include fever, chest pain, anxiety, back pain, and dyspnea. Many are masked by general anesthesia, but clues to the diagnosis include fever, hypotension, hemoglobinuria, unexplained bleeding, or failure of Hct to increase after transfusion. Table 34.2 indicates steps to take if a transfusion reaction is suspected. The incidence of fatal hemolytic transfusion reaction in the United States is approximately 1 of every 250,000 to 1,000,000 units transfused. Most reactions occur because of administrative errors, with most due to improper identification of the blood unit or patient. The importance of adhering to strict policies of checking blood and matching to the correct patient in the operating room cannot be overemphasized.

2. **Delayed hemolytic transfusion reactions** occur because of incompatibility of minor antigens (e.g., Kidd) and are characterized by extravascular hemolysis. They present 2 days to months after transfusion. Patients complain of no or minimal symptoms but may display signs of anemia and jaundice. Laboratory studies reveal a positive direct antiglobulin test, hyperbilirubinemia, decreased haptoglobin levels, and hemosiderin in the urine. Treatment is aimed at correcting the anemia.

3. **Febrile nonhemolytic transfusion reactions** (FNHTR) are the most common transfusion reactions, occurring in

approximately 1% of RBC transfusions and up to 30% of platelet transfusions. They occur when antileukocyte antibodies in a recipient react with white blood cells in a transfused blood product. Signs and symptoms include fever, chills, tachycardia, discomfort, nausea, and vomiting. Approach to treatment involves first stopping the transfusion and excluding an acute, hemolytic transfusion reaction or bacterial contamination of the donor unit. Acetaminophen and meperidine may diminish fever and rigors. Once the diagnosis of FNHTR has been made, future reactions may be avoided or diminished by administering leukocyte reduced blood products (see section IV.B.2), premedicating at-risk patients with acetaminophen and hydrocortisone (50 to 100 mg IV), and administering the transfusion slowly.

4. **Allergic transfusion reactions** are common, occurring in 1% to 3% of transfusions. They arise from recipient antibody response to donor plasma proteins. Urticaria with pruritus and erythema is the most common manifestation, but rarely bronchospasm or anaphylaxis presents. Many patients also have fever. Patients with IgA deficiency may be at increased risk of allergic transfusion reaction because of the presence of anti-IgA antibodies that react with transfused IgA. Treatment involves stopping the transfusion, excluding a more severe reaction (see above), and administering antihistamines (diphenhydramine 50 mg IV and ranitidine 50 mg IV). A significant reaction may warrant treating with a corticosteroid (methylprednisolone 80 mg IV). Bronchospasm and anaphylaxis should be treated as described in Chapter 18.

5. **Transfusion-related acute lung injury** is a condition of severe pulmonary insufficiency occurring as a result of blood, FFP, cryoprecipitate, or platelet transfusion. Signs and symptoms include fever, dyspnea, hypoxemia, hypotension, and pulmonary edema developing within 4 hours of transfusion. The pathophysiology likely involves a reaction between recipient white blood cells and leukocyte antibodies present in donor plasma. The incidence, likely underestimated, is 1 of 5,000 PRBC units transfused and is more common in transfusions of platelets and FFP. Therapy is supportive, mimicking the treatment of acute respiratory distress syndrome, from which the diagnosis may be clinically indistinguishable. Mechanical ventilation usually is required during the acute phase, but resolution often occurs within 4 days. Preventive measures have not yet been identified.

B. **Metabolic complications of blood transfusions**

1. **Potassium (K^+)** concentration changes are common with rapid blood transfusion but usually are clinically important only in massive transfusion or renal failure. With storage, red cells leak K^+ into the extracellular storage fluid. However, with transfusion and replenishment of cellular energy stores, this is rapidly corrected.

2. **Calcium.** Citrate, which binds calcium, is used as an anticoagulant in stored blood products. Consequently, rapid transfusion may cause a decreased ionized calcium level. Hypocalcemia is usually not significant because the liver

rapidly metabolizes the infused citrate, but it may become an important problem in patients with impaired liver function, during the anhepatic phase of liver transplantation, in hypothermic patients, or in patients with decreased hepatic blood flow. Ionized calcium levels should be followed, because total serum calcium measures the citrate-bound calcium and may not accurately reflect free serum calcium.

3. **Acid-base status.** Banked blood is acidic because of accumulated red cell metabolites. However, the actual acid load to the patient is minimal. Acidosis in the face of severe blood loss is more likely due to hypoperfusion and will improve with volume resuscitation. Alkalosis is frequent following massive blood transfusion because citrate is metabolized in the liver to bicarbonate.

C. **Infectious complications of blood transfusions** have decreased with improved laboratory testing for transmissible diseases. Exposure to pooled products (e.g., cryoprecipitate) increases the risk in proportion to the number of donors.

1. **Hepatitis**

   a. **Hepatitis B** (see Chapter 7, section III.A.2). The risk of hepatitis B infection from a blood transfusion has decreased since testing donated blood for hepatitis B antigen became routine in 1971. The current risk is estimated to be 1:60,000 to 1:120,000 units transfused.

   b. **Hepatitis C** (see Chapter 7, section III.A.3). Institution of routine testing for antibody to hepatitis C virus (HCV) in 1990 (and recently nucleic acid testing) has reduced the risk of transfusion-related HCV to approximately 1:800,000 to 1:1.6 million units.

2. **Human immunodeficiency virus** (HIV; see Chapter 7, section III.A.1). Because of improved screening and testing, the risk of transfusion-associated HIV has been estimated to be about 1:1.4 to 1:2.4 million units transfused in the United States.

3. **Cytomegalovirus (CMV)** (see Chapter 7, section II.A.5). The prevalence of antibodies to CMV in the general adult population is approximately 70%. The incidence of transfusion-associated CMV infection in previously non-infected patients is quite high. Usually the infection is asymptomatic, but because immunosuppressed patients and neonates can have severe reactions, CMV-negative blood or leukocyte-reduced blood may be recommended.

4. **Bacterial sepsis** caused by transfused blood products is rare. Donors with evidence of infectious disease are excluded and the storage of PRBCs at 4°C minimizes infectious risk. Nonetheless, PRBCs may become infected, most commonly with *Yersinia enterocolitica*. Platelets, which are stored at room temperature, are more problematic, with an estimated infection rate of 1:1,000 to 1:2,000 units. Organisms associated with platelet contamination are usually *Staphylococcus* (*aureus* and *epidermidis*) and diphtheroids. The risk of infection is directly related to the storage time of the product with 15% to 25% of infected transfused units causing severe

sepsis. The signs usually are apparent during transfusion and should trigger immediate halt of the transfusion and testing of the unit for contamination. The impact on the individual patient depends on the size of the bacterial inoculum and the immunocompetence of the recipient, but overall mortality from transfusion-acquired sepsis is approximately 60%.

D. Immunomodulation by blood transfusion. Transfusion of allogeneic blood is known to suppress the immune system. Although the exact mechanism is unknown, theories suggest that transfusion of donor leukocytes may induce an immune-"tolerant" state in the recipient. Thus, allogeneic blood transfusion has been used pre- and intraoperatively in renal transplant recipients to improve graft viability. Less clear and more controversial are the potential detrimental effects of intraoperative allogeneic blood transfusion on cancer recurrence rates, postoperative infections, activation of latent viral infections, and postoperative mortality. Some experts contend that many of the adverse immunomodulary effects of allogeneic blood transfusion may be diminished by universal blood product leukoreduction.

IX. Perioperative coagulopathy

A. Coagulopathy of massive transfusion is unusual before the transfusion of greater than 1.0 to 1.5 blood volumes, assuming the patient had a normal coagulation profile, platelet count, and platelet function to start.

1. **Thrombocytopenia.** Diffuse oozing and failure to form clots after massive transfusion are often at least in part due to thrombocytopenia. The decreased platelet count is due to the transfusion of platelet-poor blood products. Clinical bleeding is unlikely with platelet counts above 50,000 cells/mm^3. If loss of one blood volume or more is expected, platelets should be available and transfused to maintain a count of more than 50,000 cells/mm^3 or greater if ongoing blood loss is expected.

2. **Clotting factors.** The normal human body has tremendous reserves of clotting factors. In addition, the patient receives small amounts of the stable clotting factors in the plasma of each unit of red cells. Bleeding from factor deficiency in the face of massive transfusion is usually due to decreased levels of fibrinogen and labile factors (V, VIII, or IX). Bleeding from hypofibrinogenemia is unusual unless the fibrinogen level is below 75 mg/dL. In some patients, factor VIII levels increase with massive transfusion because of increased release from endothelial cells. Labile clotting factors are administered in the form of FFP. Six units of platelets contain the equivalent of 1 unit of FFP. Cryoprecipitate provides a source of concentrated fibrinogen for the patient who cannot tolerate FFP due to volume overload.

B. Disseminated intravascular coagulation (DIC) refers to the abnormal, diffuse systemic activation of the clotting system. The pathophysiology involves excessive formation of thrombin, resulting in fibrin formation throughout the vasculature and accompanied by platelet activation, fibrinolysis, and consumption of coagulation factors. The profound consumptive coagulopathy produced by DIC often results in hemorrhage.

1. **Causes of DIC** include infection, shock, trauma, complications of pregnancy (e.g., amniotic fluid embolism, placental abruption, or septic abortion), burns, and fat or cholesterol embolism. DIC is common in extensive head injury because of the high content of thromboplastin in brain tissue. A chronic form of DIC may accompany cirrhotic liver disease, aortic dissection, and malignancy.

2. **Clinical features** include petechiae, ecchymoses, bleeding from venipuncture sites, and frank hemorrhage from operative incisions. The bleeding manifestations of DIC are most obvious, but the diffuse microvascular and macrovascular thromboses are usually more common, more difficult to treat, and more frequently life-threatening because of ischemia to vital organs. Bradykinin release in DIC may also cause hypotension.

3. **Laboratory features** of DIC include an elevated D-dimer, indicating fibrin degradation by plasmin, in all cases. Fibrinogen degradation products (FDPs) are increased, but this is not specific to DIC because FDPs may be present from the formation of fibrin by fibrinogen or from the degradation of fibrinogen by plasmin. The PT and PTT typically are prolonged and serial measurements reveal falling fibrinogen levels and platelet counts.

4. **Treatment of DIC** involves treating the precipitating cause and transfusion of appropriate blood products (e.g., FFP, platelets, and cryoprecipitate) to correct bleeding. In cases associated with inappropriate thrombosis rather than bleeding, the use of heparin to decrease fibrin formation can be considered, although this may risk life-threatening hemorrhage in the operating room. Inhibitors of fibrinolysis (e.g., aminocaproic acid and aprotinin) are not recommended for treatment of DIC because of the possibility of diffuse intravascular thrombosis.

C. **Chronic liver disease.** With the exception of factor VIII and vWf, which are manufactured by the endothelium, the liver synthesizes coagulation factors. Patients with hepatic dysfunction may have decreased production of coagulation factors and decreased clearance of activated factors. Patients may have an ongoing consumptive coagulopathy, similar to DIC, if circulating activated clotting factors are increased. Because the liver is also instrumental in removing the byproducts of fibrinolysis, circulating fibrin degradation products may be elevated.

D. **Vitamin K deficiency.** Vitamin K is required by the liver for production of factors II, VII, IX, and X, and proteins C and S. Because vitamin K cannot be synthesized by humans, interference with vitamin K absorption will cause a coagulopathy (see Chapter 5, section IV.B.6) and a prolonged prothrombin time. These patients can be treated with vitamin K, 10 mg SC daily for 3 days. IV administration of vitamin K may result in a slightly faster correction of the PT but is accompanied by a rare risk of anaphylaxis. If used, IV vitamin K should be administered very slowly. If faster correction of PT than vitamin K is required, FFP (5 to 8 mL/kg) can be used.

E. **Pharmacologic intervention**
1. **Heparin** acts by accelerating the effect of antithrombin III. It prolongs the PTT and has a short half-life so that its anticoagulant effect is usually fully reversed approximately 4 hours after discontinuation of the infusion. If faster reversal is required, protamine, a natural antagonist, may be administered.
2. **Low-molecular-weight heparins** are commercially prepared by fractionating heparin into molecules of 2,000 to 10,000 daltons. They exert their anticoagulant effect primarily by inhibiting factor X and usually do not prolong the PTT. These drugs have a longer half-life than heparin and are incompletely reversed by protamine. Fast reversal may require FFP transfusion.
3. **Warfarin (Coumadin)** inhibits vitamin K epoxide reductase. This causes a deficiency of vitamin K, preventing the hepatic carboxylation of factors II, VII, IX, and X, and proteins C and S to the active form. The PT and the INR are prolonged in patients taking warfarin. The drug's half-life is approximately 35 hours, requiring days for reversal. If quick reversal of warfarin is required, active factors can be given in the form of FFP (5 to 15 mL/kg). Vitamin K (2.5 to 10 mg IV or SC) can also be given for warfarin reversal, but its effect requires 6 or more hours.
4. **Platelet inhibitors. Aspirin** and **nonsteroidal anti-inflammatory drugs (NSAIDs)** inhibit platelet aggregation by interfering with the cyclooxygenase pathway. Aspirin permanently inhibits the pathway for the 10-day life span of the platelet. The other NSAIDs reversibly inhibit the cyclooxygenase pathway; their effects are reversed within 3 days of discontinuing the drug. **Dipyridamole** is a phosphodiesterase inhibitor that increases platelet cAMP, thereby inhibiting platelet aggregation. **Ticlopidine** and **clopidogrel** are newer antiplatelet agents that inhibit ADP-mediated platelet aggregation. **Abciximab** is an IV monoclonal antibody against the platelet glycoprotein IIb/IIIa receptor. It causes profound platelet inhibition and produces thrombocytopenia. Although the drug's plasma half-life is short, impairment of platelet function may last for days and reversal of the effect may require multiple platelet transfusions due to absorption of the antibody to donor platelets. Immediate reversal of platelet inhibitors may require platelet transfusion and may not be effective if inhibitor is still present in the plasma.
5. **Thrombolytic agents** act by dissolving thrombi via conversion of plasminogen to plasmin, which lyses fibrin clot. They are intended to reverse thrombosis and recanalize blood vessels. Two thrombolytic agents, **tissue plasminogen activator (tPA)** and **streptokinase,** are commonly used in clinical practice, each with slightly different pharmacodynamic and side effect profiles. Each of these drugs results in a hypofibrinogenemic state and carries a substantial risk of bleeding. They are generally contraindicated perioperatively. If emergent surgery is required after thrombolytic therapy, the effect may be reversed by administration of aminocaproic or tranexamic acid. The fibrinogen

level may be restored by transfusion of cryoprecipitate or FFP.

X. **Special considerations**

A. **Hemophilia.** Hemophilia A and B are rare, sex-linked diseases affecting males almost exclusively. **Hemophilia A** is due to an abnormality in factor VIII, while **hemophilia B (Christmas disease)** is due to a factor IX abnormality. The incidence in the United States is 1:10,000 males for hemophilia A and 1:100,000 males for hemophilia B.

1. **Clinical features.** Patients usually present early in childhood with hemarthroses and soft-tissue hematomas after minor trauma. Laboratory tests demonstrate a markedly prolonged PTT with normal PT and platelet count.

2. **Treatment** with the appropriate factor (of either recombinant or lyophilized concentrate source) should be coordinated with the patient's hematologist. Hemophilia A is treated with factor VIII to achieve preoperative activity levels of 25% to 100%, depending on the extent of the procedure. Some patients with mild hemophilia A may respond to DDAVP therapy. In an emergency, if factor VIII is unavailable, cryoprecipitate transfusion can provide the deficient factor. Hemophilia B is treated with factor IX to achieve at least 30% to 50% activity before surgery.

B. **Von Willebrand disease** is caused by a deficiency or abnormality in vWf, a protein involved in anchoring platelets to injured subendothelium and stabilizing factor VIII. It is the most common inherited bleeding disorder, affecting 1% to 2% of the population. It is autosomally dominant and affects both sexes equally.

1. **Clinical presentation.** The phenotypic expression is variable so that clinical manifestations may range from very mild to severe bleeding. Usually, patients have a history of easy bruisability and bleeding from mucosal surfaces, but some patients are not diagnosed with a bleeding disorder until suffering major trauma or surgery complicated by bleeding. Laboratory tests usually reveal a prolonged bleeding time.

2. **Treatment** of von Willebrand disease depends on the subtype. Many patients respond to DDAVP treatment, but others may require cryoprecipitate or a purified, lyophilized complex of vWf and factor VIII derived from pooled human plasma (Humate-P). The lysine analogue antifibrinolytics also have been used in some patients to reduce surgical bleeding. Preoperative consultation with the patient's hematologist is recommended.

C. **Sickle cell anemia** affects 1:600 African Americans. The disease is caused by the substitution of valine for glutamic acid at the sixth position on the beta chain of hemoglobin. Homozygotes for this substitution (as well as double heterozygotes SC or β-thalassemia) have clinical sickle cell disease.

1. **Clinical features.** The abnormal hemoglobin polymerizes and causes a sickling deformity of the red cell under certain conditions (e.g., hypoxia, hypothermia, acidosis, and dehydration). Sickled cells cause microvascular occlusion with tissue ischemia and infarction. A sickle cell crisis typically presents with excruciating chest or abdominal pain,

fever, tachycardia, leukocytosis, and hematuria. Signs and symptoms may be masked by anesthesia. The RBCs have a shortened survival time of 12 days, leading to anemia and extramedullary hematopoiesis.

2. **The anesthetic management** of these patients includes avoiding conditions that promote sickling (e.g., hypoxia, hypovolemia, acidemia, and hypothermia). In addition, transfusing to a preoperative Hct of approximately 30% prevents postoperative complications as effectively as the traditional "exchange transfusions" that sought to reduce the amount of hemoglobin S to 30% of total hemoglobin.

D. **Jehovah's Witness** patients generally may refuse to receive blood or blood products because of their religious beliefs, even if such refusal results in death. Special considerations may apply if the patient is a minor, is incompetent, or has responsibilities for dependents as well as in certain emergency circumstances (see also Chapter 40, section II.F). However, under elective conditions a physician is not required to agree to treat a patient who refuses a transfusion if doing so is contrary to the physician's ethical beliefs. Blood conservation measures are crucial in these patients (see section VII). Jehovah's Witnesses may allow transfusion of intraoperatively phlebotomized blood (see section VII.B) as long as the blood remains in continuity with the body (i.e., the blood tubing must always remain connected to the patient). Erythropoietin is sometimes used to increase red cell mass perioperatively. It is incumbent on the anesthesiologist to fully discuss the patient's beliefs and decisions concerning transfusion and document these decisions clearly in the medical record as well as on operative consent forms.

E. **Recombinant factor VIIa (rFVIIa)** is FDA approved for the treatment of hemophiliacs with antibody inhibitors that prevent factor VIII or IX from normalizing their coagulation. The apparent efficacy of the drug in massive surgical or traumatic bleeding from recent case studies has generated intense interest for a wider applicability of the drug. In addition, one major trial demonstrated reduced expansion of intracerebral hematoma in cases of nontraumatic, hemorrhagic stroke, which has created enthusiastic support for the use of rFVIIa in these patients by some neurointensivists. Because of the unknown hemostatic efficacy and thrombotic risks in surgical and trauma patients, and because of the prohibitive cost of rFVIIa, randomized controlled clinical trials that include patients with traumatic brain injury, burns, complex cardiac surgical procedures, and rebleeding after neurosurgical intervention for spontaneous intracerebral hemorrhage are currently under way. Despite the lack of conclusive trials, some institutions have already included rFVIIa as part of a massive transfusion protocol, but this remains controversial.

SUGGESTED READING

American Society of Anesthesiologists Task Force on Perioperative Blood Transfusion and Adjuvant Therapies. Practice guidelines for perioperative blood transfusion and adjuvant therapies. Approved October 22, 1995, last amended

October 25, 2005. Available at http://www.asahq.org/publicationsAndServices/practiceparam.htm#blood. Accessed January 22, 2006.

Dutton RP, Hess JR, Scalea TM. Recombinant factor VIIa for control of hemorrhage: early experience in critically ill trauma patients. *J Clin Anesth* 2003;15:184–188.

Goodnough LT, Brecher ME, Kanter MH, et al. Transfusion medicine. I. Blood transfusion. *N Engl J Med* 1999;340:438–447.

Goodnough LT, Brecher ME, Kanter MH, et al. Transfusion medicine: II. Blood conservation. *N Engl J Med* 1999;340:525–533.

Goodnough LT. Risks of blood transfusion. *Crit Care Med* 2003; 31(Suppl.):S678–S686.

Gross JB. Estimating allowable blood loss: corrected for dilution. *Anesthesiology* 1983;58:277–280.

Hebert PC, Wells G, Blajchman MA, et al. A multicenter, randomized controlled clinical trial of transfusion requirements in critical care. *N Engl J Med* 1999;340:409–417.

Kopko PM, Holland PV. Transfusion-related acute lung injury. *Br J Haematol* 1999;105:322–329.

Lake CL, Moore RA, eds. *Blood: hemostasis, transfusion, and alternatives in the perioperative period.* New York: Raven Press, 1995.

O'Connell NM, Perry DJ, Hodgson AJ, et al. Recombinant FVIIa in the management of uncontrolled hemorrhage. *Transfusion* 2003;43:1711–1716.

Rao SV, Jollis JG, Harrington RA, et al. Relationship of blood transfusion and clinical outcomes in patients with acute coronary syndromes. *JAMA* 2004;292:1555–1562.

Sharma AD, Sreeram G, Erb T, et al. Leukocyte-reduced blood transfusions: perioperative indications, adverse effects, and cost analysis. *Anesth Analg* 2000;90:1315–1323.

III

Perioperative Issues

The Postanesthesia Care Unit

Dragos Diaconescu and Loreta Grecu

I. **General considerations.** For most patients, recovery from anesthesia is uneventful. Nevertheless, when postoperative complications occur, they may be sudden and life-threatening. The **postanesthesia care unit (PACU)** is designed to provide close monitoring and care to patients recovering from anesthesia and sedation, during the transition to a fully awake state, and before transfer to general hospital wards. The PACU is staffed by a dedicated team, which consists of anesthesiologists, nurses, and aides. It is located in immediate proximity to the operating room (OR), with access to radiology and the laboratory. Drugs and equipment for routine care (O_2, suction, monitors) and advanced support (mechanical ventilators, pressure transducers, infusion pumps, code cart) must be readily available.

II. **Admission to the PACU**

   A. **Transport** from the OR is carried out under direct supervision of the anesthetist, preferably with the head of the bed elevated or with the patient in the lateral decubitus position to maximize airway patency. Oxygen delivered via facemask is indicated in most patients to prevent hypoxemia due to hypoventilation or diffusion hypoxia (see section VI.A.1). Unstable patients, such as patients receiving vasopressor medications, usually require monitoring of the oxygen saturation, blood pressure, heart rate, and electrocardiogram during the transport, as deemed necessary by the anesthesia provider.

   B. **Report.** Upon arrival, vital signs are recorded and the anesthetist provides a complete report to the PACU team. The anesthetist remains in charge of the care of the patient until the PACU team is ready to take over. If deemed necessary, the anesthetist may choose to speak directly to the anesthesiologist in charge of the PACU, the surgeon, or a consultant about issues of particular importance for the patient. This report is often the only formal account of the intraoperative events between the operating team and the personnel who will carry out the immediate postoperative care.

   C. **The report includes the following:**

      1. Patient identification, age, surgical procedure, diagnosis, a summary of prior medical history, medications, allergies, and preoperative vital signs. Specific features such as deafness, psychiatric issues, language barriers, and precautions for infection control should also be mentioned.

      2. Location and size of intravascular catheters.

      3. Premedication, antibiotics, anesthetic drugs for induction and maintenance, opioids, muscle relaxants, and reversal agents. Vasoactive drugs, bronchodilators, and other relevant drugs administered should be listed.

      4. Exact nature of the surgical procedure. If relevant surgical issues exist (e.g., adequacy of hemostasis, care of drains, restrictions on positioning, etc.), the PACU staff should be informed.

      5. Anesthetic course, with emphasis on problems that may affect the immediate postoperative course including laboratory values, difficult intravenous (IV) access, difficult intubation, intraoperative hemodynamic instability, and electrocardiographic (ECG) changes.

      6. Fluid balance, including amount, type, and rationale of fluid replacement, urine output, and estimated fluid and blood loss.

III. **Monitoring.** Close observation of the patient's level of consciousness, breathing pattern, and peripheral perfusion is of utmost importance. The nurse to patient ratio for routine cases is one nurse to two or three patients and increases to 1:1 for high-acuity patients, such as those with a significant medical history and those with intraoperative complications. Vital signs are monitored and charted at regular intervals according to the patient's need. Standard monitoring includes **respiratory rate** measurement by impedance plethysmography, continuous **electrocardiogram,** manual or automated oscillometric **blood pressure,** and **pulse oximetry. Temperature** should also be monitored and recorded. When necessary, invasive monitoring can be instituted. An arterial catheter provides continuous measurement of the systemic blood pressure in patients with tenuous hemodynamics and provides access for blood sampling. Central venous and pulmonary artery catheters should be considered when the etiology of hemodynamic instability is unclear (see Chapter 10) or when there is a requirement for vasopressors that can be administered only in the central venous system. If the patient's recovery is expected to be prolonged or complicated, and/or if monitoring and care requirements are escalating, plans should be made to transfer the patient to an intensive care unit (ICU).

IV. **General complications.** The incidence of PACU complications varies with the patient population and appears to be more common in patients with mild or moderate coexisting diseases. Recent studies show that complications causing at least moderate morbidity occur in approximately 5% of the PACU admissions. Respiratory and hemodynamic issues are the most frequent complications in the PACU.

V. **Hemodynamic complications** occurred in 1.2% of the PACU admissions in a large Australian study, with hypotension, arrhythmias, myocardial ischemia, and pulmonary edema being the most common complications recorded.

    A. **Hypotension.** The differential diagnosis is aided by a review of the patient's history and the intraoperative management. The anesthetist who performed the case can be contacted to help interpret the current events. In most cases, the following differential diagnosis algorithm is helpful.

      1. **Hypovolemia** is the most common cause of hypotension in the PACU and administration of a fluid bolus during the initial assessment is generally a safe maneuver. Ongoing hemorrhage, inadequate fluid replacement, osmotic polyuria, and fluid sequestration (intestinal obstruction, ascites) are among the causes of hypovolemia in the PACU. Nonspecific signs include hypotension, tachycardia, tachypnea, decreased skin turgor, dry mucous membranes, oliguria, and thirst. A meaningful volume challenge (250 to 1,000 mL of crystalloid or an equivalent volume of synthetic colloid, blood products, or both) should be considered for specific indications. Persistent hypotension after a seemingly adequate volume replacement mandates further assessment, starting with placement of a urinary catheter and, if necessary, followed by invasive monitoring.

2. **Impaired venous return** occurs when mechanical forces decrease the venous return to the heart in the absence of a reduction of circulating blood volume. Common causes include **positive pressure ventilation,** dynamic hyperinflation of the lungs with subsequent **autopositive end-expiratory pressure (auto PEEP)** (see Chapter 36), **pneumothorax,** and **pericardial tamponade.** Signs of obstruction to venous return are similar to those of true hypovolemia except for the presence of jugular vein distention, an elevated central venous pressure, and decreased breath sounds and heart tones. Volume administration is the mainstay of symptomatic therapy, but treatment of the cause is the ultimate intervention.

3. **Vasodilation.** Neuroaxial anesthesia, residual inhalation agents, rewarming after hypothermia, transfusion reactions, adrenal insufficiency, anaphylaxis, systemic inflammation, sepsis, liver failure, and the administration of vasodilator drugs are causes of hypotension resulting from vasodilation. Hypovolemia accentuates the hypotension due to vasodilation, but volume replacement alone cannot fully restore the blood pressure. Pharmacologic treatment includes α-adrenergic receptor agonists such as **phenylephrine, norepinephrine,** and even **epinephrine,** and this management should be carried out under close monitoring. Diagnosis and treatment of the specific etiology should be concurrent with symptomatic treatment.

4. **Decreased cardiac output.** Myocardial ischemia and infarction, dysrhythmias, congestive heart failure, administration of negative inotropic drugs (anesthetics, β-adrenergic blockers, calcium-channel blockers, antidysrhythmics), sepsis, hypothyroidism, and malignant hyperthermia are some of the possible etiologies for perioperative myocardial dysfunction. Symptoms include dyspnea, diaphoresis, cyanosis, jugular vein distention, oliguria, rhythm disturbances, wheezing, dependent crackles, and an S3 gallop on auscultation. A chest radiograph (CXR), 12-lead ECG, and basic laboratory values usually help with diagnosis. Invasive monitoring generally is necessary to guide therapy (see Chapters 2 and 19), and may include the following:

   a. **Inotropic agents** such as dopamine, dobutamine, epinephrine, norepinephrine, and milrinone.

   b. **Afterload reduction** with nitrates, calcium-channel blockers, or angiotensin-converting enzyme inhibitors.

   c. **Diuresis** with furosemide for fluid overload.

   d. **Antidysrhythmics or electrical cardioversion** for rhythm disorders.

B. **Hypertension** is most commonly observed in patients with preexisting hypertensive disease, particularly if antihypertensive medications were held preoperatively. Certain types of surgery such as carotid, vascular, and intrathoracic procedures are more likely to be followed by hypertensive events. Other postoperative etiologies for hypertension may include pain, bladder distention, fluid overload, hypoxemia, hypercarbia, hypothermia, increased intracranial pressure (ICP), and administration of vasoconstrictive agents. Hypertension is usually asymptomatic, but it may present with headache, visual disturbances, dyspnea, restlessness, and even chest pain. In the initial assessment, one should verify the accuracy of blood pressure measurement, review the patient's history and operative course, and rule out correctable etiologies. The management of hypertension is aimed at restoring blood pressure close to the patient's baseline. Tight blood pressure control is extremely important after surgery for an intracranial aneurysm, creation of vascularized muscular flaps, microvascular surgery, and in patients with severe vascular disease. If possible, resumption of chronic antihypertensive oral therapy is ideal. If needed, this can be supplemented or substituted with a fast-onset, short-acting IV medication.

1. **β-Adrenergic blockers.** Labetalol (an α- and a β-blocker), 5 to 20 mg IV bolus or up to 2 mg/min as IV infusion, esmolol, 10 to 100 mg IV or as an infusion at 25 to 300 μg/kg/minute, and propranolol, 0.5- to 1.0-mg IV increments, may be used.

2. **Calcium-channel blockers.** Verapamil, 2.5- to 5-mg increments IV, or nicardipine infusion initiated at 5 to 15 mg/hour, followed by 0.5 to 2.2 mg/hour. Sublingual nifedipine is no longer recommended because it may be followed by an unpredictable, and at times severe, drop in blood pressure that may induce myocardial ischemia.

3. **Hydralazine,** 5 to 20 mg IV, is a pure vasodilator that may induce reflex tachycardia.

4. **Nitrates.** Nitroglycerin, starting at 25 μg/minute IV, is preferentially a venodilator, useful for coexisting myocardial ischemia. Sodium nitroprusside, starting at 0.5 μg/kg/minute IV, is a potent arterial and venodilator and requires invasive blood pressure monitoring.

5. **Fenoldopam,** a selective peripheral dopaminergic receptor agonist, may be administered as an IV infusion starting at 0.1 μg/kg/minute up to 1.5 μg/kg/minute. Side effects include tachycardia, headache, and increased intraocular pressure.

6. **Enalaprilat,** 0.625 to 1.25 mg IV, is useful in patients receiving long-term angiotensin-converting enzyme inhibitors or angiotensin receptor blockers as an alternative when they cannot take oral medication.

C. **Dysrhythmias.** Increased sympathetic outflow, hypoxemia, hypercarbia, electrolyte and acid-base imbalance, myocardial ischemia, increased ICP, drug toxicity, thyrotoxicosis, and malignant hyperthermia are possible etiologies of perioperative dysrhythmias. Premature atrial contractions and unifocal premature ventricular contractions (PVCs) generally do not require treatment. In the presence of more worrisome rhythm disturbances, supplemental O_2 should be delivered and proper treatment begun while the etiology is investigated (see Chapters 18 and 37).

1. **Common supraventricular dysrhythmias**
   a. **Sinus tachycardia** may be secondary to pain, agitation, hypovolemia, fever, hyperthermia, hypoxemia, hypercarbia, congestive heart failure, and pulmonary embolism. The symptomatic treatment with β-blockers should be instituted only after its etiology is addressed, unless it constitutes a risk for myocardial ischemia.
   b. **Sinus bradycardia** may result from a high neuroaxial anesthetic block, opioid administration (with the exception of meperidine), vagal stimulation, β-adrenergic blockade, and increased ICP. Symptomatic treatment with anticholinergic muscarinic agents, **atropine,** 0.2 to 0.4 mg IV, or **glycopyrrolate,** 0.2 mg IV, is indicated when hypotension is present or for severe bradycardia. (See also Chapter 37.)
   c. **Paroxysmal supraventricular tachydysrhythmias** occur with a higher incidence in patients over 70 years of age; after abdominal, thoracic, or major vascular procedures; and in patients with preoperative premature atrial contractions. They include paroxysmal atrial tachycardia, multifocal atrial tachycardia, junctional tachycardia, atrial fibrillation, and flutter. These rhythms may cause significant hypotension.
      (1) **Synchronized cardioversion** should be used if the patient is hemodynamically unstable, as per the ACLS protocol (see Chapter 37).
      (2) **Adenosine,** 6 mg followed by 12 mg IV, administered rapidly has a high success rate in converting paroxysmal atrial tachycardia to sinus rhythm.
      (3) **Verapamil,** 2.5- to 5-mg increments IV, or **diltiazem** 5- to 20-mg IV push or as an infusion (bolus: 0.25 to 0.35 mg/kg IV followed by infusion rate of 5 to 15 mg/hour IV), will slow the ventricular response.
      (4) **Amiodarone** is the antidysrhythmic of choice to ensure rate control for atrial dysrhythmias in the setting of a decreased myocardial function (congestive heart failure, ejection fraction <40%).
      (5) β-**Blockers (metoprolol, propranolol, esmolol atenolol)** (see section IV.B.1) also decrease the ventricular response to supraventricular tachydysrhythmias.
      (6) **Digoxin,** 0.25-mg IV increments up to 1.0 to 1.5 mg, slows ventricular response. Because of its delayed onset (6 hours), it is mainly used as an adjunct to a β-blocker or a calcium channel blocker.
      (7) **Ibutilide,** a class III antidysrhythmic, has been shown to be particularly effective in restoring sinus rhythm in patients with atrial fibrillation. **Procainamide** and other type I-A and I-C agents can also be used. They all have a narrow therapeutic window and require close monitoring.
2. **Stable ventricular dysrhythmias.** PVCs and stable nonsustained ventricular tachycardia generally do not require treatment. However, a search for reversible causes (hypoxemia,

myocardial ischemia, acidosis, hypokalemia, hypomagnesemia, irritation due to a central venous catheter) should be conducted. Stable sustained ventricular tachycardia can be treated with synchronized cardioversion or pharmacologic modalities (Chapter 37). PVCs that are multifocal and occur in runs, or are close to the preceding beat's T-wave, should be treated, especially in patients with structural heart disease.

  a. **Beta-blockers.** Esmolol, 10 to 100 mg IV or as an infusion 25 to 300 μg/kg/minute, metoprolol, 2.5 to 10 mg IV, and propranolol, 0.5- to 2.0-mg IV increments, may be used.

  b. **Amiodarone,** 150 mg over 10 minutes followed by 1 mg/minute for 6 hours and then 0.5 mg/min, is especially indicated in patients with a decreased myocardial function.

  c. **Procainamide,** 20 to 30 mg/minute IV, maximum total 17 mg/kg, and 1 to 2 mg/minute infusion.

  d. **Lidocaine,** 1.5 mg/kg IV, followed by an infusion at 1 to 4 mg/minute.

  3. Management for **unstable ventricular tachycardia** and **ventricular fibrillation** are described in the ACLS protocol (see Chapter 37).

D. **Myocardial ischemia and infarction**

  1. **T-wave changes** (inversion, flattening, pseudonormalization) may be associated with myocardial ischemia and infarction, electrolyte changes, hypothermia, surgical manipulation of the mediastinum, or incorrect lead placement. Isolated T-wave changes must be considered within the clinical context because they are common postoperatively and only rarely are caused by myocardial ischemia.

  2. **ST segment** elevation and depression are generally indicative of myocardial infarction and ischemia, respectively. ST segment elevation can also be a normal variant or can occur in other conditions like left ventricular hypertrophy, left bundle branch block, and hyperkalemia. Unlike the myocardial infarctions in the nonsurgical setting, in the postoperative period, most myocardial infarctions are associated with ST depression and have a non-Q-wave pattern. As supplemental O_2 is administered and a 12-lead ECG obtained, possible precipitating factors for the ST-segment changes must be reviewed and corrected. Common etiologies include hypoxemia, anemia, tachycardia, hypotension, and hypertension. Cardiac enzymes should be monitored in patients with persistent changes. If tolerated, β-**blockade** is added. IV nitroglycerin should be considered, especially for cases with ST segment elevations. Aspirin and statins may decrease the mortality of patients with acute coronary syndrome in the perioperative period. In severe cases, a cardiology consultation and transfer to an ICU are indicated, particularly when ongoing ischemia mandates the institution of invasive monitoring and/or specialized treatment (thrombolysis, percutaneous angioplasty, etc.).

  3. In patients at high risk for cardiac events (patients with ischemic heart disease, cerebrovascular disease, renal insufficiency, diabetes mellitus, and patients undergoing

intrathoracic, intraperitoneal, or suprainguinal vascular procedures), β-blockade has been found to decrease the risk for cardiac events. A **perioperative β-blockade protocol** was implemented at Massachusetts General Hospital in 2005. The recommendations for the immediate postoperative period are as follows:

   a. For patients recovering from general anesthesia, monitored anesthesia care, or peripheral blocks, metoprolol 2.5 to 5 mg IV should be administered if heart rate is greater than 80 beats per minute within 20 minutes of arrival in the PACU. It should be repeated once after 5 to 10 minutes if heart rate is greater than 80 beats per minute. If heart rate continues to be above 80, the anesthesia team should be contacted for further orders. Metoprolol should be held if heart rate is less than 50 beats per minute, systolic blood pressure is less than 100 mm Hg, bronchospasm, symptoms of congestive heart failure, third-degree heart block, or in patients with a history of previous adverse reactions to β-blockers. If the metoprolol is held for heart rate or blood pressure, it should be given later when heart rate is greater than 55 beats per minute and systolic blood pressure is greater than 110 mm Hg.

   b. Patients recovering from neuraxial blockade with or without general anesthesia:

   (1) For patients treated with metoprolol intraoperatively, use metoprolol as outlined above.

   (2) For patients who did not receive β-blockers intraoperatively, initiate metoprolol as outlined above once the surgical block has resolved and heart rate is greater than 55 beats per minute.

   (3) Patients treated with esmolol should be transitioned to metoprolol by titrating off the esmolol drip and administering metoprolol 2.5 to 5 mg IV to maintain heart rate between 50 and 80 beats per minute following the above protocol.

   (4) For patients on vasoactive agents for blood pressure support due to neuraxial blockade, the initiation of β-blockade should be done at the discretion of the PACU anesthesia team and surgical team.

   c. After discharge from the PACU, patients should resume their preoperative β-blockade regimen. Patients who were not on chronic β-blockade before surgery should continue β-blockers for 2 weeks postoperatively.

E. **The patient with a permanent pacemaker (PPM) or an intracardiac defibrillator (ICD)** requires special care in the PACU. Information about the patient's pacemaker dependency state and the features of the device must be obtained from the OR team. Continuous ECG monitoring is essential paying special attention to the patient's rhythm, rate, and hemodynamic status. Electrocautery used during the surgery can electrically reset the pacemakers, especially older models. Placement of a magnet over the PPM or ICD (frequently used during surgery) can either temporarily or permanently deactivate or reset it. Most new pacemakers have rate-adaptive capabilities that usually need to be disabled for the surgery. Therefore, interrogation of the device and communication with the electrophysiology service before and after surgery are highly recommended. Reprogramming of the device to the original parameters is often required in the PACU after the operation.

VI. Respiratory and airway complications occurred in 2.2% of 8,372 PACU admissions in a recent Australian study. The main events were inadequate oxygenation and/or ventilation, upper airway obstruction, laryngospasm, and aspiration.

   A. Hypoxemia. General anesthesia is associated with inhibition of hypoxic and hypercapnic ventilatory drive and a reduction of the pulmonary functional residual capacity (FRC). These changes may persist for a variable period of time postoperatively and predispose to hypoventilation and hypoxemia. There is no consensus in the literature regarding recommendations for the prophylactic administration of oxygen to all postoperative patients, but supplemental oxygen has been shown to mask and delay the detection of hypoventilation by pulse oxymetry. Therefore, the decision to administer supplemental oxygen should be individualized for each patient. Signs of hypoxemia include dyspnea, cyanosis, altered mental status, agitation, obtundation, tachycardia, hypertension, and arrhythmias. Specific treatment for these symptoms should be done only after hypoxemia is ruled out. Causes of hypoxemia include the following:

   1. **Atelectasis,** with subsequent increased intrapulmonary shunting, is a predictable effect of a decreased FRC caused by general anesthesia. Additional reduction of the FRC that occurs in obese patients and after thoracic or upper abdominal procedures can further aggravate the atelectasis. Patients who receive epidural anesthesia without general anesthesia have little or no atelectasis formation. Deep breathing (with or without holding) and incentive spirometry are equally effective in rapidly reexpanding small areas of alveolar collapse. Noninvasive ventilation (NIV) has been shown to further improve atelectasis and oxygenation in postoperative patients. Occasionally, hypoxemia may persist and a CXR may reveal a segmental or lobar collapse. Chest physiotherapy or fiberoptic bronchoscopy may also help with reinflation of the atelectatic segment.

   2. **Hypoventilation** causes hypoxemia by promoting alveolar collapse and increasing the CO_2 partial pressure in the alveolar air.

   3. **Diffusion hypoxia** may occur during washout of nitrous oxide upon emergence from general anesthesia. High-inspired O_2 fraction (Fio_2) by facemask can prevent hypoxemia.

   4. **Upper airway obstruction** is most often caused by inadequate recovery of the airway reflexes and tone (see section VI.C).

   5. **Bronchospasm** may cause hypoventilation, CO_2 retention, and hypoxemia (see section VI.B.2.e).

   6. **Aspiration of gastric contents** (see Chapter 18).

   7. **Pulmonary edema** may occur from either cardiac failure or increased pulmonary capillary permeability. Cardiogenic edema occurs mostly in individuals with preexisting cardiac disease and is characterized by hypoxemia, dyspnea, orthopnea, jugular venous distention, wheezing, and an S_3

gallop. It may be precipitated by fluid overload, dysrhythmias, and myocardial ischemia. A physical exam, a chest x-ray, arterial blood gas tensions, and a 12-lead ECG should be obtained. Evaluation by a cardiologist may be indicated, particularly when aggressive management of conditions such as unstable angina or acute valvular disease is being considered. Inotropic agents, diuretics, and vasodilators are the mainstay of treatment. The use of NIV can obviate the need for intubation in patients with severe hypoxia pending the response to the medical treatment. "Permeability" pulmonary edema secondary to sepsis, head injury, aspiration, transfusion reaction, anaphylaxis, or upper airway obstruction is characterized by hypoxemia without the signs of left ventricular overload. Treatment generally needs to be continued in an ICU (see Chapter 36).

8. **Pneumothorax** may cause hypoventilation, hypoxemia, and hemodynamic instability (see section VI.B.2.f).

9. **Pulmonary embolism** seldom occurs immediately postoperatively. However, it should be considered in the differential diagnosis of hypoxemia in patients with deep venous thrombosis, cancer, multiple trauma, and in those with prolonged bedrest.

B. **Hypoventilation** is characterized by inappropriately low minute ventilation and results in hypercapnea and acute respiratory acidosis. When severe, hypoventilation produces hypoxemia, CO_2 narcosis, and ultimately apnea. Supplemental oxygen may mask early detection of hypoventilation. A decline in oxygen saturation, as a sign of hypoventilation, has been found to be accurate only in patients breathing room air. Therefore, monitoring the ventilatory status of postoperative patients should not rely entirely on pulse oximetry. Etiologies of postoperative hypoventilation may be divided in two groups:

1. **Decreased ventilatory drive.**

   a. All inhaled **halogenated agents** depress ventilatory drive (see Chapter 11) and may produce hypoventilation in the postoperative period. **Opioids** are also potent respiratory depressants. All μ-receptor agonists increase the apneic threshold. Overnarcotized patients typically appear pain-free, with a slow respiratory rate and a tendency to become apneic if left unstimulated. Large doses of **benzodiazepines** may also inhibit ventilatory drive. The safest treatment of anesthetic-related hypoventilation is to continue mechanical ventilation until breathing is adequate. Alternatively, pharmacologic reversal may be considered.

      (1) Opioid-induced hypoventilation can be reversed by **naloxone,** a pure μ-receptor antagonist. Doses of 40 to 80 μg IV are titrated to effect. Reversal occurs within 1 to 2 minutes and lasts for 30 to 60 minutes. Naloxone treatment may induce significant side effects such as pain, tachycardia, hypertension, pulmonary edema. The respiratory effects of the opioids may outlast a single dose of naloxone. The patient should be monitored for recurrence of opioid-induced hypoventilation.

(2) Hypoventilation secondary to benzodiazepines can be reversed by **flumazenil** (increments of 0.2 to 1 mg IV over 5 minutes, up to a maximum of 5 mg). The onset of reversal occurs within 1 to 2 minutes with peak effect at 6 to 10 minutes. The patients should be followed closely afterward, because resedation may occur due to its short half-life. Flumazenil should be used cautiously in patients with chronic benzodiazepine use because it may precipitate seizures.

b. Less common, but potentially life-threatening, causes of decreased ventilatory drive include complications of **intracranial** and **carotid artery** surgery, **head injuries,** and intraoperative **stroke** (see section VIII).

2. **Pulmonary and respiratory muscle insufficiency**

a. **Preexisting respiratory disease** is the most important risk factor for postoperative respiratory complications. **Chronic obstructive pulmonary disease** (COPD; see Chapter 3) alters the match of ventilation and perfusion, resulting in hypoxemia and hypercapnia. Impaired gas exchange and expiratory flow limitation cause a high ventilatory workload under normal circumstances, which is worsened by surgical trauma, anesthesia, airway secretions, etc. **Restrictive disease** (e.g., pulmonary fibrosis, pleural effusions, obesity, scoliosis, massive ascites, pregnancy) is associated with fewer complications than COPD, particularly when respiratory muscle strength is preserved and the restrictive defect is extrapulmonary. Noninvasive ventilation (NIV) can be beneficial in patients with COPD and in those with restrictive pulmonary disease by decreasing the work of breathing, augmenting the ventilatory parameters, and avoiding intubation.

b. **Inadequate reversal of neuromuscular blockade** is suggested by the observation of spasmodic twitching, generalized weakness, upper airway obstruction, or by more subtle signs like hypoxemia or shallow breathing. It is generally more common with long-acting muscle relaxants than with medium- or short-acting ones and when reversal agents were not administered in the OR. Adequacy of muscle strength can be assessed clinically and with the aid of a peripheral nerve stimulator (see Chapter 12). Special situations such as myasthenia gravis and myasthenic syndromes, pseudocholinesterase deficiency, succinylcholine-induced phase II block, hypothermia, acid-base and electrolyte imbalance, and anticholinesterase overdose should be considered. If muscle weakness persists after adequate pharmacologic reversal (e.g., **neostigmine** up to 5 mg and **glycopyrrolate** up to 1 mg in an adult), it is best to institute or continue mechanical ventilation, administer adequate anxiolysis, and wait for the muscle strength to recover while the appropriate workup is performed.

c. **Upper airway obstruction** may cause hypercapnea and hypoxemia (see section VI.C).

d. **Inadequate analgesia** after thoracic or upper abdominal surgery may cause splinting and decreased minute ventilation, resulting in alveolar collapse, hypercapnia, and hypoxemia. This is preventable with early analgesia and encouragement of deep breathing and coughing. Compared with systemic opioids, epidural analgesia may have a weak tendency to reduce the incidence of respiratory complications (atelectasis, pulmonary infections, or hypoxia).

e. **Bronchospasm** is common in patients with COPD, asthma, or recent respiratory tract infection. It is often precipitated by manipulation of the airway, particularly tracheal intubation. Wheezing may also be heard upon chest examination of patients with pulmonary edema, endobronchial intubation, aspiration pneumonitis, and pneumothorax. Treatment is discussed in Chapter 3.

f. **Pneumothorax** may complicate certain procedures like thoracotomy, mediastinoscopy, bronchoscopy, high retroperitoneal dissection for nephrectomy or adrenalectomy, laparoscopic surgery, and spinal fusion. Insertion of central venous lines and nerve blocks of the upper extremities are other possible etiologies. Diagnosis is made with a portable CXR in the sitting position. In the presence of hemodynamic instability (tension pneumothorax), a tube thoracostomy must be performed even without CXR confirmation. Treatment of pneumothorax is discussed in Chapter 21.

C. **Upper airway obstruction** may occur during recovery from anesthesia. Principal signs are the lack of adequate air movement, intercostal and suprasternal retractions, and discoordinate abdominal and chest wall motion during inspiration. Complete upper airway obstruction is silent, whereas partial obstruction is accompanied by snoring (if the obstruction is above the larynx) or inspiratory stridor (if perilaryngeal). Obstruction is more commonly seen in patients with obstructive sleep apnea (OSA), obesity, or obstruction due to tonsillar or adenoidal hypertrophy. While **100% O_2** is given by mask, swift airway management is required from the PACU anesthesiologist. Oftentimes, a chin lift, with or without jaw thrust, may be all it takes to relieve the obstruction (see Chapter 13). Patients with OSA may benefit from the use of continuous positive airway pressure, especially if they use it at home on a regular basis. Common etiologies for upper airway obstruction include the following:

1. **Incomplete recovery** from general anesthesia and/or neuromuscular blockade (see section VI.B). Decreased strength and coordination of the intrinsic and extrinsic airway musculature causes the tongue to fall backward and occlude the airway. Patency is reestablished by inserting a nasal or oral airway, by manually assisting ventilation, or by intubating the trachea.

2. **Laryngospasm** may be precipitated by light anesthesia and irritation of the glottis by secretions, blood, or a foreign body (see Chapter 18).

3. **Airway edema** may occur during bronchoscopy, esophagoscopy, and surgery of the head and neck. It may also

follow a traumatic intubation, allergic reaction, the administration of large amounts of IV fluids, or prolonged prone position. Children are particularly susceptible to airway obstruction from edema because of the small diameter of their upper airway. The cuff leak test is neither sensitive nor specific and should not be used as the sole test when deciding whether to extubate a patient with suspected airway edema. Treatment of upper airway edema includes the following:

a. Administration of warmed, humidified **100% O$_2$** by face mask.

b. **Head elevation** and **fluid restriction.**

c. Nebulization of racemic **epinephrine** 2.25% solution, 0.5 to 1.0 mL in normal saline, or L-epinephrine, 2 mL of a 1:1,000 solution, which may be repeated in 20 minutes if needed.

d. **Dexamethasone,** 4 to 8 mg IV every 6 hours for 24 hours.

e. Administration of **Heliox** (helium:oxygen, 80:20) can dramatically improve gas exchange and the work of breathing while awaiting the response to other medical treatments.

f. **Reintubation** of the trachea must be considered early because distortion of airway anatomy may occur rapidly, especially with allergic reactions.

4. **Wound hematoma.** Bleeding at the surgical site may complicate thyroid, parathyroid surgery, neck dissections, and carotid endoarterectomy. The pressure caused by an expanding hematoma within the neck tissue planes causes obstruction of venous and lymphatic drainage and massive edema. Patients complain of local pain and pressure, dysphagia, and variable degrees of respiratory distress and may have drainage from the surgical site. Neck wound hematomas must be treated by emergency reexploration and evacuation in the OR. The surgeon should be notified immediately and an OR prepared. The anesthesiologist must support the airway by mask ventilation with 100% O$_2$, followed by intubation of the trachea under direct vision. If tracheal intubation cannot be rapidly accomplished, the wound must be reopened in the PACU to relieve tissue congestion and improve airway patency.

5. **Vocal cord (VC) paralysis** may occur after thyroid, parathyroid, thoracic, and tracheal surgery or a traumatic endotracheal intubation. VC paralysis may be transient, resulting from manipulation of the recurrent laryngeal nerve, or permanent, from severing the nerve. Unilateral transient VC paralysis is relatively common and the primary concern is potential aspiration of gastric contents. Permanent unilateral VC paralysis is fairly benign. With time, compensatory action of the contralateral VC minimizes the occurrence of aspiration. Bilateral VC paralysis can occur after radical surgery for thyroid or tracheal cancer when neoplastic infiltration makes identification of the recurrent laryngeal nerves virtually impossible. Bilateral VC paralysis is a serious complication that leads to complete upper airway

obstruction immediately after extubation or in the first hours after surgery. It requires emergency endotracheal intubation and, when permanent, necessitates a tracheotomy. Unilateral or bilateral lesions of the superior laryngeal nerve lead to vocal fatigue and a low-pitched voice but no respiratory distress.

D. **The intubated patient** presents special considerations. Spontaneous ventilation through a "T-piece" may be sufficient when prolonged intubation is not foreseen. Some patients require partial or full ventilatory support. The anesthesiologist in the PACU should establish a plan regarding weaning and extubation or, alternatively, possible transfer to an ICU. Conditions that could delay the extubation at the end of the surgery include the following:

1. **Delayed emergence from general anesthesia** due to volatile or IV agents. Reversal may be facilitated pharmacologically (see section VI.B.1.a), but generally it is prudent to support ventilation while the respiratory depression resolves spontaneously. The presence of a full stomach mandates additional vigilance in observing the recovery of pharyngeal reflexes and consciousness before extubation.

2. **Inadequate reversal of neuromuscular blockade.** If muscle weakness persists after adequate pharmacologic reversal (see section VI.B.2.b), the patient needs mechanical support until full recovery is achieved.

3. **Inadequate gas exchange.** Decreased O_2 and CO_2 exchange often resolves as the effects of anesthesia, surgery, and positioning fade. While supporting ventilation, possible etiologies, discussed in sections VI.A and VI.B, must be considered.

4. **Potential for airway obstruction** exists after head and neck procedures, drainage of pharyngeal abscesses, mandibular wiring, or prolonged surgeries, especially in the prone position. These patients should not be extubated until fully awake. If airway edema is suspected, the patient should be treated as outlined in section VI.C.3.

5. **Hemodynamic instability,** when severe, may be associated with a variable degree of impaired gas exchange and/or consciousness that mandate continuation of mechanical ventilation. Transfer to an ICU should be arranged for patients who fail to improve.

6. **Hypothermia** has numerous adverse effects that may make extubation undesirable immediately after surgery (see section XI.A).

E. **Guidelines for extubation.** There is no single value or ventilatory parameter that will predict a successful extubation with certainty. The following criteria may be used when assessing the readiness to resume unassisted ventilation in a postoperative patient:

1. Adequate **arterial oxygen pressure** (Pa_{O_2}) or oxygen saturation (Sp_{O_2}).

2. Adequate **breathing pattern.** Patients should be able to sustain spontaneous, unlabored breathing at a slow rate (<30 breaths per minute) and adequate tidal volume (>300 mL), as can be easily tested in a 10-minute trial of unsupported breathing.

3. Adequate **level of consciousness** for cooperation and airway protection.

4. Full **recovery of muscle strength.**

5. Before proceeding with **extubation,** the PACU anesthesiologist should be aware of preexisting airway problems in the event that reintubation is necessary. Supplemental O_2 is administered; the endotracheal tube, mouth, and pharynx are suctioned; and the tube is removed after a positive-pressure breath. Oxygen is then supplied by face-mask as indicated, SpO_2 is monitored, and the patient is assessed for signs of airway obstruction or ventilatory insufficiency.

VII. **Renal complications.** Acute renal failure in the postoperative period significantly increases the morbidity and mortality of the surgical patient. The physiology, diagnosis, and treatment of renal abnormalities are described in Chapter 4. Three main conditions may be encountered in the PACU.

A. **Oliguria** is defined as a urine output of less than 0.5 mL/kg/hour. **Hypovolemia** is the most frequent cause of postoperative oliguria. Administration of a fluid bolus (250 to 500 mL of crystalloid or a synthetic colloid), even when other etiologies are not yet excluded, is acceptable. Further diagnostic tests (e.g., plasma and urine electrolytes) and invasive monitoring should be considered when oliguria persists. **Diuretics** (see Chapter 4) should be used only when deemed necessary, such as in congestive heart failure and chronic renal insufficiency. The unwarranted use of diuretics may aggravate preexisting renal hypoperfusion and worsen kidney damage. Temporary maintenance of urine output via forced diuresis does not improve the prognosis of acute renal failure. The traditional algorithm of pre-, post-, and intrarenal causes is helpful in the approach to the postoperative patient with oliguria.

1. **Prerenal** oliguria includes conditions that decrease renal perfusion pressure. Besides **hypovolemia,** other causes of decreased cardiac output must be considered (see section V.A.4). Abdominal compartment syndrome from high intra-abdominal pressures (i.e., intraperitoneal hemorrhage, massive ascites) can also reduce renal perfusion. Analysis of urine electrolytes (see Chapter 4) will reveal a low urinary sodium concentration (<10 mEq/L).

2. **Intrarenal** causes of postoperative oliguria include acute tubular necrosis secondary to hypoperfusion (e.g., hypotension, hypovolemia, sepsis), toxins (e.g., nephrotoxic drugs, myoglobinuria), and trauma. Urinalysis may show granular casts.

3. **Postrenal** causes include urinary catheter obstruction, trauma, and iatrogenic damage to the ureters.

B. **Polyuria,** defined as a urine output disproportionately high for a given fluid intake, is less frequent. Symptomatic treatment is based on volume replacement to maintain hemodynamic stability and adequate fluid balance. Electrolyte and acid-base equilibrium may be perturbed secondary to the etiologic condition or to large volume loss. The differential diagnosis includes the following:

1. **Excessive volume** administration, requiring simple observation in healthy subjects.

2. **Pharmacologic** diuresis.

3. **Postobstructive diuresis** after resolution of urinary obstruction.

4. **Nonoliguric renal failure.** Acute tubular necrosis may cause transient polyuria due to the loss of concentrating function of the tubules.

5. **Osmotic diuresis** may be caused by hyperglycemia, hypercalcemia, alcohol intoxication, and administration of hypertonic saline, mannitol, or parenteral nutrition.

6. **Diabetes insipidus** secondary to the lack of antidiuretic hormone may follow head injury or intracranial surgery.

C. **Electrolyte disturbances.** Renal failure may induce **hyperkalemia** and acidemia that can develop within hours and need to be corrected emergently to avoid ventricular dysrhythmias and death (see Chapter 4). Polyuria may cause profound dehydration, with massive potassium losses and resulting alkalemia. **Hypokalemia,** often associated with **hypomagnesemia,** may also trigger atrial and ventricular dysrhythmias, although not as severe as those associated with hyperkalemia. Potassium should be replaced cautiously to avoid overdose. Magnesium replacement may effectively treat atrial and ventricular dysrhythmias, especially if the latter are in the form of torsades de pointes.

VIII. **Neurologic complications**

A. **Delayed awakening**

1. The most frequent cause of delayed awakening is **persistent effects of anesthetics** (see section VI.B). Less common but possibly life-threatening causes include the organic cerebral events described below.

2. **Decreased cerebral perfusion** of sufficient duration, during or after surgery, may cause diffuse or localized cerebral damage responsible for obtundation and delayed awakening. In patients with cerebrovascular disease, short periods of hypotension may cause a critical reduction of cerebral perfusion and brain damage. If such an event is suspected, a neurologic consultation should be obtained as soon as possible and specific tests (e.g., computed tomography [CT], magnetic resonance imaging [MRI], or angiography) should be considered. If cerebral edema is suspected, treatment should be started immediately (see Chapter 24).

3. **Metabolic causes** of delayed awakening include hypothermia, sepsis, preexisting encephalopathies, hypoglycemia, and electrolyte or acid-base derangements. Cerebral edema from the inadvertent infusion of hypotonic crystalloid solutions has been reported.

B. **Neurologic damage** may be the result of a **stroke** or may be due to peripheral nerve injury (see section VIII.D). Strokes in the perioperative period have an incidence of 0.08% to 2.9% and may be ischemic or hemorrhagic. Early diagnosis of a stroke may be difficult because symptoms such as slurred speech, visual changes, dizziness, agitation, confusion, psychosis, numbness, muscular weakness, and paralysis may overlap with the manifestations of residual anesthetics. **Ischemic strokes** are more common in patients with cerebrovascular disease, hypercoagulable states, and atrial fibrillation, and they may be associated with intraoperative hypotension. Fat emboli secondary to long bone fractures can also lead to strokes. **Hemorrhagic strokes** are more common in patients with coagulopathies, uncontrolled hypertension, cerebral aneurysms or arteriovenous malformations, and head trauma. Strokes are more frequent after intracranial surgery, carotid endarterectomy, cardiac surgery, and multiple traumas. Neurologic consultation followed by brain CT or MRI is mandatory to guide the possible choice for immediate, and possibly life-saving, treatment options.

C. **Emergence delirium** is characterized by excitement alternating with lethargy, disorientation, and inappropriate behavior. Delirium may occur in any patient but occurs more frequently in the elderly and in those with a history of drug dependency, dementia, or other psychiatric disorders. Many drugs used perioperatively may precipitate delirium: ketamine, opioids, benzodiazepines, large doses of metoclopramide, anticholinergics (atropine or scopolamine), and droperidol. Delirium may be a symptom of ongoing pathology like hypoxemia, acidemia, hyponatremia, hypoglycemia, intracranial injury, sepsis, severe pain, and alcohol withdrawal that must be investigated. Treatment is symptomatic: supplemental O_2, fluid and electrolyte replacement, and adequate analgesia. Antipsychotic medications such as **haloperidol** (2.5 to 5 mg IV increments every 20 to 30 minutes) may be indicated. Benzodiazepines (**diazepam,** 2.5 to 5 mg IV, **lorazepam,** 1 to 2 mg IV) may be added if agitation is severe. **Physostigmine** (0.5 to 2.0 mg IV) may reverse delirium due to anticholinergic agents.

D. **Peripheral neurologic lesions** may follow improper intraoperative positioning or direct surgical damage or may be a complication of regional anesthetic techniques. In the ASA closed-claim analysis, ulnar nerve injury accounted for about a third of the cases of nerve injury, followed by damage of the brachial plexus and the common peroneal nerve. The risk factors for nerve injury after surgery include thin body habitus, previous history of neuropathy, smoking, and diabetes. Other sites of possible nerve damage are the wrist (median and ulnar nerve), internal aspect of the arm (radial nerve), and the points of emergence of the main branches of the VII cranial nerve, which can be compressed during mask-airway cases. Lithotomy position, especially when prolonged, may result in sciatic, femoral, common peroneal, and saphenous nerve injury. Improper positioning leads to compression or stretching of the nerve with demyelination. Often, remyelination results in recovery in 6 to 8 weeks. Nevertheless, recovery may be more prolonged and, in some instances, the injuries are permanent. Early neurologic consultation for diagnosis and rehabilitation is crucial for a full recovery.

E. **Awareness and recall** are rare complications of general anesthesia (0.13% in a large multicenter trial) that can be first detected in the PACU. These are often the consequences of light anesthetic techniques and occur especially after trauma, cardiac, and obstetric surgery. Risk factors include young age, history of substance abuse, ASA physical status III to V, and the use of muscular relaxants. The use of a BIS monitor may decrease the incidence of awareness by allowing the anesthesiologist to appreciate the depth of anesthesia (see Chapter 10). The long-term effects of awareness under general anesthesia range from mild anxiety to overt posttraumatic stress disorder. A short interview (modified Brice protocol) should be conducted in the PACU to identify

Table 35.1. Modified Brice protocol

What is the last thing you remember before going to sleep for the operation?

What is the first thing you remember on waking after the operation?

Do you remember anything between going to sleep and waking up?

Did you have any dreams?

What was the most unpleasant thing you remember from the operation and anesthesia?

---

patients with recall (Table 35.1). Patients with recall should receive reassurance and sympathetic care. Referral for psychological counseling should also be considered.

IX. **Principles of pain management** are described in Chapter 38. Adequate analgesia begins in the OR and continues in the PACU.

    A. **Opioids** (IV or epidural) are the mainstay of postoperative analgesia.

        1. **Fentanyl,** a potent synthetic opioid with a rapid onset of action, is commonly limited to the operative setting. Occasionally, however, small IV doses (25 to 50 μg IV) can be titrated postoperatively to establish rapid analgesia.

        2. **Morphine,** 2 to 4 mg IV, may be repeated every 10 to 20 minutes until adequate analgesia is achieved. In children above 1 year of age, 15 to 20 μg/kg IV or IM, can be safely administered at 30- to 60-minute intervals.

        3. **Meperidine,** 25 to 50 mg IV, is similarly effective. It lacks the vagotonic effect of other opiates and may reduce postanesthetic shivering. **Meperidine must be avoided in patients taking monoamine oxidase inhibitors** and must be administered cautiously in patients with renal insufficiency.

    B. **Nonsteroidal** anti-inflammatory drugs (NSAIDs) and **acetaminophen** are effective complements to opioids. **Ketorolac,** 30 mg IV followed by 15 mg every 6 to 8 hours, provides potent postoperative analgesia. Other nonselective NSAIDs (**ibuprofen, naproxen,** and **indomethacin**) are also effective. Potential toxicities of all NSAIDs include decreased platelet aggregation, gastrointestinal bleeding, and nephrotoxicity. The cyclooxygenase-2 (COX-2) inhibitors (valdecoxib, celecoxib) offer similar analgesia but have been shown to increase the incidence of cardiovascular events (myocardial infarction, thrombotic stroke, hypertension, heart failure), especially in patients at risk for such events. In 2005, the FDA recommended increased caution in prescribing these drugs and a careful assessment of the risk-to-benefit ratio for each individual patient. The use of COX-2 inhibitors should be limited to patients for whom there are no appropriate alternatives or for whom those alternatives have been exhausted. They should be used in the lowest dose and for the shortest duration necessary. Similar to nonselective NSAIDs, COX-2 inhibitors have platelet toxicity, thus predisposing to bleeding complications, and nephrotoxicity. On the other hand, they may have a lower incidence of adverse gastrointestinal effects.

    C. **Adjuvant analgesics** include spasmolytics (**cyclobenzaprine**) and small doses of benzodiazepines and neuroleptics.

    D. **Regional sensory blocks** can be very effective postoperatively (see Chapter 17).

    E. **IV patient-controlled analgesia (PCA)** has been shown to be superior in patient satisfaction compared with intermittent analgesia administered by the medical staff.

    F. **Continuous epidural analgesia** should be continued postoperatively or promptly initiated in the PACU if not used in the OR.

X. **Postoperative nausea and vomiting (PONV)** is a common complication of general anesthesia and less often of regional anesthesia. An algorithm for managing PONV is presented in Figure 35.1. Patients are stratified preoperatively with regard to their risk of PONV. The incidence of PONV is higher in women, nonsmokers, and patients with a history of PONV or motion sickness, and when opioids, nitrous oxide, volatile anesthetics, and neostigmine are used. Certain types

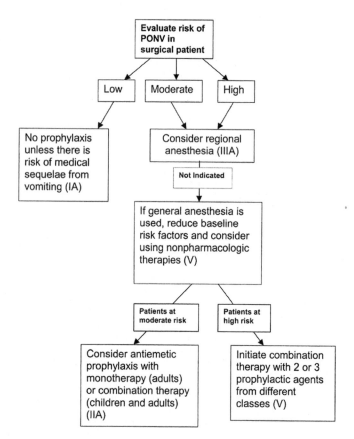

Figure 35.1. Algorithm for management of PONV.

of surgery (strabismus, abdominal, breast, ENT, and neurosurgery) as well as prolonged surgeries may also increase the risk for PONV. PONV prophylaxis is not recommended in individuals believed to be at minimal risk, such as young males undergoing minimally invasive procedures (hernia repair). Patients with higher risk for PONV should be offered, if possible, a regional anesthetic technique, or they should receive antiemesis prophylaxis before or during the surgery. Monotherapy or a combination of two or three antiemetic drugs from different classes is recommended along with measures aimed to diminish the baseline risk factors for PONV: preoperative anxiolysis, use of propofol for induction and maintenance of anesthesia, total IV anesthesia, adequate hydration, and perioperative supplemental oxygen. If PONV occurs in a patient who has not received prophylaxis, therapy should be initiated with a serotonin antagonist and supplemented, if necessary, with medications from other classes. In patients who have received prophylaxis, rescue therapy should consist of drugs from classes other than the ones already administered. Administration of drugs from the same class within the first 6 hours after surgery has not been found to be effective in treating PONV. Common agents include the following:

1. **Transdermal scopolamine** (1.5 mg) is effective in prophylaxis if applied at least 4 hours before the end of the surgery. It may cause visual changes and sedation.

2. **Dexamethasone** (2 to 8 mg IV) is most effective for prophylaxis if administered before the induction of anesthesia. It can also be used as a rescue drug.

3. **Serotonin antagonists** (**ondansetron** 4 to 8 mg IV, **granisetron** 0.35 to 1 mg IV, **dolasetron** 12.5 mg IV) are efficient as prophylactic antiemetics, especially when administered at the end of surgery. About one-quarter of the doses used for prophylaxis can be used for rescue therapy.

4. **Haloperidol** (1 mg IV) may be as effective as ondansetron 4 mg IV in preventing and treating PONV and is significantly less expensive.

5. **Phenothiazines** (**promethazine** 12.5 to 25 mg IV, **prochlorperazine** 5 to 10 mg IV) have been used for prevention and treatment of PONV. They can be associated with significant sedation.

6. **Dimenhydrinate** (1 to 2 mg /kg IV) is used for prophylaxis and treatment of PONV. The major side effect is sedation.

7. **Droperidol** (0.625 to 1.25 mg IV) is no longer used as the first-line drug for the prevention and treatment of PONV. A "black box" warning issued in 2001 by the FDA associated droperidol with QT segment prolongation and torsades de pointes in some patients. Documentation of a normal QT segment before droperidol administration and continuous ECG monitoring for 2 to 3 hours thereafter are recommended. It is now generally used only for the treatment of PONV that has been refractory to other drugs.

XI. **Body temperature changes**

   A. Postoperative **hypothermia** causes vasoconstriction with secondary elevation of blood pressure, increased myocardial contractility, and tissue hypoperfusion; it impairs platelet function and clot formation and may increase the risk of bleeding. Changes in cardiac repolarization such as prolongation of the QT interval may induce dysrhythmias. In addition, the metabolism of various drugs is slowed and may result in prolonged recovery from the neuromuscular blockade. During rewarming, shivering significantly increases O_2 consumption and CO_2 production, which may be undesirable in patients with limited cardiopulmonary reserve. Hypothermia in the postoperative period can increase length of stay in PACU, wound infection rates, and cardiac morbidity. Heated blankets, forced warm air blankets, and warm IV solutions should be used to correct hypothermia (see Chapter 18 section VII).

B. Etiologies of **hyperthermia** include infection, transfusion reaction (see Chapter 34 section VIII.A), hyperthyroidism (see Chapter 6 section III), **malignant hyperthermia** (see Chapter 18 section XVII), and neuroleptic malignant syndrome (see Chapter 18 section XVII.F). Symptomatic treatment should be limited to situations in which hyperthermia is potentially dangerous, such as in young children or patients with compromised respiratory or cardiac reserve (see Chapter 18 section VIII). **Acetaminophen** (suppositories 650 to 1,300 mg or 10 mg/kg in children) and cooling blankets are commonly used.

XII. Recovery from regional anesthesia

A. Uncomplicated regional blocks do not require recovery in the PACU. Postoperative monitoring is indicated when heavy sedation was administered, when a complication from the block occurred (e.g., intravascular injection of a local anesthetic, pneumothorax), or when required by the nature of the surgery (e.g., carotid endarterectomy).

B. Recovery from spinal and epidural anesthesia progresses from cephalad to caudad, with sensory blockade waning first (see Chapter 16). Patients should show signs of regression of both sensory and motor blockade before discharge. If recovery seems delayed, a neurologic exam should be performed to investigate the possibility of epidural hematoma or spinal cord damage.

XIII. Criteria for discharge. At the Massachusetts General Hospital, all patients who receive general anesthesia are observed until ready for discharge, with no mandatory minimum recovery time. However, at least 30 minutes of observation after the last dose of opioids (or other respiratory depressant medication) is required to ensure the adequacy of ventilation and oxygenation.

A. To be discharged from the PACU, patients must meet several criteria. They should be easily arousable and oriented or at their baseline. Vital signs should be stable and within normal limits for at least 30 minutes. Pain and nausea should be under control and appropriate IV access secured. The requirement for urination or drinking clear fluids before discharge is not part of a routine discharge protocol and may be required in selected patients only. There should be no obvious surgical complications (e.g., active bleeding) present. Patients who have received neuraxial anesthesia should show signs of regression of both sensory and motor block before discharge. Effective communication with both the surgical team and the ward to which the patient is to be transferred can expedite the discharge of patients from the PACU. Outpatients should be discharged to a responsible adult with written instructions regarding postprocedure diet, medications, etc. and with a phone number to call in case of emergency.

B. **Fast-track recovery** is used for patients who meet certain criteria when they come out of the OR and are deemed ready to bypass the traditional PACU at the discretion of the anesthesia provider. They can be transferred directly to a second-stage recovery unit if they are outpatients or to the floor if they are inpatients. Fast-track recovery criteria include the following:

1. Patient should be awake, alert, oriented (or at the baseline state).
2. Vital signs should be stable (unlikely to require pharmacologic intervention).
3. Oxygen saturation should be 94% or higher on room air (3 minutes or longer) or at baseline.
4. If a muscular relaxant has been used, the patient should be able to perform a 5-second head lift or the train-of-four monitoring should indicate no fade.
5. Nausea and pain should be minimal (unlikely to require parenteral medications).
6. There should be no active bleeding.

   The intraoperative use of short-acting pharmacologic agents (midazolam, propofol, fentanyl, mivacurium, succinylcholine, desflurane, sevoflurane) and certain surgeries (orthopedic or simple gynecological procedures) may make the fast-track recovery more likely.

XIV. **Considerations for pediatric recovery**

A. **PONV** is rare in children younger than 2 years old. After this age and until they reach puberty, children have a PONV incidence that is approximately twice as high as in adults. Certain operations (adenotonsillectomy, strabismus repair, hernia repair, orchidopexy, penile surgery) are associated with increased incidence for PONV. Risk factors, as well as the general principles for prevention and treatment, are similar to those described in adults (see section X). In some studies, serotonin antagonists (**ondansetron,** 50 to 100 μg/kg IV up to 4 mg, **dolasetron** 350 μg/kg IV up to 12.5 mg) appear to be superior to other drugs in the prevention and treatment of PONV in children. **Dexamethasone** 150 μg/kg IV (up to 8 mg), **dimenhydrinate** 0.5 mg/kg IV, **perphenazine** 70 μg/ kg IV (up to 5 mg), **promethazine** 0.25 to 0.5 mg/kg IV (up to 25 mg), and **droperidol** 50 to 75 μg/kg IV (up to 1.25 mg) are possible alternatives. Administration of droperidol requires the same precautions as in adults.

B. **Airway obstruction.** Etiology and the principles of treatment are similar to those used in adults (section VI.C). Active or recent upper respiratory infections increase the risk of postoperative laryngospasm, especially in children with a history of prematurity or reactive airway disease, or when nasal congestion and copious secretions are present. Subglottic edema after extubation (postextubation croup) is associated with concurrent upper respiratory infections, traumatic, repeated or prolonged intubations, tight-fitting endotracheal tubes, and surgeries of the head and neck. The treatment is outlined in section VI.C. Placement of the children in the lateral decubitus position after emergence from anesthesia improves the patency of the upper airway and minimizes the risk of aspiration of gastric contents should vomiting occur.

C. **Agitation** in children may be a normal response upon emergence from anesthesia in a strange, unfamiliar environment and in the absence of their parents. Intraoperative use of volatile anesthetics (especially sevoflurane), ketamine, and atropine as well as inadequately treated pain may increase the incidence of agitation and anxiety. Other causes such as hypoxemia, hypercarbia, hypothermia, hypotension, metabolic disorders, and central nervous system pathology should be considered, investigated, and treated appropriately. Adequate pain control, reassurance, cuddling, and the presence of the parents at the bedside may mitigate the symptoms in most children.

SUGGESTED READING

Amar D. Perioperative atrial tachyarrhythmias. *Anesthesiology* 2002;97:1618–1623.

Apfel CC, Korttila K, Abdalla M, Kerger H. A factorial trial of six interventions for the prevention of postoperative nausea and vomiting. *N Engl J Med* 2004;350:2441–2451.

Apfelbaum JL, Walawander CA, Grasela TH, et al. Eliminating intensive postoperative care in same-day surgery patients using short-acting anesthetics. *Anesthesiology* 2002;97:66–74.

ASA Task Force on Postanesthetic Care. Practice guidelines for postanesthetic care. *Anesthesiology* 2002;96:742–752.

Ballantyne J, Carr D, DeFerranti S, Suarez T, et al. The comparative effects of postoperative analgesic therapies on pulmonary outcome: cumulative meta-analyses of randomized controlled trials. *Anesth Analg* 1998;86:598–612.

Fu ES, Downs JB, Schweiger JW, Miguel RV. Supplemental oxygen impairs detection of hypoventilation by pulse oxymetry. *Chest* 2004;126:1552–1558.

Gan TJ, Meyer T, Apfel CC, Chung F. Consensus guidelines for managing postoperative nausea and vomiting. *Anesth Analg* 2003;97:62–71.

Kluger MT, Bullock FM. Recovery room incidence: a review of 419 reports from the Anaesthetic Incident Monitoring Study (AIMS). *Anaesthesia* 2002;57:1060–1066.

Lindenauer PK, Pekow P, Wang K. Perioperative beta-blocker therapy and mortality after major non cardiac surgery. *N Engl J Med* 2005;353:349–361.

Priebe HJ. Perioperative myocardial infarction-aetiology and prevention. *Br J Anaesth* 2005;95:3–19.

Sebel PS, Bowdle TA, Ghoneim MM, Rampil IJ. The incidence of awareness during anesthesia: a multicenter United States study. *Anesth Analg* 2004;99:833–839.

Thompson A, Balser JR. Perioperative cardiac arrhythmias. *Br J Anaesth* 2004;93:86–94.

Wang K, Asinger RW, Marriott HJL. ST-segment elevations in conditions other than acute myocardial infarction. *N Engl J Med* 2003;349:2128–2135.

Perioperative Respiratory Failure

Amy C. Lu and Luca M. Bigatello

Anesthesiologists are often consulted to assist with perioperative management of the airway (Chapter 13), pulmonary problems (Chapter 3), and ventilatory support. This chapter reviews the basic principles of acute respiratory failure within the context of postoperative care of the surgical patient.

I. **Pathophysiology of postoperative acute respiratory failure.** Gas exchange between the inspired air and the body tissues is governed by three main mechanisms: ventilation, diffusion, and blood flow. Respiratory failure can be viewed as the impairment of one or more of these functions.

   A. **Ventilatory failure: hypoventilation**

   1. **Abnormal control of ventilation**

      a. **Central control of ventilation** occurs by chemoreceptors located in the medulla. Alterations in cerebrospinal fluid (CSF) **pH** are the major stimuli for these receptors. Acute changes in arterial partial pressure of carbon dioxide (**$PaCO_2$**) rapidly affect CSF pH due to the high permeability of the blood–brain barrier to CO_2.

      b. **Peripheral chemoreceptors,** located in the carotid bodies, are sensitive to changes of the arterial partial pressure of oxygen (PaO_2) and, to a lesser extent, the $PaCO_2$. These receptors are responsible for the increase in alveolar ventilation that occurs as the PaO_2 decreases below 60 mm Hg. After bilateral carotid surgery, patients may lose a significant portion of their hypoxic ventilatory response. However, within a normal PaO_2 range, **the $PaCO_2$ is the main determinant of alveolar ventilation,** as alveolar ventilation increases by 1 to 3 L/minute for each 1 mm Hg increase in $PaCO_2$.

      c. **All halogenated inhalational agents** depress hypoxic ventilatory drive, starting with alveolar concentrations as low as 0.1% to 0.3% of the minimal alveolar concentration (see Chapters 11 and 35). Higher concentrations cause a significant decrease in the minute ventilation and generate the characteristic pattern of rapid, shallow breathing. **Opioids** are potent inhibitors of the hypercapnic ventilatory drive. Overnarcotized patients show a slow respiratory rate and tend to become apneic if not stimulated. **Benzodiazepines** also inhibit ventilatory drive, but to a lesser extent than opioids. Other **psychotropic and sedative drugs,** such as phenothiazines (compazine), butyrophenones (droperidol, haloperidol), the newer antipsychotics (quetiapine and olanzepine), major antidepressants (amitriptyline), and antihistamines (benadryl, atarax) have a minimal effect on ventilatory drive unless administered in unusually large doses.

d. **Intracranial pathology** (e.g., traumatic brain injury, neoplasm, or major cerebrovascular accidents) that causes cerebral edema or interrupts the vascular supply to the medulla may affect control of ventilation.

2. **Neuromuscular dysfunction**

a. **Upper motor neuron** lesions can disrupt phrenic nerve (spinal nerves C-3 to C-5) and intercostal and expiratory muscle function (thoracic spinal nerves), resulting in variable degrees of ventilatory dysfunction. These lesions include neoplasms, demyelinating disorders, syringomyelia, and trauma.

b. **Lower motor neurons** supplying the respiratory muscles may be interrupted by trauma or regional anesthesia or affected by diseases including polyneuritis (Guillain-Barré syndrome), amyotrophic lateral sclerosis, and various neuropathies.

c. **Disorders of the neuromuscular junction** include myasthenia gravis, Eaton-Lambert syndrome, organophosphate overdose, and residual neuromuscular blockade (see Chapter 12).

d. In patients who have been critically ill for prolonged periods of time, **malnutrition, infection,** and **polyneuropathy of critical illness** are frequently present and may be responsible for generalized and ventilatory weakness.

e. **Respiratory muscle dysfunction** in the postoperative period may result from a number of causes, including all those listed above in this section. In addition, preexisting respiratory disease may affect the function of the muscle pump in different ways. In **chronic obstructive pulmonary disease (COPD),** flattening of the diaphragm decreases the range of its contraction. In chronic restrictive disease of the chest wall, such as scoliosis, the mechanics of the respiratory muscles can be so altered as to significantly affect their function. Transient impairment of ventilatory function has been documented after upper abdominal and thoracic surgery, primarily related to diaphragmatic dysfunction. Although the extent of such compromise is generally limited, it may become significant when other factors affecting ventilation coexist.

3. **Increased ventilatory load.** Hypoventilation can also occur when the action of the respiratory muscles is hindered by either an increased airway resistance (R_{aw}) or a decreased compliance of the respiratory system (C_{rs}, see section VI).

a. **Increased R_{aw}** is commonly caused by bronchospasm, copious bronchial secretions, compression or narrowing of the airway, and inappropriately small endotracheal tubes (see Chapters 3 and 35).

b. **Decreased C_{rs}** occurs because of pathologic processes of the lung parenchyma (edema, pneumonia, and interstitial fibrosis), pleura (effusions and pneumothorax), or the musculoskeletal apparatus (kyphoscoliosis, increased intra-abdominal pressure).

B. **Diffusion impairment** of O_2 across the pulmonary capillaries is uncommon because capillary Po_2 equilibrates very rapidly with alveolar Po_2 (P_Ao_2). When diffusion is limited, in diseases such as asbestosis, sarcoidosis, collagen vascular diseases, diffuse interstitial fibrosis, and alveolar cell carcinoma, supplemental O_2 is effective to correct hypoxemia.

C. **Ventilation–perfusion ($\dot{V}/\dot{Q}$) mismatch** is the most common cause of hypoxemia associated with acute respiratory failure. Optimal gas exchange depends on the precise match of alveolar ventilation and perfusion. The resting minute ventilation in adults is 4 to 5 L/minute and cardiac output is approximately 5 L/minute, producing a typical $\dot{V}/\dot{Q}$ ratio of 0.8 to 1.0. At the two pathologic extremes of $\dot{V}/\dot{Q}$ mismatch, alveoli that are ventilated but not perfused represent **dead space,** and alveoli that are perfused but not ventilated represent **true shunt** (see section VI). Dead space ventilation causes hypercapnia, and shunt causes hypoxemia. In practice, $\dot{V}/\dot{Q}$ mismatch is far more frequent than alveolar dead space and shunt. Virtually all lung parenchymal pathology (pneumonia, pulmonary edema, acute respiratory distress syndrome, COPD, interstitial lung diseases, etc.) can result in hypoxemia and hypercapnia secondary to $\dot{V}/\dot{Q}$ mismatch.

D. **Insufficient O_2 delivery** is a less common cause of hypoxemia.

1. **Decreased cardiac output** from hypovolemia or congestive heart failure may compromise tissue O_2 supply. The subsequent increase in O_2 extraction by the tissues decreases the venous Po_2 (**mixed venous Po_2 [$P\bar{v}o_2$]**), which in turn may decrease Pao_2.

2. **Increased O_2 demand** can cause hypoxemia. Basal O_2 consumption averages 200 to 250 mL/minute in adults. Hypermetabolic conditions such as fever, increased muscle activity from shivering, seizures, hyperthyroidism, and, to a lesser degree, sepsis may increase tissue O_2 consumption 2- to 10-fold. This may result in a decrease in $P\bar{v}o_2$ and consequently a decrease in Pao_2 (see above section). In patients with limited reserve, such as those with respiratory failure, coronary artery disease, and cerebrovascular disease, this phenomenon may result in significant morbidity.

II. **Diagnosis of respiratory failure**

A. **Clinical findings.** Signs of impending respiratory failure include dyspnea, tachypnea (respiratory rate >30 breaths per minute), bradypnea (respiratory rate <6 breaths per minute), shallow respirations, use of accessory respiratory muscles, dyscoordinate motions of the chest and abdomen, cyanosis, and obtundation.

B. **Arterial blood gas analysis.** A **normal Pao_2** is 90 to 100 mm Hg, and it decreases slightly with age due to progressive worsening of $\dot{V}/\dot{Q}$ match. A Pao_2 less than 60 mm Hg requires consideration and treatment. A **normal $Paco_2$** is 40 mm Hg, and its acute increase may indicate impending respiratory failure. A **normal arterial pH** is 7.40 $\pm$ 0.02; an acute increase of the $Paco_2$ decreases the arterial pH. As a rule of thumb, for each 10 mm Hg of acute increase of $Paco_2$, the pH decreases by 0.08 unit. Longstanding CO_2 retention is associated with a nearly normal pH because of bicarbonate reabsorption by the kidneys.

C. **A portable chest radiograph (CXR)** obtained at the bedside may reveal acute pathology such as edema, pneumonia, lung collapse, pleural effusion, and pneumothorax. More accurate imaging of the thorax is provided by **computed tomography (CT).** Given the rapid time of execution of the test, its noninvasiveness, and its relatively low cost, chest CT should be performed whenever possible as an alternative or in addition to portable CXR. If pulmonary embolism is suspected, a **helical CT scan** or **pulmonary angiogram** should be obtained (see Chapter 18). In elderly patients and in those with known risk factors for coronary artery disease, a 12-lead **electrocardiogram** (ECG) may diagnose an acute coronary syndrome that may be the cause or a consequence of the respiratory distress. **Fiberoptic bronchoscopy** may diagnose airway pathology and provide samples for microbiological and pathological analysis. Bronchoscopy can also be therapeutic, by removing excessive bronchial secretions, thus facilitating ventilation and gas exchange. However, bronchoscopy in nonintubated or unstable patients should be performed by experienced clinicians to avoid hypoventilation and hypoxemia.

III. **Treatment**

A. **Supplemental O_2. Hypoxemia is life-threatening** and must always be treated promptly.

1. **Low-flow O_2 systems** are simple and readily available. They produce a limited and variable inspired O_2 concentration (FIO_2) that is inversely proportional to the patient's peak inspiratory flow rate and minute ventilation.

a. **Nasal cannulae** increase the FIO_2 by approximately 0.04 (4%) per L minute of O_2. Flows above 4 L/minute dry the nasal mucosa and may produce nasal irritation and bleeding. The nasal passages must be patent, although nose breathing is not required because of the effective anatomic reservoir of the upper airway.

b. **Simple masks** increase the FIO_2 to 0.55 or 0.60 by virtue of higher O_2 flow rates and reservoir space.

c. **Masks with reservoir bags** (nonrebreathing masks) increase FIO_2 further. With a good seal, an FIO_2 of 0.60 to 0.80 can be reached.

d. **Venturi masks** deliver a more precise FIO_2, from 0.24 to 0.50, by entraining a set ratio of room air to oxygen. The inspired FIO_2 is independent of the inspiratory flow rate at flow rates below 40 L/minute. As the FIO_2 increases above 0.40, higher oxygen flow rates are required because of the higher O_2/air entrainment ratio; thus actual FIO_2 may be lower than indicated.

2. **High-flow systems** provide gas flows to meet the patient's peak inspiratory flow rate (30 to 120 L/minute). The maximum FIO_2 depends mainly on the face mask fit and can approach 1.0. High-flow systems should always be humidified to avoid excessive drying of the airway mucosa (see below).

B. **Secretion clearance.** Retained secretions increase airway resistance and promote alveolar collapse. Secretion clearance may be facilitated in several ways.

1. **Humidification and warming of inspired gases.** Administration of dry and cold inspired gas irritates the respiratory mucosa, dries bronchial secretions, and depletes the airways of moisture and heat. **Humidified respiratory circuits** facilitate humidification of the most distal airways. Alternatively, **passive heat and moisture exchangers** can be placed between the endotracheal tube and the breathing circuit.

2. **Suctioning.** Bronchial ciliary function is compromised after anesthesia, endotracheal intubation, and respiratory infections. Pain, sedation, and general debilitation can limit patients' ability to cough and expel secretions. Blind nasotracheal suctioning effectively clears tracheal secretions and stimulates coughing but must be used with caution because it may cause hypoxemia, vagal stimulation, bronchospasm, and mucosal trauma.

3. **Chest physical therapy.** Properly performed percussion, vibration, and postural drainage are effective means of clearing secretions and preventing mucus plugging. Incentive spirometry (maximum deep inspiration with end-inspiratory hold) is also effective.

4. **Mucolytics.** Local instillation of **acetylcysteine** (mucomyst, 2 to 5 mL of 5% to 20% solution every 6 to 8 hours) may decrease mucus viscosity by reducing glycoprotein disulfide bonds. When nebulized, acetylcysteine may precipitate bronchospasm; mixing it with 0.5 mL of albuterol is helpful.

5. **Bronchoscopy** (see section II.C) is an effective way to remove secretions and thick mucus plugs from the airways.

C. **Pharmacologic therapy**

1. **Reversal of ventilatory depression.** Numerous drugs can depress alveolar ventilation (see section I.A.1.c). Although their effect can be reversed by pharmacologic antagonists (**naloxone** for opioids, **flumazenil** for benzodiazepines, see Chapters 11 and 35), they must be used with great caution. Reversal of sedation can be associated with hypertension, tachycardia, ECG changes (particularly with naloxone), acute loss of the effects of the original drug, and the possibility of later renarcotization due to their short duration of action.

2. **Reversal of residual neuromuscular blockade** should be carried out to avoid ventilatory failure and inadequate airway protection (see Chapter 12).

3. **Analgesia.** Pain from surgical incisions, trauma, and invasive procedures may hinder the effectiveness of ventilation. Numerous analgesic options are available (see Chapter 38).

4. **Bronchodilation.** Agents used to treat acute bronchospasm can be administered by inhalation, nebulization, or intravenously (see Chapters 3 and 18).

5. **Treatment of the underlying condition** must be instituted. This includes hemodynamic control, treatment of infections, dysrhythmias, myocardial ischemia, anemia, etc. Broad-spectrum **antibiotics** should be started immediately if the diagnosis of infectious pneumonia is made. Antimicrobial therapy can later be tailored on the basis of culture results.

D. Mechanical ventilation treats hypoxemia by delivering high FIO_2 and positive pressure to the alveoli and treats hypercarbia by assisting the patients' minute ventilation ($\dot{V}_E$).

1. **Noninvasive ventilation.**

   a. Mechanical ventilation can be delivered without tracheal intubation. In postoperative patients, adequate levels of support in the form of either noninvasive **continuous positive airway pressure (CPAP)** or noninvasive **positive pressure ventilation (NPPV)** are best administered through an orofacial mask. If a specialized ventilator is not available, a standard critical care ventilator is effective. CPAP or NPPV avoid the need for tracheal intubation in selected patients with acute respiratory failure, including those with transient postoperative hypoxemia, respiratory distress after pulmonary resection, acute congestive heart failure, and acute hypercarbia from hypoventilation.

   b. An experienced clinician (often a respiratory therapist) who will properly fit the mask and set the ventilator is critical to the success of noninvasive ventilation. The most common cause of failure is the inability of the patient to tolerate the discomfort of the tight face mask and high gas flow. It is important to recognize the failure of noninvasive ventilation and proceed to tracheal intubation to avoid patient exhaustion and respiratory arrest.

   c. A common side effect of noninvasive ventilation is **gastric distention** from air insufflation, which can predispose to vomiting and aspiration. The use of noninvasive ventilation immediately after abdominal surgery should be discussed with the surgeon. When deemed safe, gastric distention can be effectively treated by continuous nasogastric suction.

   d. Current evidence suggests that noninvasive ventilation **does not decrease the need for reintubation** after a failed tracheal extubation, nor does it reduce long-term mortality.

2. **Endotracheal intubation** remains the most common way to deliver positive pressure ventilation during acute respiratory failure.

E. Modes of mechanical ventilation. Many postoperative patients require a limited period of mechanical ventilation for relatively simple reasons such as airway protection, residual sedation, or neuromuscular blockade. In these patients, the management of mechanical ventilation can be kept simple. In patients with acute respiratory failure who require an extensive period on the ventilator, implementation of mechanical ventilation is complex and it is beyond the scope of this chapter. **Different terms** are used to define modes of ventilation; often, near-identical modes have completely different names. In the following sections, we propose a simple system to denote all currently used modes of ventilation (Table 36.1).

1. Three elements are necessary **to define each mechanical breath.**

Table 36.1. System to denote all common modes of mechanical ventilation

Nomenclature

	Volume	Pressure
IMV	Volume-limited IMV	Pressure-limited IMV
ACV	Volume-limited ACV	Pressure-limited ACV
PSV	—	PSV

Volume-controlled versus pressure-controlled ventilation

	Pressure-controlled	Volume-controlled
Tidal volume	Variable	Set
Inspiratory pressure	Limited by pressure control setting	Variable
Inspiratory flow	Variable, descending ramp	Set; constant flow or descending ramp
Inspiratory time	Set directly	Set (flow and volume settings)
Respiratory rate	Minimum set (patient can trigger)	Minimum set (patient can trigger)

IMV, intermittent mandatory ventilation; ACV, assist-control ventilation; PSV, pressure support ventilation.

    a. What initiates (triggers) a mechanical breath: either the ventilator or the patient.

    b. What determines the size of a mechanical breath—that is, what do we set on the ventilator to limit inspiration: a **pressure** or a **volume?**

    c. What ends (cycles off) a mechanical breath: time, flow, or volume?

    d. For example, breaths delivered during pressure support ventilation (PSV, see below) are patient-triggered, pressure-limited, and flow-cycled.

  2. Full versus partial ventilation. When the ventilator provides the entire $\dot{V}_E$ (as is often the case during general anesthesia), the terms **full** or **mandatory** ventilation are used. When the patient contributes to the $\dot{V}_E$, (as often occurs during postoperative ventilation), the terms **partial** or **assisted** ventilation are used. During **partial ventilation,** spontaneous breaths can be interspersed with mandatory breaths in different ways:

    a. Intermittent mandatory ventilation (IMV). The ventilator delivers a set number of breaths per minute of a set size, and the patient may breathe unsupported between mandatory breaths. A very simple mode of ventilation, and once the most popular, it has been largely substituted by the two modes described below.

    b. **Assist-control ventilation (ACV).** The ventilator delivers a set number of breaths per minute, of a set size. When the patient triggers additional breaths, the breath will be supported similar to the mandatory breaths.

    c. **Pressure support ventilation (PSV).** The ventilator delivers a set pressure every time the patient initiates a spontaneous breath and holds that pressure constant until the inspiratory flow rate declines to a predetermined value (generally 25% of the peak inspiratory flow), at which point, inspiration is cycled off. In many ventilators, the percentage of peak inspiratory flow at which the breath is cycled off can be adjusted (expiratory sensitivity) to optimize synchrony. This variable method of ending inspiration results in the most synchronous interaction between patient and ventilator of all three modes described here. Although there is ample discussion in the literature about whether PSV actually provides better support than the other modes, it has become very popular in postoperative patients, because of its simple and apparently effective mode of operation. It is important to note that because every breath must be triggered by the patient, PSV does not provide a baseline mandatory support; for this reason, it may be combined with IMV.

3. **Volume** versus **pressure-limited ventilation. Volume ventilation** has the advantage of guaranteeing a set $\dot{V}_E$. This, however, may at times produce dangerously high alveolar pressures. **Pressure ventilation** ensures a limit of inspiratory pressure. This, however, may occur at the expense of the $\dot{V}_E$. Hence, the choice between the two modalities may be dictated by individual patient needs. A potential advantage of pressure-limited ventilation is that it delivers a high and variable inspiratory flow rate (as high as 180 L/minute and more). This feature obviates a significant problem of traditional volume ventilation; the inspiratory flow rate often does not match the patient's demand, resulting in dysynchrony, excessive respiratory work, and fatigue.

4. The combination of the settings described above (full versus partial, volume versus pressure) generates five possible modes of ventilation, illustrated in Table 36.1. Other modes are available; however, these basic five modes should be more than sufficient to properly ventilate most patients in the initial stages of acute postoperative respiratory failure.

5. **Additional ventilator settings.**

    a. **The F_{IO_2}** is usually set at 1.0 (100%) immediately after mechanical ventilation is instituted, and then it is progressively reduced to maintain a PaO_2 above 60 mm Hg and/or an arterial O_2 saturation (SpO_2) above 90%.

    b. **Positive end-expiratory pressure (PEEP)** maintains alveolar recruitment, decreases intrapulmonary shunt, and increases functional residual capacity. A PEEP value of 5 cm H_2O provides a reasonable starting point when initiating postoperative mechanical ventilation. The term **CPAP** (see also section III.D.1) is used when PEEP is applied without additional support of patient-initiated breaths.

   c. Minute ventilation ($\dot{V}_E$ = tidal volume × respiratory rate) is the main determinant of CO_2 elimination (section I.A). A normal value of $\dot{V}_E$ is 5 to 6 L/minute. Patients with postoperative acute respiratory failure may have increased ventilation requirements because of fever, shivering, or increased dead space fraction.

F. Complications of mechanical ventilation

  1. O₂ toxicity. High FIO_2 over long periods of time causes acute tracheobronchitis, impairment of ciliary motion, and alveolar damage. However, when administered for short periods of time, such as in postoperative ventilation, toxicity does not constitute a significant issue. A possible exception may occur in patients who have been exposed to **bleomycin,** a chemotherapeutic agent that may act in synergy to a high O_2 concentration in causing alveolar damage. More relevant to the postoperative period is that a high FIO_2 causes **absorption atelectasis,** the consequence of full absorption of the alveolar gas when little or no nitrogen is present.

  2. Ventilator-induced lung injury (VILI). Mechanical ventilation can injure the lung. High alveolar pressures caused by large ventilatory volumes worsen preexistent acute lung injury (ALI) and lead to poor outcome. While the occurrence of VILI is undisputed during the course of ALI/acute respiratory distress syndrome (ARDS), the need to limit ventilating volumes and pressures in all patients with acute respiratory failure has not been clearly demonstrated. Nevertheless, it seems sensible to avoid excessive ventilatory pressures and volumes even in the absence of definite ALI/ARDS.

  3. Hemodynamic dysfunction

    a. Positive pressure ventilation increases intrathoracic pressure and decreases venous return to the heart.

     (1) Right ventricular (RV) filling is limited by the reduced venous return. High ventilatory pressures may also increase pulmonary vascular resistance and RV afterload, further decreasing RV output.

     (2) Left ventricular (LV) filling is limited by the reduced RV output. Increased RV size also affects LV performance by shifting the interventricular septum to the left and decreasing LV diastolic compliance.

     (3) Intravascular volume replacement counteracts these hemodynamic effects of positive pressure ventilation.

     (4) Conversely, **LV transmural pressure decreases,** thus increasing LV ejection and stroke volume. This beneficial effect may be especially noticeable in patients with reduced ventricular function.

    b. Decreasing intrathoracic pressure during discontinuation of positive pressure ventilation increases venous return and LV transmural pressure, with effects opposite those described above. Accordingly, in hypovolemic patients RV filling and cardiac output may increase. Conversely, patients with compromised LV function may not tolerate the sudden increase of venous return and may develop pulmonary edema and/or myocardial ischemia.

    c. **Overall,** these effects are of little importance in healthy, normovolemic patients undergoing a short period of postoperative mechanical ventilation. They become clinically relevant in patients with congestive heart failure and hypo- or hypervolemia.

G. Infection. Prolonged tracheal intubation is associated with bacterial colonization of the airways and an increased risk of **nosocomial pneumonia.** Noninvasive ventilation, appropriate use of antibiotic therapy, and good infection control practices limit the incidence of nosocomial pneumonia (see Chapter 7).

H. Miscellaneous ventilatory strategies

    1. Recruitment maneuvers. Acute respiratory failure may be associated with the development of atelectasis, particularly when a lung-protective strategy with low tidal volumes (V_T) is used (see section III.F.2). Under these circumstances, recruitment maneuvers (i.e., applying higher airway pressures for brief periods of time) can be used to recruit atelectatic areas of the lung. Recruitment maneuvers can be carried out in different ways:

        a. Sustained insufflations (SI) of 30 to 60 seconds at pressures higher than the inflating pressure increase the Pao_2 in more than half of the patients with ALI. **Extreme care must be exercised** in selecting candidates for a SI, because the generation of high alveolar pressure may cause severe complications such as hypotension and pneumothorax. We recommend continuous hemodynamic and respiratory monitoring during a SI.

        b. Sighs are periodic large breaths interspersed among the breaths of a set V_T.

        c. When a positive response (an increased Pao_2) to a SI or sighs is observed, increasing the PEEP level will tend to stabilize the lung at a higher inflation status and prolong the beneficial effect. Nevertheless, most of the time the effect of a recruitment maneuver is transient, and no study has demonstrated a benefit beyond a transient increase in Pao_2.

    2. Neuromuscular blockade can facilitate mechanical ventilation by increasing chest wall compliance and enhancing patient-ventilator synchrony. Nondepolarizing muscle relaxants can be given by continuous infusion, and their effects can be monitored clinically and with a peripheral nerve stimulator (see Chapter 12). The prolonged use of muscle relaxants has been associated with an increased incidence of polyneuropathy of critical illness.

    3. Inhaled nitric oxide (NO) transiently increases Pao_2 by improving $\dot{V}/\dot{Q}$ match. Currently, the use of inhaled NO in adult patients with hypoxemia is limited to a role of rescue therapy, as a bridge to more permanent interventions.

IV. Weaning from mechanical ventilation. Most patients with postoperative respiratory failure wean rapidly from ventilatory support once the etiologic condition is treated. For a small number of patients, withdrawing ventilatory support is difficult. Most of these patients have associated conditions that may compromise their ability to breathe unsupported, including preexistent pulmonary disease, heart disease, neuromuscular disease, infection, and malnutrition. Successful withdrawal of mechanical ventilation depends on the ability to tailor the process to the needs of the individual patient by avoiding muscle atrophy, fatigue, distress, and hemodynamic compromise.

A. **Weaning techniques include the following:**

1. **Progressive withdrawal of ventilatory support.** The patient's contribution to minute ventilation is gradually increased until he or she reaches a level where mechanical support is no longer necessary. This method of withdrawal of ventilatory support seems to be accomplished best by progressively decreasing the level of **PSV** (see section III.E.2.c).

2. **Alternating full ventilation with unsupported breathing.** Full ventilatory support, generally delivered with ACV (see section III.E.2.b), provides muscle rest, ideal gas exchange, and hemodynamic stability. Ventilatory support is interrupted at least once a day, and the patient is allowed to breathe unsupported, either on a **T-piece** or on the ventilator with 0 inspiratory pressure and 0 PEEP **(spontaneous breathing trial, SBT).** The latter permits continuous evaluation of the respiratory parameters on the ventilator display. **SBTs** provide the clinician the opportunity to observe the patient's response to withdrawal of mechanical support without removing the endotracheal tube. Extubation should proceed when judged safe. This strategy may decrease the chance of premature extubation while avoiding unnecessary prolongation of mechanical ventilation.

3. Both techniques have been proven effective, with the key to success being the **SBT.** Although initially described only in combination with full support (see section IV.A.2), SBTs are currently used as the endpoint of any weaning strategy. Studies have shown that a weaning protocol including daily SBTs carried out by respiratory therapists resulted in earlier successful tracheal extubation than a withdrawal guided by traditional physician's orders.

B. **Measures of weaning potential.**

1. **To initiate the process of withdrawal from mechanical ventilation,** there should be evidence of clearing of the underlying pathology, acceptable gas exchange, stabilization of acute and chronic respiratory problems (bronchospasm, edema, tracheo-bronchial secretions), stability of concurrent medical conditions, and a neurologic status that ensures protection of the airway once the trachea is extubated.

2. **Subjective symptoms of failure** to sustain unsupported ventilation include dyspnea, fatigue, chest discomfort, anxiety, confusion, and restlessness.

3. **Objective evaluation** includes assessment of the ventilatory pattern, associated hemodynamics, and of the general appearance of the patient during an SBT. Many predictors of successful extubation have been suggested, but their applicability to each individual patient is limited. Nevertheless, desirable clinical parameters in adults include a $V_T > 300$ mL with a respiratory rate <30 breaths per minute, a vital capacity sufficient to generate an effective cough (ideally ≥ 700 to 800 mL), a $\dot{V}_E$ <10 L/minute, and a maximum negative inspiratory pressure of 30 cm H_2O or more.

V. **Thoracostomy tubes (Fig. 36.1).** Commercial "three-bottle" systems are commonly used to drain the pleural space. The proximal bottle traps the drainage, the middle bottle is the water seal that prevents air and fluid from being drawn into the thorax, and the distal bottle regulates the level of suction applied to the pleural cavity. The negative pressure is independent of the strength of the wall suction and depends only on the height of the water column in the suction-control chamber. Chest tubes are connected to water seal if minimal air or fluid drainage is expected (e.g., immediately after pneumonectomy) or to suction (usually 10 to 20 cm H_2O) when significant drainage is expected or a pneumothorax needs to be drained.

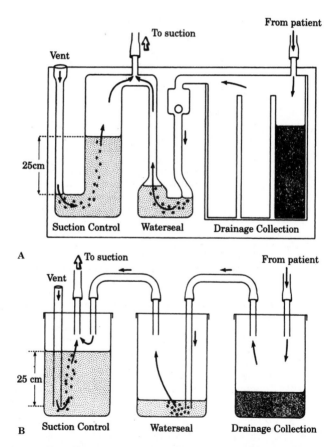

Figure 36.1. Chest tube drainage system. A: Commercial apparatus. The proximal chamber is for pleural drainage, the middle chamber (the water seal) prevents air or fluid from being drawn into the thorax, and the distal chamber regulates the level of suction. B: Traditional three-bottle system is shown for comparison.

When examining a chest tube drainage system, the water seal level should vary with respiration if the chest tube is patent. Bubbling in the water seal chamber with inspiration indicates a bronchopleural leak.

VI. **Respiratory function calculations**

A. **The flow of air** in and out of the lungs during spontaneous as well as mechanical ventilation is opposed by two mechanical variables, the **compliance of the respiratory system (C_{rs}),** and the **resistance of the airways (R_{aw}).**

1. **Measurement of C_{rs} and R_{aw}.** C_{rs} is defined as the change in volume that occurs with a change in the pressure applied. A clinically acceptable way to measure compliance is:

$$C_{rs} = V_T/(P_{plat} - PEEP)$$

where P_{plat} is the end-inspiratory pressure measured at the airway after an end-inspiratory pause. By applying an end-inspiratory pause (generally 1 second), the flow rate is decreased to zero or near zero, thereby eliminating the resistive component of breathing. A **normal value of C_{rs} is 80 to 100 mL/cm H_2O.** Patients with chronic restrictive disorders or acute respiratory failure (e.g., from ARDS) can have C_{rs} values as low as 25 mL/cm H_2O or less. At the same time, the R_{aw} can be calculated as:

$$R_{aw} = (P_{ip} - P_{plat})/\dot{V}$$

where P_{ip} is the peak inspiratory pressure, the pressure reached at end-inspiration just before the end-inspiratory pause maneuver. **Normal values of R_{aw} range from 1 to 3 cm H_2O/L/second** and can increase well above 10 cm H_2O/L/second in patients with asthma and/or COPD.

2. **A practical way to measure C_{rs} and R_{aw}** at the bedside in a mechanically ventilated patient is as follows. The patient should be either very cooperative or sedated. Set the ventilator on volume-limited ACV, V_T of 500 mL with a square-wave flow pattern at a flow rate of 60 L/minute (these settings are chosen to simplify the calculations). Once the patient appears comfortable with minimal spontaneous breathing effort, an end-inspiratory pause is applied; this can be accomplished by pushing the appropriate button on most modern ventilators. Figure 36.2 shows a representative tracing of airway pressure over time during an end-inspiratory pause maneuver.

3. **C_{rs} is made up of the individual compliances of the lung and the chest wall** (rib cage and diaphragm), which are nearly equal under normal circumstances. A decrease in the C_{rs} in a patient with acute respiratory failure is generally due to a decrease in the lung component (e.g., from pneumonia, edema, aspiration, etc.). At times, however, a decrease in the compliance of the chest wall rather than the lung may be significant enough to compromise respiration (e.g., from increased intra-abdominal pressure due to severe abdominal distention, tight chest, or abdominal bandages, burn scars, etc.).

B. **The alveolar gas equation** calculates the alveolar Po_2 (P_AO_2). A clinically acceptable version is:

$$P_AO_2 = [(P_{baro} - P_{H_2O}) \times (F_IO_2)] - [Paco_2/RQ]$$

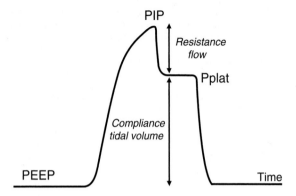

Figure 36.2. Airway pressure over time trace during an end-inspiratory pause maneuver to measure respiratory compliance and resistance at the bedside. P_{IP} = peak inspiratory pressure; P_{plat} = end-inspiratory plateau pressure.

where P_{baro} is the barometric pressure (760 mm Hg at sea level), P_{H_2O} is the water vapor pressure (47 mm Hg when fully saturated), and RQ is the respiratory quotient (usually 0.8). Accordingly, a normal P_{AO_2} while breathing air (0.21 F_{IO_2}) at a normal $\dot{V}_E$ (i.e., normal P_{aCO_2}) is 100 to 105 mm Hg which, with the normal minimal physiologic shunt fraction, results in a P_{aO_2} of approximately 100 mm Hg. This equation is useful for understanding the effects of breathing different O_2 mixtures on gas exchange at different P_{aCO_2} levels.

C. Oxygen content (CaO_2) of arterial blood. CaO_2 = O_2 bound to hemoglobin + O_2 dissolved in blood:

$$CaO_2 = (1.36 \text{ mL } O_2/\text{g hemoglobin}) \times (\text{g hemoglobin/dL})$$
$$\times (SaO_2) + (PaO_2 \times 0.003 \text{ mL } O_2/\text{mm Hg/dL})$$

D. The shunt equation estimates the venous admixture of arterial blood:

$$\dot{Q}_S/\dot{Q}_T = (CcO_2 - CaO_2)/(CaO_2 - C\bar{v}O_2)$$

where CcO_2 is the O_2 content of pulmonary capillary blood and is calculated from the P_{AO_2} (estimated from the alveolar air equation described above).

E. P_{aCO_2} and $\dot{V}_E$ relationship:

$$P_{aCO_2} = P_{ACO_2} = \dot{V}CO_2/\text{alveolar ventilation}$$

where $\dot{V}CO_2$ is the CO_2 production. In normal subjects, the P_{ACO_2} and P_{aCO_2} can be considered identical. The relationship between alveolar ventilation and P_{aCO_2} is of practical importance. For example, if the alveolar ventilation is halved, the P_{aCO_2} will double, if CO_2 production is constant.

Dead space ventilation occurs where ventilation is wasted. This occurs in the proximal airways (**anatomic dead space**) and in those alveoli that are ventilated and not perfused (**alveolar dead space**). The term

physiologic dead space includes anatomic and alveolar dead space and is the ultimate determinant of the $Paco_2$ at constant $\dot{V}co_2$ and $\dot{V}_E$. Expressed as a fraction of the tidal volume (**V_D /V_T**), physiologic dead space is a useful measure of lung dysfunction. Values of 0.7 or more can be seen in patients with severe ALI/ARDS.

$$V_D/V_T = (Paco_2 - P_{\overline{E}}co_2)/Paco_2$$

where $P_{\overline{E}}co_2$ is the mean expired CO_2. If the $P_{\overline{E}}co_2$ is substituted in the equation by the **end-tidal CO_2 ($P_{et}CO_2$)**, the alveolar dead space can be estimated. Under normal circumstances, $P_{et}co_2$ and $Paco_2$ are almost equal, indicating that there is minimal alveolar dead space. $P_{et}co_2$ can be measured by capnography when a clear and steady end-expiratory plateau is present.

SUGGESTED READING

ARDS-*Net* Investigators. Ventilation with lower tidal volumes as compared with traditional tidal volumes for acute lung injury and the acute respiratory distress syndrome. *N Engl J Med* 2000;342:301–308.

Artigas A, Bernard G, Carlet J, et al. The American-European Consensus Conference on ARDS. Part II. *Am J Respir Crit Care Med* 1998;157:1332–1347.

Ware LB, Matthay MA. The acute respiratory distress syndrome. *N Engl J Med* 2000;342:1334–1349.

Lumb AB, Nunn JF. *Nunn's applied respiratory physiology,* 6th ed. Boston: Butterworth-Heinemann, 2005.

West JB. *Respiratory physiology: the essentials,* 7th ed. Philadelphia: Lippincott Williams & Wilkins, 2004.

Metha S, Hill NS. Noninvasive ventilation. *Am J Respir Crit Care Med* 2001;163:540–577.

Meade M, Guyatt G, Cook D, et al. Predicting success in weaning from mechanical ventilation. *Chest* 2001;120:400s–424s.

37

Adult, Pediatric, and Newborn Resuscitation

Bradley E. Randel and Richard M. Pino

I. **Overview. Cardiopulmonary resuscitation (CPR)** in the operating room (OR) is the responsibility of the anesthesiologist, who knows the location and function of resuscitation equipment, delegates tasks, and instills calmness in assisting personnel. The protocols described below have been modified as appropriate for the anesthesiologist in a hospital setting but closely follow the evidenced-based *2005 American Heart Association Guidelines for Cardiopulmonary Resuscitation and Emergency Cardiovascular Care.* These guidelines emphasize the importance of the prompt delivery of effective, uninterrupted chest compressions, even before checking that a defibrillation has been successful, to deliver oxygen and energy substrates to the myocardium. An additional major change in the guidelines is the reduction of ventilation that may decrease venous return to the heart and diminish cardiac output. Table 37.1 lists the classifications for the quality of evidence used to support most of the protocol interventions presented in this chapter.

II. **Cardiac arrest**
   A. **Diagnosis.** The absence of a palpable pulse in a major peripheral artery (carotid, radial, or femoral) in an unconscious, unmonitored patient is diagnostic of a cardiac arrest. An electrocardiogram (ECG) may reveal asystole, ventricular fibrillation (VF), ventricular tachycardia (VT), or even an organized rhythm (as in pulseless electrical activity).
   B. **Etiologies.** Common causes of cardiac arrest are as follows:
      1. Hypoxemia.
      2. Acid-base disturbances.
      3. Derangements of potassium, calcium, and magnesium.
      4. Hypovolemia.
      5. Adverse drug effects.
      6. Pericardial tamponade.
      7. Tension pneumothorax.
      8. Pulmonary embolus.
      9. Hypothermia.
      10. Myocardial infarction.
   C. **Pathophysiology.** With the onset of a cardiac arrest, effective blood flow ceases, and tissue hypoxia, anaerobic metabolism, and accumulation of cellular wastes result. Organ function is compromised, and permanent damage ensues unless resuscitation measures are instituted within minutes. Acidosis from anaerobic metabolism may cause systemic vasodilation, pulmonary vasoconstriction, and decreased responsiveness to catecholamines.

III. **Adult resuscitation**
   A. **Basic life support** includes basic techniques taught to the general public but applies equally to OR situations. A cardiac

Table 37.1.   Evidence classification for interventions

Class	Evidence	Clinical Use
I	Excellent	Definitely recommended
IIa	Good/very good	Acceptable, safe, useful
IIb	Fair/good	Acceptable, safe, useful
Indeterminate	Preliminary research stage	May be used
III	Positive evidence absent or strongly suggests or confirms harm	None

arrest should be suspected in any person unexpectedly found unconscious. If the subject is unarousable, the "ABCDs" (**a**irway, **b**reathing, **c**irculation, **d**efibrillation) of resuscitation should be followed after first calling for assistance. For lone rescuers, the lay public is taught the "phone first/phone fast" rule (evidence class indeterminate). For adults, children beyond the onset of adolescence or puberty (12 to 14 years of age), and all children known to be at high risk for dysrhythmias, the emergency medical system (EMS) should be activated (phone 911) or an automatic external defibrillator (AED) located before CPR is started by a lone rescuer ("phone first"). An initial resuscitation attempt followed by the activation of EMS ("phone fast") is indicated for children aged younger than the onset of puberty because cessation of respiration is the usual etiology of a cardiac arrest in this population. In cases of submersion, near drowning, arrest secondary to trauma, and drug overdose, the "phone fast" rule applies. Healthcare providers can tailor the sequence of rescue actions as deemed appropriate for the likely etiology of the arrest based on any additional information or evidence they may be aware of regarding the patient or the nature of the arrest.

1. **Airway and breathing.** Spontaneous ventilation is evaluated by observation and auscultation and is aided by repositioning or insertion of an oropharyngeal or nasopharyngeal airway. In the absence of effective spontaneous ventilation, rescue breathing is begun (or ventilation by bag-valve-mask with 100% O_2). Two slow breaths at low airway pressures (to limit gastric distention) are delivered initially, followed by 8 to 10 breaths per minute. If ventilation is not possible after these maneuvers, efforts to clear the airway of a suspected foreign body (e.g., Heimlich maneuver, chest compressions, or manual removal) should be attempted.

2. **Circulation.** The circulation is assessed by palpation of the carotid artery pulse for 5 to 10 seconds. In the absence of a palpable pulse, artificial circulation should be instituted with external chest compressions. (The presence of a pulse does not necessarily mean that an adequate mean arterial pressure is present. Lay rescuers no longer perform pulse checks but are taught to initiate chest compressions in the absence of signs

of circulation such as moving, coughing, and breathing.) The patient should be on a firm surface (e.g., backboard) with the head on the same level as the thorax. The rescuer (surgeon in the OR) should compress the lower half of the sternum by placing the heel of one hand on the patient's sternum in the center of the chest, between the nipples, and the heel of the other hand on top of the first so that the hands are overlapped and parallel (class IIa). The rescuer's shoulders should be positioned directly over the patient, with the elbows locked for effective compressions. Sternal depression during CPR is to a depth of 1.5 to 2.0 inches in a normal-sized adult. A 1:1 compression–relaxation ratio at a rate of 100 compressions per minute is recommended. For a prone patient in the OR who cannot be quickly turned supine for CPR, one rescuer can place a clenched fist between the subxiphoid area and the OR table while compressions are administered over the corresponding region of the back. The chest compression-to-ventilation ratio is 30:2. This ratio is used for the resuscitation of adults and children when only one rescuer is present. If an advanced airway (i.e., endotracheal tube or laryngeal mask airway) is in place during two-person CPR, there is no need to synchronize breaths between compressions. Ventilations should be given at a rate of 8 to 10 breaths per minute, and chest compressions should be given at a rate of 100 per minute without pauses for ventilation.

3. **Defibrillation** within 3 minutes in the hospital (evidence class I) and 5 minutes after calling the EMS (along with immediate high-quality CPR) is the major determinant of a successful resuscitation because VF is the most likely etiology of a cardiac arrest in adults. Public-access defibrillation programs have now enabled "level I" responders (e.g., fire personnel, police, security guards, and airline attendants) to employ readily accessible AEDs. AEDs are small, lightweight defibrillators that use adhesive electrode pads for sensing and for delivering shocks. The AED, after analysis of the frequency, amplitude, and slope of the ECG signal, advises either "shock indicated" or "no shock indicated." The AED is manually triggered and does not automatically defibrillate the patient.

4. **Reassessment.** CPR should be resumed immediately after shock delivery without pausing for a pulse or rhythm check, and it should be continued for five cycles (or about 2 minutes if an advanced airway is in place) before the rhythm is rechecked. Healthcare providers should also check for a pulse if an organized rhythm has established. In the absence of a pulse or a "no shock indicated" with an AED, CPR should be resumed with rhythm checks every five cycles.

B. **Advanced cardiac life support** (ACLS), including endotracheal intubation, electrical defibrillation, and pharmacologic intervention, is the definitive treatment for cardiac arrest. Specific protocols are found in Figures 37.1 through 37.3:

1. **Intubation.** Swift control of the airway (with minimal interruptions in chest compressions and no delay in defibrillation) will optimize oxygenation and removal of carbon dioxide during resuscitation. Endotracheal intubation (confirmed by

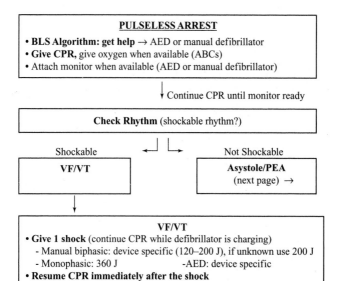

PULSELESS ARREST
- **BLS Algorithm: get help** → AED or manual defibrillator
- **Give CPR,** give oxygen when available (ABCs)
- Attach monitor when available (AED or manual defibrillator)

↓ Continue CPR until monitor ready

Check Rhythm (shockable rhythm?)

Shockable   Not Shockable

VF/VT   **Asystole/PEA**
(next page) →

VF/VT
- **Give 1 shock** (continue CPR while defibrillator is charging)
  - Manual biphasic: device specific (120–200 J), if unknown use 200 J
  - Monophasic: 360 J   -AED: device specific
- **Resume CPR immediately after the shock**

Give 5 cycles/2 minutes of CPR: 30 chest compressions, then 2 breaths/cycle*
Intubated patients: continuous compressions without pause for breaths
Check rhythm every 2 minutes

Check Rhythm (shockable rhythm?)
- If VF/VT → VF/VT protocol (above)
- If asystole → Asystole/PEA protocol (next page)
- If organized rhythm check pulse: no pulse → Asystole/PEA protocol
- If pulse, begin post-resuscitation care

↓ Continue CPR/rhythm checks as above

Give Vasopressor when IV/IO established
- **Epinephrine 1 mg IV, repeat every 3 to 5 min**
- May give 1 dose **vasopressin** 40 U IV in place of 1st or 2nd dose of epinephrine

↓ Continue CPR/rhythm checks as above

Consider Antiarrhythmics
- **Amiodrone** 300 mg IV once, may give additional 150 mg once, or **lidocaine**, 1–1.5mg/kg, then 0.5–0.75mg/kg q 5–10 min (max 3 mg/kg)
- Consider **magnesium**, loading dose 1–2 g IV for torsades de pointes
- Continue cycles of CPR/rhythm checks as above, shock if indicated

Figure 37.1. Protocol for pulseless arrest in adults. IABP, postoperative intra-aortic balloon pump; IO, intraosseous; MI, myocardial infarction; PE, pulmonary embolism; PEA, pulseless electrical activity; PTX, pneumothorax.

Asystole/PEA

- **Resume CPR immediately**

    Give vasopressor when IV/IO established
- **Epinephrine 1 mg IV, repeat every 3 to 5 min**
- May give 1 dose **vasopressin** 40 U IV in place of 1st or 2nd dose of epinephrine

    Consider **Atropine** 1 mg IV
- For asystole or PEA rate that is slow
- Repeat every 3 to 5 min (up to 3 doses)

$\downarrow$ Give 5 cycles/2 minutes of CPR

Check Rhythm (shockable rhythm?)
- If VF/VT $\rightarrow$ VF/VT protocol (previous page)
- If asystole $\rightarrow$ Asystole/PEA protocol (above)
- If organized rhythm check pulse: no pulse $\rightarrow$ Asystole/PEA protocol
- If pulse, begin post-resuscitation care

---

*One cycle of CPR = 30 chest compressions, then 2 breaths. If intubated, give compressions continuously without pausing to give breaths, give 8–10 breaths/minute, check rhythm every 2 minutes

During CPR

- Push hard and fast (100 chest compression/min)
- Minimize interruptions in chest compressions
- Avoid hyperventilation and large tidal volumes

- Search for and treat possible contributing factors:
    - **Hypovolemia** $\rightarrow$ give volume
    - **Hypoxia** $\rightarrow$ improve oxygenation
    - **H^+** (bicarb-responsive metabolic acidosis) $\rightarrow$ give bicarbonate
    - **Hypo/hyperkalemia** $\rightarrow$ give K^+ or Ca^{++}/insulin/glucose, etc.
    - **Hypoglycemia** $\rightarrow$ give dextrose
    - **Hypothermia** $\rightarrow$ warm patient; may be refractory to shock until warm and need prolonged CPR
    - **Toxins** $\rightarrow$ treatment appropriate to substance
    - **Tamponade**, cardiac $\rightarrow$ perform pericardiocentesis
    - **Tension pneumothorax** $\rightarrow$ relieve pressure, chest tube
    - **Thrombosis**: coronary (MI) $\rightarrow$ IABP, thrombolysis/cath, heparin
        pulmonary (PE) $\rightarrow$ inotrope, heparin
    - **Trauma** $\rightarrow$ consider occult injury: bleeding, tamponade, PTX, etc.

Figure 37.1. (*Continued*)

TACHYCARDIA WITH PULSES
- Assess and support ABCs, give oxygen
- Monitors: ECG (identify rhythm), blood pressure, oximetry
- Identify and treat reversible causes

↓ Symptoms persist

Is patient stable?
- Unstable signs: ↓ BP, chest pain, SOB, shock, mental status change (rate-related symptoms uncommon if heart rat <150 bpm)

Stable | **Unstable**

- Establish IV access
- Obtain 12-lead ECG (when available) or rhythm strip

Perform **immediate synchronized cardioversion**
- Establish IV access and give sedation if conscious; don't delay cardioversion
- Consider expert consultation
- If pulseless arrest develops, see Figure 37.1

Is QRS wide or narrow? (< or ≥0.12 sec)
→ appropriate section below

Wide QRS
- Is rhythm regular or irregular? (Expert consultation advised)

Regular | **Irregular**

- **If ventricular tachycardia** or uncertain rhythm:
  - **Amiodarone**: 150 mg IV over 10 min, repeat as needed to max dose of 2.2 g in 24 hours
  - Prepare for elective **synchronized cardioversion**

- **If SVT with aberrancy:**
  - **Adenosine** (go to Narrow QRS/Regular rhythm on next page)

- **If AF with aberrancy**
  - Go to Narrow QRS/Irregular rhythm on next page
- **If pre-excited AF** (AF + WPW)
  - Expert consulation advised
  - Avoid AV nodal–blocking agents (e.g., **adenosine, digoxin, diltiazem, verapamil**)
  - Consider antiarrhythmics (e.g., **amiodarone** 150 mg/10 min)
- **If recurrent polymorphic VT:**
  - Seek expert consultation
- **If torsades de pointes:**
  - **Magnesium** (load with 1–2 g over 5–60 min, then start infusion)

Figure 37.2. Protocol for tachycardia with pulses in adults. CHF, congestive heart failure; MAT, multifocal atrial tachycardia; PE, pulmonary embolism; PEA, pulseless electrical activity; SOB, shortness of breath.

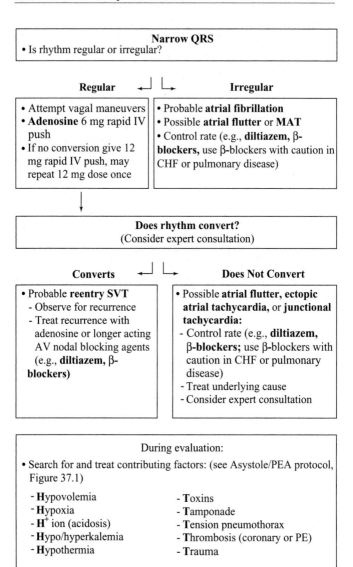

Narrow QRS
• Is rhythm regular or irregular?

Regular ⟵⌐ ⌐⟶ **Irregular**

• Attempt vagal maneuvers
• **Adenosine** 6 mg rapid IV push
• If no conversion give 12 mg rapid IV push, may repeat 12 mg dose once

• Probable **atrial fibrillation**
• Possible **atrial flutter** or **MAT**
• Control rate (e.g., **diltiazem, β-blockers,** use β-blockers with caution in CHF or pulmonary disease)

Does rhythm convert?
(Consider expert consultation)

Converts ⟵⌐ ⌐⟶ **Does Not Convert**

• Probable **reentry SVT**
  - Observe for recurrence
  - Treat recurrence with adenosine or longer acting AV nodal blocking agents (e.g., **diltiazem, β-blockers**)

• Possible **atrial flutter, ectopic atrial tachycardia,** or **junctional tachycardia:**
  - Control rate (e.g., **diltiazem, β-blockers;** use β-blockers with caution in CHF or pulmonary disease)
  - Treat underlying cause
  - Consider expert consultation

During evaluation:
• Search for and treat contributing factors: (see Asystole/PEA protocol, Figure 37.1)

  - Hypovolemia
  - Hypoxia
  - H^+ ion (acidosis)
  - Hypo/hyperkalemia
  - Hypothermia

  - Toxins
  - Tamponade
  - Tension pneumothorax
  - Thrombosis (coronary or PE)
  - Trauma

Figure 37.2. (*Continued*)

BRADYCARDIA

Heart rate <60 bpm and inadequate for clinical condition

↓

- Assess and support ABCs, give oxygen
- Monitors: EGG (identify rhythm), blood pressure, oximetry
- Establish IV access

↓

- **Are there signs or symptoms of poor perfusion caused by the bradycardia?**
  - (e.g., acute altered mental status, ongoing chest pain, hypotension, other signs of shock)

Adequate Perfusion

- Observe/monitor

Poor Perfusion

- **Prepare for transcutaneous pacing:**
  - Use without delay for high-degree block (type-II second-degree block or third-degree block)
- Consider **atropine** 0.5 mg while awaiting pacer
  - May repeat to a total dose of 3 mg. If ineffective, begin pacing
- Consider **epinephrine** (2–10 μg/min) or **dopamine** (2–10 μg/kg/min) infusion while awaiting pacer or if pacing ineffective

↓

- Prepare for **transvenous pacing**
- Treat contributing causes
- Consider expert consultation

Reminders

- If pulseless arrest develops, go to Pulseless Arrest Algorithm (Fig. 37.1)
- Search for and treat contributing factors: (see Asystole/PEA protocol, Fig. 37.1)

- **H**ypovolemia	- **T**oxins
- **H**ypoxia	- **T**amponade
- **H**$^+$ ion (acidosis)	- **T**ension pneumothorax
- **H**ypo/hyperkalemia	- **T**hrombosis (coronary or PE)
- **H**ypothermia	- **T**rauma

Figure 37.3. Protocol for bradycardia in adults. bpm, beats per minute; PE, pulmonary embolism; PEA, pulseless electrical activity.

capnography) by the most experienced person present should minimally disrupt the resuscitative measures. The endotracheal tube may be used to deliver certain drugs if intravenous (IV) access has not been established. Examples are naloxone, atropine, vasopressin, epinephrine, and lidocaine ("NAVEL"). Because peak drug concentrations are lower with the endotracheal route compared with IV administration, higher doses (two to three times) diluted in 10 mL of sterile saline should be used.

2. **Defibrillation.** VT and VF (see Fig. 37.1) are the most common arrhythmias associated with a cardiac arrest. As the duration of a VF/VT arrest increases, the cardiac activity deteriorates and becomes more difficult to convert to a viable rhythm. Therefore, early defibrillation is the priority and can often be administered by the anesthetist without compromising the surgical field. It is the responsibility of the person operating the defibrillator to ensure that members of the resuscitation team are not in contact with the patient during defibrillation.

   a. **Biphasic waveform defibrillators** are used in virtually all AEDs and manual defibrillators sold in the United States today. They function by delivering an energy that flows in a positive direction for specified milliseconds followed by a reversal in the negative direction. The optimal energy needed to terminate VF is device specific, depends on the manufacturer and the type of waveform used, and ranges from 120 to 200 J. If the optimum energy is not indicated on the front of the defibrillator, 200 J should be used. If VF is at any time terminated by a shock and then recurs, subsequent shocks should be given at the previously successful energy level.

   b. **Monophasic waveform defibrillators,** still used in many institutions, deliver energy in a unidirectional manner. The initial and subsequent defibrillations should be given at 360 J.

   c. **Cardioversion** for atrial flutter, other supraventricular dysrhythmias such as paroxysmal supraventricular tachycardia (PSVT), and hemodynamically stable VT generally require less energy (50 to 100 J monophasic) than what is necessary for atrial fibrillation (AF) (100 to 120 J). The optimal energy for cardioversion with biphasic waveforms has not yet been established, but experience with elective cardioversion of AF indicates that an initial energy of 100 to 120 J will be efficacious and can be extrapolated to other tachyarrhythmias. Cardioversion will not be effective for the treatment of junctional tachycardia or ectopic or multifocal atrial tachycardia because these rhythms are caused by an automatic focus rather than reentry. In fact, delivery of a shock to a heart with a rapid automatic focus may actually increase the rate of the tachyarrhythmia.

3. **Pacing.** High-grade heart block with profound bradycardia is an etiology of cardiac arrest (see Fig. 37.3). Temporary pacing should be used when the heart rate does not increase with

pharmacologic therapy. Transcutaneous pacing is the easiest method to increase the ventricular rate. Transesophageal atrial pacing is efficacious for sinus bradycardia with maintained atrioventricular (A-V) conduction and is useful intraoperatively for bradycardia-related hypotension in otherwise stable patients. Transvenous pacing via a temporary wire into the right heart is a third option to increase heart rate while CPR continues. Special pacing pulmonary artery catheters are capable of A-V pacing.

4. **Intravenous access** is imperative for a successful resuscitation. The most desirable route is into the central circulation. Central lines can be achieved via internal jugular, external jugular, subclavian, or femoral veins and sometimes via peripheral veins (long lines). Choice of route is predicated on the anatomy of the patient, experience of the physician, and what is the least disruptive to the resuscitation. Short (peripheral) catheters in antecubital veins are adequate when an appropriate volume is used to flush medications toward the central circulation. Fluid replacement is indicated for patients with known or suspected intravascular volume depletion.

5. **Drugs.** The drugs described below are used in ACLS protocols for the treatment of hemodynamic instability, myocardial ischemia or infarction, and arrhythmias. The doses of drugs used for **pediatric advanced life support (PALS)** are in parentheses following discussion of adult doses.

   a. **Adenosine,** an endogenous purine nucleotide with a half-life of 5 seconds, slows A-V nodal conduction and interrupts A-V node reentry pathways to convert a PSVT to a sinus rhythm. It also assists in the differential diagnosis of supraventricular tachycardia (e.g., atrial flutter with a rapid ventricular response versus PSVT). Dosing is based on peripheral administration and should be halved if given through central venous access. The initial dose is a 6-mg rapid IV bolus. A brief asystole ensues that is followed by P waves, flutter waves, or fibrillation waves that are initially without ventricular responses. PSVT is sometimes converted to a sinus rhythm by the 6-mg dose of adenosine. A second injection of 12 mg may terminate PSVT if the first dose is unsuccessful. Recurrent PSVT, AF, and atrial flutter will require longer-acting drugs for definitive treatment. The dose of adenosine should be increased in the presence of methylxanthines (competitive inhibition) and decreased if dipyridamole (potentiation via blockage of nucleoside transport) has been administered. (PALS: 0.1 mg/kg; repeat dose 0.2 mg/kg; maximum dose 12 mg.)

   b. **Amiodarone** is the most versatile drug in the ACLS algorithms. It has the properties of all four classes of antiarrhythmics (lengthening of action potential, sodium channel blockade at high frequencies of stimulation, noncompetitive antisynaptic actions, and negative chronotropism). Because of its high efficacy and low incidence of prodysrhythmic effects, it is the preferred antidysrhythmic for patients with severely impaired cardiac function. The dose for the treatment of unstable VT or VF is 300 mg diluted in 20 to 30 mL of saline or 5% dextrose in water (D5W) and administered rapidly. For the treatment of more stable disorders, the dose is 150 mg administered over 10 minutes, followed by an infusion of 1 mg/minute for 6 hours and then 0.5 mg/minute. The maximum daily dose is 2 g. Immediate side effects can be bradycardia and hypotension. With chronic use, hypothyroidism, elevation of hepatic enzymes, alveolar pneumonitis, and pulmonary fibrosis may occur. (PALS: loading dose, 5 mg/kg; maximum dose, 15 mg/kg/day.) Amiodarone is indicated in the following dysrhythmia situations.

   (1) Unstable VT (evidence class IIb).
   (2) VF after failed electrical defibrillation and epinephrine treatment (class IIb).
   (3) Rate control during stable monomorphic VT, polymorphic VT (class IIb), or AF (class IIa).
   (4) Ventricular rate control of rapid atrial arrhythmias when digitalis is ineffective (class IIb) or when the tachycardia is secondary to accessory pathways (class IIb).
   (5) Adjunct to electrical cardioversion of refractory PSVTs (class IIa) or atrial tachycardia (class IIb).

c.   **Atropine** is useful in the treatment of hemodynamically significant bradycardia (evidence class I) or A-V block occurring at the nodal level (evidence class IIa). It increases the rate of sinus node discharge and enhances A-V node conduction by its vagolytic activity. The dose of atropine for bradycardia or A-V block is 0.5 mg repeated every 3 to 5 min to a total dose of 0.04 mg/kg. For asystole, atropine is given as a 1-mg bolus repeated in 3 to 5 minutes if needed. Full vagal blockade is obtained at a cumulative dose of 3 mg. (PALS: 0.02 mg/kg; minimum dose, 0.1 mg; maximum single dose, 0.5 mg in child, 1.0 mg in adolescent.)

d.   **β-Adrenergic blocking drugs** (atenolol, metoprolol, and propranolol) have established utility (evidence class I) for patients with unstable angina or myocardial infarction. These drugs reduce the rates of recurrent ischemia, nonfatal reinfarction, and postinfarction VF. In contrast to calcium channel blockers, β-blockers are not direct negative inotropes. Esmolol, in addition to other β-blockers, is useful for the acute treatment of PSVT, AF, atrial flutter (evidence class I), and ectopic atrial tachycardia (evidence class IIb). Initial and subsequent IV doses, if tolerated, are as follows: atenolol, 5 mg over 5 minutes, repeated once at 10 minutes; metoprolol, three doses of 5 mg every 5 minutes; propranolol, 0.1 mg/kg divided into three doses given every 2 to 3 minutes; esmolol, 0.5 mg/kg over 1 minute followed by an infusion starting at 50 μg/minute and titrated as needed up to 200 μg/minute. Contraindications include second- or third-degree heart block, hypotension, and severe congestive heart failure. Atenolol and metoprolol, because of their relatively specific β_1-adrenergic blockade, are preferable to propranolol in patients with a history of reactive airway disease. A small number of patients will exhibit bronchospasm with the administration of any beta-blocker. Most patients with chronic obstructive pulmonary disease, however, are able to tolerate beta-blockers.

e. **Calcium** is indicated during cardiac arrest only when hyperkalemia, hypermagnesemia, hypocalcemia, or toxicity from calcium channel blockers is suspected. Calcium chloride, 5 to 10 mg/kg IV, can be repeated as necessary. (PALS: 20 mg/kg.)

f. **Calcium-channel blockers.** Verapamil and diltiazem slow conduction and increase refractoriness in the A-V node. They are used to treat hemodynamically stable, narrow complex PSVTs that are unresponsive to vagal maneuvers or adenosine. They can also be used to control the rate of ventricular response in AF or atrial flutter. The initial verapamil dose is 2.5 to 5.0 mg IV, with subsequent doses of 5 to 10 mg IV administered every 15 to 30 minutes. Diltiazem is given as an initial bolus of 0.25 mg/kg. An additional dose of 0.35 mg/kg and an infusion of 5 to 15 mg/hour can be administered if needed. Their vasodilator and negative inotrope properties can cause hypotension, exacerbation of congestive heart failure, bradycardia, and enhancement of accessory conduction in patients with Wolff-Parkinson-White syndrome. The hypotension can often be reversed with calcium chloride, 0.5 to 1.0 g IV.

g. **Dopamine** has dopaminergic (evident at doses less than 2 μg/kg/minute), β-adrenergic (evident at 2 to 5 μg/kg/minute), and a-adrenergic (at 5 to 10 μg/kg/minute) activities. Although the above are "traditional" doses, the adrenergic effects can manifest at the lowest dosage levels. Therefore, the drug should be started at a low dose (e.g., 150 μg/minute) and titrated up until the desired effect (e.g., increased urine output, increased heart rate/inotropy, or increased blood pressure) is seen or undesired side effects (e.g., tachyarrhythmia) occur.

h. **Epinephrine** continues to be the mainstay of pharmacologic therapy for cardiac arrest, although there is little evidence that it improves survival. Its α-adrenergic vasoconstriction of noncerebral and noncoronary vascular beds produces compensatory shunting of blood toward the brain and the heart. High doses may contribute to myocardial dysfunction and are not recommended. However, high doses may be indicated in specific situations, such as beta-blocker or calcium channel blocker overdose. The recommended dose is 1.0 mg IV, repeated every 3 to 5 minutes, or administration as an infusion of 1 to 4 μg/minute. Epinephrine used for symptomatic bradycardia is evidence class IIb. (PALS: bradycardia, 0.01 mg/kg; pulseless arrest, 0.01 mg/kg.)

i. **Ibutilide** is used for the acute conversion of AF or atrial flutter, either alone or with electrical cardioversion. It prolongs the duration of the action potential and increases the refractory period. The dose of 1 mg given over 10 minutes can be repeated in 10 minutes. The dose for patients weighing less than 60 kg is 0.01 mg/kg. Continuous monitoring of the patient is required during its administration and for at least 6 hours thereafter because the major side effect of ibutilide is polymorphic VT (including torsade de pointes).

j. **Isoproterenol** is a β_1- and β_2-adrenergic agonist. It is a second-line drug used to treat hemodynamically significant bradycardia that is unresponsive to atropine and dobutamine in the event that a temporary pacemaker is not available (evidence class IIb). Its β_2 activity can cause hypotension. Isoproterenol is administered by IV infusion at 2 to 10 μg/minute, titrated to achieve the desired heart rate.

k. **Lidocaine** may be useful for the control (not prophylaxis) of ventricular ectopy during an acute myocardial infarction. The initial dose during a cardiac arrest is 1.0 to 1.5 mg/kg IV, and this may be repeated as a 0.5- to 0.75-mg/kg bolus every 3 to 5 minutes to a total dose of 3 mg/kg. A continuous infusion of lidocaine at a rate of 2 to 4 mg/minute is instituted after successful resuscitation. The lidocaine dose should be decreased for patients with reduced cardiac output, hepatic dysfunction, or advanced age. (PALS: 1 mg/kg; infusion, 20 to 50 μg/kg/minute.)

l. **Magnesium** is a cofactor in a variety of enzyme reactions, including Na^+,K^+-ATPase. Hypomagnesemia can precipitate refractory VF as well as exacerbate hypokalemia. Magnesium replacement is effective for the treatment of drug-induced torsade de pointes. The dose for emergent administration is 1 to 2 g in 10 mL of D5W over 1 to 2 minutes. Hypotension and bradycardia are side effects of rapid administration. (PALS: 25 to 50 mg/kg; maximum dose, 2 g.)

m. **Oxygen** (100%) should be administered to all cardiac arrest victims whether or not ventilation requires assistance.

n. **Procainamide** may be considered in patients with preserved ventricular function. The loading dose is a continuous infusion of 20 mg/minute that is terminated when the arrhythmia is suppressed, hypotension occurs, the QRS complex is widened by 50% of its original size, or a total dose of 17 mg/kg is reached. When the arrhythmia is suppressed, a maintenance infusion of 1 to 4 mg/minute should be initiated, with a reduced dose considered in the presence of renal failure. It should be used with caution if at all in patients with preexisting QT prolongation or if used in combination with other drugs that prolong the QT interval. An ECG should be examined for QRS widening at least daily. (PALS: 15 mg/kg.) It is indicated in the follow situations:

(1) Treatment of stable monomorphic VT (Class IIa).

(2) Ventricular rate control in AF and atrial flutter.

(3) Control of the heart rhythm in AF or atrial flutter in patients with known preexcitation (WPW) syndrome.

(4) For reentrant, narrow-complex tachycardias that are unable to be controlled by adenosine or vagal maneuvers.

o. **Sodium bicarbonate** administration is detrimental in most cardiac arrests because it creates a paradoxical intracellular acidosis (evidence class III). It may be considered when the standard ACLS protocol has failed in the presence of severe preexisting metabolic acidosis, and it may assist in the treatment of hyperkalemia or tricyclic antidepressant overdose. The initial dose of bicarbonate is 1 mEq/kg IV, with subsequent doses of 0.5 mEq/kg given every 10 minutes (as guided by arterial blood pH and partial pressure of carbon dioxide [$Paco_2$]). (PALS: 1 mEq/kg.)

p. **Vasopressin,** an antidiuretic and pressor produced in the neurohypophysis, may be substituted for either the first or second dose of epinephrine in the treatment of pulseless arrest (40 units IV, class indeterminate). It constricts vascular smooth muscle when used in high doses. It is more effective than epinephrine in maintaining the coronary perfusion pressure and has a longer half-life of 10 to 20 minutes.

6. **Open-chest direct cardiac compression** is an intervention used at institutions with appropriate resources to manage penetrating chest trauma, abdominal trauma with cardiac arrest, pericardial tamponade, hypothermia, or pulmonary embolism. Direct cardiac compressions also are indicated for individuals with anatomic deformities of the chest that prevent adequate closed-chest compression.

7. **Termination of CPR.** There are no absolute guidelines to determine when to stop an unsuccessful resuscitation, but there is a very low probability of survival after 30 minutes. It is at the discretion of the physician in charge to determine when the failure of the cardiovascular system to respond to adequately applied basic life support and ACLS indicates that the patient has died. There should be a meticulous documentation of the resuscitation, including the reasons for terminating the effort.

8. The advanced directive "**do not resuscitate**" (**DNR**) places the anesthesiologist in a key position with respect to intraoperative and postoperative care. It should not be *assumed* that a DNR order is suspended in the perioperative period. Institution-specific written guidelines should be reviewed. In advance of a procedure, physicians and the patient with the DNR status (or the patient's health care proxy) should clarify what resuscitative measures would be compatible with the patient's wishes—i.e., goal-directed care. For example, the use of a pressor to control hypotension after induction of general anesthesia might be permitted while defibrillation and CPR for spontaneous VF might be prohibited. When asked to perform an emergent intubation outside of the OR, the anesthesiologist should ask about the patient's code

status and is ethically and legally bound to a known decision to limit treatment.

IV. **Pediatric resuscitation**

A. **Basic life support.** The need for CPR in the pediatric age group is rare after the neonatal period. Pediatric cardiac arrests usually result from hypoxemia linked to respiratory failure or airway obstruction. Initial efforts should be directed toward the establishment of a secure airway and adequate ventilation. The pediatric guidelines apply to infants (1 month after the perinatal period to 1 year) and children (1 to 8 years of age. For children greater than 8 years old, resuscitation is the same as for adults including the application of the "phone first" rule. "Phone fast" applies to resuscitation of infants and children before the start of puberty and to resuscitation of any child with suspected drowning, traumatic arrest, or drug overdose. The lone rescuer should perform five cycles (about 2 minute) of CPR before phoning 911. Exceptions to this rule include situations when the arrest of a child is witnessed and sudden (e.g., an athlete who collapses on the playing field) or situations in which a child is known to be at high risk for a sudden arrhythmia. Modifications of the rate and magnitude of compressions and ventilations, as well as of the hand position for compressions, are necessary because of anatomic and physiologic differences (Table 37.2). Differences between pediatric and adult resuscitation techniques are detailed below.

1. **Airway and breathing.** Maneuvers to establish an airway are the same as in the adult, with a few caveats. For children less than 1 year of age, abdominal thrusts are not used because the gastrointestinal tract can be damaged easily. Hyperextension of an infant's neck for the head tilt/chin lift may lead to airway obstruction because of the small diameter and ease of compression of the immature airway. Submental compression while performing the chin lift can also lead to airway obstruction by pushing the tongue into the pharynx. Ventilations should be given slowly with low airway pressures to avoid gastric distention and should be of sufficient volume to cause the chest to rise and fall.

2. **Circulation.** The brachial or femoral artery is used for pulse assessment in infants because the carotid artery is difficult to palpate. In the absence of a pulse, chest compressions should be initiated at a compression/relaxation ratio of 1:1. These are delivered to infants by using two fingertips applied to the sternum or by encircling the chest with both hands and using the thumbs to depress the sternum one fingerbreadth below the intermammary line. In older children, the correct hand position is determined as for adults but with only one hand depressing the sternum to about one-third to one-half of the anterior-posterior depth of the chest. The compression/ventilation ratio is 30:2 for one-rescuer CPR of infants and children and 15:2 when two rescuers are available. Ventilations should be given at a rate of 8 to 10 breaths per minute, and chest compressions should be given at a rate of 100 per minute. If an advanced airway is in place during two-rescuer CPR, there is no need to synchronize breaths between compressions.

Table 37.2. Adult and pediatric cardiopulmonary resuscitation

Age	Ventilations/ min	Compressions/ min	Ventilation: Compression Ratio	Depth of Compressions
Neonate	30	90	$3{:}1^{a,b}$	1/3 depth of chest
Infant (<1 yr)	12–20	100	$30{:}2^{a}/15{:}2^{b}$	1/3–1/2 depth of chest
Child (1–8 yr)	12–20	100	$30{:}2^{a}/15{:}2^{b}$	1/3–1/2 depth of chest
Adult and child >8 yr	10–12	100	$30{:}2^{a,b}$	1.5–2 inches

[a]One-person rescue.
[b]Two-person rescue.

B. Pediatric advanced life support. Most pediatric cardiac arrests present as asystole or bradycardia rather than ventricular arrhythmias. In infants less than 1 year old, respiratory and idiopathic (sudden infant death syndrome) etiologies predominate. Anatomic and physiologic differences from the adult require defibrillator settings and drug doses to be weight based. Specific PALS algorithms are illustrated in Figures 37.4 through 37.6.

   1. **Intubation.** The endotracheal tube size is based on the patient's age (uncuffed tube size [mm inner diameter] = 4 + (age/4) for children over 2 years old. Use one half-size smaller for a cuffed tube). Atropine, epinephrine, lidocaine, or naloxone can be administered via the endotracheal tube before establishment of IV access.

   2. **Defibrillation.** Defibrillator paddles used for infants are 4.5 cm in diameter, and those used for older children are 8 cm in diameter. For either monophasic or biphasic devices, the energy level is 2 J/kg for the initial shock and 4 J/kg, or the lowest level that was previously successful, for any subsequent shocks. Hypoxemia, acidosis, and hypothermia should be considered as treatable causes of an arrest if the defibrillation attempts are unsuccessful. For cardioversion, the starting energy is 0.2 J/kg, with escalation to 1.0 J/kg if needed. The configuration for pediatric paddles varies among defibrillators.

   3. **Intravenous access.** Central venous access is preferred, but existing peripheral IVs should be used without delay. The femoral vein can be used with a catheter of suitable length. The intraosseous route may also be used in children. A bone marrow biopsy needle or spinal needle is inserted into the tibial shaft away from the epiphyseal plates to gain access to the large venous sinuses of the bone marrow. If none of the above is available, the endotracheal tube may be used to deliver essential medications if they are diluted in 2 to 5 mL of normal saline to ensure their delivery to the pulmonary vasculature.

   4. **Medications.** Most of the drugs described in the adult ACLS section (III.B.6) apply to PALS with doses adjusted to the child's weight.

V. Neonatal resuscitation. The neonatal period extends through the first 28 days of life. Someone who is skilled in resuscitation of newborns should be present at every delivery. Resuscitation is divided into four phases: stimulation and suctioning, ventilation, chest compressions, and delivery of resuscitation drugs and fluids. Resuscitation is often needed during an emergent cesarean section for fetal distress. In the event that the anesthesiologist is the only one available to treat the newborn, the neonatal warmer should be brought to the head of the OR table to facilitate the treatment and monitoring of the mother and child until the pediatrician arrives.

   A. Assessment. Immediate neonatal resuscitation is crucial, because profound hypoxemia occurs rapidly and will be exacerbated by respiratory acidosis, which contributes to the persistence of fetal circulation and right-to-left shunting. A neonate who requires resuscitation will likely have a significant right-to-left shunt.

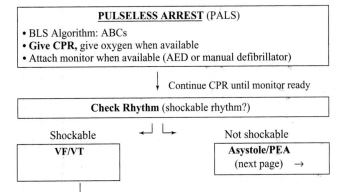

PULSELESS ARREST (PALS)

- BLS Algorithm: ABCs
- **Give CPR,** give oxygen when available
- Attach monitor when available (AED or manual defibrillator)

↓ Continue CPR until monitor ready

Check Rhythm (shockable rhythm?)

Shockable — ⌐ ⌐→ Not shockable

VF/VT

Asystole/PEA
(next page) →

↓

VF/VT

- **Give 1 shock** (continue CPR while defibrillator is charging)
  - Manual (biphasic or monophasic): 2 J/kg for the 1st attempt, 4 J/kg for subsequent attempts
  - AED: use pediatric system for 1 to 8 years of age if available
- **Resume CPR immediately after the shock**

↓ Give 5 cycles/2 minutes of CPR*

Check Rhythm (shockable rhythm?)
- If VF/VT → VF/VT protocol (above)
- If asystole → Asystole/PEA protocol (next page)
- If organized rhythm check pulse: no pulse → Asystole/PEA protocol
- If pulse, begin post-resuscitation care

↓ Continue CPR/rhythm checks as above

Give Epinephrine when IV/IO established
- IV/IO: 0.01 mg/kg (1:10,000; 0.1 mL/kg), **repeat every 3 to 5 min**
- Endotracheal tube: 0.1 mg/kg (1:1,000; 0.1 mL/kg)

↓ Continue CPR/rhythm checks as above

Consider Antiarrhythmics[1]
- **Amiodarone** 5 mg/kg IV/IO or lidocaine 1 mg/kg IV/IO
- Consider **magnesium** 25–50 mg/kg for torsades de pointes, max 2 g
- Continue cycles of CPR/rhythm checks as above, shock if indicated

[1]When VF/VT persist after 2–3 shocks plus CPR and a vasopressor

Figure 37.4. Protocol for pulseless arrest in infants and children. IABP, postoperative intra-aortic balloon pump; **IO,** intraosseus; **MI,** myocardial infarction; **PE,** pulmonary embolism; **PEA,** pulseless electrical activity; **PTX,** pneumothorax.

Asystole/PEA
- **Resume CPR immediately**

    Give **Epinephrine** when IV/IO established
- **Repeat every 3 to 5 min**
- IV/IO: 0.01 mg/kg (1:10,000; 0.1 mL/kg)
- Endotracheal tube: 0.1 mg/kg (1:1,000; 0.1 mL/kg)

↓ Give 5 cycles/2 minutes of CPR*

Check Rhythm (shockable rhythm?)

- If VF/VT → VF/VT protocol (previous page)
- If asystole → Asystole/PEA protocol (above)
- If organized rhythm check pulse: no pulse → Asystole/PEA protocol
- If pulse, begin post-resuscitation care

---

*One cycle of CPR = 15 chest compressions, then 2 breaths. If
intubated give compressions continuously without pausing to give
breaths, give 8–10 breaths/minute, check rhythm every 2 minutes

During CPR

- Push hard and fast (100 chest compressions/min)
- Minimize interruptions in chest compressions
- Avoid hyperventilation and large tidal volumes

- Search for and treat possible contributing factors:
  - **H**ypovolemia → give volume
  - **H**ypoxia → improve oxygenation
  - **H**$^+$ (bicarb-responsive metabolic acidosis) → give bicarbonate
  - **H**ypo/hyperkalemia → give K$^+$ or Ca^{++}/insulin/glucose, etc.
  - **H**ypoglycemia → give dextrose
  - **H**ypothermia → warm patient; may be refractory to shock until
    warm and need prolonged CPR
  - **T**oxins → treatment appropriate to substance
  - **T**amponade, cardiac → perform pericardiocentesis
  - **T**ension pneumothorax → relieve pressure, chest tube
  - **T**hrombosis: coronary (MI) → IABP, thrombolysis/cath, heparin
                    pulmonary (PE) → inotrope, heparin
  - **T**rauma → consider occult injury: bleeding, tamponade, PTX, etc.

Figure 37.4. (*Continued*)

TACHYCARDIA (PALS)

With Pulses and Poor Perfusion

- Assess and support ABCs as needed
- Give oxygen
- Attach monitors/defibrillator

↓ Symptoms persist

Evaluate QRS duration

→ appropriate section below or Narrow QRS on next page

Wide QRS
(>0.08 sec)

↓

Possible **Ventricular Tachycardia**

- Perform **synchronized cardioversion**
  - 0.5 to 1 J/kg; if not effective, increase to 2 J/kg
  - Sedate if possible but do not delay cardioversion
- May attempt **adenosine** if it does not delay electrical cardioversion`

↓

Expert Consultation Advised

- **Amiodarone** 5 mg/kg IV over 20 to 60 minutes

or

- **Procainamide** 15 mg/kg IV over 30 to 60 minutes

(Do not routinely administer amiodarone and procainamide together)

Figure 37.5. Protocol for tachycardia in infants and children. bpm, beats per minute; HR, heart rate; PE, pulmonary embolism; PEA, pulseless electrical activity.

Narrow QRS (≤0.08 sec)
- Evaluate rhythm with 12-lead ECG or monitor

Probable Sinus Tachycardia

- Compatible history consistent with known cause
- P waves present/normal
- Variable R-R; constant P-R
- Infants: rate usually <220 bpm
- Children: rate usually <180 bpm

Probable Supraventricular Tachycardia

- Compatible history (vague, nonspecific)
- P waves absent/abnormal
- HR not variable
- History of abrupt rate changes
- Infants: rate usually ≥220 bpm
- Children: rate usually ≥80 bpm

Search For and Treat Cause

Consider Vagal Maneuvers (no delays)

- **If IV access readily available:**
  - Give **adenosine** 0.1 mg/kg (maximum 1st dose 6 mg) by rapid bolus
  - May double first dose and give once (maximum 2nd dose 12 mg)
- Evaluate rhythm with 12-lead ECG or monitor

or

- **Synchronized cardioversion:** 0.5 to 1 J/kg; if not effective, increase to 2 J/kg
  - Sedate if possible but do not delay cardioversion

Expert Consultation Advised

- **Amiodarone** 5 mg/kg IV over 20 to 60 minutes

or

- **Procainamide** 15 mg/kg IV over 30 to 60 minutes

(Do not routinely administer amiodarone and procainamide together)

During evaluation:

- Search for and treat contributing factors: (see Asystole/PEA protocol, Fig. 37.4)

  - **H**ypovolemia
  - **H**ypoxia
  - **H**+ ion (acidosis)
  - **H**ypo/hyperkalemia
  - **H**ypothermia

  - **T**oxins
  - **T**amponade
  - **T**ension pneumothorax
  - **T**hrombosis (coronary or PE)
  - **T**rauma

Figure 37.5. *(Continued)*

BRADYCARDIA (PALS)

With a Pulse

Causing cardiorespiratory compromise

↓

- Support ABCs as needed
- Give oxygen
- Attach monitor/defibrillator

↓

Bradycardia still causing cardiorespiratory compromise?

No ← ↓ → **Yes**

• Support ABCs; give oxygen if needed • Observe • Consider expert consultation	• Perform CPR if, despite oxygenation and ventilation, HR <60/min with poor perfusion

↑ ← **No** ← • Persistent symptomatic bradycardia?

↓ **Yes**

Give Epinephrine
- IV/IO: 0.01 mg/kg (1:10,000; 0.1 mL/kg)
- Endotracheal tube: 0.1 mg/kg (1:1,000; 0.1 mL/kg)
- **Repeat every 3 to 5 min**

If increased vagal tone or primary AV block:
- Give **atropine**: 0.02 mg/kg, may repeat (minimum dose: 0.1 mg; maximum total dose for child: 1 mg)
- Consider cardiac pacing

↓

- If pulseless arrest develops, go to Pulseless Arrest Algorithm (Fig. 37.4)

During evaluation:

- Search for and treat possible contributing factors (see Asystole/PEA protocol, Figure 37.4)

-**H**ypovolemia	-**T**oxins
-**H**ypoxia	-**T**amponade
-**H**+ ion (acidosis)	-**T**ension pneumothorax
-**H**ypo-/hyperkalemia	-**T**hrombosis (coronary or PE)
-**H**ypothermia	-**T**rauma

Figure 37.6. Protocol for bradycardia in infants and children. HR, heart rate; PE, pulmonary embolism; PEA, pulseless electrical activity.

1. The **Apgar score** is an objective assessment of the physiologic well-being of the child and is done 1 and 5 minutes after birth (Table 28.2).

2. An Apgar score of 0 to 2 mandates immediate CPR. Neonates with scores of 3 to 4 will need bag and mask ventilation and may require more extensive resuscitation. Supplemental oxygen and stimulation are normally sufficient for newborns with Apgar scores of 5 to 7. Respiratory activity should be evaluated by watching chest excursions and by auscultation. The heart rate is assessed by auscultation or by palpation of the umbilical pulse.

B. **Four phases of newborn resuscitation.** Each step is allotted approximately 30 seconds, including reevaluation after the step is completed. The decision whether to proceed to the next step is determined by assessment of three vital signs: respiration, heart rate, and color (Fig. 37.7).

1. **Stimulation and suctioning.** The cold-intolerant neonate should be dried thoroughly after birth and placed in a prewarmed environment to minimize heat loss and the exacerbation of acidosis. Placement in the lateral Trendelenberg position with the head in a "sniffing" position to open the airway will assist with the drainage of secretions. The mouth and nose should be suctioned with a bulb syringe to remove blood, mucus, and meconium. Suctioning should be limited to 10 seconds, with oxygen supplied between attempts. During suctioning, the heart rate should be monitored, because bradycardia can occur from hypoxemia or from vagal reflexes to pharyngeal stimulation. Drying and suctioning usually provide adequate respiratory stimulation. Additional measures include gently rubbing the newborn's back and slapping the soles of the feet. For infants born to mothers with meconium staining of amniotic fluid, the airway is traditionally suctioned by the obstetrician after delivery of the head but before delivery of the thorax (intrapartum suctioning). Routine intrapartum suctioning has not been shown to be effective at decreasing the risk of aspiration syndrome and is no longer advised (class I). Intubation for suctioning does not offer any benefit for the infant who is vigorous with strong respiratory efforts, good muscle tone, and a heart rate >100 beats per minute (class I). Endotracheal suctioning should be performed immediately after birth for infants with meconium and repeated until the trachea is clear. Each period of suctioning is kept brief to avoid bradycardia.

2. **Ventilation.** After the initial steps of stimulation and stabilization, babies who are breathing and have a heart rate greater than 100 beats per minute but exhibit central cyanosis (determined by examining the face, trunk, and mucous membranes) should be administered supplemental free-flow oxygen. Acrocyanosis (blue color of the hands and feet alone) is usually normal and is not a reliable indicator of hypoxemia. Positive pressure ventilation with 100% oxygen is used for apnea, cyanosis, and heart rates below 100 beats per minute. Bag and mask ventilation should be attempted initially. The initial breath may require airway pressures as

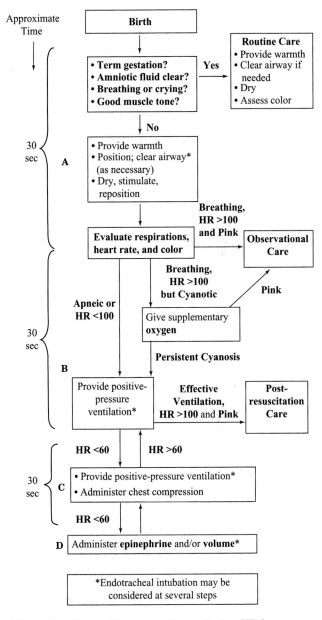

Figure 37.7. Protocol for neonatal resuscitation. HR, heart rate.

high as 30- to 40-cm H_2O held for 2 seconds to permit adequate lung expansion. All breaths should be at the lowest pressure possible (while ensuring adequate chest expansion) to prevent gastric distention that may lead to further respiratory compromise. Assisted ventilation is continued until there are adequate spontaneous breaths and a heart rate greater than 100 beats per minute. Endotracheal intubation is used when mask ventilation is ineffective, tracheal suctioning is needed (e.g., meconium aspiration), or prolonged ventilatory assistance is anticipated.

3. **Chest compressions.** For initial heart rates less than 100 beats per minute, the heart rate is reassessed after adequate ventilation with 100% oxygen has been performed for 30 seconds. If the heart rate is less than 60 beats per minute, chest compressions are required in addition to continued assisted ventilation. They should be delivered on the lower third of the sternum, and the chest should be compressed approximately one-third of its anterior-posterior depth. Compressions and ventilations should be coordinated to avoid simultaneous delivery and delivered at a 3:1 ratio, with 90 compressions and 30 breaths to achieve approximately 120 events per minute. The compressions are stopped about every 30 seconds to reassess respirations, heart rate, and color and should continue until the spontaneous heart rate is greater than 60 beats per minute.

4. **Delivery of resuscitation drugs and fluids.** Resuscitation drugs should be administered when the heart rate remains below 60 beats per minute despite adequate ventilation with 100% oxygen and chest compressions. The umbilical vein, the largest and thinnest of the three umbilical vessels, provides the best vascular access for resuscitation of the newborn. It is cannulated with a 3.5- to 5.0-French umbilical catheter after the umbilical cord stump has been prepped with an antiseptic and trimmed. Sterile umbilical tape placed at the base of the cord will prevent bleeding. The catheter should be placed below the skin level with blood aspirated freely, and care must be taken not to permit air into the system. If vascular access is unavailable, the endotracheal tube can be used to administer epinephrine, atropine, lidocaine, or naloxone. The drugs may be diluted in 1 to 2 mL of normal saline to ensure their delivery to the pulmonary vasculature.

5. **Drug and fluid dosages**
   a. Supplementary **oxygen** is recommended whenever positive pressure ventilation is used, and free-flow oxygen should be administered to babies who are breathing but have central cyanosis (class indeterminate). Undiluted oxygen is typically used for assisted ventilation, but some recent clinical studies have raised new concerns about its potential adverse effects on respiratory physiology and cerebral circulation. There is also the concern of potential tissue damage from oxygen free radicals. Some clinicians begin resuscitation with an oxygen concentration that is less than 100%, and the latest recommendations state that it is "reasonable" to do so.

b. **Epinephrine.** The β-adrenergic effect of epinephrine increases the intrinsic heart rate during neonatal resuscitation. Epinephrine should be used for asystole and for heart rates less than 60 beats per minute despite adequate oxygenation and chest compressions. The dose is 0.01 to 0.03 mg/kg of a 1:10,000 (1 mg/mL) solution IV. While access is being obtained, a higher dose (up to 0.1 mg/kg) may be administered through the endotracheal tube. Doses can be repeated every 3 to 5 minutes, as needed.

c. **Naloxone** is a specific opiate antagonist used for neonatal respiratory depression secondary to narcotics administered to the mother. The initial dose is 0.1 mg/kg. The respiratory status of the child should be monitored for an extended period of time after narcotic reversal because the duration of action of naloxone is shorter than that of many narcotics. An acute withdrawal reaction may be precipitated in the child of a narcotic-addicted mother.

d. The routine use of **sodium bicarbonate** is not recommended. The use of bicarbonate may be considered during prolonged arrests in an attempt to relieve depression of myocardial function and reduced action of catecholamines induced by marked acidosis. Intraventricular hemorrhage in premature infants has been associated with the osmolar load occurring with bicarbonate administration. A neonatal preparation of sodium bicarbonate (4.2% or 0.5 mEq/mL) should be used to prevent this from occurring. The initial dose is 1 mEq/kg IV given over 2 minutes. Subsequent doses of 0.5 mEq/kg may be given every 10 minutes and should be guided by arterial blood pH and $Paco_2$.

e. **Atropine, calcium, and glucose** are not recommended for use in neonatal resuscitation unless specifically indicated.

f. **Fluids.** Hypovolemia should be considered in the setting of peripartum hemorrhage or when hypotension, weak pulses, and persistent pallor are present despite adequate oxygenation and chest compressions. The fluid of choice for volume expansion in the delivery room is an isotonic crystalloid rather than albumin (class IIb). The volume infused should be 10 mL/kg and repeated as necessary. The administration of volume expanders such as albumin rapidly to premature infants has been associated with intraventricular hemorrhage.

SUGGESTED READING

2005 American Heart Association guidelines for cardiopulmonary resuscitation and emergency cardiovascular care. *Circulation* 2005;12(suppl. 24).

38

Pain

Adrian K. Hamburger and Salahadin Abdi

I. **Definitions**
   A. **Pain** (per the International Association for the Study of Pain): An unpleasant sensory and emotional experience associated with actual or potential tissue damage, or described in terms of such damage. The pain system provides information on noxious stimuli that allows the body to respond to the injury (immediate, withdrawal from a noxious source; long-term, protection of the injured part by guarding). Pain may be somatic, visceral, neuropathic, or sympathetically maintained.
   B. **Allodynia:** Pain resulting from a stimulus that does not normally provoke pain.
   C. **Analgesia:** Absence of pain in response to stimulation that normally would be painful.
   D. **Anesthesia dolorosa:** An anesthetic area that develops pain.
   E. **Central pain:** Pain initiated or caused by a primary lesion or dysfunction in the central nervous system.
   F. **Dysesthesia:** An unpleasant abnormal sensation, whether spontaneous or evoked.
   G. **Hyperalgesia:** An increased response to a stimulus that is normally painful.
   H. **Neuralgia:** Pain in the distribution of a nerve or nerves.
   I. **Neuropathy:** Pain initiated or caused by a primary lesion or dysfunction in the peripheral nervous system.
   J. **Radiculopathy:** Dysfunction of a nerve root leading to either motor manifestations (weakness) or sensory manifestations (pain, numbness, paresthesias), or both, along a dermatomal segment.

II. **Types of Pain**
   A. *Somatic pain* is described as aching, gnawing, and/or sharp in quality. It is generally well localized and initiated by nociceptor activation in cutaneous and deep tissues. Examples of somatic pain include acute postoperative pain and bone fractures.
   B. *Visceral pain* is also associated with tissue injury, specifically infiltration, compression, and distention of viscera. It is usually described as dull and aching in quality and poorly localized, and it may be referred to other sites. Examples include abdominal pain due to constipation.
   C. *Neuropathic pain* results from injury to the peripheral or central nervous system (CNS). Shooting, electrical, or burning pain often is superimposed on a chronic background of burning and aching sensations. Examples include postherpetic neuralgia (PHN) and diabetic neuropathy.

III. **Neural basis for pain**
   A. *Nociceptors:* Sensory information about stimuli that may cause tissue damage is conveyed to the CNS by nociceptors, free nerve endings located within cutaneous and noncutaneous tissue. The

information is relayed to the dorsal horn of the spinal cord by way of small-diameter, unmyelinated C-fibers and thinly myelinated A-delta-fibers. C-fiber responses are polymodal and allow the individual to discriminate among mechanical, thermal, and chemical stimuli. When tissue damage occurs, a host of chemical mediators are released in the area of damage, leading to inflammation. Nociceptors in this area demonstrate decreased threshold responses, increased responses to suprathreshold stimuli, and both basal and spontaneous fiber discharge. The resulting pain state is referred to as primary hyperalgesia. Often, the tissue surrounding the area of damage is also sensitive, and this is referred to as secondary hyperalgesia.

B. *Primary afferent fibers:* The nociceptive input to the CNS is carried by unmyelinated C-fibers and myelinated A-delta-fibers. The cell bodies of these primary afferent neurons are located within the dorsal root ganglion (DRG). A-delta-fibers conduct relatively rapidly (5 to 25 m/second), while C-fibers have a slower conduction velocity (<2 m/second). The next key step in nerve transmission occurs at the synapse between these primary afferent fibers and neurons found within the dorsal horn. Cutaneous pain fibers travel in the sensory nerves. Visceral afferent pain fibers travel in the parasympathetic and sympathetic nerves (the cell bodies of these are also located in the DRG).

C. *Dorsal horn:* Nociceptive afferents enter the spinal cord by way of the dorsal root ganglion to terminate on neurons within the dorsal horn. The gray matter of the dorsal horn is divided into 10 layers referred to as Rexed's laminae. C-fibers terminate principally within lamina II (substantia gelatinosa), while A-delta-fibers terminate within lamina I and V. These fibers synapse onto interneurons and second-order neurons; the latter forming the ascending tracts. These neurons have been divided into categories based on their responses to pain.

1. Wide–dynamic-range neurons respond to mechanical as well as noxious stimuli and are located mainly in Rexed's laminae I, II, and V.

2. Nociceptive-specific neurons are activated only by painful stimuli and are found in a number of laminae.

3. The axons from these second-order neurons cross the spinal cord to the anterolateral segment and ascend to higher brain structures. The classic tract is the spinothalamic tract; however, other tracts including the spinohypothalamic, spinoreticular, and spinopontoamygdala tracts exist as well.

D. *Ascending tracts:* Of the four ascending tracts listed above, the spinothalamic tract, located in the ventrolateral aspect of the spinal cord, is the most important. Most of the peripheral afferents cross the spinal cord within one or two segments of entry and, after synapsing within the dorsal horn, ascend to the higher centers within the CNS. The first cortical synapse is within the thalamus; from there third-order neurons send axons to the somatosensory cortex (from the lateral thalamus) or regions of the brain involved in affective responses to pain (from the medial thalamus or limbic system including the cingulate cortex). Other tracts involved in the autonomic response to pain project to the hypothalamus (e.g., stress response and sleep-wake response). In this way, the CNS is "wired" to allow for a sensory and emotional response to an acute, painful stimulus.

E. ***Pain modulation and descending tracts:*** The periaqueductal gray (located in the midbrain) and raphe magnus (located in the medulla) are not the only areas involved in pain modulation. Stimulation of specific thalamic and hypothalamic nuclei also produce analgesia via opioid, central noradrenergic, and serotonergic systems. Receptors for these mediators have been found within pain modulating areas and, when stimulated, cause analgesia that is effectively reversed by pharmacologic antagonists. Axons descend in the dorsolateral funiculus to terminate in the dorsal horn where they modulate afferent input from the periphery.

F. ***Changes producing chronic neuropathic pain*** may result from minor or major trauma, medical disease, or nerve injury. Various anatomic and/or functional neuronal abnormalities have been proposed as the mechanism underlying this type of chronic pain. Some of these changes are as follows:

1. **Ephaptic cross-talk** is the development of abnormal contacts (ephapsis) between axons after injury. Activity in one nerve leads to the activation of another.

2. **Altered adrenergic receptors:** After injury, regenerating nociceptors become sensitive to norepinephrine and the number of α_1-adrenergic receptors on the axons increases. This mechanism has been implicated in the development of sympathetic pain states.

3. **Altered neural connectivity:** A-delta and C-fibers make contacts predominantly within laminae I and II. Light touch is carried by A-beta-fibers that normally synapse within laminae III and IV. However, after injury, A-beta-fibers sprout, making new connections within the superficial laminae and synapsing on the pain projecting neurons. Thus, pain can be produced by light touch in neuropathic pain conditions.

4. **Ectopic impulses:** Under normal conditions, neuromodulators keep pain fibers quiescent. Following damage, abnormal spontaneous activity develops within these nerves. This spontaneous activity may be due to the release of excitatory neuromodulators such as glutamate and substance P.

5. **Sympathetic-afferent coupling:** Under normal conditions, the sympathetic system has no effect on primary afferent neurons. After nerve injury, noradrenergic axons sprout within the DRG and form basket-like structures around injured neurons. As described above, the injured neurons develop adrenergic receptors, which completes the coupling of the two systems. Now, with sympathetic activation the pain system becomes activated. Conversely, with sympathetic blockade, pain is inhibited (hence, sympathetically maintained pain).

IV. **Acute pain**

A. **Basics**

1. Acute pain follows injury to the body and generally disappears with wound healing. It often is associated with physical signs of autonomic hyperactivity. Unfortunately, the most common reason for unrelieved pain is the failure of medical staff to routinely and systematically evaluate the patient's pain and provide adequate pain relief.

2. Visual analog scale: The visual analogue scale (0 to 10 scale) is critical in assessing a patient's pain; in general, a pain level of less than 5 out of 10 is acceptable for many patients and correlates with increased activity, sleep, and so forth. Ideal pain control (0 out of 10) is often an unrealistic goal.

3. Acute (somatic) pain usually is responsive to opioids. Acetaminophen and nonsteroidal anti-inflammatory drugs (NSAIDs) are normally given in addition to opioids as a multimodal treatment approach and also to have an opioid sparing effect.

4. A patient's underlying anxiety can play a major role in the perception of acute pain, and therefore adjuvant anxiolytics or sedatives can be helpful.

B. Preemptive analgesia. Animal and clinical experiments suggest that analgesic intervention before a noxious stimulus will reduce or eliminate subsequent pain. Noxious impulses from deep tissues can trigger prolonged changes in spinal cord excitability, which result in pain that is more resistant to treatment. Hyperexcitability may be prevented if small doses of local anesthetic or opioid are administered before the stimulus. A part of this effect may also be behavioral: a patient who experiences satisfactory analgesia is likely to have a good response to subsequent analgesic treatment.

C. Postoperative pain management. Patients expected to have significant postoperative pain should be given adequate treatment before emergence from general anesthesia. The sudden onset of severe pain during recovery can lead to emergence delirium, undesirable cardiovascular effects, and impaired ventilation. Reestablishing analgesia can be more difficult in this circumstance. Patients tolerant or dependent on opioids should be treated similarly to any other acute pain patient, except that tolerance will increase the amount of opioid that needs to be given to manage baseline requirements. Postoperative analgesia can be provided with intravenous (IV) boluses or infusions of opioids (nurse or patient-controlled), oral and parenteral NSAIDs, or neuraxial infusion of opioids and/or local anesthetics. Initial analgesia is most often established by titration with incremental IV or epidural bolus doses. Some of the pharmacologic agents often used to treat acute pain are as follows:

1. **Nonopioid analgesics (Table 38.1)**
   a. Aspirin, acetaminophen, and NSAIDs are all useful in the management of acute and chronic pain. These agents differ significantly from opioid analgesics because the intensity of the analgesic effect is more limited; they do not produce tolerance or physical dependence, and they are antipyretic. Both ASA and the NSAIDs work by inhibiting the cyclooxygenase pathway, which in turn stops the production of various prostaglandins that can sensitize free nerve endings to painful stimuli. The mechanism of analgesia produced by acetaminophen is not known. As a general rule, severe pain will require treatment with opioid analgesics, but most patients will do better if a nonopioid agent is also administered as an adjuvant.
      (1) **Aspirin (ASA):** Gastritis and bleeding are common with therapeutic doses of ASA, and the presence of bleeding is poorly correlated with symptoms.

Table 38.1. Selected nonopioid analgesics: dosages and comparative efficacy to standards

Drug	Proprietary Names (not all-inclusive)	Special Nonopioid Analgesic Dosage and Comparative Efficacy to Standards						
		Average Analgesic Dose (mg)	Dose Interval (hrs)	Maximal Daily Dose (mg)	Pediatric Dose (mg/kg)	Analgesic Efficacy Compared with Standards	Plasma Half-life (hrs)	Comments
Acetaminophen	Numerous	500–1,000 PO	4–6	4,000	10–15 PO q4–6h	Comparable to aspirin 650 mg	2–3	Rectal suppository available for children and adults
Salicylates Aspirin	Numerous	500–1,000 PO	4–6	4,000	10–15 PO q4–6h	xx	0.25	Because of risk of Reye syndrome, do not use in children under 12 yr with possible viral illness; rectal suppository available for children and adults

Diflunisal	Dolobid	1,000 PO initial, 500 PO subsequent	8–12	1,500	xx	500 mg superior to aspirin 650 mg, with slower onset and longer duration; initial dose of 1,000 mg significantly shortens time to onset	8–12	xx
Choline magnesium trisalicylate	Trilisate	100–1,500 PO	12	2,000–3,000	25 PO bid	Longer duration of action than aspirin 650 mg	9–17	xx
NSAIDs *Propionic acids* Ibuprofen	Motrin, Rufen, Nuprin, Advil, Medipren	200–400 PO	4–6	2,400	10 PO q6-8h	Superior at 200 mg to aspirin at 650 mg	2–2.5	xx
Naproxen	Naprosyn	500 PO initial; 250 PO	6–8	1,250	5 PO bid	xx	12–15	xx

continued

Table 38.1. *Continued.*

Drug	Proprietary Names (not all-inclusive)	Average Analgesic Dose (mg)	Dose Interval (hrs)	Maximal Daily Dose (mg)	Pediatric Dose (mg/kg)	Analgesic Efficacy Compared with Standards	Plasma Half-life (hrs)	Comments
						Special Nonopioid Analgesic Dosage and Comparative Efficacy to Standards		
Naproxen sodium	Anaprox	550 initial; 275 PO subsequent	6–8	1,375	5 PO bid	275 mg comparable to aspirin 650 mg, with longer slower onset and duration; 550 mg superior to aspirin 650 mg	xx	xx
Fenopren	Nalfon	200 PO	4–6	800	xx	Comparable to aspirin 650 mg	2–3	xx
Ketoprofen	Orudis	25–50 PO	6–8	300	xx	Superior at 25 mg to aspirin 650 mg	1.5	xx

Indolacetic acids

Indomethacin	Indocin	25 PO	8–12	100	xx	Comparable to aspirin 650 mg	2	Not routinely used because of high incidence of side effects; rectal, IV forms available for adults

Pyrrolacetic acids

Ketorolac	Toraldol	30 mg IM initial; 15 or 30 mg IM subsequent	6	150 first day, 120 thereafter	xx	In the range of 6–12 mg morphine	6	Not >5 days PO

COX II Inhibitors

Celecoxib	Celebrex	100–200 mg PO	q12	400 mg	xx	xx	11	Not to be taken if sulfa allergic

Anthranilic acids

Mefenamic acid	Ponstel	500 mg PO initial; 250 mg PO subsequent	6	1,500	xx	Comparable to aspirin 650 mg	2	In U.S. use is restricted to interval of 1 week

COX, cyclooxygenase; h, hour(s); bid, twice a day; IM, intramuscularly; IV, intravenous; NSAIDs, nonsteroidal anti-inflammatory drugs; PO, orally; q, every.

Because of the risk of Reyes syndrome, ASA is usually avoided in children less than 12 years of age in the setting of a viral syndrome (particularly varicella). Hypersensitivity to ASA is well described. Patients may develop respiratory symptoms with rhinitis, asthma, and nasal polyps. They may also develop urticaria, angioneurotic edema, and shock. Patients who are sensitive to ASA may also be sensitive to NSAIDs.

(2) Acetaminophen has no antiplatelet effects, minimal anti-inflammatory effects, and minimal effects on gastric mucosa. Patients with liver disease or significant alcohol intake may develop hepatic failure when usual therapeutic doses of acetaminophen are taken.

(3) NSAIDs: These agents are useful analgesics in most acute pain states but often are overlooked in the postoperative period. Unless there is a specific contraindication, these drugs should be routinely considered. NSAIDs are a useful first line of therapy in cancer pain, particularly because metastatic lesions to bone often cause prostaglandin-mediated inflammation and pain. Some of the effects and side effects of these agents are discussed as follows:

(a) Analgesic effects: Cyclooxygenase (Cox) I and II nonselective inhibitors (ibuprofen, naproxyn, and ketorolac) are the most commonly used. NSAIDs with short half-lives (ibuprofen, diclofenac) or parenteral preparations (ketorolac) are most useful for rapid control of perioperative pain. Ketorolac may take 45 minutes for the onset of significant analgesia, and this should be considered when dosing. Patients vary in their response to these agents, and a second drug may work if the first is unsuccessful.

(b) Hematologic effects: Unlike ASA, NSAIDs reversibly inhibit platelet aggregation. This inhibition lasts only as long as there is an effective serum drug concentration. NSAIDs cause an excessive prolongation of the prothrombin time in those individuals taking oral anticoagulants. Ketorolac has a somewhat longer effect on hemostasis and its cumulative dosing over a few days has been associated with a higher incidence of postoperative hemorrhage. Published data suggest that NSAIDs treatment does not increase the risk for bleeding from epidural catheters.

(c) Gastrointestinal effects: Dyspepsia, gastritis, and duodenitis have been reported. The concomitant use of a prophylactic regimen such as antacids, H2 antagonists, or proton-pump inhibitors is recommended. The use of alcohol should also be avoided, because the risk of gastrointestinal bleeding and hepatitis are increased.

(d) Renal effects: Renal insufficiency has been described in patients taking NSAIDs, although large-scale trials suggest this is unlikely unless there are other significant risk factors (hypovolemia, congestive heart failure, chronic renal insufficiency, cirrhosis with ascites, systemic lupus erythematosus, diuretic use, peripheral vascular disease, multiple myeloma). The putative mechanism of the renal insufficiency is decreased synthesis of renal vasodilator prostaglandins, impaired renin secretion, and enhanced tubular water and sodium reabsorption. NSAIDs have also been associated with allergic nephritis, renal tubular acidosis with hyperkalemia, and enhanced secretion of antidiuretic hormone with significant hyponatremia.

b. COX II selective inhibitors (coxibs): The only coxib that is still marketed in the United States is celecoxib. It unquestionably produces fewer gastrointestinal symptoms and bleeding than nonselective NSAIDs, but this class definitely increases the risk of thrombosis, myocardial infarction, and stroke. Coxibs and NSAIDs produce similar analgesic effects, so coxib use should be restricted to those select patients in whom the risk of gastrointestinal toxicity offsets the cardiovascular risk.

2. Opioids (Table 38.2). Systemic opioids have long been the treatment of choice for acute postoperative pain and for severe chronic pain in combination with adjuvant medications. The general properties of opioids are reviewed in Chapter 11, section I.F. Individualization of analgesic therapy is essential for rapid and safe pain control. Routes of administration include the following:

a. Oral: In patients who can take oral medications immediately after surgery, rapid-acting opioids (oxycodone/acetaminophen, hydrocodone, codeine) may be sufficient and provide a good transition to analgesic therapy at home. The oral route is optimal for patients with chronic pain because of its convenience and flexibility. For patients who cannot swallow tablets, some can be crushed and put into concentrated emulsion, and many are also available as elixirs. For chronic pain, it is best to keep the patient on long-acting medication. Most of the oral opioids reach peak effect within 30 to 60 minutes, and it may take longer for sustained-release formulations. This may not be fast enough for patients with rapidly fluctuating pain, and "rescue" doses of short-acting medications may be required. Opioid dosage should be increased until pain is under reasonable control or side effects interfere. In the chronic pain setting, sedation is a common dose-limiting side effect. This can sometimes be treated with the addition of a stimulant like methylphenidate (5 to 10 mg once a day; rarely this dose could be given every 12 hours).

b. Intramuscular: Although commonly used, painful intramuscular (IM) injections are rarely necessary in a

Table 38.2. Opioid analgesics

Name	Equianalgesic Dose (mg) Oral	Equianalgesic Dose (mg) Parenteral[a]	Starting Oral Dose Adults (mg)	Starting Oral Dose Children (mg/kg)	Time (h)
Morphine	30	10	15–30	0.3	2–3.5
Hydromorphone (Dilaudid)	7.5	1.5	4–8	0.06	
Oxycodone	30	xx	15–30	0.3	2–3
Methadone (Dolophine)	20	10	5–10	0.2	
Fentanyl	xx	0.1	xx	xx	3–12
Oxymorphone (Numorphan)	xx	1	xx	xx	
Meperidine (Demerol)	300	75	Not recommended		3–4[a]

[a]These are standard intramuscular (IM) doses for acute pain in adults and also may be used to convert doses for intravenous (IV) infusions and repeated small IV boluses. For single IV boluses, use half the IM dose. IV doses for children <6 months of age = parenteral equianalgesic dose x weight (kg)/100.

postoperative patient and even less so in the chronic pain patient. In addition, IM injections may cause subcutaneous inflammation, muscular fibrosis, and/or abscesses.

c. **Rectal:** Although not commonly used, rectal administration is a good alternative that permits rapid absorption and avoids hepatic first-pass metabolism. However bioavailability is very variable, depending on the amount of stool in the rectum as well as blood flow. Frequently, rectal dosing is equivalent to oral dosing.

d. **IV:** This is the most commonly used route for immediate postoperative pain control. Parenteral opioids are also used when oral medications fail. The appropriate parenteral dosage is calculated using available oral to parenteral conversion data (see Table 38.2). Because patients may develop significant physical dependence on opioids during prolonged IV therapy, changing to a route with lower bioavailability may lead to withdrawal. This can almost always be managed by avoiding abrupt changes. For outpatients with severe cancer pain, a patient-controlled analgesia (PCA) system can be used but requires the help of skilled nurses. In acute pain states, bolus administration is the fastest way to achieve adequate analgesia. Time to onset or peak effect is determined by the lipid solubility of the drug. Onset time ranges from 3 to 5 minutes with fentanyl and 10 to 30 minutes with morphine or hydromorphone. Titration to adequate pain relief is commonly provided by a physician or nurse and then maintained with a PCA system.

(1) **PCA:** This device will deliver a preset dose of opioid on demand as an IV bolus. The prescription must specify an incremental dose, a lock-out interval, and a maximum 1-hour total dose (Table 38.3). This is a

Table 38.3. Patient-controlled analgesia (PCA) for adults

Requirements	Drug		
	Morphine	Hydromorphone	Meperidine
Concentration (mg/mL)	1	0.5	10
Demand dose (mL)	1	0.5	1
Range (mL)	0.5–2.0	0.5–2.0	0.5–2.0
Lockout interval	6 min	10 min	6 min
Basal rate (mL/hr)			
Day	0	0	0
Night	0.5	0.5	0.5
Hourly limit (mL)	<12	<6	<10
Loading dose (mg) (every 5 min until comfortable)	2 mg	0.5 mg	20 mg
Maximum loading dose (mg)	10–15 mg	2–4 mg	75–150 mg

safe tool for postoperative pain management, and it also provides patients with a sense of control. PCA is not appropriate for use in very young children or patients with cognitive impairment. However, PCA may be used in children who understand the relationship between a stimulus (pain), a response (pushing the button), and a delayed result (pain relief) for PCA to be effective (Table 38.4).

(a) Morphine is the most commonly used opioid, and its behavior in PCA is well understood. For nontolerant patients, we generally start with a 1-mg/mL concentration, a demand/bolus dose of 1 mL, a lockout interval of 6 minutes, and a basal rate of 0 to 1 mL/hour during sleep. For babies and infants with acute

Table 38.4. Patient-controlled analgesia (PCA) or continuous infusion of morphine for pediatric patients

Children Under 7 Years of Age (Use Dilute Solution: 0.2 mg/mL)

Requirements	Dose (mg/kg)	Example: For a 10 kg Child, Using 0.2 mg/mL
Basal rate (per hour)	0.01–0.05	0.1 mg = 0.5 mL
Hourly limit	0.03	0.3 mg = 1.5 mL
Initial bolus (every 5 min until comfortable)	0.02	0.2 mg = 1 mL
Maximum bolus	0.1	1 mg = 5 mL
For increasing pain	2 to 3 times basal rate	

Children 7 to 11 Years of Age (These Children Can Usually Cope With Patient-Controlled Dosing: Use Dilute Solution : 0.2 mg/mL)

Age Range (yr)	Approximate Weight (kg)	PCA Setting[a] Using 0.2 mg/mL
7–8	20	1/6/0
9–11	30	2/6/0

Children 12 to 15 Years of Age (These Children Cope Well With PCA; Use Standard Solution (1 mg/mL); Over 15 Years of Age, Treat as Adults)

Age Range (yr)	Approximate Weight (kg)	PCA Setting[a] Using 1 mg/mL
12–14	40–50	0.5/6/0
15	>50	1/6/0

[a]PCA setting: demand dose mL/lockout interval (min)/basal rate (mL/h).

postoperative pain, continuous morphine infusions (10 to 50 μg/kg/hour) without a bolus are used.

   (b) Hydromorphone (dilaudid) is the second drug of choice for PCA. It is more potent than morphine and is sometimes tolerated in patients who have side effects from morphine. Its metabolites are inactive, so it may be a better choice than morphine for patients with renal failure. A typical PCA starting concentration is 0.5 mg/mL, a demand/bolus dose of 0.5 to 1 mL, a lockout interval of 10 minutes, and a basal rate of 0 to 1 mL/hour during sleep.

   (c) Meperidine continues to be widely used for acute pain and is useful in some patients. Its onset is faster than that of morphine (5 to 7 min), but the duration is shorter. Meperidine is N-demethylated to an epileptogenic metabolite, normeperidine, which may accumulate in patients with renal dysfunction. It inhibits serotonin reuptake and may create toxic interactions in patients taking monoamine oxidase inhibitors or selective serotonin reuptake inhibitors. A typical PCA concentration is 10 mg/mL, a demand dose of 1 mL, a lockout interval of 6 min, and a basal rate of 0 to 1 mL/hour during sleep. Due to its sporadic toxicity and its relatively short duration, this drug is less desirable for management of long-term pain.

  e. **Transdermal:** Fentanyl is lipid soluble and is readily absorbed through skin. A fentanyl patch is extremely convenient because steady blood levels are attained with a system that is changed only every 3 days. A 25-μg/hour patch is equivalent to 10 mg of IV morphine administered every 8 hours. Peak effect after the initial application occurs at 24 to 72 hours. After removal, fentanyl continues to be absorbed from the depot remaining in the subcutaneous tissue, so serum drug levels drop by 50% after an average of 17 hours. Transdermal delivery of fentanyl is an alternative to the oral route for the treatment of chronic pain. Given the lag time to peak effect, this method of drug delivery is not commonly used in the acute pain setting. The advantage of the patch is the production of a steady, consistent blood concentration of fentanyl, while avoiding the need for needles or a functioning gastrointestinal tract. Unfortunately, transdermal fentanyl appears to induce tolerance as quickly as continuous infusions, and nausea remains a frequent side effect.

  f. **Epidural:** Narcotics can be deposited in the epidural space. This is most safely done in the perioperative setting if the patient is monitored with oximetry. Most commonly, patients are given local anesthetic-opioid infusions, but a bolus dose of preservative-free morphine can be used (2 to 5 mg) and provides analgesia up to 18 to 22 hours. If a patient receives epidural opioids, great care must be taken before administering any other supplemental opioids. The risk of opioid accumulation and subsequent respiratory depression is greatly increased.

3. **Opioid agonist-antagonist.** These include pentazocine, nalbuphine, and butorphanol. Only pentazocine is available orally. They are less abusable than morphine but may cause dysphoria, so they are not commonly used. Nalbuphine (0.05 to 0.1 mg/kg IV/IM) is an effective antagonist for the management of opioid-related pruritus but may reverse some analgesia.

a. **Opioid conversion:** IV to oral: Equivalent oral and parenteral doses and approximate relative potency for opioids are given in Table 38.2. An IV infusion of 1 mg of morphine per hour is equivalent to 25 μg of fentanyl per hour. During prolonged dosing, it is sometimes necessary to practice "opioid rotation" (see Tolerance below). When rotating one opioid to another, it is safest to administer 25% to 50% of the calculated equivalent dose and titrate higher as needed.

b. **Side effects:** The side effects of acute opioid administration are described in Chapter 11, section F. Chronic administration can lead to the problems of tolerance and physical dependence.

c. *Tolerance* is a reduced effect on repeated exposure to a drug at a constant dose. Often the first manifestation is reduced duration of analgesic effect. Tolerance develops most rapidly to analgesia, euphoria, nausea, and respiratory depression but very slowly to constipation. For this reason, patients receiving long-term opioid treatment almost always need stool softeners or laxatives. Two quaternary opioid antagonists, alvimopan and methylnalterexone, are nearing FDA approval, and these can reverse or prevent constipation but do not affect analgesia. Urinary retention can occur and may require catheterization or administration of a cholinergic agonist like bethanecol.

d. *Cross-tolerance.* When a patient becomes tolerant to one mu-opioid agonist, there is simultaneous development of cross-tolerance to all other mu opioids. This cross-tolerance is often incomplete, and it is the basis for so-called "opioid rotation." When a patient is no longer obtaining adequate relief from one opioid, changing to another may increase efficacy. The basis for this may be actions of the drugs on different subtypes of mu receptors.

e. *Physical dependence* is a physiological state that appears with continued exposure to opioids. Stopping the drug causes a withdrawal syndrome characterized by sympathetic activation, drug seeking, gooseflesh, mydriasis, runny nose, hyperpyrexia, diarrhea, and hyperalgesia. Cross dependence occurs between opioids, so one opioid will prevent withdrawal from another. Weaning a dependent patient from opioids is commonly done by switching to methadone, which produces a mild, but protracted, withdrawal. The opioid is then tapered over 7 to 21 days. Symptoms may be managed with sedatives and an α_2-agonist like clonidine.

    f. *Addiction* is a biological and behavioral disorder involving serious compulsive use of a substance despite adverse consequences: Fear of patient addiction is widespread among health care providers and among patients and their families. Although most patients who take opioids daily for more than a month develop some degree of tolerance and physical dependence, the available data suggest that the risk of addiction is extremely low and should not be a primary concern in the treatment of acute or chronic pain. There is some risk of diversion and abuse during chronic opioid therapy, and this should be discussed frankly with the patient upon initiating such a treatment plan.

    4. Local anesthetics. Epidural catheters: Epidural analgesia can provide excellent intraoperative as well as postoperative analgesia. They are commonly placed for the following surgeries: thoracic or abdominal surgery, especially in patients with significant underlying pulmonary disease; lower limb surgery where early progression to ambulation is important; lower extremity vascular surgery where a sympathectomy would be advantageous.

        a. Common infusions (Table 38.5): A commonly used (in our institution) infusion for postoperative epidural therapy is a mixture of 0.1% bupivacaine with hydromorphone at 0.02 mg/mL. In elderly patients, patients with marginal respiratory status, and patients aged 1 through 7 years, a mixture of 0.1% bupivacaine with fentanyl at 2 μg/mL is

Table 38.5. Suitable regimens for epidural infusions in adults and children

Solutions

<1 yr old: 0.1% bupivacaine *without* fentanyl

1 to 7 yr of age: 0.1% bupivacaine with fentanyl at 2 μg/mL fentanyl

>7 yr of age or adult: 0.1% bupivacaine with hydromorphone at 20 μg/mL

Special indications: fentanyl or hydromorphone without bupivacaine

Rate of infusion

Adults

    Starting rate, 2 to 10 mL/hour

    For increasing pain, increase in increments of up to 10 mL/hour

    For decreasing pain or for side effects, decrease in increments down to 1 mL/hour

Children

    Starting rate, 0.1 mL/kg/hour of appropriate solution (see above)

    For increasing pain, increase in increments up to 0.3 mL/kg/hour

    For bolusing catheter:

        ≥6 kg, 1 mL of 1% lidocaine with 1:200,000 epinephrine

        6 to 15 kg, 2 mL of 1% Lidocaine with 1:200,000 epinephrine

        >15 kg, 5 mL of 1% lidocaine with 1:200,000 epinephrine

Note: Pediatric mixtures of bupivacaine and fentanyl may be indicated in special circumstances for adult patients.

commonly used. Infants under 1 year of age should not have fentanyl added to the epidural mixture (unless they will be monitored in an ICU), because this age group is particularly sensitive to the depressant effects of opioids. Fentanyl is much more lipophilic than morphine or hydromorphone, so it is shorter acting and produces a more segmental analgesic effect. The very low concentrations of fentanyl in CSF are less likely to reach respiratory centers in the brainstem. Other drugs may be used for epidural analgesia, including morphine and the α_2-adrenergic agonist, clonidine (2 to 10 μg/kg for a normal adult as a bolus, and 10 to 40 μg/hour continuous infusion).

b. Epidural management issues: Many problems can be avoided with attention to the details of epidural catheter placement and management. It should typically be 3 to 5 cm in the epidural space. When the catheter is placed before a general anesthetic, proper function should ideally be demonstrated before anesthesia is induced. Epidural catheter insertion sites should be inspected daily for signs of infection. Catheters are usually removed after 4 to 7 days of use.

c. Inadequate analgesia: If pain is not well controlled, the infusion rate or concentration can be increased, or a bolus of 5 to 10 mL of the patient's epidural solution can be administered. If the patient is receiving epidural opioids, supplemental parenteral opioids should be given cautiously and generally in a monitored setting (operating room, postanesthesia care unit, or intensive care unit). Concentrated local anesthetics (usually 3 to 5 mL of 1% lidocaine with epinephrine) can be administered to test the catheter. If there is no response within 10 to 20 minutes, the catheter should be replaced or the patient should be started on alternative systemic analgesia.

d. Catheter disconnection: After a witnessed "disconnect," the distal inch of the catheter can be cleaned with an alcohol swab, cut off, and a new sterile adapter hub attached to the freshly cut end. After an unwitnessed disconnection, the catheter should be removed and replaced, or the patient should be switched to systemic analgesics.

e. Side effects: As with any epidural, those placed for postoperative analgesia carry the risks of bleeding, infection, and neural damage. The use of dilute local anesthetic solutions can minimize the risks of weakness and injury to unprotected limbs. Epidural opioids can cause pruritus, urinary retention, and nausea. These may be treated with the opioid antagonist naloxone (1 μg/kg up to 100 μg IV). A continuous infusion of naloxone is sometimes necessary. Profound sedation and respiratory depression will usually require higher doses of naloxone (0.1 to 0.4 mg IV as needed), and these doses may also partially reverse analgesia. A continuous, naloxone infusion (5 to 10 μg/kg/hour) is often useful to reverse respiratory depression while permitting continued analgesia. The risk of delayed respiratory depression after epidural opioids is greatest for a hydrophilic opioid like morphine, but it is still a rare event. The risk of delayed respiratory depression after epidural opioids is increased by coadministered CNS depressants such as parenteral opioids, barbiturates, and benzodiazepines. Additional risk factors include advanced age, respiratory disease, and factors that encourage the cephalad spread of drug such as increased intrathoracic and abdominal pressure, a more cephalad level of injection, and a larger dose of opioid.

    f. Discontinuing treatment: Epidural analgesia can either be converted to parenteral analgesics or directly to oral if the patient is tolerating oral intake.

  5. Miscellaneous analgesia techniques: Several other single shot or catheter techniques that may be used for short- and/or long-term analgesia include the following: intrathecal, intercostal, and interpleural analgesia as well as peripheral nerve blocks (e.g., "3 in 1," lumbar plexus, and brachial plexus blocks). It is critical to understand their indication, contraindication, and complications to be able to use these techniques safely and effectively (see Chapter 17).

V. Chronic pain. While acute pain that normally occurs after trauma or surgery lasts for a limited time, chronic pain persists for months or even years. Common chronic pain complaints include low back pain, neuropathic pain (pain resulting from damage to the peripheral nerves and/or to the central nervous system), complex regional pain syndrome, post herpetic neuralgia, cancer pain, and myofascial pain.

  A. Low back pain occurs in almost all adults due to multiple, often coexistent mechanisms. Usually it is acute in nature and will resolve within 6 weeks. Chronic low back pain is present in up to 50% of adults. Occult disease (e.g., retroperitoneal tumor) must be excluded, anatomic derangements (e.g., bony fragments) must be characterized, and possible surgical options (e.g., decompression foraminotomy) must be considered with orthopedic surgeons or neurosurgeons before selecting nonsurgical management. Sensorimotor function, including tenderness and pain on flexion or extension of the spine and extremities, should be documented at each stage of treatment. Bowel or bladder dysfunction argues for aggressive surgical intervention, as does a persistent decrease in motor or sensory function. Two of the most commonly used interventional procedures for the treatment of low back pain are as follows:

    1. Epidural steroid injection

      a. Indications. When a patient with low back pain fails more conservative treatment and there has been no progression of neurologic symptoms (e.g., foot drop or bowel and bladder dysfunction), epidural steroid injection is indicated. Indications for epidural steroid therapy for low back pain include patients with disk herniation and postlaminectomy syndrome. Each of these conditions may cause nerve root irritation with subsequent edema and swelling. Epidural steroid administration will decrease pain and inflammation in many patients and is especially attractive when coexistent disease places the patient at increased operative and anesthetic risk.

        (1) Protrusion: Protrusion of the intervertebral disk may lead to nerve compression or cauda equina syndrome. Pain and paresthesias in the lower extremities may ensue and progress to muscle weakness and paralysis as well as loss of sexual function, bowel, and bladder control. Acute nerve entrapment leading to sudden progression of neurologic symptoms should be considered a neurosurgical emergency, and immediate consultation must be obtained.

(2) Stenosis: congenital, traumatic, or degenerative narrowing of the spinal canal produces spinal stenosis. This narrowing usually is accompanied by painless bilateral leg weakness and/or neurogenic claudication relieved with rest.

b. Technique

(1) Interlaminar: With the patient in the prone position, a 22-gauge $3\frac{1}{2}$-inch spinal needle (Quincke point) is advanced under fluoroscopic guidance into the epidural space. Nonionic contrast is injected to verify epidural spread. Local trauma due to needle insertion may exacerbate back pain for a few days after the injection. Patients are reevaluated in 2 weeks. If the patient is substantially improved and satisfied with this level of improvement, no further therapy is needed. If there is only some improvement or the symptoms have returned, a repeat block may be indicated. If pain is worse after the first injection, a different modality (e.g., substitution of one brand of glucocorticoid for another, injection at a different site, or a different epidural approach) should be tried. No more than three injections in a 12-week period should be performed, because significant blunting of the hypothalamic-pituitary axis may take place.

(2) Transforaminal technique allows for a more lateral and ventral spread of the medication and is obtained with an oblique fluoroscopic view, using a 25-gauge, $3\frac{1}{2}$-inch spinal needle. This approach is preferred if there has been previous surgery at that level, as it decreases the likelihood of intrathecal entry. Typically, we use 40 mg of triamcinolone and a low dose of local anesthetic (1 mL of 1% lidocaine or 0.25% bupivacaine is sufficient). The steroid component takes 2 to 6 days before the patient notices improvement.

(3) Caudal technique is especially useful in our experience for patients after failed back surgery. We normally use about 20 mL of a mixture of triamnicolone (80 mg), 5 mL of 0.25% bupivacaine, and 13 mL of preservative-free normal saline. Furthermore, this approach is widely used to do epidural adhesiolysis.

2. Facet joint injection

a. Indications: Lumbar facet joint pathology is suspected when low back pain is referred to the buttock or thighs in a nondermatomal pattern, and the patient is able to perform forward flexion but is limited in extension and rotation of the spine. Cervical facet joint arthropathy is suspected usually after acceleration-deceleration injury to the cervical spine, associated with a classical referred pain pattern, worsened with rotation of the neck.

- b. **Technique**
    - (1) **Intra-articular:** With the patient prone, a $3\frac{1}{2}$-inch 25-gauge spinal needle is advanced into the facet joint under fluoroscopic guidance. A characteristic change in resistance is felt when penetration of the joint is achieved. The correct needle position is verified by injecting a small amount of contrast dye under fluoroscopy and then a dose of 1 mL of 0.25% bupivacaine is administered. A corticosteroid is often added for therapeutic effect.
    - (2) **Medial branch block:** While the intra-articular approach can provide short-term relief, the medial branch block serves as a good diagnostic maneuver before a more permanent radiofrequency lesioning. These are most effective in the cervical and the lumbar region. For the lumbar approach, a 10-cm ($3\frac{1}{2}$-inch) 25-gauge spinal needle is advanced, under fluoroscopic guidance, to the junction of the superior articulating process and the transverse process. For the cervical approach, the same size needle is advanced toward the midsection of the articular pillar until contact with bone is made. Typically, we use 0.25 to 0.5 mL of local anesthetic and expect a significant improvement in pain for this type of block to have a diagnostic use. If this block is successful, then the patient is a candidate for radiofrequency lesioning.

B. **Neuropathic pain** results from an aberration of nerve physiology or anatomy (examples include alcoholic or diabetic neuropathy, amputation, and partial spinal cord damage). Commonly described as either a lancinating or burning pain, neuropathic pain is often treated with tricyclic antidepressant drugs (amitriptyline, nortriptyline, desipramine) or anticonvulsants (gabapentin, pregabalin, carbamezapine, oxcarbazepine, topiramate).

1. **Oral medications.** Among the antidepressants, **nortriptyline** has a better side-effect profile than amitriptyline. The starting dose for nortriptyline is 10 to 25 mg orally QHS, and it can be escalated slowly. Common side effects include sedation, dry mouth, and constipation. This class of drugs should be avoided in patients with preexisting dysrhythmias or cardiac dysfunction. On the other hand, **gabapentin** is relatively safe and has minimal side effects other than sedation. Commonly this drug is started at a low dose of 100 to 300 mg QHS and slowly escalated to relief or 1,200 mg orally TID as tolerated. These medications can also be used in combination relatively safely. The sedating side effect of both tricyclic antidepressants and anticonvulsive agents is often beneficial for the management of insomnia (commonly seen with neuropathic and other forms of chronic pain). Further, opioids are sometimes helpful in combination with the adjuvant neuropathic pain medications as described above. For intractable neuropathic pain that is localized to one or two extremities, dorsal column stimulation can be tried.

2. **Infusions for intractable neuropathies:** IV infusion of local anesthetic may be used as a diagnostic test or to treat

neuropathic pain. If an IV infusion of 100 to 300 mg of 1% lidocaine over 20 to 30 minutes provides long-lasting relief, the patient may benefit from a trial of oral mexiletine hydrochloride. Careful follow-up with periodic blood levels is prudent. Some patients will respond only to IV lidocaine, without much response to mexiletine, in which case they can use a continuous subcutaneous lidocaine infusion.

C. **Complex regional pain syndrome (CRPS),** formerly known as reflex sympathetic dystrophy (RSD), typically occurs after a trivial injury or obvious nerve trauma and is associated with an alteration of the nervous system, often resulting in heightened sympathetic outflow. **CRPS I (RSD):** Most often initiated by trauma, and sometimes can be iatrogenic (surgery, poorly fit cast). **CRPS II (Causalgia):** Similar pattern of symptoms to CRPS I, except that a direct causal relationship can be implied by damage to a specific nerve.

1. **Symptoms:** The hallmark of this syndrome is an exquisitely painful body part (usually a limb). The pain is characterized as a burning sensation with extreme sensitivity to stimuli (hyperesthesia) and progression of pain with repetitive innocuous stimuli (hyperpathia). Innocuous stimuli (e.g., light touch) may also produce pain (allodynia). Typically starting in a small, discrete area, the pain intensifies over time and spreads proximally from its origin. Characteristic changes are noted when RSD becomes progressive. The skin, which is typically cold, adopts a smooth, glassy appearance and has decreased hair growth and sweating. The end stage is significant for disuse atrophy and marked osteoporosis.

2. **Diagnostics:** Diagnosis is based on the whole clinical picture. If the pain is sympathetically mediated, it will often respond to a sympathetic block using local anesthetic. Some have advocated the use of quantitative sensory testing for diagnosis, but this is controversial.

3. The **pharmacologic management** of this syndrome is very similar to the treatment of neuropathic pain as described above in (b).

4. The following interventional procedures are commonly performed as part of the treatment of this syndrome.

   a. **Stellate ganglion block (SGB)**

      (1) **Indications:** SGB is used by pain specialists for treating sympathetically mediated or maintained pain syndromes. Some of the pain syndromes that are successfully treated with this procedure are complex regional pain syndrome types I, and II (CRPS) of upper extremity, peripheral vasospastic disease, atypical facial pain, and pain associated with intractable angina.

      (2) **Technique.** With the patient in the supine position, a 22-gauge 1- or 2-inch needle is advanced under fluoroscopic guidance posteriorly between the trachea and carotid artery. The target is the prevertebral fascia on the anterolateral surface of the C-6 and preferably C-7 vertebra. After confirmation of the correct needle position by injecting contrast dye and negative aspiration for blood, air, CSF, 5 to 10 mL of 1% lidocaine or 0.25% bupivacaine is slowly

injected. Using lower volumes could minimize cervical plexus, phrenic, superficial, or recurrent laryngeal nerve anesthesia. Horner's syndrome (ptosis, enophthalmos, miosis, and anhidrosis) is typically seen, although this sign alone is not pathognomonic for successful sympathetic blockade of the upper extremity. More frequently, there will be evidence of vasodilation in the intended limb as well as possibly some nasal congestion ipsilaterally.

b. Lumbar sympathetic block (LSB)

    (1) Indications: This block is indicated for diagnosis and treatment of sympathetically maintained pain of the lower extremities, peripheral vascular disease and complex regional pain syndrome type I and II (CRPS) of the lower extremity.

    (2) Technique. The L-2 vertebra is identified with fluoroscopy. A 10- to 15-cm, 22- or 20-gauge needle is inserted just below the 12th rib and directed toward the body of the L-2 vertebra with the needle bevel facing laterally. When the transverse process is encountered, the needle is redirected cephalad to slide off the edge and contact the vertebral body. The needle tip is advanced slightly beyond the anterior projection of the vertebral body and confirmed with fluoroscopy. A total of 15 to 20 mL of 1% lidocaine, or 0.25% bupivacaine is given in divided doses after negative aspiration for blood and CSF and the limb is monitored for effect. This technique may also be performed by a catheter technique to provide intermittent injections (10 to 20 mL of 0.25% bupivacaine four times a day) or a continuous infusion (4 to 8 mL/hour of 0.125% to 0.25% bupivacaine). This type of block should be followed by aggressive physical therapy.

c. IV regional sympathetic block: Alternative to the above described sympathetic nerve block techniques; adrenergic antagonist drugs (e.g. guanethidine, reserpine, labetatol) with lidocaine can be IV administered to a tourniquet-isolated limb. Typically, we use a combination of 100 mg of lidocaine and 20 mg of labetatol with normal saline to a total volume of 20 mL for the upper extremity and 200 mg of lidocaine and 30 mg of labetatol with normal saline to a total volume of 40 mL for the lower extremity. It is imperative that the patient is monitored appropriately for any evidence of systemic leakage (especially cardio-CNS side effects). A minimum of 20 minutes tourniquet time is recommended to minimize systemic side effects and complications. Furthermore, the tourniquet should be released slowly or intermittently to avoid the sudden rash of the local anesthetics into the systemic circulation. This type of block should be followed by aggressive physical therapy.

d. Spinal cord stimulation (SCS)

    (1) Indications: Also known as dorsal column stimulation is a useful device for the management of medically nonresponsive neuropathic pain. The more distal the neuropathy the greater the likelihood of success with the stimulator. Before permanent implantation, the patient will be trialed first. Of note, spinal cord stimulators are not magnetic resonance imaging (MRI) compatible because of the long conducting lead that lies against the spinal cord.

(2) **Technique:** Using an interlaminar approach to the epidural space, a special lead is placed along the dorsal column. This lead in turn is connected to an external pulse generator, which provides electrical stimulation. Often the patients will find that the neuropathic pain in their limb is replaced with a gentle, throbbing, buzzing sensation, which is far more tolerable. If the patient wishes to proceed, an internal pulse generator and permanent catheter are implanted in the operating room.

D. **PHN** is an extremely painful complication of acute varicella zoster infection, occurring most commonly in the elderly and immunocompromised patients. The patient experiences persistent severe burning pain in the same distribution as the original infection. It is imperative that antivirals be initiated immediately upon diagnosis of shingles as this reduces the likelihood of progression to PHN. Typically, patients experience some relief with neuropathic pain medications as well as with topical local anesthesia (cream/ointment versus transdermal applicator patch). Currently, medical therapies appear to be more beneficial than interventional procedures (e.g., nerve blocks, epidural steroid injections), although these procedures can produce long-lasting effects in some patients.

E. **Cancer pain:** Treatment of cancer pain is multifaceted and may require pharmacologic intervention combined with counseling, nursing care, pastoral and social services, nerve blockade, surgery, radiation therapy, chemotherapy, and hospice care. Cancer pain often is a dynamic process with remissions and exacerbations paralleling the disease course. Because of the terminal character of most chronic cancer pain, narcotics are considered the mainstay of treatment. Long-acting continuous-release preparations of opioids are useful in providing basal analgesia, and short-acting preparations (immediate-release morphine, oral transmucosal fentanyl) can be used to treat episodic "breakthrough" pain. Often the side effects of the narcotics (especially constipation) can start affecting quality of life, and these need to be treated aggressively. However, in patients who cannot tolerate escalation of systemic opioids because of the side effects, the following techniques can sometimes provide excellent control while minimizing side effects.

1. **Intrathecal drug delivery system**

a. **Indications.** Most commonly used for chronic cancer pain, this device allows the use of narcotics while avoiding some of the significant side effects, such as constipation and sedation. A trial is mandatory and may consist of an inpatient admission.

b. **Technique.** Either an epidural or an intrathecal trial catheter is placed and an infusion is started, and titrated to effect, or a single shot intrathecal dose of narcotic is administered. A permanent implant is performed in the operating room under sterile conditions. Intrathecal pump devices are MRI compatible but may need to be interrogated post-MRI to verify maintenance of normal function.

2. **Celiac plexus block** is one of the most commonly performed interventional pain procedures for the management of cancer pain.

   a. **Indications.** Visceral pain from the upper abdominal organs is transmitted via the celiac ganglia. Even though pancreatic cancer ranks among the top indications for a neurolytic celiac plexus block, other upper abdominal malignancies may also benefit from this block. Interestingly, chronic pancreatitis does not seem to be very responsive to this type of block.

   b. **Technique.** Under fluoroscopic guidance and with the patient prone, 15-cm, 20-gauge needles are inserted bilaterally just below the 12th rib and directed medially to contact the body of the L-1 vertebra. The left-sided needle is advanced cephalad to the transverse process 1 to 2 cm anterior to the L-1 vertebral body or until aortic pulsations are felt. Ideally, we place one needle anterior to and the other one posterior to the aorta. The correct needle position is verified by injecting contrast dye (make sure there is no psoas muscle injection or tracking of dye under the diaphragm or toward spinal nerve roots. Then 10 to 20 mL of 0.25% bupivacaine or a 50:50 mixture of 1% lidocaine and 0.5% bupivacaine is injected in divided doses through each needle after a negative aspiration for blood or CSF. If pain is relieved, this may be followed after 24 hours (or earlier if necessary) by 10 to 20 mL of 50% alcohol through each needle. Alternatively, 6% aqueous phenol can be used instead of alcohol. Complications include temporary (although sometimes persistent) hypotension and diarrhea. Intrathecal, epidural, or IM injection of a neurolytic agent may result in sexual dysfunction, lower-extremity dysesthesias, or paraplegia secondary to spinal artery syndrome. Pneumothorax, bowel perforation, kidney or liver puncture, and retroperitoneal hemorrhage may occur. For patients who cannot tolerate the prone position, the same technique can be used in the lateral position. Otherwise, the block could be performed supine with ultrasound or CT guidance.

F. **Myofascial pain** is a relatively common pain process. It is usually seen with trauma or repetitive motion injury. Pain is often described as deep, aching, and worsening with activity. Hyperirritable sites in muscle and connective tissue, termed trigger points, result from trauma, fatigue, or tension and can produce reflex muscle spasm, pain, and, in some circumstances, ischemia. It is important to distinguish discrete trigger points from a diffuse myofascial pain syndrome, because the latter may be a symptom of systemic disease. Treatment options for trigger points include the following:

1. **Trigger point injection.** Local anesthetic, 1 to 2 mL (either 1% lidocaine or 0.25% bupivacaine), is generally injected into the trigger point(s) with a 25-gauge 5/8-inch needle and the area is massaged. It is important to start physical therapy shortly

thereafter. Patients generally respond quickly to this type of therapy. The need for frequent treatments may indicate misdiagnosis or concomitant psychological dysfunction.

2. Use of **NSAIDs, muscle relaxants (benzodiazepines), or physical therapy techniques** (cooling and stretching of trigger points) also may be used. **Botox** may benefit patients with recurring trigger points, often providing 3 to 5 months of pain relief.

SUGGESTED READING

Acute Pain Management. *Anesthesiology.* 2004;100(6):1573–1581.

Anand KJ, Arnold JH. Opioid tolerance and dependence in infants and children. *Crit Care Med* 1994;22:334–342.

Ballantyne J, Fishman SM, Abdi S. *The Massachusetts General Hospital handbook of pain management,* 2nd ed. Philadelphia: Lippincott Williams & Wilkins, 2002.

Brown DL. *Atlas of regional anesthesia,* 2nd ed. Philadelphia: WB Saunders, 1999.

Carr DB, Goudas LC. Acute pain. *Lancet* 1999;353:2051–2058.

Collins JJ, Grier HE, Kinney HC, et al. Control of severe pain in children with terminal malignancy. *J Pediatr* 1995;126:653–657.

Ferrante FM. Principles of opioid pharmacotherapy: practical implications of basic mechanisms. *J Pain Symptom Manage* 1996;11:265–273.

Galer BS. Neuropathic pain of peripheral origin: advances in pharmacologic treatment. *Neurology* 1995;45:S17–S25, S35–S36.

Latarjet J, Choinere M. Pain in burn patients. *Burns* 1995;21:344–348.

Mather CM, Ready LB. Management of acute pain. *Br J Hosp Med* 1994;51:85–88.

McQuay H, Carroll D, Jadad AR, et al. Anticonvulsant drugs for management of pain: a systematic review. *BMJ* 1995;311:1047–1052.

McQuay H. Opioids in pain management. *Lancet* 1999;353:2229–2232.

Portenoy RK, Kanner RM. Pain management: theory and practice. Philadelphia: FA Davis Co, 1996.

Portenoy RK. Tolerance to opioid analgesics: clinical aspects. *Cancer Surv* 1994;21:49–65.

Practice guidelines for acute pain management in the perioperative setting: Section. Practice guidelines for cancer pain management. *Anesthesiology.* 1996;84(5):1243–1257.

Section. Practice guidelines for chronic pain management. *Anesthesiology.* 1997;86(4):995–1004.

Stanton-Hicks M, Janig W, Hassenbusch S, et al. Reflex sympathetic dystrophy: changing concepts and taxonomy. *Pain* 1995;63:127–133.

Waldman SD. *Interventional pain management,* 2nd ed. Philadelphia: WB Saunders, 2001.

Wall PD, Melzak R. *Textbook of pain,* 4th ed. Philadelphia: WB Saunders, 1999.

Woolf CJ, Mannion RJ. Neuropathic pain: aetiology, symptoms, mechanisms, and management. *Lancet* 1999;353:1959–1964.

Woolf CJ, Salter MW. Neuronal plasticity: increasing the gain in pain. *Science* 2000;288:1765–1769.

39

Complementary and Alternative Medicine

Margaret Gargarian, P. Grace Harrell, and
Meraj M. Mohiuddin

I. **Complementary and alternative medicine (CAM).** Complementary and alternative therapies encompass a broad range of therapeutic modalities that can be integrated into Western medicine. CAM offers patients treatment options, especially when dealing with chronic illness and symptom alleviation. As physicians, the more comfortable and informed we are about CAM, the more effectively we can help our patients make safe and intelligent decisions. As anesthesiologists, we should ask about CAM use during our standard history taking, especially the use of herbs. Knowledge of CAM use can help prevent potential hazards during surgery and can assist with the management of pain, anxiety, and nausea and vomiting.

A. **Definitions of CAM**

1. Practices that are not accepted as correct or in conformity with the beliefs of the dominant group of medical practitioners in a society.

2. Interventions neither taught widely in medical schools nor generally available in hospitals.

B. **Categories of CAM practices.** The National Center for Complementary and Alternative Medicine, a subdivision of the National Institutes of Health, has grouped CAM practices into five major subdivisions:

1. **Alternative medical systems** are complete systems of theory and practice that have evolved in various cultures, mostly before the inception of conventional medicine. An example is traditional oriental medicine, which uses acupuncture, herbal medicine, massage, and qi gong.

   a. **Acupuncture** involves the insertion of fine, solid needles into specific points on the body to produce a therapeutic result. Acupuncture influences the nervous system at multiple levels and causes release of endorphins, serotonin, norepinephrine, and cortisol. Many of these substances reduce inflammation and pain sensation.

   b. **Ayurveda** is India's traditional system of medicine, which emphasizes the equal importance of body, mind, and spirit. It utilizes diet, exercise, meditation, herbs, massage, and controlled breathing.

2. **Mind–body interventions** use techniques to facilitate the mind's ability to affect bodily functions. Examples include hypnosis, meditation, prayer, and mental healing.

3. **Biologically based treatments** overlap with conventional medicine's use of dietary supplements. They include herbal

therapy (see section III), special diets, shark cartilage to treat cancer, and bee pollen to treat autoimmune diseases.
4. **Manipulative and body-based methods** use movement or manipulation of the body to restore health. An example is chiropractic medicine, which proposes that realigning the spine allows the "innate intelligence" of the body to restore itself to health. Other examples are massage therapy and osteopathic manipulation.
5. **Energy therapies** focus on energy fields originating within the body (biofields) or from other sources (electromagnetic fields). Examples are qi gong, reiki, and therapeutic touch. **Qi gong** combines movement, meditation, and regulation of breathing to enhance the flow of qi (a vital energy) and improve circulation. **Reiki** is based on channeling spiritual energy through the practitioner to heal the spirit and in turn heal the body. **Therapeutic touch** involves a practitioner focusing on the intent to heal, while lightly touching or passing hands over the patient, to identify energy imbalances.
C. **Prevalence of CAM**
1. Researchers at Harvard Medical School have found that 35% of adults in the United States use at least one form of CAM. This prevalence has remained stable from 1997 to 2002, signifying its importance in modern day health care. The most commonly used modality in 2002 was herbal therapy, representing 18.6% of U.S. adults. Herbal therapy has increased by 50% from 1997 to 2002. Total out-of-pocket expense for CAM represents billions of dollars and compares with the money spent on traditional physicians.
2. Most CAM therapies are used for chronic conditions, especially back and neck problems, depression, anxiety, and chronic fatigue. Symptom relief is the main benefit reported. The vast majority of people use CAM in conjunction with conventional therapies.
3. Seventy-five U.S. medical schools offer coursework in alternative medicine, and many U.S. hospitals now have complementary medicine departments.
4. **Disclosure rates.** Only 40% of patients tell their doctors about the CAM therapies they are using. This places the burden on physicians to elicit this information from their patients. A physician informed about alternative medicine can help patients avoid dangerous side effects and also help them make safe and intelligent choices.
II. **Herbal therapy and anesthesia**
A. **Herbal medicines and phytopharmaceuticals** are plants or parts of plants that contain biologically active components. There is tremendous variability in the purity and potency of herbal preparations. The amount of active component can vary widely within the same species depending on growing conditions. Herbal products are sometimes adulterated with foreign substances, including pharmaceuticals, bacteria, and toxic metals. **Dietary supplements** contain "concentrate, metabolite, constituent, extract, or combination of any ingredient of a vitamin, mineral, amino acid, enzyme or herb." Vitamins are supplements that contain essential organic compounds or nutrients that are required in small amounts to maintain body functions. **Homeopathic medications** are derived from

plant, animal, or mineral sources. It is thought that they stimulate natural defenses in very diluted doses.

B. Herbal medicines are currently regulated by the U.S. Food and Drug Administration in the category of "dietary supplements" along with compounds such as vitamins and amino acids. The manufacturer does not have to prove efficacy or safety of a compound before it is marketed, and products are not scrutinized via the same stringent testing placed on drugs. Some companies are now using techniques such as chromatography to identify and standardize herbal preparations.

C. **Herbal medications may be dangerous** when used in combination with prescription or over-the-counter drugs. They can alter the metabolism of important medications and may have anticoagulant effects. The sale of Ephedra (Ma Huang) was banned by the federal government after a review of adverse events including heart attack, stroke, and death. The American Society of Anesthesiologists recommends discontinuing herbal remedies 2 weeks before elective surgery.

D. It has been estimated that one in five Americans taking prescription drugs is also taking vitamins or herbal supplements. The most frequently used herbs are echinacea, gingko biloba, St. John's wort, garlic, and ginseng.

E. **Commonly used herbs** and possible anesthetic interactions

    1. **Echinacea** (*Echinacea purpura*, purple cone flower)

        a. Uses: for common colds, wounds and burns, urinary tract infections, coughs, and bronchitis (immunostimulation via enhanced phagocytosis and nonspecific T-cell stimulation).

        b. Problems and interactions: may cause hepatotoxicity or potentiate hepatotoxic effects of anabolic steroids, amiodarone, ketoconazole, and methotrexate. By inhibiting microsomal enzymes, can precipitate the toxicity of drugs dependent on hepatic metabolism (e.g., phenytoin, rifampin, and phenobarbital). May decrease effectiveness of corticosteroids and cyclosporine.

    2. **Ephedra** (*Ephedra sinica*, Ma Huang) **not approved by FDA**

        a. Uses: in over-the-counter diet aids; for bacteriostatic, antitussive actions (sympathomimetic with positive inotropic/chronotropic effects; α- and β-adrenergic agonist).

        b. Problems and interactions: potential interactions with cardiac glycosides and halothane (arrhythmias); guanethidine (enhanced sympathomimetic effects); monoamine oxidase inhibitors (MAOIs; enhanced sympathomimetic effects); oxytocin (hypertension); intraoperative hypotension better treated with phenylephrine than ephedrine.

    3. **Feverfew** (*Tanacetum parthenium*)

        a. Uses: as migraine prophylactic and antipyretic (inhibits serotonin release from aggregating platelets via inhibition of arachidonic acid release).

        b. Problems and interactions: can inhibit platelet activity (potentiate anticoagulants); rebound headache with sudden cessation; 5% to 15% develop aphthous ulcers or gastrointestinal irritation. Like other tannin-containing herbs, feverfew can interact with iron preparations and decrease bioavailability.

4. **GBL, BD, and GHB** (γ-butyrolactone; butyrolactone γ; 1,4-butanediol; γ-hydroxybutyrate) **not approved by FDA.**
   a. Uses: bodybuilding, weight loss aid, sleep aid.
   b. Problems and interactions: death, seizures, unconsciousness, bradycardia, slowed respirations.

5. **Garlic** (*Allium sativum*)
   a. Uses: lipid lowering, vasodilatory, antihypertensive, antiplatelet, antioxidant, and antithrombotic/fibrinolytic qualities.
   b. Problems and interactions: may potentiate effects of warfarin. A case of spontaneous epidural hematoma has been reported.

6. **Ginger** (*Zingiber officinalis*)
   a. Uses: for antiemetic, antivertigo, and antispasmodic effects.
   b. Problems and interactions: potent inhibitor of thromboxane synthetase; can potentiate anticoagulant effects of other medications.

7. **Ginkgo** (*Ginkgo biloba*, maidenhair tree)
   a. Uses: as a circulatory stimulant; antioxidant; for intermittent claudication, tinnitus, vertigo, memory loss, dementia, and sexual dysfunction (inhibits platelet-activating factor, modulates nitric oxide, has anti-inflammatory effects).
   b. Problems and interactions: may enhance bleeding in patients already on anticoagulant or antithrombotic therapy (e.g., aspirin, nonsteroidal anti-inflammatory drugs, warfarin, heparin). Cases of spontaneous subarachnoid hemorrhage and subdural hematomas have been reported. May decrease effectiveness of anticonvulsant drugs (e.g., carbamazepine, phenytoin, and phenobarbital).

8. **Ginseng** (*Panax ginseng*)
   a. Uses: to enhance energy level, and for antioxidant and reported aphrodisiac effects (thought to augment adrenal steroidogenesis via a centrally mediated mechanism).
   b. Problems and interactions: "ginseng abuse syndrome" (more than 15 g per day) characterized by sleepiness, hypertonia, and edema. May see tachycardia or hypertension with other stimulants, hypotension intraoperatively, mastalgia, postmenopausal bleeding, mania in patients on MAOIs (phenelzine), and decreased effectiveness of warfarin. Hypoglycemic effect may necessitate monitoring in diabetics or neurosurgical patients receiving steroids.

9. **Goldenseal** (*Hydrastis canadensis*, turmeric root)
   a. Uses: as diuretic, anti-inflammatory, laxative.
   b. Problems and interactions: functions as an oxytocic, overdose may cause paralysis (amount not known), free water diuresis (no sodium excreted, just free water), electrolyte abnormalities, hypertension.

10. **Kava-kava** (*Piper methysticum*)
    a. Uses: as anxiolytic, treatment for gonorrhea, skin diseases.
    b. Problems and interactions: thought to inhibit norepinephrine; potentiates sedating effects of barbiturates,

benzodiazepines; can potentiate ethanol effects. Increased suicide risk in patients with endogenous depression.

11. **Licorice** (*Glycyrrhiza glabra*)
    a. Uses: for gastritis, gastric and duodenal ulcers, cough, and bronchitis.
    b. Problems and interactions: glycyrrhizic acid in licorice may cause hypertension, hypokalemia, and edema. Contraindicated in many chronic liver conditions, renal insufficiency, hypertonia, hypokalemia.

12. **Saw palmetto** (*Serenoa repens*, cabbage palm)
    a. Uses: for treatment of benign prostatic hypertrophy; has an antiandrogenic effect.
    b. Problems and interactions: may see additive effects with other hormone therapies (including oral contraceptives and estrogen replacement therapy).

13. **St. John's wort** (*Hypericum perforatum*, goat weed)
    a. Uses: for depression, anxiety, sleep disorders, vitiligo (may inhibit monoamine oxidase, γ-aminobutyric acid, and serotonin receptors).
    b. Problems and interactions: possible interaction with MAOIs, may prolong effects of anesthesia, and may photosensitize. Potential serotonergic syndrome (tremors, hypertonicity, autonomic dysfunction, and hyperthermia) with concomitant use of beta-sympathomimetic amines or selective serotonin reuptake inhibitors, including fluoxetine, paroxetine.

14. **Valerian** (*Valeriana officinalis*, all-heal, vandal root)
    a. Uses: has mild sedative and anxiolytic properties.
    b. Problems and interactions: potentiates effects of barbiturates, may decrease symptoms of benzodiazepine withdrawal, and prolong anesthetic actions.

15. **Vitamin E** (Vitamin E)
    a. Uses: to slow aging process, prevention of stroke and pulmonary emboli, prevention of atherosclerosis, promotion of would healing, effective against fibrocystic breast syndrome
    b. Problems and interactions: May increase bleeding.

III. **Perioperative acupuncture**
   A. **Preoperative use:** acupuncture might help prepare patients for surgery by creating a sense of calm and relaxation. In two double-blinded studies, preoperative auricular acupuncture reduced anxiety up to 48 hours compared with sham acupuncture. Another small study using acupuncture as an adjunct for colonoscopy found better procedure acceptability than control and sham groups.
   B. **Intraoperative use:** acupuncture creates analgesia and sedation but does not provide muscle relaxation, suppress autonomic reflexes, or provide unconsciousness. Available data show that acupuncture has little or no effect on anesthetic requirements.
   C. **Postoperative use**
      1. **Pain control:** although the findings are controversial, several good studies reveal substantial reduction in postoperative pain with acupuncture. This probably requires a well-trained practitioner who can design a complex treatment plan that treats varieties of pain, such as visceral and dermatomal pain.

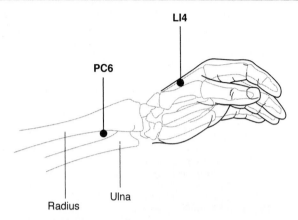

Figure 39.1. PC6 helps relieve anxiety, nausea, and travel sickness. LI4 is good for headaches, toothache, sinusitis, colds, and pain in the upper body. (From Kuhn MA. *Complementary therapies for health care providers.* Philadelphia: Lippincott Williams & Wilkins, 1999:296.)

2. Postoperative nausea and vomiting: The use of acupuncture to treat postoperative nausea and vomiting has been well studied. Acupuncture appears effective as an antiemetic, especially when administered before induction of general anesthesia. Laser stimulation of PC6 (Fig. 39.1) after induction of general anesthesia in children will still effectively reduce postoperative nausea and vomiting. Acupuncture may be used with or without conventional antiemetics.

IV. **Hypnosis**
   A. **Definition:** hypnosis involves the induction of a state of mind, allowing for a heightened receptivity for suggestions. It is generally a state of relaxation in which critical thought is bypassed.
   B. **Possible applications**
      1. **Pain relief:** Numerous studies show benefits of hypnosis for pain relief. The analgesic mechanism differs from a placebo effect in that the pain is not perceived, rather than experienced with greater tolerance. Studies using positron emission tomography scans show a decrease in both subjective and objective pain perception under hypnosis.
      2. **Anesthesia:** hypnosis as a sole anesthetic has been rejected because of easily available and effective pharmacologic agents. It could be combined with other agents for conscious sedation rather than general anesthesia for operations such as breast biopsies. It has been used effectively for dressing changes in burn patients, with the concurrent suggestions of improved appetite and nutrition.
      3. **Postoperative recovery:** a meta-analysis published in 2002 states that hypnosis as an adjunct to surgery was beneficial for most patients in areas such as postoperative pain, nausea, anxiety, and recovery time. Positive suggestions to anesthetized patients may also promote fewer postoperative complications.

SUGGESTED READING

American Society of Anesthesiologists. What you should know about your patient's use of herbal medicines. http://www.asahq.org. Accessed April 29, 2002.

Astin JA. Why patients use alternative medicine: results of a national study. *JAMA* 1998;279:1548–1553.

Chernyak GV, Sessler D. Perioperative acupuncture and related techniques. *Anesthesiology* 2005;102(5):1031–1049.

Jonas W, Levin J, eds. *Essentials of complementary and alternative medicine.* Philadelphia: Williams & Wilkins, 1999.

Kaye AD, Kucera I, Sabar R. Perioperative anesthesia clinical considerations of alternative medicines. *Anesthesiol Clin North Am* 2004;22:125–139.

Kuhn M. *Complementary therapies for health care providers.* Baltimore, MD: Lippincott Williams & Wilkins, 1999.

Meurisse M, Hamoir E, Defechereaux T, et al. Bilateral neck exploration under hypnosedation: a new standard of care in primary hyperparathyroidism. *Ann Surg* 1999;229:401–408.

Miller LG. Herbal medicinals: selected clinical considerations focussing on known or potential drug-herb interactions. *Arch Intern Med* 1998;158:2200–2211.

National Center for Complementary and Alternative Medicine. Major domains of complementary and alternative medicine. http://www.nccam.nih.gov. Accessed April 29, 2002.

Stewart JH. Hypnosis in contemporary medicine (review). *Mayo Clin Proc* 2005;80(4):511–524.

Tindle HA, Davis RB, Phillips RS, Eisenberg DM. Trends in use of complementary and alternative medicine by US adults: 1997–2002. *Altern Ther Health Med* 2005;11(1):42–49.

Tsen LC, Segal S, Pothier M, et al. Alternative medicine use in presurgical patients. *Anesthesiology* 2000;93:148–151.

40

Ethical and End-of-Life Issues

Rae M. Allain and Aalok Agarwala

This chapter explores ethical issues that frequently arise in anesthetic practice. Customs, laws, ethical beliefs, and religious practices vary among cultures and societies. This chapter describes the prevailing practice at the Massachusetts General Hospital in Boston, Massachusetts.

I. **Decisions concerning treatment**
   A. **Patient autonomy** (i.e., respect for an individual's preferences) is a highly valued guiding ethical principle in U.S. medicine. Competent adult patients can and may choose to accept or refuse medical therapies. If a patient's competence is questionable, a psychiatrist should evaluate the patient to determine whether he or she has decision-making capacity. This requires an ability to receive and understand medical information, to discern the various options presented, and to choose a course based on the information offered and one's values.
   B. Autonomy is best preserved by involving the patient in medical decision making whenever possible. Obtaining **informed consent** for procedures and therapies is an ethical responsibility of the treating physician (see Chapter 1). Rarely, a patient's condition and emergent circumstances may prevent the discussion involved in the informed consent process. Many critically ill patients are incompetent to make medical decisions because of the gravity of their illness or because of sedative/analgesic medications used to diminish suffering. In these circumstances, an advance directive and/or surrogate may be helpful.
      1. An **advance directive (or "living will"),** a document specifying the types of treatment that the patient wishes to receive or reject should future need arise, is very useful in this circumstance.
      2. In addition to or in the absence of an advance directive, a patient may designate a **surrogate** (health care proxy or health care power of attorney) who is charged with executing the patient's wishes should he or she become incompetent. The surrogate offers **substituted judgment** for the patient, providing decisions that the patient would make if competent. If the patient has not designated a surrogate before becoming incompetent, the next of kin may become the de facto surrogate. In some circumstances where no family is living or available, a trusted friend may act as the patient's surrogate.
      3. A court-appointed legal **guardian** may be necessary in rare instances in which no family member or friend is able to make decisions in the best interest of the patient.
   C. **Conflict** is best resolved via ongoing discussion with the individuals involved. The anesthetist must recognize and respect cultural differences that influence a patient's decisions. Irresolvable conflict

among family members, health care team members, or between the family and the medical care team often is best addressed by the institutional ethics committee (see below).

D. **The institutional ethics committee** is generally composed of a group of health care professionals trained in medical ethics.

   1. **The purpose** of the ethics committee is to educate and advise clinicians about ethical dilemmas and to enable resolution of ethical conflicts. The ethics committee offers an objective analysis of the patient's case and may draw upon basic ethical principles to guide the patient, physician, and family to a consensus about the therapeutic course. Ideally, the ethics committee should be accessible to all members of the health care team and to the patient and family. This diminishes inequalities of power present in the hospital environment and promotes a climate of respect for all viewpoints.

   2. When the ethics committee is requested to consult on a case, the question to be answered or the nature of the conflict should be clearly stated. The patient's condition and prognosis should be documented. Members of the ethics committee may help organize and/or attend a family meeting to facilitate decision making.

   3. The ethics committee uses guiding ethical principles to make recommendations to the health care team, the patient, and/or the family. The role is one of expert consultant, not arbiter in a dispute. In rare situations in which irreconcilable differences exist between the physician and the patient and/or family, care of the patient may be transferred to another accepting attending physician. It is even more extraordinary for ethical conflicts to reach resolution by judicial intervention.

E. **The pediatric patient** deserves special consideration when ethical issues are confronted. Legally, such decisions are deferred to the parents. Ethically, the child may participate in these decisions depending on his or her developmental level and decision-making capacity. If the child is too immature to participate in decisions, parents are relied upon to make decisions in the child's best interest by weighing the benefit versus burden of the planned therapy. Pediatric anesthetists must be sensitive to individual family dynamics and parenting styles when approaching such discussions.

F. **Jehovah's Witness** patients generally may refuse to receive blood or blood products (e.g., fresh frozen plasma, platelets, cryoprecipitate, or albumin) based on their religious beliefs, even if such refusal results in death. Some patients may accept autotransfused or chest tube–salvaged autologous blood, especially if it remains in contiguous circulation with their vasculature. Special considerations regarding homologous transfusion may apply if the patient is a minor, is incompetent, or has responsibilities for dependents, and in certain emergency circumstances. An ethical dilemma may present when unexpected hemorrhage is encountered after a preoperative agreement not to transfuse. Careful documentation of preoperative discussions and informed consent is mandatory. Legal precedent generally supports patient autonomy regarding the acceptance of transfusion.

G. **"Do not resuscitate (DNR)" orders in the operating room** should not be automatically suspended. Rather, the institution's written policy regarding this situation should be followed. The

American Society of Anesthesiologists recognizes a patient's right to self-determination and recommends that preexisting advance directives be discussed with the patient (or surrogate) and other involved parties (e.g., surgeon, primary physician) before initiating anesthetic care for the proposed procedure. Specific aspects of the anesthetic that might be considered resuscitation in another setting (e.g., endotracheal intubation) should be frankly discussed, including the anesthesiologist's judgment of the relative necessity of the intervention toward providing a successful anesthetic as well as the patient's preference regarding the intervention. Decisions that arise from these communications should be documented in the chart and used to guide the anesthetic care. Three general courses of action may usually be agreed upon:

1. A "full resuscitation" status is implemented for the perioperative period, suspending the "DNR" status.
2. A "limited resuscitation" with respect to certain procedures is implemented for the perioperative period. For example, a patient may accept endotracheal intubation, but reject chest compressions in the event of cardiac arrest.
3. A "limited resuscitation," which is goal-directed based on the patient's values is implemented for the perioperative period. For example, the patient may allow resuscitation for events that are deemed to be reversible and known complications of the anesthetic (e.g., hypotension) but not allow resuscitation for events that in the judgment of the anesthesiologist are likely irreversible (e.g., ventricular fibrillation due to myocardial ischemia). Similarly, a patient may define a priori based on his/her values circumstances what would result in an unacceptable quality of life and from which he/she would prefer not to receive resuscitation.

Regardless of which course of resuscitation is agreed upon preoperatively, the duration of the resuscitation plan into the postoperative period should be defined. Time-limited courses of therapy with an evaluation of effectiveness (or lack thereof) may be helpful in deciding whether to continue or limit ongoing treatments. If the anesthesiologist disagrees with either the patient or the surgeon on moral grounds about the level of perioperative resuscitation, then he/she should withdraw from participating in the care of the patient and seek to provide a colleague who will provide anesthetic care.

II. **Determination of death using brain criteria**
   A. **"Brain death"** is a term used to connote that death had been determined via evaluation of brain function. Brain death must be understood to be no different from a diagnosis of death made by cardiac criteria. Practically, the diagnosis of brain death means that a patient can potentially become an organ donor on the conditions of consent and medical acceptability. **Locally accepted guidelines** are used to establish the diagnosis of brain death. Diagnostic criteria for the clinical diagnosis of brain death in adults, adapted from those used at the Massachusetts General Hospital, are summarized below. Other institutions may have different criteria.
   B. **Brain death is a clinical syndrome** of coma or unresponsiveness, absence of brain stem reflexes, and apnea in which the proximate cause is known and demonstrably irreversible. Prerequisites include the following:

1. Evidence of an acute central nervous system catastrophe that is compatible with brain death.
2. Exclusion of complicating medical conditions that may confound clinical assessment (e.g., severe electrolyte, acid-base, or endocrine disturbance).
3. No evidence of drug intoxication or poisoning.
4. Demonstrated absence of neuromuscular blockade if the patient has had recent or prolonged use of muscle relaxants.
5. Core temperature greater than $32°C$ ($90°F$).
6. In the presence of confounding variables, brain death may still be determined with the aid of ancillary testing (see below). A period of observation of at least 24 hours without clinical neurologic change is necessary if the cause of the coma is unknown.

C. **Many clinical conditions may interfere** with the clinical diagnosis of brain death, so that the diagnosis cannot be made with certainty on clinical grounds alone. In such cases, confirmatory tests are recommended.

D. **Confirmatory laboratory tests** that may support the diagnosis of brain death include angiography, electroencephalography, transcranial Doppler ultrasonography, and technetium 99m hexamethyl-propyleneamine oxime brain scanning.

III. **Organ donation.** Patients who are declared brain dead and whose surrogates provide consent may be considered for organ or tissue donation. In addition, recent attempts to increase the number of organs available for transplantation has resulted in considering critically ill patients who depend on life-sustaining treatments for donation after cardiac death **(DCD).** For DCD donations, death should be expected to occur imminently (within minutes) upon withdrawal of life-sustaining measures.

A. **Conversations with the family** regarding organ donation must be done tactfully and in consultation with trained professionals from the regional organ procurement agency. Ideally, a physician with whom the family has developed a rapport should coordinate the discussion. The topic may be introduced by asking the family if the deceased had ever expressed an opinion regarding use of his or her organs after death. Many families are consoled by the thought that their loved one's body parts may be lifesaving to another individual and may in some sense carry on the life that has been lost.

B. **Early contact** with the organ procurement agency is important in cases of potential organ donors. Organ procurement agencies generally have specific preferences regarding medications (such as vasopressors and diuretics), mechanical ventilator settings, and laboratory blood work to be performed. The anesthetist should know these.

C. **Care of the brain-dead patient** for organ donation is challenging (see Chapter 20, section IV.N). Problems frequently encountered include hypotension, arrhythmias, hypoxemia, and diabetes insipidus. If a successful donation is to occur, a vigilant anesthetist, in concert with direction from the organ procurement agency, is necessary.

D. **DCD organ procurement** is challenging and demands adherence to guiding ethical principles. The institutional policy for DCD procurement should be reviewed and followed when DCD organ procurement is planned. Care of the dying patient, including provision of analgesic and amnestic medications by the ICU team caring for the patient, supersedes the goal of organ procurement. The institutional policy should clearly define the following:

1. The nonoverlapping roles of caregivers to the donor and the recipient to avoid a conflict of interest.
2. The physician (usually the intensivist) responsible for pronouncing cardiac death.
3. The time interval after asystole at which death is cleared. Currently at the Massachusetts General Hospital (MGH), this is 5 minutes.
4. The process for obtaining consent for and administering medications or treatments necessary for organ procurement but not of benefit (and potentially harmful) to the patient. Examples include heparin administration or femoral arterial cannula placement.
5. The process for allowing family presence at the time of death (in the ICU or operating room).
6. The time interval after which organ procurement will not be attempted in the case of unexpected patient survival after the withdrawal of life-sustaining therapies and the process of return to the ICU. Currently this time interval is 2 hours after extubation at the MGH.

E. If the institutional transplant team will participate in harvesting or transplanting organs, it is prudent to establish contact with the team and immediately apprise them of any change in the donor's condition that might warrant expedited harvest.

IV. **Supporting survivors**
   A. **Support** of the patient's survivors after a death begins with honest, frequent, and compassionate communication from the medical team.
   B. **Cultural background and individual values** will affect each conversation. The medical team should strive for flexibility when presented with each situation.
      1. The medical social worker may be an important source for understanding the family's religious and cultural background.
      2. Many patients and families find solace in the presence of clergy. If so, arrangements should be made for the patient's own religious representative or a hospital-based chaplain to be available.

V. **Legal considerations.** Physicians who engage in honest, open communication with patients and their families about ethical and end-of-life issues should rarely find themselves resolving such issues in a court of law. Nevertheless, several recent judicial rulings have implications that may prove useful to the clinician when confronted with ethical issues.
   A. **Patient autonomy is primary in decision-making.** That patients may refuse life-sustaining or other therapies has been repeatedly affirmed. Wishes of the patient may be expressed via advance directives or, lacking this, via prior voiced opinion. The role of a surrogate in providing substituted judgment has been supported.
   B. **Human life has qualification beyond mere biologic existence.** Thus, a surrogate's decision to withdraw care may be based on the potential for meaningful existence (**"quality of life"**).
   C. **Care once rendered may be withdrawn.** The idea that a life-sustaining therapy that has been implemented can never be stopped is not valid.

D. **End-of-life decisions are best addressed by the physician and the patient and/or family** with help from institutional facilitators (e.g., ethics committee) as needed. Permission to withdraw or withhold a therapy does not require a "court order."

E. **Withdrawal of hydration or nutritional support is not legally different from withdrawal of other life support.** In addition to legal decisions, this stance has been supported by numerous medical societies, including the American Medical Association and the American Academy of Neurology.

F. **Physicians are not bound to provide care that they deem futile.** While still somewhat controversial, the latter was supported by a jury decision involving a patient at MGH from whom ventilatory support was withdrawn despite the objection of one family member. It is advisable for a physician, however, to pursue every avenue of conflict resolution, including removing herself or himself from the care of a patient, before exercising this dictum against a family's wishes.

G. **For unusual or questionable cases,** it is appropriate to seek the advice of the institutional legal counsel before acting on decisions.

SUGGESTED READING

American Society of Anesthesiologists. Guidelines of the ethical practice of anesthesiology. Approved October 3, 1967, amended October 15, 2003. Available at www.asahq.org/publicationsAndServices/sgstoc.htm. Accessed February 21, 2006.

American Society of Anesthesiologists. Ethical guidelines for the anesthesia care of patients with do-not-resuscitate orders. Approved October 13, 1993, amended October 17, 2001. Available at www. asahq.org/publicationsAnd Services/sgstoc.htm. Accessed February 21, 2006.

Jenkins K, Baker AB. Consent and anaesthetic risk. *Anaesthesia* 2003;58:962–984.

Meisel A. Legal myths about terminating life support. *Arch Intern Med* 1991; 151:1497–1502.

Van Norman, GA. Another matter of life and death: what every anesthesiologist should know about the ethical, legal, and policy implications of the non-heart-beating cadaver organ donor. *Anesthesiology* 2003;98:763–773.

Appendix A

Supplemental Drug Information

Jonathan G. Hsiao and Eric Corey Matten

ABCIXIMAB (REOPRO)

Indications	Prevents thrombus formation after percutaneous coronary intervention (PCI).
Dosage	Bolus (0.25 mg/kg) administered 10–60 min prior to PCI, then 10 μg/min IV infusion.
Effect	Inhibits glycoprotein IIB/IIIA; prevents platelet adhesion and aggregation.
Clearance	Remains in circulation for $\geq$10 days in a platelet-bound state, but platelet function recovers in about 48 hours.
Comments	Anaphylaxis may occur; hypotension with bolus dose. Bleeding complications and thrombocytopenia are common side effects.

ACETAZOLAMIDE (DIAMOX)

Indications	Respiratory acidosis with metabolic alkalosis. Increased intraocular and intracranial pressures.
Dosage	125–500 mg IV over 1 to 2 min or PO not to exceed 2 g in 24 h.
Effect	Inhibits carbonic anhydrase, which results in increased renal excretion of bicarbonate.
Clearance	70% to 100% excreted unchanged in the urine within 24 h.
Comments	May increase insulin requirements in diabetic patients; cause renal calculi in patients with past history of calcium stones; cause hypokalemia, thrombocytopenia, aplastic anemia, increased urinary excretion of uric acid, and hyperglycemia. Initial dose may produce marked diuresis. Tolerance to desired effects of acetazolamide occurs in 2 to 3 days. Rare hypersensitivity reaction in patients with sulfa allergies.

ADENOSINE (ADENOCARD)

Indications	Paroxysmal supraventricular tachycardia.
Dosage	Adult: 6–12 mg IV bolus. Pediatric: 50 μg/kg IV.
Effect	Slows or temporarily blocks AV node conduction and conduction though reentrant pathways (especially those involving the AV node).
Clearance	RBC and endothelial cell metabolism.
Comments	The effects of adenosine are antagonized by methylxanthines such as theophylline. Adenosine is contraindicated in patients with second- or third-degree heart block or sick sinus syndrome. When large doses are given by infusion, hypotension can occur. Not effective in terminating atrial flutter or fibrillation, but may aid in diagnosis by slowing ventricular response. Asystole for 3–6 s after administration is common. May cause bronchospasm in patients with reactive airways disease. Use with caution in patients with preexcitation syndromes (e.g., Wolff-Parkinson-White).

ALBUTEROL (PROVENTIL, VENTOLIN)

Indications	Bronchospasm.
Dosage	Aerosolized: 2.5 mg in 3 mL saline via nebulizer; 180 or 200 μg (2 puffs) via inhaler. PO: 2.5 mg. Pediatric: 0.1 mg/kg (syrup 2 mg/5 mL).
Effect	Beta$_2$-receptor agonist.
Comments	Possible β-adrenergic overload, tachydysrhythmias.

AMINOCAPROIC ACID (AMICAR)

Indications	Hemorrhage due to fibrinolysis.
Dosage	5 g/100–250 mL of NS IV to load, followed by 1 g/hr infusion.
Effect	Stabilizes clot formation by inhibiting plasminogen activators and plasmin.
Clearance	Primarily renal elimination.
Comments	Contraindicated in disseminated intravascular coagulation.

AMINOPHYLLINE (THEOPHYLLINE ETHYLENEDIAMINE)

Indications	Bronchospasm, infantile apneic spells.
Dosage	Adult: LOAD—5.0 mg/kg IV at <25 mg/min; MAINT—0.5–0.7 mg/kg/h IV. Lower dose in elderly, CHF, hepatic disease. Pediatric: 1 mo–1 yr, 0.16–0.7 mg/kg/h; 1–9 yr, 0.8 mg/kg/h.
Effect	Inhibits phosphodiesterase, antagonizes adenosine, resulting in bronchodilation and positive inotropic and chronotropic effects.
Clearance	Hepatic metabolism; renal elimination (10% unchanged).
Comments	May cause tachydysrhythmias. Therapeutic concentration, 10–20 μg/mL. Aminophylline 100 mg = Theophylline 80 mg.

AMIODARONE (CORDARONE)

Indications	Refractory or recurrent atrial and ventricular tachydysrhythmias.
Dosage	LOAD: 800–1,600 mg/day PO × 1–3 weeks, then 600–800 mg/day PO × 4 weeks; MAINT: 100–400 mg/day PO. IV: 150 to 300 mg over 10 min (15 mg/min), 360 mg over the next 6 h (1 mg/min), then 540 mg over the next 18 h (0.5 mg/min).
Effect	Depresses the sinoatrial node and prolongs the PR, QRS, and QT intervals; produces α- and β-adrenergic blockade.
Clearance	Biliary elimination.
Comments	May cause severe sinus bradycardia, ventricular arrhythmias, AV block, liver and thyroid function test abnormalities, hepatitis, and cirrhosis. Pulmonary fibrosis can result from long-term use. Increases serum levels of digoxin, oral anticoagulants, diltiazem, quinidine, procainamide, and phenytoin.

AMRINONE (INOCOR)

Indication	Acute ventricular failure.
Dosage	0.75 mg/kg IV bolus over several minutes, then infuse at 5–15 μg/kg/min. Infusion mixtures (usually 100 mg in 250 mL) must not contain dextrose.
Effect	Inhibits phosphodiesterase, which results in increased cardiac output, increased contractility, and direct vasodilation.
Clearance	Variable hepatic metabolism; renal/fecal excretion.
Comments	May cause hypotension, thrombocytopenia, and anaphylaxis (contains sulfites).

APROTININ (TRASYLOL)

Indications	Prophylactic reduction in perioperative blood loss in patients undergoing cardiopulmonary bypass.
Dosage	Supplied as 10,000 KIU (Kallikrein inhibitor units)/mL or 1.4 mg/mL. One-milliliter test dose followed by LOAD: 1–2 million KIU (100–200 mL) IV over 20–30 min; pump prime": 1–2 million KIU; MAINT: 250,000–500,000 KIU/h (25–50 mL/h).
Effect	Protease inhibitor of trypsin, plasmin, and kallikrein. Antifibrinolytic. Protects glycoprotein Ib receptor on platelets during cardiopulmonary bypass.
Clearance	Renal elimination.
Comments	Rapid administration may cause transient hypotension. Anaphylactic reaction in <0.5% of patients. Recent data indicate a significantly increased risk of renal failure, MI, congestive heart failure, and stroke when this drug is used in coronary artery surgery.

ARGATROBAN

Indications	1. Treatment or prophylaxis of thrombosis in heparin-induced thrombocytopenia. 2. Percutaneous coronary intervention in patients with or at risk for heparin-induced thrombocytopenia.
Dosage	1. 2 μg/kg/min IV continuous infusion, MAX 10 μg/kg/min, adjust until steady-state aPTT is 1.5–3 times the initial baseline value (not to exceed 100 seconds). 2. 350 μg/kg IV over 3–5 min and 25 μg/kg/min IV continuous infusion, maintain ACT between 300 and 450 seconds. Safety and efficacy in children less than 18 years old have not been established.
Effect	Direct, highly selective thrombin inhibitor. Inhibits fibrin formation; activation of factors V, VIII, and XIII; protein C; and platelet aggregation.
Clearance	Hepatic metabolism with 65% biliary excretion and 22% renal (16% excreted as unchanged drug).
Comments	Bleeding is the major adverse effect. Not to be administered with other parenteral anticoagulants. Caution when switching to or from other anticoagulants: allow heparin's effect on the aPTT to decrease; loading doses of warfarin should not be used. Caution in patients with severe hypertension, recent lumbar puncture, or major surgery. Reduce dose in hepatic dysfunction.

ATENOLOL (TENORMIN)

Indications	Hypertension, angina, postmyocardial infarction (MI).
Dosage	PO: 50–100 mg/day. IV: 5 mg prn.
Effect	Beta$_1$-selective adrenergic receptor blockade.
Clearance	Renal, intestinal elimination.
Comments	High doses block β_2-adrenergic receptors. Relatively contraindicated in acute congestive heart failure, asthma, and heart block. Caution in patients on calcium-channel blockers and other agents prolonging AV conduction. Rebound angina can occur with abrupt cessation.

ATROPINE

Indications	1. Antisialagogue. 2. Bradycardia.
Dosage	Adult: 1. 0.2–0.4 mg IV. 2. 0.4–1.0 mg IV. Pediatric: 1. 0.01 mg/kg/dose IV/IM (<0.4 mg). 2. 0.02 mg/kg/dose IV (<0.4 mg).

Effect	Competitive blockade of acetylcholine at muscarinic receptors.
Clearance	50%–70% hepatic metabolism; renal elimination.
Comments	May cause tachydysrhythmias, AV dissociation, premature ventricular contractions, dry mouth, or urinary retention. CNS effects occur at high doses.

BICARBONATE, SODIUM (NaHCO$_3$)

Indications	Metabolic acidosis.
Dosage	IV dose in mEq NaHCO$_3$ = (base deficit × weight [kg] × 0.3) (subsequent doses titrated against patient's pH).
Effect	H$^+$ neutralization.
Clearance	Plasma metabolism; pulmonary, renal elimination.
Comments	May cause metabolic alkalosis, hypercarbia, and hyperosmolality. In neonates, can cause intraventricular hemorrhage. Crosses placenta. An 8.4% solution is approximately 1.0 mEq/mL; a 4.2% solution is approximately 0.5 mEq/mL.

BUMETANIDE (BUMEX)

Indications	Edema, hypertension, intracranial hypertension.
Dosage	0.5–1.0 mg IV, repeated to a maximum of 10 mg/day.
Effect	Loop diuretic with principal effect on the ascending limb of the loop of Henle. Causes increased excretion of Na$^+$, K$^+$, Cl$^-$, and H$_2$O.
Clearance	Hepatic metabolism; 81% renal excretion (45% unchanged).
Comments	May cause electrolyte imbalance, dehydration, and deafness. Patients who are allergic to sulfonamides may show hypersensitivity to bumetanide. Effective in renal insufficiency.

CALCIUM CHLORIDE (CaCL$_2$); CALCIUM GLUCONATE (KALCINATE)

Indications	Hypocalcemia, hyperkalemia, hypermagnesemia.
Dosage	Calcium chloride: 5–10 mg/kg IV prn (10% CaCl$_2$ = 1.36 mEq Ca^{2+}/mL). Calcium gluconate: 15–30 mg/kg IV prn (10% calcium gluconate = 0.45 mEq Ca^{2+}/mL).
Effect	Maintains cell membrane integrity, muscular excitation–contraction coupling, glandular stimulation–secretion coupling, and enzyme function. Increases blood pressure.
Clearance	Incorporated into muscle, bone, and other tissues. Renal excretion.
Comments	May cause bradycardia or arrhythmia (especially with digitalis). Irritating to veins. Ca^{2+} less available with calcium gluconate than with calcium chloride due to binding of gluconate.

CAPTOPRIL (CAPOTEN)

Indications	Hypertension, congestive heart failure.
Dosage	LOAD: 12.5–25.0 mg PO tid; MAINT: 25–100 mg PO tid.
Effect	Angiotensin I-converting enzyme inhibition decreases angiotensin II and aldosterone levels. Reduces both preload and afterload in patients with congestive heart failure.
Clearance	Hepatic metabolism; 95% renal elimination (40%–50% unchanged).
Comments	May cause neutropenia, agranulocytosis, hypotension, or bronchospasm. Avoid in pregnant patients. Exaggerated response in renal artery stenosis and with diuretics.

CHLOROTHIAZIDE (DIURIL)

Indications	Edema in heart failure, acute or chronic renal failure; hypertension.
Dosage	Adult: 250–500 mg IV bolus at 50–100 mg/min, 2 g maximum over 24 h. Pediatric: oral, 20 mg/kg/day in two divided doses every 12 h.
Effect	Thiazide diuretic.
Clearance	Renal elimination.
Comments	Enhances activity of antihypertensives, digoxin. May enhance activity of loop diuretics in renal failure. May increase insulin requirements in diabetic patients.

CIMETIDINE (TAGAMET)

Indications	Pulmonary aspiration prophylaxis (reduction of gastric volume and acidity), gastroesophageal reflux, gastric acid hypersecretion, anaphylaxis prophylaxis.
Dosage	300 mg q6h IV/IM/PO (q12h in renal failure).
Effect	Antagonizes action of histamine on H_2 receptors, with inhibition of gastric acid secretion.
Clearance	Hepatic metabolism; 75% renal elimination (unchanged) (IV dose).
Comments	May cause small increases in creatinine levels, increases concentration of many drugs due to inhibition of oxidative drug metabolism. Can produce confusion or somnolence with repeated dosing. Venous irritation.

CITRATE, SODIUM DIHYDRATE/CITRIC ACID MONOHYDRATE (BICITRA)

Indications	Gastric acid neutralization.
Dosage	15 mL in 15 mL water PO (500 mg sodium citrate, 334 mg citric acid per 5 mL).
Effect	Absorbed and metabolized to sodium bicarbonate.
Clearance	Oxidation; 5% excreted in urine (unchanged).
Comments	Contraindicated in patients with sodium restriction or severe renal impairment. Do not use with aluminum-based antacids.

CLONIDINE (CATAPRES)

Indications	Hypertension; autonomic hyperactivity secondary to drug withdrawal.
Dosage	0.1–1.2 mg/day PO in divided doses (2.4 mg/day maximum dose). Also available as a transdermal patch delivering 0.1, 0.2, or 0.3 mg/day for 7 days.
Effect	Central α_2-adrenergic agonist; decreases systemic vascular resistance and heart rate.
Clearance	50% hepatic metabolism; elimination 20% biliary, 80% renal.
Comments	Abrupt withdrawal may cause rebound hypertension or arrhythmias. Can cause drowsiness, nightmares, restlessness, anxiety, or depression. Intravenous injection may cause transient peripheral α-adrenergic stimulation.

CLOPIDOGREL (PLAVIX)

Indications	Antiplatelet agent. **1.** Acute coronary syndrome. **2.** Percutaneous coronary intervention. **3.** Recent MI, recent thromboembolic stroke, or established arterial disease.

Dosage	**1 and 2.** PO: LOAD: 300 mg; MAINT: 75 mg qd. **3.** PO: 75 mg qd.
Effect	ADP receptor blocker: prevents fibrinogen binding, thus reducing the possibility of platelet adhesion and aggregation.
Clearance	Hepatic metabolism; renal excretion.
Comments	Major side effect is bleeding. Concurrent use with heparin and aspirin is accepted, particularly in treatment of ACS. Caution in bleeding states. Gastrointestinal intolerance in >20% of patients. Reduce dose in hepatic insufficiency. Recommend discontinuing 7 days prior to neuraxial anesthesia.

DALTEPARIN (FRAGMIN)

Indications	**1.** Prophylaxis of deep venous thrombosis. **2.** Acute coronary syndromes. **3.** Deep venous thrombosis.
Dosage	**1.** 2,500–5,000 units SC qd. **2.** 120 units/kg (maximum dose 10,000 units) SC q12h × 5–8 days with concurrent aspirin therapy. **3.** 100 units/kg SC bid or 200 units/kg SC qd.
Effect	Anticoagulant; inhibits both factor Xa and factor IIa. See heparin.
Clearance	Hepatic; renal excretion.
Comments	Equally effective as unfractionated heparin; more predictable dose–response characteristics. Spinal and epidural hematomas have been associated with neuraxial anesthesia and lumbar punctures. Risk of hematoma is increased with indwelling epidural catheters. Safety and efficacy in pediatric patients not established. Rarely causes thrombocytopenia.

DANTROLENE (DANTRIUM)

Indications	Malignant hyperthermia (MH); skeletal muscle spasticity.
Dosage	Mix 20 mg in 60 mL of sterile water. At first signs of MH, 2.5 mg/kg IV bolus; if signs persist after 30 min, repeat dose, up to 10 mg/kg. Prophylactic IV treatment is not recommended.
Effect	Reduces Ca^{2+} release from sarcoplasmic reticulum.
Clearance	Hepatic metabolism; renal elimination.
Comments	Dissolves slowly into solution. May cause muscle weakness, gastrointestinal upset, drowsiness, sedation, or abnormal liver function (chronically). Additive effects with neuromuscular blocking agents. Tissue irritant.

DESMOPRESSIN ACETATE (DDAVP)

Indications	**1.** Treatment of coagulopathy in von Willebrand disease, hemophilia A, renal failure. **2.** Antidiuretic.
Dosage	Adult: **1.** 0.3 μg/kg IV (diluted 50 mL NS), infused over 15–30 min. **2.** 2–4 μg/day usually in two divided doses. Pediatric: <10 kg, dilute adult dose in 10 mL NSS; >10 kg, see adult dose.
Effect	Increases plasma levels of factor VIII activity by causing release of von Willebrand's factor from endothelial cells; increases renal water reabsorption.
Clearance	Renal elimination.
Comments	Chlorpropamide, carbamazepine, and clofibrate potentiate the antidiuretic effect. Repeat doses q12–24h will have diminished effect compared with initial dose.

DEXAMETHASONE (DECADRON)

Indications	**1.** Cerebral edema from CNS tumors; airway edema. **2.** Prophylaxis of postoperative nausea and vomiting.

Dosage	**1.** LOAD: 10 mg IV. MAINT: 4 mg IV q6h (tapered over 6 days). **2.** 4 mg IV.
Effect	See hydrocortisone. Has 20 to 25 times the glucocorticoid potency of hydrocortisone. Minimal mineralocorticoid effect.
Clearance	Primarily hepatic metabolism; renal elimination.
Comments	See hydrocortisone.

DEXMEDETOMIDINE (PRECEDEX)

Indications	ICU sedation.
Dosage	Adult ICU Sedation: LOAD: 1 μg/kg over 10 minutes; MAINT: 0.2–0.7 μg/kg/hour; not indicated for infusions lasting >24 hours. Safety and efficacy in children less than 18 years of age have not been established.
Effect	Selective alpha-2-adrenoreceptor agonist; alpha-1 activity observed at high doses or after rapid infusion. Produces sedation and potentiates effects of sedative-hypnotics, anesthetics and opioids. Minimal effects on ventilation.
Clearance	Hepatic metabolism; 95% renal excretion.
Comments	Labeled use for sedation of intubated and mechanically ventilated patients during treatment in an intensive care setting. Nausea and dry mouth are common. Episodes of bradycardia, atrial fibrillation, hypotension, and sinus arrest have occurred, especially after IV bolus. Use with caution in patients with cardiovascular dysfunction and those receiving vasodilators or negative chronotropic agents. Transient vasoconstriction and hypertension may occur with initial loading dose.

DEXTRAN 40 (RHEOMACRODEX)

Indications	Inhibition of platelet aggregation; improvement of blood flow in low-flow states (e.g., vascular surgery); intravascular volume expansion.
Dosage	Adult: LOAD: 30–50 mL IV over 30 min; MAINT: 15–30 mL/hr IV (10% solution). Pediatric: <20 mL/kg/24 hr of 10% dextran.
Effect	Immediate, short-lived plasma volume expansion; adsorption to RBC surface prevents RBC aggregation, decreases blood viscosity and platelet adhesiveness.
Clearance	Renal elimination.
Comments	May cause volume overload, anaphylaxis, bleeding tendency, interference with blood cross-matching, or false elevation of blood sugar. Renal failure has been reported.

DIGOXIN (LANOXIN)

Indications	Heart failure, tachydysrhythmias, atrial fibrillation, atrial flutter.
Dosage	Adult: LOAD: 0.5–1.0 mg/d IV or PO in divided doses; MAINT: 0.125–0.5 mg IV or PO qd. Pediatric (IV/IM in divided doses): LOAD: Total daily doses usually divided into two or more doses. Neonates: 15–30 μg/kg/day; 1 month–2 yr: 30–50 μg/kg/day; 2–5 yr: 25–35 μg/kg/day; 5–10 yr: 15–30 μg/kg/day; >10 yr: 8–12 μg/kg/day. MAINT: 20%–35% of LOAD qd (reduce in renal failure).
Effect	Increases myocardial contractility; decreases conduction in AV node and Purkinje fibers.
Clearance	Renal elimination (50%–70% unchanged).

Comments   May cause gastrointestinal intolerance, blurred vision, ECG changes, or dysrhythmias. Toxicity potentiated by hypokalemia, hypomagnesemia, hypercalcemia. Use cautiously in Wolff–Parkinson–White syndrome and with defibrillation. Heart block potentiated by beta blockade and calcium-channel blockade.

DILTIAZEM (CARDIZEM)

Indications   Angina pectoris, variant angina from coronary artery spasm, atrial fibrillation/flutter, paroxysmal supraventricular tachycardia, hypertension.

Dosage   PO: 30–60 mg q6h. IV: 20 mg bolus then 10 mg/h infusion.

Effect   Calcium channel antagonist that slows conduction though sinoatrial and AV nodes, dilates coronary and peripheral arterioles, and reduces myocardial contractility.

Clearance   Primarily hepatic metabolism; renal elimination.

Comments   May cause bradycardia and heart block. May interact with beta-blockers and digoxin to impair contractility. Causes transiently elevated liver function tests. Avoid use in patients with accessory conduction tracts, AV block, IV beta-blockers, or ventricular tachycardia. Active metabolite has 1/4–1/2 of the coronary dilation effect.

DIPHENHYDRAMINE (BENADRYL)

Indications   Allergic reactions, drug-induced extrapyramidal reactions; sedation.

Dosage   Adult: 25–50 mg IV q6–8h. Pediatric: 5.0 mg/kg/day IV in 4 divided doses (maximum 300 mg).

Effect   Antagonizes action of histamine on H_1 receptors; anticholinergic; CNS depressant.

Clearance   Hepatic metabolism; renal excretion.

Comments   May cause hypotension, tachycardia, dizziness, urinary retention, seizures.

DOBUTAMINE (DOBUTREX)

Indications   Heart failure.

Dosage   Infusion mix: 250 mg in 250 mL of D5W or NS. Adult: Begin infusion at 2 μg/kg/min and titrate to effect. Pediatric: 5–20 μg/kg/min.

Effect β_1-Adrenergic agonist.

Clearance   Hepatic metabolism; renal elimination.

Comments   May cause hypotension, arrhythmias, or myocardial ischemia. Can increase ventricular rate in atrial fibrillation.

DOPAMINE (INTROPIN)

Indications   1. Hypotension, heart failure. 2. Oliguria.

Dosage   Infusion mix: 200–800 mg in 250 mL of D5W or NS. 1. Infusion at 5–20 μg/kg/min IV titrate to effect. 2. Infusion at 1–3 μg/kg/min IV.

Effect   Dopaminergic; α- and β-adrenergic agonist.

Clearance   MAO/COMT metabolism.

Comments   May cause hypertension, dysrhythmias, or myocardial ischemia. Primarily dopaminergic effects (increased renal blood flow) at 1–5 μg/kg/min. Primarily α- and β-adrenergic effects at $\geq$10 μg/kg/min.

DOXAZOSIN (CARDURA)

Indications	Hypertension.
Dosage	Start 1 mg PO qd, may be slowly increased (over weeks) to 4 to 16 mg PO qd depending on individual patient's response.
Effect	Alpha$_1$ (postjunctional) adrenergic antagonist.
Clearance	Hepatic metabolism predominates.
Comments	Significant "first-dose" effect with marked postural hypotension and dizziness. Maximum reductions of blood pressure within 2 to 6 hr of dosing.

DROPERIDOL (INAPSINE)

Indications	**1.** Nausea, vomiting. **2.** Agitation; adjunct to anesthesia.
Dosage	Adult: **1.** 0.625–2.5 mg IV prn. **2.** 2.5–10 mg IV prn. Pediatric: **1.** 0.05–0.06 mg/kg q4–6h.
Effect	Dopamine (D$_2$) receptor antagonist. Apparent psychic indifference to environment, catatonia, antipsychotic, antiemetic.
Clearance	Hepatic metabolism; renal excretion.
Comments	Given alone, may cause dysphoria. Causes dose-related prolongation of QTc interval. Weak evidence for cardiac toxicity (torsades de pointes) at doses used for prophylaxis of nausea and vomiting. FDA recommends avoiding droperidol in patients with QTc prolongation, reserving the drug for patients failing other therapies, and monitoring ECG for 2 to 3 hours after treatment.

ENALAPRIL/ENALAPRILAT (VASOTEC)

Indications	Hypertension, congestive heart failure.
Dosage	PO: LOAD: 2.5–5.0 mg qd; MAINT: 10–20 mg bid. IV: 0.625–5.0 mg q6h (as enalaprilat).
Effect	Angiotensin-converting enzyme inhibitor; synergistic with diuretics.
Clearance	Hepatic metabolism of enalapril to active metabolite (enalaprilat); renal and fecal elimination.
Comments	Causes increased serum potassium, volume-responsive hypotension. Subsequent doses are additive in effect. Can cause angioedema, blood dyscrasia, cough, lithium toxicity, or worsening of renal impairment.

ENOXAPARIN (LOVENOX)

Indications	**1.** Prophylaxis of deep venous thrombosis. **2.** Acute coronary syndromes. **3.** Treatment of deep venous thrombosis.
Dosage	**1.** 30 mg SC bid or 40 mg SC qd. **2.** 1 mg/kg SC bid for a minimum of 2 days, in conjunction with aspirin therapy. **3.** 1 mg/kg SC q12h or 1.5 mg/kg SC qd.
Effect	Anticoagulant; inhibits both factor Xa and factor IIa. See heparin.
Clearance	Hepatic; renal excretion.
Comments	More predictable dose–response characteristics than unfractionated heparin. Appears superior to unfractionated heparin in aspirin-treated patients with unstable angina or non–Q-wave myocardial infarction. Spinal and epidural hematomas have been associated with neuraxial anesthesia and lumbar punctures. Risk of hematoma is increased with indwelling epidural catheters. Safety and efficacy in pediatric patients not established. Rarely causes thrombocytopenia.

EPHEDRINE

Indication	Hypotension.
Dosage	5–50 mg IV prn.
Effect	α- and β-adrenergic stimulation; norepinephrine release at sympathetic nerve endings.
Clearance	Mostly renal elimination (unchanged).
Comments	May cause hypertension, dysrhythmias, myocardial ischemia, CNS stimulation, decrease in uterine activity, and mild bronchodilation. Minimal effect on uterine blood flow. Avoid in patients taking MAO inhibitors. Tachyphylaxis with repeated dosing.

EPINEPHRINE (ADRENALIN)

Indications	**1.** Heart failure, hypotension, cardiac arrest. **2.** Bronchospasm, anaphylaxis.
Dosage	Infusion mix: 1 mg in 250 mL of D5W or NS. Adult: **1.** 0.1–1 mg IV or 1 mg intratracheal q5 min prn. **2.** 0.1–0.5 mg SC, 0.1–0.25 mg IV, or 0.25–1.5 μ/min IV infusion. Pediatric: **1.** Neonates: 0.01–0.03 mg/kg IV or intratracheal q3–5 min; children: 0.01 mg/kg IV or intratracheal q3–5h (up to 5 mL 1:10,000). **2.** 0.01 mg/kg IV up to 0.5 mg. 0.01 mg/kg SC q15 min × 2 doses up to 1 mg/dose.
Effect	α- and β-adrenergic agonist.
Clearance	MAO/COMT metabolism.
Comments	May cause hypertension, arrhythmias, or myocardial ischemia. Dysrhythmias potentiated by halothane. Topical or local injection (1:80,000–1:500,000) causes vasoconstriction. Crosses the placenta.

EPINEPHRINE, RACEMIC (VAPONEFRIN)

Indications	Airway edema, bronchospasm.
Dosage	Adult: Inhaled via nebulizer—0.5 mL of 2.25% solution in 2.5–3.5 mL of NS q1–4h prn. Pediatric: Inhaled via nebulizer—0.5 mL of 2.25% solution in 2.5–3.5 mL of NS q4h prn.
Effect	Mucosal vasoconstriction (see also epinephrine [adrenalin]).
Clearance	See epinephrine.
Comments	See epinephrine.

EPTIFIBATIDE (INTEGRILIN)

Indications	Prevents thrombus formation after percutaneous coronary intervention (PCI).
Dosage	Bolus (180 μg/kg), then 0.5–2 μg/kg/min continuous infusion.
Effect	Inhibits glycoprotein IIb/IIIa; prevents platelet adhesion and aggregation.
Clearance	Platelet function recovers within 4 to 8 hours after discontinuation of infusion.
Comments	Bleeding complications and thrombocytopenia are common side effects.

ERGONOVINE (ERGOTRATE)

Indication	Postpartum hemorrhage due to uterine atony.
Dosage	For postpartum hemorrhage: IV (emergency only), 0.2 mg in 5 mL of NS $\geq$1 min; IM, 0.2 mg q2–4h prn for $\leq$5 doses, then PO: 0.2–0.4 mg q6–12h for 2 days or prn.

Effect   Constriction of uterine and vascular smooth muscle.
Clearance   Hepatic metabolism; renal elimination.
Comments   May cause hypertension from systemic vasoconstriction (especially in eclampsia and hypertension), dysrhythmias, coronary spasm, uterine tetany, or gastrointestinal upset. Intravenous route is only used in emergencies. Overdosage may cause convulsions or stroke.

ESMOLOL (BREVIBLOC)

Indications Supraventricular tachydysrhythmias, myocardial ischemia.
Dosage   Start with 5–10 mg IV bolus and increase q3 min prn to total 100–300 mg; infusion 1–15 mg/min.
Effect   Selective β_1-adrenergic blockade.
Clearance   Degraded by RBC esterases; renal elimination.
Comments   May cause bradycardia, AV conduction delay, hypotension, congestive heart failure; beta$_2$ activity at high doses.

ETHACRYNIC ACID (EDECRIN)

Indications Edema, congestive heart failure, acute/chronic renal failure.
Dosage   Adult: PO: 50–200 mg/day in 1–2 divided doses; IV: 25–100 mg IV over 5–10 min; 24-h cumulative dose, 400 mg. Pediatric: PO: 25 mg/day to start, increase by 25 mg/day until response is obtained (maximum, 3 mg/kg/day); IV: 1 mg/kg/dose (repeat doses with caution due to potential for ototoxicity).
Effect   Diuretic.
Clearance   Hepatically metabolized to active cysteine conjugate (35% to 40%); 30% to 60% excreted unchanged in bile and urine.
Comments   May potentiate the activity of antihypertensives, neuromuscular blocking agents, digoxin, and increase insulin requirements in diabetic patients.

FAMOTIDINE (PEPCID)

Indications Pulmonary aspiration prophylaxis, peptic ulcer disease.
Dosage   20 mg IV/PO q12h (dilute in 1–10 mL of D5W or NS).
Effect   Antagonizes action of histamine on H$_2$ receptors.
Clearance   30%–35% hepatic metabolism; 65%–70% renal elimination.
Comments   May cause confusion. Rapid IV administration may increase risk of cardiac dysrhythmias and hypotension.

FLUMAZENIL (MAZICON)

Indication   **1.** Reversal of benzodiazepine sedation. **2.** Reversal of benzodiazepine overdose.
Dosage   **1.** 0.2–1.0 mg IV q20 min at 0.2 mg/min. **2.** 3–5 mg IV at 0.5 mg/min.
Effect   Competitive antagonism of CNS benzodiazepine receptor.
Clearance   100% hepatic metabolism; 90%–95% renal elimination of metabolite.
Comments   Duration of action shorter than midazolam and other agonists. May induce CNS excitation including seizures, acute withdrawal, nausea, dizziness, and agitation. Only partial reversal of midazolam-induced ventilatory depression. Does not reverse nonbenzodiazepine induced CNS depression.

FUROSEMIDE (LASIX)

Indications	Edema, hypertension, intracranial hypertension, renal failure, hypercalcemia.
Dosage	Adult: 2–40 mg IV (initial dose, dosage individualized). Pediatric: 1–2 mg/kg/day.
Effect	Increases excretion of Na^+, Cl^-, K^+, PO_4^{3-}, Ca^{2+}, and H_2O by inhibiting reabsorption in loop of Henle.
Clearance	Hepatic metabolism; 88% renal elimination.
Comments	May cause electrolyte imbalance, dehydration, transient hypotension, deafness, hyperglycemia, or hyperuricemia. Sulfa-allergic patients may exhibit hypersensitivity to furosemide.

GLUCAGON

Indications	1. Duodenal or choledochal relaxation. 2. Refractory β-adrenergic blocker toxicity.
Dosage	1. 0.25–0.5 mg IV q20 min prn. 2. 5 mg IV bolus, with 1–10 mg/h titrated to patient response.
Effect	Catecholamine release. Positive inotrope and chronotrope.
Clearance	Hepatic and renal proteolysis.
Comments	May cause anaphylaxis, nausea, vomiting, hyperglycemia, or positive inotropic and chronotropic effects. High doses potentiate oral anticoagulants. Use with caution in presence of insulinoma or pheochromocytoma.

GLYCOPYRROLATE (ROBINUL)

Indications	1. Decrease gastrointestinal motility, antisialagogue. 2. Bradycardia.
Dosage	Adult: 1. 0.1–0.2 mg IV/IM/SC; 1–2 mg PO. 2. 0.1–0.2 mg/dose IV. Pediatric: 0.004–0.008 mg/kg IV/IM up to 0.1 mg.
Effect	See atropine.
Clearance	Renal elimination.
Comments	See atropine. Longer duration, possibly less chronotropic effect than atropine. Does not cross blood–brain barrier or placenta. Unreliable oral absorption.

HALOPERIDOL (HALDOL)

Indications	Psychosis, agitation, postoperative nausea and vomiting.
Dosage	0.5–10 mg PO/IM/IV prn (dosage individualized).
Effect	Antipsychotic effects due to dopamine (D_2) receptor antagonism. CNS depression.
Clearance	Hepatic metabolism; renal/biliary elimination.
Comments	May cause extrapyramidal reactions or mild α-adrenergic antagonism. Can prolong QT interval and produce ventricular arrhythmias, notably torsade de pointes, and lower seizure threshold. May precipitate neuroleptic malignant syndrome. Contraindicated in Parkinson disease. Recent data indicate haloperidol 1 mg IV is efficacious for the prevention of postoperative nausea and vomiting.

HEPARIN-UNFRACTIONATED

Indications	Anticoagulation for: 1. Thrombosis, thromboembolism. 2. Cardiopulmonary bypass. 3. Disseminated intravascular coagulation. 4. Thromboembolism prophylaxis.

Dosage	Adult: **1.** LOAD: 50–150 units/kg IV; MAINT: 15–25 units/kg/h IV. Titrate dosage with partial thromboplastin time or activated clotting time. **2.** LOAD: 300 units/kg IV; MAINT: 100 units/kg/h IV, titrate with coagulation tests. **3.** LOAD: 50–100 units/kg IV; MAINT: 15–25 units/kg/h IV; titrate with coagulation tests. **4.** 5,000 units q8–12h SC.
Effect	Potentiates action of antithrombin III; blocks conversion of prothrombin and activation of other coagulation factors.
Clearance	Primarily by reticuloendothelial uptake, hepatic biotransformation.
Comments	May cause bleeding, thrombocytopenia, allergic reactions, and diuresis (36–48 h after a large dose). Half-life increased in renal failure and decreased in thromboembolism and liver disease. Does not cross placenta. Reversed by protamine. Spinal and epidural hematomas have been associated with neuraxial anesthesia and lumbar punctures. Risk of hematoma is increased with indwelling epidural catheters.

HYDRALAZINE (APRESOLINE)

Indication	Hypertension.
Dosage	2.5–20 mg IV q4h or prn (dosage individualized).
Effect	Reduces vascular smooth muscle tone (arteriole more than venule).
Clearance	Extensive hepatic metabolism; renal elimination.
Comments	May cause hypotension (diastolic more than systolic), reflex tachycardia, systemic lupus erythematosus syndrome. Increases coronary, splanchnic, cerebral, and renal blood flows.

HYDROCORTISONE (SOLU-CORTEF)

Indications	Adrenal insufficiency, inflammation and allergy, cerebral edema from CNS tumors, asthma.
Dosage	10–100 mg IV q8h. Physiologic replacement: IV: 0.25–0.35 mg/kg/day; PO: 0.5–0.75 mg/kg/day.
Effect	Anti-inflammatory and antiallergic effect; mineralocorticoid effect; stimulates gluconeogenesis; inhibits peripheral protein synthesis; has membrane stabilizing effect.
Clearance	Hepatic metabolism; renal elimination.
Comments	May cause adrenocortical insufficiency (Addisonian crisis) with abrupt withdrawal, delayed wound healing, CNS disturbances, osteoporosis, or electrolyte disturbances.

HYDROXYZINE (VISTARIL, ATARAX)

Indications	Anxiety, nausea and vomiting, allergies, sedation.
Dosage	PO: 25–200 mg q6–8h; IM: 25–100 mg q4–6h. Not an IV drug.
Effect	Antagonizes action of histamine on H_1 receptors. CNS depression, antiemetic. Some evidence for analgesic effect.
Clearance	Hepatic (P-450) metabolism; renal elimination.
Comments	May cause dry mouth. Minimal cardiorespiratory depression. Intravenous injection may cause thrombosis. Crosses the placenta.

INDIGO CARMINE

Indications	Evaluation of urine output. Localization of ureteral orifices during cystoscopy.
Dosage	40 mg IV slowly (5 mL of 0.8% solution).

Effect	Rapid glomerular filtration produces blue urine.
Clearance	Renal elimination.
Comments	Hypertension from α-adrenergic stimulation, lasts 15–30 min after IV dose.

INDOCYANINE GREEN (CARDIO-GREEN)

Indications	Cardiac output measurement by indicator dye dilution.
Dosage	5 mg IV (diluted in 1 mL of normal saline) rapidly injected into central circulation.
Effect	Almost complete binding to plasma proteins, with distribution within plasma volume.
Clearance	Hepatic elimination.
Comments	May cause allergic reactions or transient increases in bilirubin levels. Absorption spectra changed by heparin. Cautious use in patients with iodine allergy (contains 5% sodium iodide).

INSULIN (REGULAR, CZI)

Indications	1. Hyperglycemia. 2. Diabetic ketoacidosis.
Dosage	1. (Individualized): usually 5–10 units IV/SC prn. 2. LOAD: 10–20 units IV; MAINT: 0.05–0.1 units/kg/h IV, titrated against plasma glucose level.
Effect	Facilitates glucose transport intracellularly. Shifts K^+ and Mg^{2+} intracellularly.
Clearance	Hepatic and renal metabolism; 30%–80% renal elimination. Unchanged insulin is reabsorbed.
Comments	May cause hypoglycemia, allergic reactions, or synthesis of insulin antibodies. May be absorbed by plastic in IV tubing.

ISOPROTERENOL (ISUPREL)

Indications	Heart failure, bradycardia.
Dosage	Adult: 2 μg/min titrated up to 20 μg/min. Pediatric: Start at 0.1 μg/kg/min; titrate to effect.
Effect	β-Adrenergic agonist; positive chronotrope and inotrope.
Clearance	Hepatic and pulmonary metabolism; 40%–50% renal excretion (unchanged).
Comments	May cause dysrhythmias, myocardial ischemia, hypertension, or CNS excitation.

ISOSORBIDE DINITRATE (ISORDIL)

Indications	Angina, hypertension, myocardial infarction, congestive heart failure.
Dosage	5–20 mg PO q6h.
Effect	See nitroglycerin.
Clearance	Nearly 100% hepatic metabolism; renal elimination.
Comments	See nitroglycerin. Tolerance may develop.

KETOROLAC (TORADOL)

Indications	Nonsteroidal, anti-inflammatory analgesic (NSAID) for moderate pain. Useful adjunct for severe pain when used with parenteral or epidural opioids.
Dosage	PO: 10 mg q4–6h. IM/IV: 30–60 mg, then 15–30 mg q6h.
Effect	Limits prostaglandin synthesis by cyclooxygenase inhibition.
Clearance	Less than 50% hepatic metabolism, renal metabolism; 91% renal elimination.

Comments Adverse effects are similar to those with other NSAIDs: peptic
ulceration, bleeding, decreased renal blood flow. Duration of
treatment not to exceed 5 days.

LABETALOL (NORMODYNE, TRANDATE)

Indications Hypertension, angina, controlled hypotension.
Dosage IV: 5–10-mg increments at 5-min intervals, to 40–80 mg/dose.
Infusion: titrate to desired response, 10–180 mg/hr.
Effect Selective α_1-adrenergic blockade with nonselective β-adrenergic
blockade. Ratio of α/β blockade = 1:7.
Clearance Hepatic metabolism; renal elimination.
Comments May cause bradycardia, AV conduction delays, bronchospasm in
some asthmatics, and postural hypotension. Crosses the
placenta.

LEVOTHYROXINE (SYNTHROID)

Indications Hypothyroidism.
Dosage Adjust according to individual requirements and response. Adults:
PO: 0.1–0.2 mg/day; IV: 75% of adult oral dose. Pediatric:
PO: 0–6 months: 25–50 μg/day or 8–10 μg/kg/day;
6–12 months: 50–75 μg/day or 6–8 μg/kg/day; 1–5 years:
75–100 μg/day or 5–6 μg/kg/day; 6–12 years: 100–150 μg/
day or 4–5 μg/kg/day; >12 years: over 150 μg/day or 2–3 μg/
kg/day. IV: 75% of oral dose.
Effect Exogenous thyroxine.
Clearance Metabolized in the liver to triiodothyronine (active); eliminated in
feces and urine.
Comments Contraindicated with recent myocardial infarction, thyrotoxicosis,
or uncorrected adrenal insufficiency. Phenytoin may decrease
levothyroxine levels. Increases effects of oral anticoagulants.
Tricyclic antidepressants may increase toxic potential of both
drugs.

LIDOCAINE (XYLOCAINE)

Indications 1. Ventricular dysrhythmias. 2. Cough suppression. 3. Local
anesthesia.
Dosage Adult: 1. LOAD: 1 mg/kg IV × 2 (2nd dose 20–30 min after
1st dose); MAINT: 15–50 μg/kg/min IV (1–4 mg/min).
2. 1 mg/kg IV. 3. 5 mg/kg maximum dose for infiltration or
conduction block. Pediatric: 1. LOAD: 0.5–1 mg/kg IV (2nd
dose 20–30 min after 1st dose); MAINT: 15–50 μg/kg/min IV.
2. 1 mg/kg IV. 3. 5 mg/kg maximum dose for infiltration or
conduction block.
Effect Decreases conductance of sodium channels. Antiarrhythmic
effect; sedation; neural blockade.
Clearance Hepatic metabolism to active/toxic metabolites; renal elimination
(10% unchanged).
Comments May cause dizziness, seizures, disorientation, heart block (with
myocardial conduction defect), or hypotension. Crosses the
placenta. Therapeutic concentration = 1 –5 mg/L. Caution in
patients with Wolff–Parkinson–White syndrome.

LOW MOLECULAR WEIGHT HEPARIN

Please see individual entries for dalteparin (Fragmin) and enoxaparin(Lovenox).

MAGNESIUM SULFATE

Indications	**1.** Preeclampsia/eclampsia. **2.** Hypomagnesemia. **3.** Polymorphic ventricular tachycardia (torsade de pointes).
Dosage	**1.** LOAD: 1–8 g IV; MAINT: 1–4 g/hr. **2.** 1–2 g q6–8 h, prn. **3.** 1–2 g in 10 mL D5W over 1–2 min; 5–10 g may be administered for refractory arrhythmias.
Effect	Repletes serum magnesium; prevents and treats seizures or hyperreflexia associated with preeclampsia/eclampsia.
Clearance	100% renal elimination for IV route.
Comments	Potentiates neuromuscular blockade (both depolarizing and nondepolarizing agents). Potentiates CNS effects of anesthetics, hypnotics, and opioids. Toxicity occurs with serum concentration ≥ 10 mEq/L. May alter cardiac conduction in digitalized patients. Avoid in patients with heart block. Caution in patients with renal failure.

MANNITOL (OSMITROL)

Indications	**1.** Increased intracranial pressure. **2.** Oliguria or anuria associated with acute renal injury.
Dosage	Adult: **1.** 0.25–1.0 g/kg IV as 20% solution over 30–60 min (in acute situation, can give bolus of 1.25–25.0 g over 5–10 min). **2.** 0.2 g/kg test dose over 3–5 min, then 50–100 g IV over 30 min if adequate response. Pediatric: **1.** 0.2 g/kg test dose, then 2 g/kg over 30–60 min.
Effect	Increases serum osmolality, which reduces cerebral edema and lowers intracranial and intraocular pressure; also causes osmotic diuresis and transient expansion of intravascular volume.
Clearance	Renal elimination.
Comments	Rapid administration may cause vasodilation and hypotension. May worsen or cause pulmonary edema, intracranial hemorrhage, systemic hypertension, or rebound intracranial hypertension.

METHYLENE BLUE (METHYLTHIONINE CHLORIDE, UROLENE BLUE)

Indications	**1.** Surgical marker for genitourinary surgery. **2.** Methemoglobinemia.
Dosage	**1.** 100 mg (10 mL of 1% solution) IV. **2.** 1–2 mg/kg IV of 1% solution over 10 min; repeat q1h, prn.
Effect	Low dose promotes conversion of methemoglobin to hemoglobin. High dose promotes conversion of hemoglobin to methemoglobin.
Clearance	Tissue reduction; urinary and biliary elimination.
Comments	May cause RBC destruction (prolonged use), hypertension, bladder irritation, nausea, diaphoresis. May inhibit nitrate-induced coronary artery relaxation. Interferes with pulse oximetry for 1–2 min. Can cause hemolysis in patients with glucose-6 phosphate-dehydrogenase deficiency.

METHYLERGONOVINE (METHERGINE)

Indication	Postpartum hemorrhage.
Dosage	IV (*emergency only*, after delivery of placenta): 0.2 mg in 5 mL of NS, dose over ≥ 1 min IM: 0.2 mg q2–4h, prn (<5 doses). PO (after IM or IV doses): 0.2–0.4 mg q6–12h × 2–7 days.

Clearance   Hepatic metabolism; renal elimination.
Comments   See ergonovine. Hypertensive response less marked than with ergonovine.

METHYLPREDNISOLONE (SOLU-MEDROL)

Indications   See hydrocortisone. Spinal cord injury.
Dosage   Adult: 40–60 mg IV q6h. Higher doses in transplant patients. Pediatric: 0.16–0.8 mg/kg/day. Status asthmaticus: LOAD: 2 mg/kg; MAINT: 0.5–1 mg/kg q6h. Spinal cord injury: LOAD: 30 mg/kg IV over 15 min; after 45 min begin MAINT: 5.4 mg/kg/h × 23 or 47 h.
Effect   See hydrocortisone; has five times the glucocorticoid potency of hydrocortisone. Almost no mineralocorticoid activity.
Clearance   Hepatic metabolism; renal elimination (dose and route dependent).
Comments   See hydrocortisone.

METOCLOPRAMIDE (REGLAN)

Indications   Gastroesophageal reflux, diabetic gastroparesis, pulmonary aspiration prophylaxis, antiemetic.
Dosage   Adult: 10 mg IV or PO q6–8h. Pediatric: 0.1 mg/kg IV or PO.
Effect   Facilitates gastric emptying by increasing gastric motility; relaxes pyloric sphincter and increases peristalsis in the duodenum and jejunum. Increases resting tone of the lower esophageal sphincter. Weak antiemetic effects appear secondary to antagonism of central and peripheral dopamine receptors.
Clearance   Hepatic metabolism; renal elimination.
Comments   Avoid in patients with GI obstruction, pheochromocytoma, or Parkinson disease. Extrapyramidal reactions occur in 0.2%–1% of patients. May exacerbate depression.

METOPROLOL (LOPRESSOR)

Indications   Hypertension, angina pectoris, dysrhythmia, hypertrophic cardiomyopathy, myocardial infarction, pheochromocytoma.
Dosage   50–100 mg PO q6–24h. 2.5–5 mg IV boluses q2 min, prn, up to 15 mg.
Effect β_1-Adrenergic blockade (β_2-adrenergic antagonism at high doses).
Clearance   Hepatic metabolism, renal elimination.
Comments   May cause bradycardia, clinically significant bronchoconstriction (with doses >100 mg/day), dizziness, fatigue, insomnia. Can increase risk of heart block. Crosses the placenta and blood–brain barrier.

MILRINONE (PRIMACOR)

Indications   Congestive heart failure.
Dosage   LOAD: 50 μg/kg IV over 10 min; MAINT: titrate 0.375–0.75 μg/kg/min to effect.
Effect   Phosphodiesterase inhibition causing positive inotropy and vasodilation.
Clearance   Renal elimination.
Comments   Short-term therapy. May increase ventricular ectopy, may aggravate outflow tract obstruction in IHSS. May cause hypotension. Not recommended for acute MI.

NADOLOL (CORGARD)

Indications	Angina pectoris, hypertension.
Dosage	40–240 mg/day PO.
Effect	Prolonged (approximately 24 h) nonselective β-adrenergic blockade.
Clearance	No hepatic metabolism; renal elimination.
Comments	May cause bronchospasm in susceptible patients (see propranolol).

NALOXONE (NARCAN)

Indications	Reversal of systemic opioid effects.
Dosage	Adult: 0.04- to 0.4-mg doses IV, titrated q2–3 min. Pediatric: 1–10 μg/kg IV (in increments) q2–3 min (up to 0.4 mg).
Effect	Antagonizes effects of opioids by competitive inhibition.
Clearance	Hepatic metabolism (95%); primarily renal elimination.
Comments	May cause hypertension, dysrhythmias, rare pulmonary edema, delirium, reversal of analgesia, or withdrawal syndrome (in opioid-dependent patients). Renarcotization may occur because antagonist has short duration. Caution in hepatic failure.

NIFEDIPINE (PROCARDIA)

Indications	Coronary artery spasm, hypertension, myocardial ischemia.
Dosage	10–40 mg PO tid.
Effect	Blocks slow calcium channels, which produces systemic and coronary vasodilation and can increase myocardial perfusion.
Clearance	Hepatic metabolism.
Comments	May cause reflex tachycardia, gastrointestinal upset, and mild negative inotropic effects. Little effect on automaticity and atrial conduction. May be useful in asymmetric septal hypertrophy. Drug solution is light sensitive. May rapidly produce severe hypotension in some patients, especially with sublingual administration.

NITROGLYCERIN (GLYCEROL TRINITRATE, NITROSTAT, NITROL, NITRO-BID, NITROLINGUAL)

Indications	Angina, myocardial ischemia or infarction, hypertension, congestive heart failure, controlled hypotension, esophageal spasm.
Dosage	IV infusion initially at 50 μg/min. Titrate to effect, 25–1,000 μg/min. Customary mix: 30–50 mg in 250 mL of D5W or NS. SL: 0.15–0.6 mg/dose. Topical: 2% ointment, 0.5–2.5 inches q6–8h.
Effect	Produces smooth muscle relaxation by enzymatic release of NO, causing systemic, coronary, and pulmonary vasodilatation (veins more than arteries); bronchodilation; biliary, gastrointestinal, and genitourinary tract relaxation.
Clearance	Nearly complete hepatic metabolism; renal elimination.
Comments	May cause reflex tachycardia, hypotension, or headache. Tolerance with chronic use may be avoided with a 10- to 12-h nitrate-free period. May be absorbed by plastic in IV tubing. May cause methemoglobinemia at very high doses.

NITROPRUSSIDE (NIPRIDE, NITROPRESS)

Indications	Hypertension, controlled hypotension, congestive heart failure.
Dosage	IV infusion initially at 0.1 μg/kg/min, then titrated to patient response to maximum 10 μg/kg/min. Lower doses often

adequate during general anesthesia. Customary mix: 50 mg in 250 mL of D5W or NS.

Effect   Direct NO donor causing smooth muscle relaxation in both arterioles and veins.

Clearance   RBC and tissue metabolism; renal elimination.

Comments   May cause excessive hypotension, reflex tachycardia. Accumulation of cyanide with liver dysfunction; thiocyanate with kidney dysfunction. Cyanide/thiocyanate buildup with prolonged infusion. Avoid with Leber's hereditary optic atrophy, hypothyroidism, or vitamin B_{12} deficiency. Solution and powder are light sensitive and must be wrapped in opaque material.

NOREPINEPHRINE (LEVARTERENOL, LEVOPHED)

Indication   Hypotension.

Dosage   1–30 μg/min IV, titrated to desired effect. Customary mix: 4 mg in 250 mL of D5W or NS. If possible, should be administered through central venous catheter.

Effect   Both α- and β-adrenergic activity, with α-adrenergic activity predominating.

Clearance   MAO/COMT metabolism.

Comments   May cause hypertension, dysrhythmias, myocardial ischemia, increased uterine contractility, constricted microcirculation, or CNS stimulation.

OCTREOTIDE (SANDOSTATIN)

Indication   Upper gastrointestinal tract bleeding, acute variceal hemorrhage.

Dosage   **1.** 25–50 μg IV bolus followed by continuous IV infusion of 25–50 μg/h.

Effect   Somatostatin analogue that suppresses release of serotonin, gastrin, vasoactive intestinal peptide, insulin, glucagon, and secretin.

Clearance   Hepatic and renal (32% eliminated unchanged); decreased in renal failure.

Comments   May cause nausea, decreased GI motility, transient hyperglycemia. Duration of therapy should be no longer than 72 h because of lack of documented efficacy beyond this time.

OMEPRAZOLE (PRILOSEC)

Indications   Gastric acid hypersecretion or gastritis, gastroesophageal reflux.

Dosage   20–40 mg PO qd.

Effect   Inhibits H^+ secretion by irreversibly binding H^+/K^+ ATPase.

Clearance   Extensive hepatic metabolism; 72% to 80% renal elimination; 18% to 23% fecal elimination.

Comments   Increases secretion of gastrin. More rapid healing of gastric ulcers than with H_2 blockers. Effective in ulcers resistant to H_2 blocker therapy. Inhibits some cytochrome P450 enzymes.

ONDANSETRON (ZOFRAN)

Indications   Prophylaxis and treatment of perioperative nausea and vomiting.

Dosage   Adult: 4 mg IV over >30 s or 8 mg PO. Pediatric: 4 mg PO.

Effect   Selective 5-HT_3 receptor antagonist.

Clearance   Hepatic, 95%; 5% renal excretion.

Comments   Used in much higher doses for chemotherapy-induced nausea. Mild side effects include headache and reversible transaminase elevation.

OXYTOCIN (PITOCIN, SYNTOCINON)

Indications	**1.** Postpartum hemorrhage, uterine atony. **2.** Augmentation of labor.
Dosage	**1.** 10 units IM or 10–40 units in 1,000 mL of crystalloid-infused IV at rate necessary to control atony (e.g., 0.02–0.04 units/min). **2.** Labor induction: 0.0005–0.002 units/min, increasing until contraction pattern established or maximum dose of 20 milliunits/min reached.
Effect	Reduces postpartum blood loss by contraction of uterine smooth muscle. Renal, coronary, and cerebral vasodilation.
Clearance	Tissue metabolism; renal elimination.
Comments	May cause uterine tetany and rupture, fetal distress, or anaphylaxis. Intravenous bolus can cause hypotension, tachycardia, dysrhythmia.

PHENOBARBITAL

Indications	**1.** Sedation, hypnosis. **2.** Seizures.
Dosage	**1.** Adult and pediatric: 1–3 mg/kg PO, IM, or IV. **2.** Adult and pediatric: LOAD: 10–20 mg/kg IV, additional 5 mg/kg doses q15–30 min for control of status epilepticus, maximum 30 mg/kg; MAINT: 3–5 mg/kg/day PO or IV in divided doses.
Clearance	Hepatic metabolism; 25%–50% renal elimination (unchanged).
Comments	May cause hypotension. Multiple drug interactions through induction of hepatic enzyme systems. Therapeutic anticonvulsant concentration 15–40 μg/mL at trough (just before next dose).

PHENOXYBENZAMINE (DIBENZYLINE)

Indication	Preoperative preparation for pheochromocytoma resection.
Dosage	10–40 mg/day PO (start at 10 mg/day and increase dosage by 10 mg/day every 4 days prn).
Effect	Nonselective, noncompetitive α-adrenergic antagonist.
Clearance	Hepatic metabolism; renal/biliary excretion.
Comments	May cause orthostatic hypotension (which may be refractory to norepinephrine), reflex tachycardia.

PHENTOLAMINE (REGITINE)

Indications	**1.** Hypertension from catecholamine excess as in pheochromocytoma. **2.** Extravasation of alpha-agonist.
Dosage	**1.** 1–5 mg IV prn for hypertension. **2.** 5–10 mg in 10 mL of NS SC into affected area within 12 h of extravasation.
Effect	Nonselective, competitive α-adrenergic antagonist.
Clearance	Unknown metabolism; 10% renally eliminated (unchanged).
Comments	May cause hypotension, reflex tachycardia, cerebrovascular spasm, dysrhythmias, stimulation of gastrointestinal tract, or hypoglycemia.

PHENYLEPHRINE (NEO-SYNEPHRINE)

Indication	Hypotension.
Dosage	10 μg/min IV initially, then titrated to response; IV bolus 40–100 μg/dose. Customary mix: 10–30 mg in 250 mL of D5W or NS.
Effect	α_1-Adrenergic agonist.
Clearance	Hepatic metabolism; renal elimination.
Comments	May cause hypertension, reflex bradycardia, microcirculatory constriction, uterine contraction, or uterine vasoconstriction.

PHENYTOIN (DILANTIN)

Indications   1. Seizures. **2**. Digoxin-induced dysrhythmias.

Dosage   Adult: **1**. LOAD, 10–15 mg/kg IV at <50 mg/min (up to 1,000 mg cautiously, with ECG monitoring); for neurosurgical prophylaxis, 100–200 mg IV q4h (at <50 mg/min). **2**. 50–100 mg IV at <50 mg/min q10–15 min until dysrhythmia is abolished, side effects occur, or a maximal dose of 10–15 mg/kg is given.

Effect   Anticonvulsant effect via membrane stabilization. Antidysrhythmic effect similar to those of quinidine or procainamide.

Clearance   Hepatic metabolism; renal elimination (enhanced by alkaline urine).

Comments   May cause nystagmus, diplopia, ataxia, drowsiness, gingival hyperplasia, gastrointestinal upset, hyperglycemia, or hepatic microsomal enzyme induction. Intravenous bolus may cause bradycardia, hypotension, respiratory arrest, cardiac arrest, or CNS depression. Tissue irritant. Crosses the placenta. Significant interpatient variation in dose needed to achieve therapeutic concentration of 7.5–20.0 μg/mL. Determination of unbound phenytoin levels may be helpful in patients with renal failure or hypoalbuminemia.

PHOSPHORUS (PHOSPHO-SODA, NEUTRA-PHOS, POTASSIUM PHOSPHATE, SODIUM PHOSPHATE)

Indications   1. Treatment and prevention of hypophosphatemia. **2**. Short-term treatment of constipation. **3**. Evacuation of the colon for rectal and bowel exams.

Dosage   **1**. Mild to moderate hypophosphatemia: children <4 years: 250 mg (phosphorus) PO 3–4 times/day; >4 years and adults: 250–500 mg (phosphorus) PO 3 times/day or 0.08–0.15 mmol/kg IV over 6 h. Moderate to severe hypophosphatemia: children <4 years: 0.15–0.3 mmol/kg IV over 6 h; >4 years and adults: 0.15–0.25 mmol/kg IV over 6–12 h. **2**. Laxative (Phospho-Soda): children 5–9 years: 5 mL PO as a single dose; 10–12 years: 10 mL PO as a single dose; children >12 years and adults: 20–30 mL PO as a single dose. **3**. Colonoscopy preparation (Phospho–Soda): oral, adults, 45 mL diluted to 90 mL with water PO the evening prior to the examination and repeated the following morning.

Effect   Electrolyte replacement.

Clearance   Kidneys reabsorb 80% of dose.

Comments   Infuse doses of IV phosphate over a 4- to 6-h period; risks of rapid IV infusion include hypocalcemia, hypotension, muscular irritability, calcium deposition, renal function deterioration, and hyperkalemia. Orders for IV phosphate preparations should be written in mmol (1 mmol = 31 mg). Use with caution in patients with cardiac disease and renal insufficiency. Do not give with magnesium- and aluminum-containing antacids or sucralfate, which can bind with phosphate.

PHYSOSTIGMINE (ANTILIRIUM)

Indications   Postoperative delirium, tricyclic antidepressant overdose, reversal of CNS effects of anticholinergic drugs.

Dosage	0.5–2.0 mg IV q15 min prn.
Effect	Central and peripheral cholinergic effects; inhibits cholinesterase.
Clearance	Cholinesterase metabolism.
Comments	May cause bradycardia, tremor, convulsions, hallucinations, CNS depression, mild ganglionic blockade, or cholinergic crisis. Crosses blood–brain barrier. Antagonized by atropine. Contains sulfite.

POTASSIUM (KCl)

Indication	Hypokalemia, digoxin toxicity.
Dosage	Adult: 20 mEq of KCl administered IV over 30–60 min. Usual infusion 10 mEq/h. Pediatric: 0.02 mEq/kg/min.
Effect	Electrolyte replacement.
Clearance	Renal.
Comments	Intravenous bolus administration may cause cardiac arrest; infusion rate should not exceed 1 mEq/min in adults. A central venous line is preferable for administration of concentrated solutions.

PROCAINAMIDE (PRONESTYL)

Indications	Atrial and ventricular dysrhythmias.
Dosage	Adult: LOAD: 20 mg/min IV, up to 17 mg/kg, until toxicity or desired effect occurs. Stop if $\geq$50% QRS widening, or PR lengthening occurs; MAINT: 1–4 mg/min. Pediatric: LOAD: 3–6 mg/kg over 5 min, not to exceed 100 mg/dose; repeat q5–10 min to maximum dose of 15 mg/kg; MAINT: 20–80 μg/kg/min; maximum of 2 g/24 hr.
Effect	Blocks sodium channels; class I-A antidysrhythmic.
Clearance	Hepatic conversion of 25% to active metabolite N-acetylprocainamide (NAPA), a class-III antidysrhythmic; renal elimination (50% to 60% unchanged).
Comments	May cause increased ventricular response with atrial tachydysrhythmias unless receiving digitalis; asystole (with AV block); myocardial depression; CNS excitement; blood dyscrasia; lupus syndrome with +ANA; liver damage. Intravenous administration can cause hypotension from vasodilation, accentuated by general anesthesia. Decrease LOAD by one-third in congestive heart failure or shock. Reduce doses in hepatic or renal impairment. Therapeutic concentration 4–10 μg/mL (procainamide); 15–25 μg/mL (NAPA); 10–30 μg/mL (combined). Contains sulfite.

PROCHLORPERAZINE (COMPAZINE)

Indications	Nausea and vomiting.
Dosage	5–10 mg/dose IV ($\leq$40 mg/day); 5–10 mg IM q2–4h prn; 25 mg PR q12h prn.
Effect	Central dopamine (D_2) antagonist with neuroleptic and antiemetic effects. Also antimuscarinic and antihistaminic (H_1) effects.
Clearance	Hepatic metabolism; renal and biliary elimination.
Comments	May cause hypotension (especially when given IV), extrapyramidal reactions, neuroleptic malignant syndrome, leukopenia, and cholestatic jaundice. Contains sulfites. Caution in liver disease. Less sedating than chlorpromazine.

PROMETHAZINE (PHENERGAN)

Indications   Allergies, anaphylaxis, nausea and vomiting, sedation.

Dosage   Adult: 12.5–25 mg IV q4–6h prn. Pediatric: 0.1–1 mg/kg IV, IM, PO, PR q4–6h prn.

Effect   Antagonist of H_1, and muscarinic receptors. Antiemetic and sedative.

Clearance   Hepatic metabolism; renal elimination.

Comments   Lower doses (3–6 mg) may be effective in immediate postoperative period for nausea and vomiting. May cause mild hypotension or mild anticholinergic effects. Crosses the placenta. May interfere with blood grouping. Contains sulfite. Intraarterial injection can cause gangrene.

PROPRANOLOL (INDERAL)

Indications   Hypertension, atrial and ventricular dysrhythmias, myocardial ischemia or infarction, hypertension, thyrotoxicosis, hypertrophic cardiomyopathy, migraine headache.

Dosage   Adult: Test dose of 0.25–0.5 IV, then titrate ≤1 mg/min to effect. PO: 10–40 mg q6–8h, increased prn. Pediatric: 0.05–0.1 mg/kg IV over 10 min.

Effect   Nonspecific β-adrenergic blockade.

Clearance   Hepatic metabolism; renal elimination.

Comments   May cause bradycardia, AV dissociation, and hypoglycemia. Bronchospasm, congestive heart failure, and drowsiness can occur. Crosses the placenta and blood–brain barrier. Abrupt withdrawal can precipitate rebound angina.

PROSTAGLANDIN E_1 (ALPROSTADIL, PROSTIN VR)

Indications   Pulmonary vasodilator, maintenance of patent ductus arteriosus.

Dosage   Starting dose 0.05–0.1 μg/kg/min. Titrate to effect or maximum or 0.6 μg/kg/min. Customary mix: 500 μg/250 mL of NS or D5W.

Effect   Vasodilation, inhibition of platelet aggregation, vascular smooth muscle relaxation, and uterine and intestinal smooth muscle stimulation.

Clearance   Pulmonary metabolism; renal elimination.

Comments   May cause hypotension, apnea, flushing, and bradycardia.

PROTAMINE

Indication   Reversal of the effects of heparin.

Dosage   1 mg/100 units of heparin activity IV at ≤5 mg/min.

Effect   Polybasic compound forms complex with polyacidic heparin.

Clearance   Fate of the heparin–protamine complex is unknown.

Comments   May cause myocardial depression and peripheral vasodilation with sudden hypotension or bradycardia. May cause severe pulmonary hypertension, particularly in the setting of cardiopulmonary bypass. Protamine–heparin complex antigenically active. Transient reversal of heparin may be followed by rebound heparinization. Can cause anticoagulation if given in excess relative to amount of circulating heparin (controversial). Monitor response with activated partial thromboplastin time or activated clotting time.

RANITIDINE (ZANTAC)

Indications	Duodenal and gastric ulcers, esophageal reflux; reduction of gastric volume, increasing gastric pH.
Dosage	IV: 50 mg q8h. PO: 150–300 mg q12h.
Effect	Histamine H_2-receptor antagonist. Inhibits basal, nocturnal, and stimulated gastric acid secretion.
Clearance	Renal elimination of 70% (unchanged).
Comments	Doses should be reduced by 50% with renal failure.

SCOPOLAMINE (HYOSCINE)

Indications	Antisialagogue, sedative, antiemetic, motion sickness.
Dosage	0.3–0.6 mg IV/IM, 1.5-mg transdermal patch.
Effect	Peripheral and central cholinergic (muscarinic) antagonism.
Clearance	Hepatic metabolism; renal elimination.
Comments	Excessive CNS depression can be reversed by physostigmine. May cause excitement, delirium, transient tachycardia, hyperthermia, or urinary retention. Care when handling patch because contact with eyes may cause long-lasting mydriasis and cycloplegia. Crosses the blood–brain barrier and placenta.

STREPTOKINASE (STREPTASE)

Indications	**1.** Thrombolytic agent used in treatment of recent severe or massive deep-vein thrombosis; pulmonary emboli. **2.** Myocardial infarction. **3.** Occluded arteriovenous cannulas.
Dosage	Adult: **1.** Thromboses: 250,000 units IV over 30 min, then 100,000 units/h for 24–72 h. **2.** Myocardial infarction: 1.5 million units IV over 1 h; if hypotension develops, decrease infusion rate by 50%; standard concentration is 1.5 million units/250 mL. **3.** Cannula occlusion: 250,000 units into cannula, clamp for 2 h, then aspirate contents and flush with normal saline. Use with caution, considering risk of potentially life-threatening adverse reactions (e.g., hypersensitivity or bleeding). Pediatric: Safety and efficacy not established; limited studies have used 3,500–4,000 units/kg over 30 min followed by 1,000–1,500 units/kg/h.
Effect	Thrombolytic agent.
Clearance	Eliminated by circulating antibodies and via the reticuloendothelial system.
Comments	Best results are realized if used within 5–6 h of myocardial infarction; has been demonstrated to be effective up to 12 h after coronary artery occlusion and onset of symptoms; give aspirin (325 mg) at the start of streptokinase infusion; begin heparin therapy (800–1,000 units/h) at the end of streptokinase infusion. Avoid intramuscular injections and vascular punctures at noncompressible sites before, during, and after therapy. Contraindicated with recent administration of streptokinase (antibodies to streptokinase remain for 3–6 months after initial dose), recent *Streptococcus* infection, active internal bleeding, recent CVA (within 2 months), or intracranial or intraspinal surgery. Relatively contraindicated following major surgery within the last 10 days, GI bleeding, recent trauma, or severe hypertension. Fibrinolytic effects last only a few hours, while anticoagulant effects can persist for 12–24 h.

TERBUTALINE (BRETHINE, BRICANYL)

Indications	1. Bronchospasm. 2. Tocolysis (inhibition of premature labor).
Dosage	1. Adult: 0.25 mg SC; repeat in 15 min prn (use <0.5 mg/4 h); 2.5–5.0 mg PO q6h prn (<15.0 mg/day). Pediatric: 3.5–5.0 μg/kg SC. 2. 2.5–10 μg/min IV infusion. Titrate upward as necessary; usually maximal dose of 17.5–30 μg/min.
Effect	β_2-Selective adrenergic agonist.
Clearance	Hepatic metabolism; renal elimination.
Comments	May cause dysrhythmias, pulmonary edema, hypertension, hypokalemia, or CNS excitement.

TISSUE PLASMINOGEN ACTIVATOR (ALTEPLASE, ACTIVASE, t-PA)

Indications	1. Lysis of coronary arterial thrombi in hemodynamically unstable patients with acute myocardial infarction. 2. Management of acute massive pulmonary embolism in adults. 3. Acute embolic stroke.
Dosage	1. LOAD: 15 mg (30 mL of the infusion) IV over 1 min followed by 0.75 mg/kg (not to exceed 50 mg) given over 30 min. MAINT: 0.5 mg/kg IV up to 35 mg per hour for 1 h immediately following the loading dose. Total dose not to exceed 100 mg. 2. 100 mg IV continuous infusion over 2 h. 3. Total dose of 0.9 mg/kg IV (maximum 90 mg); administer 10% as a bolus and the remainder over 60 min.
Effect	Tissue plasminogen activator.
Clearance	Rapid hepatic clearance.
Comments	Doses above 150 mg have been associated with an increased incidence of intracranial hemorrhage. Contraindicated with active internal bleeding, history of hemorrhagic stroke, intracranial neoplasm, aneurysm, or recent (within 2 months) intracranial or intraspinal surgery or trauma. Should be used with caution in patients who have received chest compressions and in patients who are currently receiving heparin, warfarin, or antiplatelet drugs.

UROKINASE (ABBOKINASE)

Indications	1. Recent myocardial infarction. 2. Deep vein thrombosis. 3. Severe or massive pulmonary embolism. 4. Occluded intravenous cannulas. 5. Loculated pleural effusions and empyemas.
Dosage	Adults: 1. Myocardial infarction: 6,000 units/min intracoronary for up to 2 h. 2. Deep-vein thrombosis: 4,400 units/kg/h IV for 12 h. 3. Clot lysis (large-vessel thrombi): LOAD: 4,000 units/kg/dose IV over 10 min; MAINT: 4,400–6,000 units/kg/h adjusted to achieve clot lysis or patency of affected vessel; doses up to 50,000 units/kg/h have been used. Therapy should be initiated as soon as possible after diagnosis of thrombi and continued until clot is dissolved (usually 24–72 h). 4. Occluded IV catheters: 5,000 units into the catheter, then aspirate; may repeat every 5 min for 30 min; if still occluded, cap and leave in catheter for 30 min to 1 h, then aspirate contents and flush with normal saline. 5. 80,000 units/50 mL instilled into a chest tube.
Effect	Thrombolytic agent.
Clearance	Hepatic; a small amount is excreted in urine and bile.

Comments   Contraindicated with recent *Streptococcus* infection, any internal bleeding, CVA (within 2 months), and brain carcinoma. Use with caution in patients with severe hypertension, recent lumbar puncture, and patients receiving intramuscular injections. Increased bleeding with anticoagulants, antiplatelet drugs, aspirin, indomethacin, and dextran. Avoid intramuscular injections and vascular punctures at noncompressible sites before, during, and after therapy.

VASOPRESSIN (ANTIDIURETIC HORMONE, PITRESSIN)

Indications   **1.** Diabetes insipidus. **2.** Upper GI hemorrhage. **3.** Pulseless ventricular tachycardia or ventricular fibrillation. **4.** Shock refractory to fluid and vasopressor therapy.

Dosage   **1.** 5–10 units IM/SC q8–12h. **2.** 0.1–0.4 units/min IV infusion. **3.** 40 units IV bolus (single dose). **4.** 0.04 units/min IV infusion.

Effect   Increases urine osmolality and decreases urine volume; smooth muscle constriction; vasoconstriction of splanchnic, coronary, muscular, and cutaneous vasculature.

Clearance   Hepatic and renal metabolism; renal elimination.

Comments   May cause oliguria, water intoxication, pulmonary edema; hypertension, arrhythmias, myocardial ischemia; abdominal cramps (from increased peristalsis); anaphylaxis; contraction of gallbladder, urinary bladder, or uterus; vertigo or nausea. Patients with coronary artery disease are often treated with concurrent nitroglycerin.

VERAPAMIL (ISOPTIN, CALAN)

Indications   Supraventricular tachycardia, atrial fibrillation or flutter, Wolff–Parkinson–White syndrome.

Dosage   Adult: 2.5–10 mg IV over $\geq$2 min. If no response in 30 min, repeat 10 mg (150 μg/kg). Pediatric: 0–1 yr, 0.1–0.2 mg/kg IV; 1–15 yr, 0.1–0.3 mg/kg IV. Repeat once if no response in 30 min.

Effect   Blocks slow calcium channels in heart. Prolongs PR interval. Negative inotrope and chronotrope; systemic and coronary vasodilator.

Clearance   Hepatic metabolism; renal elimination.

Comments   May cause severe bradycardia, AV block (especially with concomitant β-adrenergic blockade), excessive hypotension, or congestive heart failure. May increase ventricular response to atrial fibrillation or flutter in patients with accessory tracts. Active metabolite has 20% of the antihypertensive effect of the parent compound.

VITAMIN K (PHYTONADIONE, AQUAMEPHYTON)

Indication   Deficiency of vitamin K-dependent clotting factors, reversal of warfarin anticoagulation.

Dosage   2.5–10 mg IM/SC/PO, or 1–10 mg IV at $\leq$1 mg/min (with caution). If prothrombin time is not improved 8 h after initial dose, repeat prn.

Effect   Promotion of synthesis of clotting factors II, VII, IX, X.

Clearance   Hepatic metabolism.

Comments   Excessive doses can make patient refractory to further oral anticoagulation. May fail with hepatocellular disease. Rapid IV bolus can cause profound hypotension, fever, diaphoresis, bronchospasm, anaphylaxis, and pain at injection site. Crosses the placenta.

WARFARIN (COUMADIN)

Indication   Anticoagulation.

Dosage   LOAD: 5 mg PO × 2–5 days; MAINT: 2–10 mg PO, titrated to prothrombin time (international normalized ratio [INR] should be 2 to 3, based on indication).

Effect   Interferes with utilization of vitamin K by the liver, and inhibits synthesis of factors II, VII, IX, X.

Clearance   Hepatic metabolism; renal elimination.

Comments   May be potentiated by ethanol, antibiotics, chloral hydrate, cimetidine, dextran, thyroxine, diazoxide, ethacrynic acid, glucagon, methyldopa, monoamine oxidase inhibitors, phenytoin, prolonged use of narcotics, quinidine, sulfonamides, congestive heart failure, hyperthermia, liver disease, malabsorption. May be antagonized by barbiturates, chlordiazepoxide, haloperidol, oral contraceptives, hypothyroidism, hyperlipidemia. Crosses the placenta.

KEY TO ABBREVIATIONS

AV, atrioventricular; CNS, central nervous system; COMT, catechol-O-methyltransferase; D5W, 5% dextrose in water; ECG, electrocardiogram; GI, gastrointestinal; IM, intramuscularly; IV, intravenously; LOAD, loading dose; MAINT, maintenance dose; MAO, monoamine oxidase; NS, normal saline; PO, orally; prn, as needed or indicated; RBCs, red blood cells; SC, subcutaneously; SL, sublingually.

Common intravenous antibiotics

Drug	Usual adult IV Dose	Usual Dose Interval	Comments
Amikacin	300 mg	q8h	Preferred for infections resistant to other aminoglycosides.
Amphotericin B (Fungizone)	Initial dose: 0.25 mg/kg administered over 6 h; dose should be gradually increased, ranging up to 1 mg/kg/d or 1.5 mg/kg on alternate days	q1–2d	Broad-spectrum antifungal. Initial test dose: 1 mg infused over 30 min to 1 h. Do not exceed 1.5 mg/kg/d. Because of the nephrotoxic potential of amphotericin, other nephrotoxic drugs should be avoided.
Ampicillin	1 g	q4h	May induce interstitial nephritis combined with sulbactam is Unasyn.
Ampicillin–sulbactam (Unasyn)	3 g	q6h	Not effective against *Pseudomonas* spp.
Aztreonam	1 g	q8h	Can be used for patients allergic to penicillins or cephalosporins.
Cefazolin (Ancef, Kefzol)	1 g	q4–8h	First generation cephalosporin. Adjust dosage in renal disease.
Cefotetan (Cefotan)	1–2 g	q12h	Second generation cephalosporin. Possible disulfiram-like reaction.
Ceftazidime	1 g	q8h	Preferred for *Pseudomonas aeruginosa* infections and neutropenic patients with fever.

Drug	Dose	Interval	Notes
Cefriaxone	1 g	q24h	Preferred for empiric coverage for bacterial meningitis,
Cefuroxime	750 mg	q8h	Preferred for community-acquired pneumonia.
Chloramphenicol	0.25–1 g	q6h	Adjust dose according to serum concentration.
Ciprofloxacin	400 mg	q12h	Good absorption via oral route (500 mg q12h).
Clindamycin (Cleocin)	600 mg	q8h	Associated with *C. difficile* colitis. May prolong neuromuscular blockade.
Doxycycline	100 mg	q12h	Possible hepatoxocity. Can cause benign intracranial hypertension with vitamin A. See tetracycline.
Erythromycin	0.5–1 g	q6h	Bacteriostatic. Gastritis with oral route. Venous irritation.
Fluconazole	200–400 mg	q24h	Well absorbed orally.
Gentamicin	60–120 mg (3–5 mg/kg/d)	q8–12h	Decrease dosage in renal failure. Renal toxicity and ototoxicity. Precipitates with heparin. May cause/prolong neuromuscular blockade.
Imipenem-cilastatin	500 mg	q6h	Preferred for multiple-drug resistant gram-negative bacterial infections. May cause seizures, expecially in renal failure.
Levofloxacin	500 mg	qd	Pure L-isomer of ofloxacin. Well absorbed orally.

(continued)

Common intravenous antibiotics (*Continued*)

Drug	Usual adult IV Dose	Usual Dose Interval	Comments
Linezolid (Zyvox)	600 mg	q12h	Treatment of vancomycin-resistant enterococcus. Good oral bioavailability. Many cause myelosuppression. Exhibits mild MAO inhibitor properties has potential to have same interactions as other MAO inhibitors.
Meropenem	0.5–1 g	q8h	Less likely to cause seizures than imipenem.
Metronidazole (Flagyl)	500 mg	q8h	Possible disulfiram-like reaction, leukopenia, convulsions, acute toxic psychosis with disulfram.
Nafcillin	1–2 g	q4h	Preferred for antistaphlyococcal coverage.
Penicillin G[a]	500,000–2,000,000 U	q4h	Hypersensitivity is common. May induce seizures at high doses and induce interstitial nephritis.
Piperacillin	4 g	q6h	Usually combined with aminoglycoside for treatment of *Pseudomonas*.
Piperacillin-tazobactam	3.375 g	q6h	Tazobactam expands activity of piperacillin to include beta-lactamase producing strains of *S. aureus, H. influenzae, Enterobacteriaceae, Pseudomonas, Klebsiella, Citrobacter, Serratia, Bacteroides,* and other gram-negative anaerobes.

Drug	Dose	Frequency	Comments
Tetracycline	250–500 mg	q12h	Contraindicated in pediatrics (tooth discoloration). Antagonism with penicillins. Crosses placenta.
Ticarcillin	3 g	q4h	Anti-Pseudomonal penicillin of choice. May cause bleeding abnormalities.
Ticarcillin-clavulanate	3.1 g	q4h	—
Trimethoprim/ sulfamethoxazole (Bactrim, Septra)	8–10 mg/kg/d (based on trimethoprim component)	q6–12h	Allergic reactions common. Interferes with elimination of creatinine and potassium; values may increase.
Tobramycin	60–120 mg (3–5 mg/kg/d over 15–20 min)	q8h	See gentamicin.
Vancomycin (Vancocin)	500 mg–1 g over 30–60 min	q6–12h	Preferred for oxacillin-resistant staphylococcal infections and patients with penicillin allergy. Decrease dose in renal disease. Histamine release ("red man syndrome"), renal damage, deafness. May precipitate with other medications.

Note: Adult doses are those usually given to healthy 70-kg patients and may vary with the patient's condition or concomitant drug intake. Older or debilitated patients may require smaller doses.

[a]Five to ten parcent of penicillin-allergic patients will react to cephalosporins.

Appendix B

Normal Adult Laboratory Values for Blood Tests Commonly Ordered at the Massachusetts General Hospital

Jonathan G. Hsiao and Eric Corey Matten

CHEMISTRY

Albumin: 3.5–5.5 g/dL
Alkaline phosphatase: 30–120 U/L
Ammonia, plasma: 6–47 μmol/L
Amylase, serum: 60–180 U/L
Anion gap (calculated): 7–16 mmol/L
Arterial blood gases and pH
   PaO_2: 80–100 mmHg
   $PaCO_2$: 35–45 mmHg
   pH: 7.38–7.44
Bicarbonate (HCO_3^-): 21–30 mEq/L
Bilirubin, direct: <0.4 mg/dL
Bilirubin, total: <1.0 mg/dL
Blood urea nitrogen (BUN): 10–20 mg/dL
Calcium: 9.0–10.5 mg/dL
Calcium, ionized: 1.1–1.4 mmol/L
Chloride: 98–106 mmol/L
Creatine kinase (CK)
   Female: 40–150 U/L
   Male: 60–400 U/L
Creatine kinase isoenzyme index: 0% to 2.5% relative index
Creatine kinase isoenzymes, MB fraction: 0–7 ng/mL
Creatinine: 0.6–1.5 mg/dL
Globulin: 2.0–3.5 g/dL
Glucose (fasting): 75–115 mg/dL
Iron, serum: 50–150 μg/dL
Lactate dehydrogenase (LDH): 100–190 U/L
Lactic acid, plasma: 0.6–1.7 mmol/L
Lipase: 0–16 U/dL
Magnesium: 1.8–3.0 mEq/L
Osmolality: 285–295 mOsm/kg
Phosphorus: 3.0–4.5 mg/dL
Potassium: 3.5–5.0 mmol/L
Protein, total: 5.5–8.0 g/dL
SGOT (aspartate aminotransferase [AST]): 0–35 U/L
SGPT (alanine aminotransferase [ALT]): 0–35 U/L
Sodium: 136–145 mmol/L
Thyroid-stimulating hormone (TSH): 0.5–4.7 μU/mL

Troponin T: <0.1 ng/mL
Uric acid
    Female: 1.5–6.0 mg/dL
    Male: 2.5–8.0 mg/dL

HEMATOLOGY AND COAGULATION VALUES

Activated clotting time (ACT): 70–180 seconds
D-dimer: 0.0–0.5 μg/mL
Erythrocyte count (RBC)
    Female: 4.0–5.2 (10^6/mm^3
    Male: 4.5–5.9 (10^6/mm^3
Erythrocyte sedimentation rate (ESR)
    Female: 1–25 mm/h
    Male: 0–17 mm/h
Fibrin degradation products (FDP): 0–2.5 μg/mL
Fibrinogen: 150–400 mg/dL
Hematocrit
    Female: 36% to 46%
    Male: 41% to 53%
Hemoglobin
    Female: 12–16 g/dL
    Male: 13.5–17.5 g/dL
Iron: 30–160 μg/dL
Iron binding capacity (TIBC): 228–428 μg/dL
Leukocyte count (WBC): 4.5–11 $\times$ 10^3/mm^3
    Neutrophils: 40% to 70%
    Band forms: 0% to 10%
    Lymphocytes: 22% to 44%
    Monocytes: 4% to 11%
    Eosinophils: 0% to 8%
    Basophils: 0% to 3%
Mean corpuscular hemoglobin (MCH): 26–34 pg/cell
Mean corpuscular hemoglobin concentration (MCHC): 31–37 g/dL
Mean corpuscular volume (MCV): 80–100 μm^3
Partial thromboplastin time, activated (aPTT): 22.1–3 .1 sec
Platelet count: 150–350 $\times$ 10^3/mm^3
Prothrombin time (PT): 11.1–13.1 sec (laboratory specific)
Reticulocyte count: 0.5% to 2.5%

Data from Kratz A, Ferraro M,Sluss PM, and Lewandrowski KB. Case records
of the Massachusetts General Hospital. Weeklyclinicopathological exercises.
Laboratory reference values. *N Engl J Med* 2004;351:1548–1563.

Index

Page numbers followed by f indicate figure; those followed by t indicate table.